Pediatric Nurse Practitioner Certification Review Guide

FOURTH EDITION

EDITORS

Virginia Layng Millonig, Ph.D, R.N., C.P.N.P.
President
Health Leadership Associates, Inc.
Germantown, Maryland

Caryl E. Mobley, Ph.D., R.N., C.P.N.P.
Professor
Associate Dean,
College of Nursing
Texas Woman's University
Dallas, Texas

Health Leadership Associates
Potomac, Maryland

Health Leadership Associates

First in Certification Review

Also offers these publications for your review and clinical practice needs:

STUDY QUESTION BOOKS

Question books are designed in a multiple choice, self testing question and answer format. Answers are provided with rationales and a reference source. The Question Books are a great companion to the Certification Review Books.

Acute Care Nurse Practitioner Certification Study Question Book
300 Test Questions, ISBN 1-878028-25-1

Adult Nurse Practitioner Certification Study Question Book (Second Edition)
300 Test Questions, ISBN 1-878028-32-4

Pediatric Nurse Practitioner Certification Study Question Book (Second Edition)
300 Test Questions, ISBN 1-878028-29-4

Women's Health Nurse Practitioner Certification Study Question Book
300 Test Questions, ISBN 1-878028-22-7

Family Nurse Practitioner Certification Study Question Book Set
(The set consists of the Adult and Pediatric NP Study Question Books)
ISBN# 1-878028-33-2

CERTIFICATION REVIEW BOOKS

Comprehensive content outline format with emphasis on major theories, diagnoses, treatment modalities and nursing interventions. Test questions and a complete bibliography follow each chapter.

Adult Nurse Practitioner Certification Review Guide (Fourth Edition)
ISBN 1-878028-31-6, 734 pages

Family Nurse Practitioner Certification Review 2 Volume Set (Fourth Edition)
Consists of Adult and Pediatric Certification Review Guides
ISBN 1-878028-35-9, 1646 pages

Midwifery/Women's Health Nurse Practitioner Certification Review Guide
ISBN 1-878028-18-9, 800 pages

Pediatric Nurse Practitioner Certification Review Guide (Fourth Edition)
ISBN 1-878028-30-8, 912 pages

Psychiatric Certification Review Guide for the Generalist and Clinical Specialist in Adult, Child, and Adolescent Psychiatric and Mental Health Nursing (Second Edition)
ISBN 1-878028-19-7, 646 pages

To Order, *Call 800-435-4775*
or visit us on the web at:
www.healthleadership.com

For information on Certification Review Courses, Home Study Programs and Review Books contact:

Health Leadership Associates, Inc.
Post Office Box 1784
Germantown, Maryland 20875

1-800-435-4775
www.healthleadership.com
hlacert@aol.com

Health Leadership Associates, Inc.
Managing Editor: Virginia Layng Millonig
Cover and Design: Merrifield Graphics
Composition: Mike Rasel, Port City Press, Inc.
Design and Production: Port City Press, Inc.

Printed in the United States of America

Health Leadership Associates, Inc.
P.O. Box 59153
Potomac, Maryland 20859

Library of Congress Cataloging-in-Publication Data

Pediatric nurse practitioner certification review guide / editors, Virginia Layng Millonig, Caryl E. Mobley;
contributing authors Beverly Ruth Bigler ... [et al.]. — 4th ed.
     p. cm.
   Includes bibliographical references and index.
   ISBN 1-878028-30-8
   1. Pediatric nursing—Outlines, syllabi, etc. 2. Examinations—Study guides. I. Millonig, Virginia Layng. II. Baroni,
Mary A. III. Bigler, Beverly.
   RJ242.P43 2004
   618.92'00231—dc22

                                                          2004005826

10 9 8 7 6 5 4 3 2

This new addition to Health Leadership Associates' certification review books is dedicated to my daughters Martha, Mary and Bridget and their families. Their contributions and commitment to the success, quality and integrity of Health Leadership Associates has been immeasurable.

Through their dedication and hard work Health Leadership Associates has become the first and foremost provider of certification review in the country and a major player in continuing education.

But most important is the joy and love they have brought to my life and the support they have provided through it all!

And finally to my mother and father, Camilla and Earle Layng who will never know how indebted I am to them for the inspiration, love and faith they instilled in me.

Virginia Layng Millonig

To the future PNPs who have completed strenuous educational programs and will now be taking their certification exams. Best wishes to all of you; with study and hard work you will become caring, competent PNPs who will be a wonderful resource to children and their families. Be strong diagnosticians and manage children's health and illness well, never forgetting that you are nurses first. And to my fellow faculty members at Texas Woman's University College of Nursing. You are an excellent team to work with and your nurturing of students in the same way you care for patients is extraordinary.

Caryl Erhardt Mobley

Contributing Authors

Beverly Ruth Bigler, Ed.D., R.N., C.P.N.P.
Professor of Nursing
School of Nursing
California State University, Los Angeles
Los Angeles, California
Nurse Practitioner\School Nurse
Alhambra School District
Alhambra, California

Mary A. Baroni, Ph.D., R.N., C.P.N.P.
Professor
Nursing Program Director
University of Washington, Bothell
Bothell, Washington

Leanne C. Busby, D.S.N., R.N.,C.S., F.A.A.N.P.
State Director
Tennessee Professional Assistance Program
Nashville, Tennessee

Juanita Conkin Dale, Ph.D., R.N., C.P.N.P.
Pediatric Nurse Practitioner
Center for Cancer and Blood Disorders
Children's Medical Center of Dallas
Dallas, Texas

Jacalyn Peck Dougherty, Ph.D-C., M.A., M.S., R.N., C.P.N.P.
Asthma Project Manager
National Association of School Nurses
Castle Rock, Colorado

Sandra L. Elvik, M.S., R.N., C.P.N.P.
Associate Professor of Pediatrics
UCLA School of Medicine
Assistant Medical Director
Child Abuse Crisis Center
Harbor-UCLA Medical Center
Torrance, California

Nancy Dickenson Hazard, M.S.N., R.N., C.P.N.P., F.A.A.N.
Executive Officer
Sigma Theta Tau International
Indianapolis, Indiana

Susan M. Heighway, M.S., R.N.,C.S. P.N.P.
Clinical Professor
Nurse Practitioner
University Center for Excellence in Developmental Disabilities
Waisman Center UAP
School of Nursing
University of Wisconsin Madison
Madison, Wisconsin

Janet Johnston, M.S.N., R.N., C.P.N.P.
Assistant Professor/Nursing Faculty
Pediatric Pulmonary Center
Pulmonary Division
Department of Pediatrics
Children's Hospital
University of Alabama at Birmingham
Birmingham, Alabama

Nancy E. Kline, Ph.D., R.N., C.P.N.P., F.A.A.N.
Director
Center for Innovation and Clinical Scholarship
Children's Hospital, Boston
Boston, Massachusetts

Bernadette Mazurek Melnyk, PhD., R.N.,C.S., P.N.P.
Professor
Associate Dean for Research
Director, Center for Research and Evidence-Based Practice
Director, Pediatric Nurse Practitioner & Dual PNP/Psychiatric Mental
    Health Nurse Practitioner Programs
University of Rochester School of Nursing and School of Medicine & Dentistry
Rochester, New York
Pediatric Nurse Practitioner and Nurse Practitioner of Psychiatry
Children and Youth In-Patient Unit
Elmira Psychiatric Center
Elmira, New York

Connie Paczkowski, M.S.N., R.N., C.S., P.N.P.
Pediatric Nurse Practitioner
Hunterdon Pediatric Associates
Flemington, New Jersey

Virginia Richardson, D.N.S., R.N., C.P.N.P.
Associate Professor
Assistant Dean for Student Affairs
Indiana University School of Nursing
Pediatric Nurse Practitioner
Clarian Health Partners
Indianapolis, Indiana

Alison W. Schultz, Ed.D., R.N., C.P.N.P.
Retired
Waynesboro, Virginia
Formerly
Associate Professor
School of Nursing
University of Rochester
Rochester, New York

Leigh Small, Ph.D., R.N., C.P.N.P.
Assistant Professor of Clinical Nursing
University of Rochester School of Nursing
Rochester, New York
Pediatric Nurse Practitioner
Genesee Health Services
Rochester, New York

Karen Uzark, Ph.D., R.N., C.P.N.P.
Director of Process Improvement
and Outcomes Research
Heart Transplant Nurse Practitioner
Pediatric Cardiology
Children's Hospital Medical Center
Cincinnati, Ohio

Victoria A. Weill, M.S.N., R.N.,C.S., C.P.N.P.
Clinical Coordinator
Pediatric Primary Care Program
School of Nursing
University of Pennsylvania
Pediatric Nurse Practitioner
Division of Emergency Medicine
Children's Hospital of Philadelphia
Philadelphia, Pennsylvania

Preface

Health Leadership Associates is pleased to introduce the fourth edition of the Pediatric Nurse Practitioner Certification Review Guide. The book has been developed especially for Pediatric Nurse Practitioners and Family Nurse Practitioners preparing to take certification examinations.

The purpose of the book is twofold and will assist individuals engaged in self-study preparation for certification examinations, and may be used as a reference guide in the practice setting.

The book has been organized to provide the reader with test taking strategies first. This is followed by the chapters on growth and development and health maintenance and promotion. The remaining address common disorders of the various body systems and provide succinct summaries of definitions, etiology, signs and symptoms, clinical findings, differential diagnoses, diagnostic tests/findings and management/treatment. The final chapter addresses PNP role development, current trends and health policy issues including topics such as credentialing, legal issues, legislation, reimbursement and delivery systems.

Following each chapter are test questions, which are intended to serve as an introduction to the testing arena. In addition a bibliography is included for those who need a more in depth discussion of the subject matter in each chapter. These references can serve as additional instructional material for the reader.

Many nurses preparing for certification examinations find that reviewing an extensive body of scientific knowledge requires a very difficult search of many sources that must be synthesized to provide a review base for the examination. This publication provides a succinct, yet comprehensive review of the core material.

The editors and contributing authors are certified pediatric nurse practitioners. They have designed this book to assist potential examinees to prepare for success in the certification examination process.

CONTENTS

1   **Test Taking Strategies**   *Nancy A. Dickenson Hazard*
                                                     Virginia Layng Millonig

2   **Human Growth And Development**   *Mary A. Baroni*

3.   **Health Promotion and Well Child Care for Infants, Children and Adolescence**   *Bernadette Mazurek Melnyk*
                                                           Leigh Small

4.   **Head, Eye, Ear, Nose, Mouth and Throat Disorders**   *Connie Paczkowski*

5. Cardiovascular Disorders

Karen Uzark

6. Lower Respiratory Disorders

Janet Johnston

7. Dermatologic Conditions

Beverly Bigler

8. Gastrointestinal Disorders

Victoria A. Weil

9. Infectious Diseases

Nancy E. Kline

10. Musculoskeletal Disorders

Susan Heighwayy

11. Neurological Disorders

Susan Heighway

12. Genitourinary And Gynecologic Disorders Adolescent Pregnancy

Sandra Elvik
Mary A. Baroni

13. Hematological\Oncologic\Immunologic Disorders

Juanita Conkin Dale

14. Endocrine Disorders

Jacalyn Peck Dougherty

15. Multisystem And Genetic Disorders

Alison W. Schultz
Virginia Richardson

16. Advanced Practice, Role Development, Current Trends And Health Policy

Leanne C. Busby
Mary A. Baroni

Test Taking Strategies and Techniques

Nancy A. Dickenson Hazard
Virginia L. Millonig

We all respond to testing situations in different ways. What separates the successful test taker from the unsuccessful one is knowing how to prepare for and take a test. Preparing yourself to be a successful test taker is as important as studying for the test. Each person needs to assess and develop individual test taking strategies and skills. The primary goal of this chapter is to assist potential examinees in knowing how to study for and take a test. Of equal importance to this study preparation is a basic understanding of how certification examinations are developed. They are based upon a universal knowledge foundation. Test items are selected from generally recognized resources available to the examinee, and specific to the type of specialty area.

STRATEGY #1 Know Yourself

When faced with an examination, do you feel threatened, experience butterflies or sweaty palms, have trouble keeping your mind focused on studying or on test questions? These common symptoms of test anxiety plague many of us, but can be used advantageously if understood and handled correctly. Over the years of test taking, each of us has developed certain testing behaviors, some of which are beneficial, while others present obstacles to successful test taking. You can take control of the test taking situation by identifying the undesirable behaviors, maintaining the desirable ones and developing skills to improve test performance.

Technique #1:   From the following descriptions of test taking personalities, find yourself (Table 1). Write down those characteristics which describe you even if they are from different personality types. Carefully review the problem list associated with your test taking personality characteristics. Write down the problems which are most troublesome. Then make a list of how you can remedy these problems from the improvement strategies list. Be sure to use these strategies as you prepare for and take examinations.

STRATEGY #2 Develop Your Thinking Skills

Understanding Thought Process: In order to improve your thinking skills and subsequent test performance, it is best to understand the types of thinking as well as the techniques to enhance the thought process.

Everyone has a personal learning style, but we all must proceed through the same process to think. Thinking occurs on six levels—the lower level of memory and comprehension and the higher levels of application, analysis, synthesis and evaluation (Sides & Korchek, 1994). Memory is the ability to recall facts. Without adequate retrieval of facts, progression through the higher levels of thinking cannot occur easily. Comprehension is the ability to understand memorized facts. To be effective, comprehension skills must allow the person to translate recalled information from one context to another. Application, or the process of using information to know why something occurs, is a higher form of learning. Effective application relies on the use of understood, memorized facts to verify intended action. Analysis is the ability to use abstract or logical forms of thought to show relationships and to distinguish the cause and effect between the variables in a situation.

Table 1

Test Taker Profile

Type	Characteristics	Pitfalls	Improvement Strategies
The Rusher	• Rushes to complete the test before the studied facts are forgotten	• Unable to read question and situation completely	• Practice progressive relaxation techniques
	• Arrives at test site early and waits anxiously	• At high risk for misreading, misinterpreting and mistakes	• Develop a study plan with sufficient time to review important content
	• Mumbles studied facts	• Difficult items heighten anxiety	• Avoid cramming and last minute studying
	• Tense body posture	• Likely to make quick, not well-thought-out guesses	• Take practice tests focusing on slowing down and reading and answering each option carefully
	• Accelerated pulse, respiration and neuromuscular excitement		• Read instructions and questions slowly
	• Answers questions rapidly and is generally one of the first to complete		
	• Experiences exhaustion once test is over		
The Turtle	• Moves slowly, methodically, deliberately through each question	• Last to finish; often does not complete the exam	• Take practice tests focusing on time spent per item
	• Repeated rereading, underlining and checking	• Has to quickly complete questions in last part of exam, increasing errors	• Place watch in convenient place to keep track of time
	• Takes 60 to 90 seconds per question versus an average of 45 to 60 seconds	• Has difficulty completing timed examinations	• Mark answer sheet in paper/pencil examination indicating where one should be halfway through exam based on total number of questions and total amount of time for exam
			• Study concepts not details
			• Attempt to answer each question as you progress through the exam
The Personalizer	• Mature person who has personal knowledge and insight from life experiences	• Risk in relying on what has been learned through observation and experience since one may develop false understandings and stereotypes	• Focus on principles and standards that support nursing practice
		• Personal beliefs and experiences are frequently not the norm or standard tested	• Avoid making connections between patients in exam clinical situations and personal clinical experience
		• Has difficulty identifying expected standards measured by standardized examination	• Focus on generalities not experiences
The Squisher	• View exams as threat, rather than an expected event in education	• Procrastinates studying for exams	• Establish a plan of progressive, disciplined study
	• Preoccupied with grades and personal accomplishment	• Unable to study effectively since waits until last minute	• Use defined time frames for studying content and taking practice exams
	• Attempts to avoid responsibility and accountability associated with testing in order to reduce anxiety	• Increased anxiety over test since procrastinating study impairs ability to learn and perform	• Use relaxation techniques • Return to difficult items • Read carefully

(Table continued on next page)

Type	Characteristics	Pitfalls	Improvement Strategies
The Philosopher	• Academically successful person who is well disciplined and structured in study habits • Displays great intensity and concentration during exam • Searches questions for hidden or unintended meaning • Experiences anxiety over not knowing everything	• Over analysis causes loss of sight of actual intent of question • Reads information into questions answering with own added information rather than answering the actual intent of question	• Focus on questions as they are written • Work on self confidence and not on question. Initial response is usually correct • Avoid multiple rereadings of questions • Avoid adding own information and unintended meanings • Practice, practice, practice with sample tests
The Second Guesser	• Answers questions twice, first as an examinee, second as an examiner • Believes second look will allow one to find and correct errors • Frequently changes initial responses (i.e., grades own test)	• Altering an initial response frequently results in an incorrect answer • Frequently changes answers because the pattern of response appears incorrect (i.e., too many "true" or too many correct responses)	• Reread only the few items of which one is unsure. Avoid changing initial responses • Take exam carefully and progressively first time, allowing little or no time for rereading • Study facts • Avoid reading into questions
The Lawyer	• Attempts to place words or ideas into the question (leads the witness) • Occurs most frequently with psychosocial or communication questions which ask for the most appropriate response	• Veers from the obvious answer and provides response from own point of view • Reads a question, jumps to a conclusion then finds a response that leads to predetermined conclusion	• Focus on distinguishing what is said in question and not on what is read into question • Avoid formulating responses aimed at obtaining certain information • Choose responses that allow expression of feelings which encourage hope, not catastrophe, those which are intended to clarify, which identify feeling tones or which avoid negating or confronting feelings • Carefully read entire question before selecting a response

From: "Making the grades as a test-taker," by N. Dickenson-Hazard, (1989) *Pediatric Nursing, 15,* p. 303. Adapted from: *Nurse's guide to successful test-taking* by M. B. Sides and N. B. Cailles, 1989. Philadelphia: J. B. Lippincott, Co., pp 59–70, 199–203. Copyright 1989 by A. J. Jannetti, Inc. Reprinted by permission.

As related to testing situations, the thought process from memory to analysis occurs quite quickly. Some examination items are designed to test memory and comprehension while others test application and analysis. An example of a memory question is as follows:

A normal child is expected to walk by:

    a)   6 months
    b)   10 months
    c)   *14 months*
    d)   18 months

To answer this question correctly, the individual has to retrieve a memorized fact. Understanding the fact, knowing why it is important or analyzing what should be done in this situation is not needed. An example of a question which tests comprehension is as follows:

The mother of an otherwise healthy 11-month-old boy voices concern that her son is not walking yet because her older daughter walked at this age. You should know that:

a) Girls generally walk before boys
b) *Her son should be walking by 14 months of age*
c) The mother is demonstrating overanxious behaviour
d) Her son is delayed developmentally

To answer this question correctly, an individual must retrieve the fact that walking well is not always achieved until 14 months of age, and understand that in this situation, a child of 11 months would not necessarily be expected to have achieved this developmental milestone.

In answering an examination question that requires a higher level of thought, an individual must be able to recall a fact, understand that fact in the context of the question, and apply this understanding to determine why one answer is correct, after analyzing possible answer choices as they relate to the situation (Sides & Korchek, 1994). An example of an application analysis question is as follows:

After administering the Denver Developmental Screening Test (Denver II), you note that an 18-month-old boy is not walking. The child's mother is voicing concern about this. Your most appropriate action is to:

a) Repeat the Denver II in 6 months
b) *Consult with pediatrician*
c) Reassure the mother that the child's not walking is normal at this age
d) Recommend exercises to strengthen the lower extremities

To answer this question correctly, the individual must recall the fact at which age walking should be achieved; understand if it is normal or abnormal for an 18-month-old child not to walk as depicted in this situation; apply this knowledge to each option, understanding why it may or may not be correct; and analyze each option for what action is most apropriate for this situation. Application/ analysis questions require the examinee to use logical rationale, based on a well defined principle or fact. Problem solving ability becomes important as the examinee must think through each question option, determining its relevance and importance to the situation in the question.

Building your thinking skills: Effective memorization is the cornerstone to learning and building thinking skills (Olney, 1989). We have all experienced ''memory power outages'' at some time, due in part to trying to memorize too much, too fast, too ineffectively. Developing skills to improve memorization is important to increasing the effectiveness of your thinking and subsequent test performance.

Technique #1: Quantity is NOT quality, so concentrate on learning important content. For example, it is important to know the various pharmacologic agents appropriate for the management of chronic obstructive pulmanary disease (COPD), not the specific dosages for each medication.

Technique #2: Memory from repetition, or saying something over and over again to remember it, usually fades. Developing memory skills which trigger retrieval of needed facts is more useful. Such skills are as follows:

Acronyms: These are mental crutches which facilitate recall. Some are already established such as PERRLA (pupils equal, round, react to light, and accommodation), C.H.F. for (congestive heart failure), or T.I.A. for (transient ischemic attack). Developing your own acronyms can be particularly useful since they are your own word association arrangements in a singular word. Nonsense words or funny, unusual ones are often more useful since they attract your attention.

Acrostics: This mental tool arranges words into catchy phrases. The first letter of each word stands for something which is recalled as the phrase is said. Your own acrostics are most valuable in triggering recall of learned information since they are your individual situation associations. An example of an acrostic is as follows:

<u>M</u>om <u>C</u>arried <u>N</u>ell <u>E</u>very <u>P</u>lace <u>S</u>he <u>W</u>ent stands for the areas of assessment for a cast check: movement, color, numbness, edema, pulse, sensation and warmth.

ABCs: This technique facilitates information retrieval by using the alphabet as a crutch. Each letter stands for a symptom, which when put together creates a picture of the clinical presentation of the disease. The clinical picture of acute epiglottitis using the ABC technique is as follows:

a) Aphonia
b) Brassy cough
c) Complaint of sore throat initially
d) Dysphagia
e) Expiratory and inspiratory stridor
f) Forward leaning position

Imaging: This technique can be used in two ways. The first is to develop a nickname for a clinical problem which when said produces a mental picture. For example, the nickname "bloated blue baby" might be used to trigger visualization of an infant with a congenital heart defect who is cyanotic, edematous and having breathing difficulty. A second form of imaging is to visualize a specific patient while you are trying to understand or solve a clinical problem when studying or answering a question. For example, imagine a child with cerebral palsy. You are trying to understand the most appropriate feeding position for this child. In your mind, visualize the various positions of supine, prone and semi-prone, imaging what will happen to the child in each position.

Rhymes, music & links: The absurd is easier to remember than the most common. Rhymes, music or links can add absurdity and humor to learning and remembering (Olney, 1989). These retrieval tools are developed by the individual for specific content. For example, making up a rhyme about diabetes may be helpful in remembering the predominant female incidence, origin of disease, primary symptoms and management as illustrated by:

> There once was a girl
> whose beta cells failed
> She grew quite thirsty
> and her glucose levels sailed
> Her lack of insulin caused her to
> increase her intake
> And her increased urinary output
> was certainly not fake
> So she learned to watch her diet
> and administer injections
> That kept her healthy, growing
> and free of complications.

Setting content to music is sometimes useful to remembering. Melodies which are repetitious jog the memory by the ups and downs of the notes and the rhythm of the music.

Links connect key words from the content by using them in a story. An example given by Olney (1989) for remembering the parts of an eye is IRIS watched a PUPIL through the LENS of a RED TIN telescope while eating CORN-EA on the cob.

Additional memory aids may also include the use of color or drawing for improving recall. Use different colored pens or paper to accentuate the material being learned. For example, highlight or make notes in blue for content about respiratory problems and in red for cardiovascular content. Drawing assists with visualizing content as well. This is particularly helpful for remembering the pathophysiology of the specific health problem.

The important thing to remember about remembering is to use good recall techniques.

Technique #3: Improving higher level thinking skills involves exercising the application and analysis of memorized facts. Small group review is particularly useful for enhancing these high level skills. Small group interaction allows verbalization of thought processes and receipt of input about content and thought process from others (Sides & Korchek, 1994). Individuals not only hear how they think, but how others think as well. This interaction allows individuals to identify flaws in their thought process as well as to strengthen their positive points.

Taking practice tests are also helpful in developing application/analysis thinking skills. Practice tests permit the individual to analyze thinking patterns as well as the cause and effect relationships between the question and its options. The problem solving skills needed to answer application/analysis questions are tested, giving the individual more experience through practice (Dickenson-Hazard, 1990).

STRATEGY #3 Know The Content

Your ability to study is directly influenced by organization and concentration (Dickenson-Hazard, 1990). If effort is spent on both of these aspects of exam preparation, examination success can be increased.

Preparation for studying: Getting organized. Study habits are developed early in our education experiences. Some of our habits enhance learning while others do not. To increase study effectiveness, organization of study materials and time is essential. Organization decreases frustration, allows for easy resumption of study and increases concentrated study time.

Technique #1: Create your own study space. Select a study area that is yours alone, free from distractions, comfortable, with good lighting. The ventilation and room temperature should be comfortable since a cold room makes it difficult to concentrate and a warm room may make you sleepy (Burkle & Marshak, 1989). All study materials should be left in a specific study space. The basic premise of a study space is that it facilitates a mind set that you are there to study. When study is interrupted, it is best to leave study materials just as they are. Don't close books or put away notes as they will have to be relocated, wasting valuable time, when study is resumed.

Technique #2: Define and organize the content. Secure an outline or the content parameters which are to be examined from the examining body. If outline is sketchy, develop a more detailed one for yourself using the recommended texts as a guideline. Next, identify available study resources: class notes, old exams, handouts, textbooks, review courses and books, home study programs, or study groups. For national standardized exams, such as initial licensing or certification, it is best to identify a few resources which cover the content being tested and stick to them. Attempting to review all available resources is not only mind boggling, but increases anxiety and frustration as well. Make your selections and stay with them.

Technique #3: Conduct a content assessment. Using a simple rating scale of:

    1 = requires no review
    2 = requires minimal review
    3 = requires intensive review
    4 = start from the beginning

Read through the content outline and rate each content area (Dickenson-Hazard, 1990). Table 2 provides a sample exam content assessment. Be honest with your assessment. It is far better to recognize your content weaknesses when you can study and remedy them, rather than wishing during the exam that you had studied more. Likewise with content strengths: If you know the material, don't waste time studying it.

Technique #4: Develop a study plan. Coordinate the content which needs to be studied with the time available (Sides & Korchek, 1994). Prioritize your study needs, starting with weak areas first. Allow for a general review at the end of the study plan. Finally, establish an overall goal for yourself; something that will motivate you when brought to mind.

Table 3 illustrates a study plan developed on the basis of the exam content assessment in Table 2. Conducting an assessment and developing a study plan should require no more than 50 minutes. It is a wise investment of time with potential payoffs of reduced study stress and exam success.

Technique #5: Begin now and use your time wisely. The smart test taker begins the study process early (Olney, 1989). Sit down, conduct the content assessment and develop a study plan as soon as you know about the exam. DON'T PROCRASTINATE!

Table 2

Sample Content Assessment

Exam Content: Health Problems of Adolescents	
Category: Provided by Test Giver	*Rating: Provided by Examinee*

I. Acne
  A. Pathophysiology 2
  B. Management 2
    1. General hygiene
    2. Medications
    3. Cleansing
    4. Expression of comedones
  C. Nursing Management 1
    1. Education
    2. Support
    3. Need for follow-up
II. Dysmenorrhea
  A. Etiology 4
  B. Pathophysiology 3
  C. Symptomatology 3
  D. Management 4
  E. Nursing Interventions 3
III. Infectious Mononucleosis
  A. Definition 1
  B. Pathophysiology 2
  C. Clinical Signs 1
  D. Diagnostic Tests 2
  E. Management 2
  F. Nursing Interventions 1
IV. Sports Injuries
  A. Types of Injuries 4
    1. Acute
    2. Chronic
  B. Management of Injuries 4
    1. Acute
    2. Chronic
  C. Injury prevention education 3
  D. Related health problems 4
    1. Nutrition
    2. Menstrual dysfunction
    3. Eating disorders
    4. Substance abuse
  E. Nursing Interventions 3

From "Study Smart" by N. Dickenson-Hazard, 1990, *Pediatric Nursing, 16,* p. 66 Copyright 1990 by A. J. Jannetti, Inc. Reprinted by permission.

Getting Down To Business—The Actual Studying: There is no better way to prepare for an examination than individual study (Dickenson-Hazard, 1989). The responsibility to achieve the goal you set for this exam lies with you alone. The means you employ to achieve this goal do vary and should begin with identifying your peak study times and using techniques to maximize them.

Technique #1: Study in short bursts. Each of us have our own biologic clock which dictates when we are at our peak during the day. If you are a morning person, you are generally active and alert early in the day, slowing down and becoming drowsy by evening. If you are an evening person, you don't completely wake up until late morning and hit your peak in the afternoon and evening. Each person generally has several peaks during the day. It is best to study during those times when your alertness is at its peak (Dickenson-Hazard, 1990).

During our concentration peaks, there are mini peaks, or bursts of alertness (Olney, 1989). These alertness (''mini'') peaks occur during a concentration peak because levels of concentration are at

Table 3

Sample Study Plan
Goal: Master content on the adolescent health problem test
Test Time Available: 2 Weeks

Objective	Activity	Date Accomplished
Master sports injury content	Read Chapter 26. Take notes on chapter content according to outline	Feb. 5 & 6, 1 hour
	Review class notes and combine with notes taken from text	Feb. 7, 1 hour
	Review combined notes and sample test questions	Feb. 8, 1 hour
Understand content on dysmenorrhea	Read Chapter 23. Take notes on chapter content according to content outline provided	Feb. 9 & 10 1 hour each day
	Review class notes combined with text notes.	Feb. 11, 1 hour
	Review combined notes and sample test questions	Feb. 12, 1 hour
Know material on infectious mononucleosis	Scan Chapter 27. Review class notes, supplementing class notes with text content	Feb. 13, 1½ hours
Know material on acne	Scan Chapter 24. Review class notes supplementing class notes with text content	Feb. 15, 1½ hours
Demonstrate understanding of all material	Review with another person	Feb. 16, 2 hours
	Review all notes	Feb. 18, 2 hours
	Take sample test questions	Feb. 19, 2 hours
Think positively	SMILE • Take frequent breaks • Reward myself after each study session	ON GOING

From "Study Smart" by N. Dickenson-Hazard, 1990, *Pediatric Nursing, 16*, p. 316 Copyright 1990 by A. J. Jannetti, Inc. Reprinted by permission.

their highest during the first part and last part of a study period. These bursts can vary from ten minutes to one hour depending on the extent of concentration. If studying is sustained for one hour there are only two mini peaks; one at the beginning and one at the end. There are eight mini peaks if that same hour is divided into four, 10-minute intervals. Hence it is more helpful to study in short bursts (Olney, 1989). More can be learned in less time.

Technique #2: Cramming can be useful. Since concentration ability is highly variable, some individuals can sustain their mini peaks for 15, 20 or even 30 minutes at a time. Pushing your concentration beyond its peak is fruitless and verges on cramming, which in general is a poor study technique. There are, however, times when cramming, a short term memory tool, is useful. Short term memory generally is at its best in the morning. A quick review or cram of content in the morning can be useful the day of the exam (Olney, 1989). Most studying, however, is best accomplished in the afternoon or evening when long term memory functions at its peak.

Technique #3: Give your brain breaks. Regular times during study to rest and absorb the content is needed by the brain. The best approach to breaks is to plan them and give yourself a conscious break (Dickenson-Hazard, 1990). This approach eliminates the "day dreaming" or "wandering thought" approach to breaks that many of us use. It is better to get up, leave the study area and do something non-study related for longer breaks. For shorter breaks of five minutes or so, leave your desk, gaze out the window or do some stretching exercises. When your brain says to give it a rest, accommodate it! You'll learn more in less stress free time.

Technique #4:   Study the correct content. It is easy for all of us to become bogged down in the detail of the content we are studying. However, it is best to focus on the major concepts or the "state of the art" content. Leave the details, the suppositions and the experience at the door of your study area. Concentrate on the major textbook facts and concepts which revolve around the subject matter being tested.

Technique #5:   Fit your studying to the test type. The best way to prepare for an objective test is to study facts, particularly anything printed in italics. Memory enhancing techniques are particularly useful when preparing for an objective test. If preparing for an essay test, study generalities, examples and concepts. Application techniques are helpful when studying for this type of an exam (Burkle & Marshak, 1989).

Technique #6:   Use your study plan wisely. Your study plan is meant to be a guide, not a rigid schedule. You should take your time with studying. Don't rush through the content just to remain on schedule. Occasionally study plans need revision. If you take more or less time than planned, readjust the plan for the time gained or lost. The plan can guide you, but you must go at your own pace.

Technique #7:   Actively study. Being an active participant in study rather than trying to absorb the printed word is also helpful. Ways to be active include taking notes on the content as you study; constructing questions and answering them; taking practice tests and discussing the content with yourself. Also, using your individual study quirks is encouraged. Some people stand, others walk around and some play background music. You should use whatever helps you to concentrate and study better.

Technique #8:   Use study aids. While there is no substitute for individual studying, several resources, if available, are useful in facilitating learning. Review courses are an excellent means for organizing or summarizing your individual study. They generally provide the content parameters and the major concepts of the content which you need to know. Review courses also provide an opportunity to clarify not-well-understood content, as well as to review known material (Dickenson-Hazard, 1990). Study guides/certification review books and home study programs are useful for organizing study. They provide detail on the content which is important to the exam. Study groups are an excellent resource for summarizing and refining content. They provide an opportunity for thinking through your knowledge base, with the advantage of hearing another person's point of view. Each of these study aids increases understanding of content and when used correctly, increases effectiveness of knowledge application.

Technique #9:   Know when to quit. It is best to stop studying when your concentration ebbs. It is unproductive and frustrating to force yourself to study. It is far better to rest or unwind, then resume at a later point in the day. Avoid studying outside your A.M. or P.M. concentration peaks and focus your study energy on your right time of day or evening.

STRATEGY #4 Become Test-wise

Most nursing examinations are composed of multiple choice questions (MCQ). This type of question requires the examinee to select the best response(s) for a specific circumstance or condition. Successful test taking is dependent not only on content knowledge but on test taking skill as well. If you are unable to impart your knowledge through the vehicle used for its conveyance, i.e., the MCQ, your test taking success is in jeopardy.

Computer based examinations are a new method of testing for some certification examinations. Eventually all of the certification paper and pencil examinations will be replaced with the computer method. Computer based testing has several advantages such as flexibility in taking the examinations at your convenience and earlier notification of test results. If the certification examination you are planning to take is computerized, the instructions will be provided both prior to the examination as well as at the time of the examination. No computer experience is required, and tutorials or introductory lessons precede the computer-based testing to familiarize you with the process.

Moreover, the strategies used to develop effective test-taking skills are applicable to both the traditional paper/pencil and computerized forms of the certification examinations (Sides & Korchek, 1994).

Technique #1:   Recognize the purpose of a test question. Most test questions are developed to examine knowledge at two separate levels: memory and comprehension or application and analysis. A memory question requires the examinee to recall facts from their knowledge base while an application question requires the examinee to use and apply the knowledge. Memory questions test recall while application questions test synthesis and problem-solving skills. When taking a test, you need to be aware when you are being asked to recall a fact, and when you are being asked to use that fact.

Technique #2:   Recognize the components of a test question. Multiple choice questions may include the basic components of a background statement, a stem and a list of options. The background statement presents information which facilitates the examinee in answering the question. The stem asks or states the intent of the question. The options are 3 to 5 possible responses to the question. The correct option is called the keyed response and all other options are called distractors (ABP, 1989). Knowing the components of a test question helps you sift through the information presented and focus on the question's intent (see Table 4).

Technique #3:   Identify the key word(s) in a test question. Don't jump to conclusions when you read the stem. Key words are generally included in the stem of a test question, whereas key concepts or conditions appear in the background statement. You should pay particular attention to the key words in the stem and their impact on the intent of the question (See Table 5). Never "read" into a question or make assumptions beyond the information given.

Technique #4:   Recognize the item types. Basically two styles of MCQs are used for examinations. One requires the examinee to select the one best answer; the other requires selection of multiple correct answers. Among the one best answer styles there are three types. The A type requires the selection of the best response among those offered. The B type requires the examinee to match the options with the appropriate statement. C type items require the examinee to compare or contrast two related conditions. The X type asks the examinee to respond either true or false to each option (ABP, 1989). Table 6 illustrates these item types. Many standardized tests such as those used for certification are composed of three to five option-A type questions.

Technique #5: Read the directions to the questions carefully. Since an examination may have several types of questions, it is imperative to read the directions carefully. If different item types are used on an exam, they are generally grouped together by type and marked clearly with directions. Be on the lookout for changing item types and be sure you understand how you are to answer before you begin reading the question.

Technique #6: Apply the basic rules of test taking. Examination candidates can avert many problems associated with test taking if they give thought to the answers are all techniques that can improve performance. Table 7 provides helpful hints for the basic rules of test-taking. Review these and apply them to the testing situation.

Table 4

Anatomy Of A Test Question

Background Statement:	A 20-year-old women brings her 3-week-old infant to the clinic because she is concerned about the child's crying, especially at night, and the infant's constant feeding demands.
Stem:	Which of the following histories would be most helpful in planning your management?
Options:	(A) Developmental (B) Family (C) Social (D) *Dietary*

Table 5

Test Question Key Words And Phrases

First	Priority	True Statements
Best	Advice	Correct Statements
Most	Approach	Contributing to
Initial	Consideration	Of the following
Important	Management	Which of the following
Major	Expectation	Each of the following
Common	Intervention	
Least	Assessment	
Except	Contraindication	
Not	Evaluation	
Greatest	Counseling	
Earliest	Facilitative	
Useful	Indicative	
Leading	Suggestive	
Significant	Appropriate	
Immediate	Accurately	
Helpful	Likely	
Closely	Characteristics	

From "Anatomy of a test question" by N. Dickenson-Hazard, 1989, *Pediatric Nursing 15*, p. 395. Copyright 1989 by A. J. Jannetti, Inc. Reprinted by permission.

Technique #7   Make educated guesses. This type of guessing is the selection of an option (answer) when certainty of the correct answer is questionable. Elimination of all options except for two of them, followed by a reevaluation of these options based upon your correct knowledge base then allows you to make an educated guess.

There are some examinations that will give credit when correct answers are selected and give no credit for incorrect answers. Directions for this type of examination may state that credit will be given for correct answers, therefore all questions should be answered and you will not be penalized for guessing.

Other kinds of examinations will only give credit for correct answers, and subtract credit for incorrect answers. Directions for this type of examination will instruct you not to guess, or that there is a penalty for guessing. However, even with this kind of an examination, it is still to your advantage to make an educated guess if you can reduce your possibilities to two options and then select the best of the two. **WILD GUESSING** should be avoided since it may not be to your advantage (Nugent & Vitale, 1997).

Technique #8:   Practice, practice, practice. Taking practice tests can improve performance. While they can assist in evaluation of your knowledge, *their primary benefit is to assist you with test taking skills.* You should use them to evaluate your thinking process, your ability to read, understand and interpret questions, and your skills in completing the mechanics of the test.

Technique #9:   Be prepared for exam day. It is important to familiarize yourself with the test site, the building, the parking and travel route prior to the exam day. If you must travel, arrive early to allow time for this familiarization. It is helpful to make a list of things you need on the exam day: pencils, admission card, watch and a few pieces of hard candy as a quick energy source. On exam day allow yourself plenty of time to arrive at the site. Wear comfortable clothes and have a good breakfast that morning. The night before the exam, go to bed at a reasonable hour, and avoid excessive drinking or eating (Sides & Korchek, 1994). The idea is to arrive on time at the test site, prepared and as rested as possible.

STRATEGY #5 Psych Yourself Up: Taking tests is stressful

While a little stress can be productive, too much can incapacitate you in your studying and test taking (Divine & Kylen, 1979). Your attitude and approach to test taking and studying can influence your outcomes. Psyching yourself up can have a positive effect and make examinations a non-anxiety laden experience (Dickenson-Hazard, 1990). The following techniques are based on the principles of successful test taking as presented by Sides & Cailles (1989). Incorporation of these techniques can improve response and performance in examination situations.

Technique #1:   Adopt an ''I can'' attitude. Believing you can succeed is the key to success. Self belief inspires and gives you the power to achieve your goals. Without a success attitude, the road to your goal is much harder. We all stand an equal chance of success in this world. It is those who believe they can who achieve it. This ''I can'' attitude must permeate all your efforts in test taking from studying to improving your skills, to actually writing the test.

TABLE 6

Item Type Examples

A TYPE
Directions for One Best Choice Items: This item-type requires that you indicate the one best answer from the lettered alternatives offered for each item. After you have decided on the one BEST answer, completely blacken the corresponding lettered circle on the answer sheet.

    #1 You have recommended that a 6-month-old infant receive a DPT immunization. His mother reports that he had a tender red thigh for three days after his last shot and a hard knot that is still there. The infant should receive:

        a. No further DPT
        b. Adult Td
        c. Tetanus toxoid alone
        d. *The recommended DPT*

B TYPE
Directions: Each group of questions below consists of five lettered headings followed by a list of numbered words or statements. For each numbered word or statement, select the one lettered heading that is most closely associated with it and fill in the circle beneath the corresponding letter on the answer sheet. Each lettered heading may be selected once, more than once, or not at all.

    #2-#4
Blood test
        a. Direct Coombs test
        b. Direct serum bilirubin concentration
        c. Hemoglobin electrophoresis
        d. Heterophil antibody titer
        e. Osmotic fragility test
Important in the diagnosis of:
        2. Blood group incompatibility (A)
        3. Mononucleosis (D)
        4. Sickle cell disease (C)

C TYPE
Directions: Each set of lettered headings below is followed by a list of numbered words or phrases. For each numbered word or phrase fill in the circle on the answer sheet under A if the item is associated with (A) only, B if the item is associated with (B) only, C if the item is associated with both (A) and (B), D if the item is associated with neither (A) nor (B).

        (A) Diabetic acidosis
        (B) Insulin shock
        (C) Both
        (D) Neither
  #5 — Elevated bicarbonate level in serum (D)
  #6 — The duration of the condition before proper treatment is begun may influence the prognosis (C)
  #7 — Deep breathing (A)
  #8 — Coma (C)
  #9 — Moist skin characteristic (B)

X TYPE
Directions: Each of the questions or incomplete statements below is followed by five suggested answers or completions. For EACH lettered alternative completely blacken one lettered circle in either column T or F on the answer sheet.

    True statements about fractures in school aged children include:
        (A) Assessment of fractures is less difficult in school aged children than adults
        (B) *The initial treatment for sprains and fractures is elevation and application of an ice pack*
        (C) After a plaster cast is applied, little care is necessary
        (D) *Fractures in children heal faster than fractures in adults*
        (E) Clavicular fractures are generally benign

Adapted from "Anatomy of a test question." by N. Dickenson-Hazard, 1989, *Pediatric Nursing 15*, p. 396. Copyright 1989 by A. J. Jannetti, Inc. Adapted by permission.

Technique #2: Take control. By identifying your goal, deciding how to accomplish it and developing a plan for achieving it, you take control. Do not leave your success or failure to chance; control it through action and attitude.

Technique #3: Think positively. Examinations are generally based on a standard which is the same for all individuals. Everyone can potentially pass. Performance is influenced not only by knowledge and skill but attitude as well. Those individuals who regard an exam as an opportunity or challenge will be more successful.

TABLE 7

Basic Rules For Test Taking

Basic Rule	Helpful Hints
Use time wisely and effectively	Allow no more than 1 minute per question—if you can't answer question, make an intelligent guess

Know the parts of a question
    Background statement: Informational scenario
    Stem: Specific question or intent statement
	Select the option that best completes question or solves the problem
	Relate options to question and balance against each other
	Consider all options

Read question carefully	Understand stem first, then look for answer Underline key words in background information and stem (i.e., first, best, initial, early, most, appropriate, except, least, not)
Identify intent of item based on information given	Don't assume any information not given Don't read in or add any information not given Actively reason through question
Answer difficult questions by eliminating obviously incorrect options first	Select the best of the viable, available options using logical thought Reread stem; select strongest option Skip difficult questions and return to them later or make an educated guess
Select responses guided by principles of communication	Choose therapeutic, respectful, communication enhancing options Avoid inappropriate, punitive responses
Know the principles of nursing practice	Select options that relate to common need or the population in general Select options that are correct without exception Select options which reflect nursing judgement
Know and use test-taking principles	Avoid changing answers without good reason Attempt every question Don't rely on flaws in test construction Be systematic and use problem-solving techniques in answering questions

From "Making the grade as a test-taker" by N. Dickenson-Hazard, 1989. *Pediatric Nursing 15*, p. 304. Adapted from *How to take tests.* (pp 15-57) by J. Millman and W. Paul, 1969, New York: McGraw-Hill Co. and from *Nurses's guide to successful test taking.* (pp 43-53) by M. B. Sides and N. B. Cailles, 1989, Philadelphia: J. B. Lippincott Co. Copyright 1989 A. J. Jannetti, Inc. Reprinted and adapted by permission.

Technique #4: Project a positive self-fulfilling prophecy. While preparing for an examination, project thoughts of the positive outcomes you will experience when you succeed. Self-talk is self-fulfilling. Expect success, not failure, of yourself.

Technique #5: Feel good about yourself. Without feeling a sense of positive self worth, passing an examination is difficult. Recognize your professional contributions and give yourself credit for your accomplishments. Think ''I will pass,'' not ''I suppose I can.''

Technique #6: Know yourself. Focus exam preparation and test taking on your strengths. Try to alter your weaknesses instead of becoming hung up on them. If you tend to overanalyze, study and read test questions at face value. If you're a speed demon when taking a test, slow down and read more carefully.

Technique #7: Failure is a possibility. We all have failed at something at some point in our lives. Rather than dwelling on the failure, making excuses and believing you'll fail again, recognize your mistakes and remedy them. Failure is a time to begin again; use it as a motivator to do better. It is not the end of the world unless you allow it to be. It is best to deal with the failure and move on, otherwise it interferes with your success.

Technique #8: Persevere, persevere, persevere! Endurance must underlie all your efforts. Call forth those reserve energies when you've had all you think you can take. Rely upon yourself and your support systems to help you maintain a sense of direction and keep your goal in the forefront.

Technique #9: Motivation is muscle. Most individuals are motivated by fear or desire. The fear in an exam situation may be one of failure, the unknown or discovery of imperfection. Put your fear into perspective; realize you are not the only one with fear and that all have an equal opportunity for success. Develop strategies to reduce fear and use fear to your advantage by improving the imperfections. Desire is a powerful motivator and you should keep the rewards of your desire foremost in your mind. Whatever motivates you, use it to make you successful. Reward yourself during your exam preparation and once the exam has been completed. You alone hold the key to success; use what you have wisely.

Technique #10: Overprepare. One of the best ways to reduce test anxiety is to overprepare. The more prepared you are the more confident you will be. Overpreparation requires you to study the same information over again even when you know the information. This activity will reinforce your learning and will build confidence and reduce anxiety when it comes time to take the examination.

Overpreparation can not occur unless adequate time is allowed for this process. A last minute cramming approach will not lead to an overprepared test taker. Being over prepared definitely places an individual in control and in a position of power and confidence (Nugent & Vitale, 1997).

This chapter has provided concepts, strategies and techniques for improving study and test taking skills. Your first task in improvement is to know yourself, how you study and how you take a test. You should use your strengths and remedy the weaknesses. Next you need to develop your thinking skills. Work on techniques to improve memory and reasoning. Now you need to organize your study and concentrate on using these new and used skills to be successful. Create a study space, develop a plan of action, then implement that plan during your periods of peak concentration. Before taking the exam be sure you understand the components of a test question, can identify key words and phrases and have practiced. Apply the test taking rules during the exam process. Finally, believe in yourself, your knowledge and your talent. Believing you can accomplish your goal facilitates the fact that you will.

BIBLIOGRAPHY

American Board of Pediatrics. (1989). *Developing questions and critiques.* Unpublished material.

Burke, M. M., & Walsh, M. B. (1992). *Gerontologic nursing.* St. Louis: Mosby Year Book.

Burkle, C. A., & Marshak, D. (1989). *Study program: Level 1.* Reston, VA: National Association of Secondary School Principals.

Dickenson-Hazard, N. (1989). Making the grade as a test taker. *Pediatric Nursing, 15,* 302–304.

Dickenson-Hazard, N. (1989). Anatomy of a test question. *Pediatric Nursing, 15,* 395–399.

Dickenson-Hazard, N. (1990). The psychology of successful test taking. *Pediatric Nursing, 16,* 66–67.

Dickenson-Hazard, N. (1990). Study smart. *Pediatric Nursing, 16,* 314–316.

Dickenson-Hazard, N. (1990). Study effectiveness: Are you 10 a.m. or p.m. scholar? *Pediatric Nursing, 16,* 419–420.

Dickenson-Hazard, N. (1990). Develop your thinking skills for improved test taking. *Pediatric Nursing, 16,* 480–481.

Divine, J. H., & Kylen, D. W. (1979). *How to beat test anxiety.* New York: Barrons Educational Series, Inc.

Goroll, A., May, L., & Mulley, A. (Eds.). (1988). *Primary care medicine* (2nd ed.). Philadelphia: J. B. Lippincott.

Millman, J., & Pauk, W. (1969). *How to take tests.* New York: McGraw-Hill Book Co.

Nugent, P. M., & Vitale, B. A. (1997). *Test success.* (2nd ed.). Philadelphia: F. A. Davis.

Olney, C. W. (1989). *Where there's a will, there's an A.* New Jersey: Chesterbrook Educational Publishers.

Sides, M., & Cailles, N. B. (1989). *Nurse's guide to successful test taking.* Philadelphia: J. B. Lippincott Co.

Sides, M., & Korchek, N. (1994). *Nurse's guide to successful test taking* (2nd ed.). Philadelphia: J. B. Lippincott.

Human Growth and Development

Mary A. Baroni

Human Growth and Development: Underlying Theory and Science of Child Health

- Definition: How and why a person changes and/or stays the same over time (Berger, 2000)
  1. Nature (heredity and genetic predisposition) vs. nurture (environmental influence)
  2. Continuity (continual process) vs. discontinuity (distinct stages)
- Three Fundamental Domains: Conceptual distinctions but overlapping processes in reality
  1. Physical domain
     a. Genetic factors
     b. Physical stature and appearance
     c. Nutritional status
     d. Physical health and well-being
     e. Fine and gross motor abilities
  2. Cognitive domain
     a. Perception, thinking, information processing and memory
     b. Communication—receptive and expressive language
  3. Psychological and social domain
     a. Temperament and personality
     b. Interpersonal relationships
     c. Home environment and other social contexts

Classic Developmental Theories and Theorists

- Nature Positions: Emphasis on heredity and maturational process
  1. Jacque Rousseau (1712–1778)
     a. *Emile—Treatise on Education*
     b. Child as an "untamed savage"
  2. Charles Darwin (1809–1882)
     a. *Origin of the Species*—human evolution (phylogeny)
     b. First use of "baby journal" as systematic method to document observed behavioral development
  3. Alfred Binet (1857–1911) and Theophile Simon (1873–1961)
     a. First standardized measurement of intelligence
     b. Intention was to identify "mentally defective" children needing specialized education
  4. G. Stanley Hall (1844–1924)

a. *Adolescence* (1904)—classic work that first described adolescence as a critical developmental period of "Sturm und Drang" or "Storm and Stress."

b. Development of questionnaires as method for the study of child development via adult retrospective recall

5. Arnold Gesell (1880–1961)

   a. Maturational-organismic theory—biological basis of development

   b. *The Atlas of Infant Behavior* (1934)—developmental milestones

   c. Developed one of the earliest infant tests

6. Sigmund Freud (1856–1939)

   a. *Three Contributions to the Sexual Theory* (1905)

   b. Stage theory of psychosexual development

      (1) Infancy: Oral stage

      (2) Toddler: Anal stage

      (3) Preschool: Phallic stage

      (4) School age: Latency stage

      (5) Adolescence: Genital stage

   c. Key principles

      (1) Id: Principle of pleasure

      (2) Ego: Principle of reality and/or self-interest

      (3) Superego: Principle of morality or conscience

7. Neo-Freudian: Erik Erikson (1902–)—stage theory of life span psychosocial development

   a. Infancy: Trust vs. Mistrust

   b. Toddler: Autonomy vs. shame and doubt

   c. Preschool: Initiative vs. guilt

   d. School age: Industry vs. inferiority

   e. Adolescence: Identity vs. role confusion

   f. Young Adult: Intimacy vs. isolation

   g. Middle-age: Generativity vs. stagnation

   h. Older Adulthood: Integrity vs. despair

8. Neo-Freudian: Margaret Mahler—psychological birth of the infant

   a. Psychological birth of the child with emerging sense of self as separate from mother

     b.   Inadequate early mothering and "psychological birth" results in mental illness

     c.   Phases of "psychological birth"

        (1)   Autism from 0 to 2 months—no real social awareness or concept of self

        (2)   Symbiosis from 2 to 5 months—mother-infant dependency

        (3)   Separation-individuation from 6 to 36 months

            (a)   Differentiation and practicing (6 to 12 months)— beginning awareness of self as separate from mother

            (b)   Rapproachment (12 to 24 months)—exploration, emotional refueling, and ability to sustain brief separations

            (c)   Consolidation (24 to 36 months)—increased ability to cope with separations through symbolic play

   9.   Jean Piaget (1896–1980)

     a.   Interactionist—structuralist stage theory of cognitive development

     b.   Sensori-motor stage: Birth to 2 years

     c.   Preoperational thinking: 2 to 7 years

     d.   Concrete operational thinking (7 to 12 years)

     e.   Formal operational thinking (12 years +)

- Nurture Positions: Emphasis on learning and environment

   1.   John Locke (1632–1704)

     a.   *Essay Concerning Human Understanding and Some Thoughts Concerning Education*

     b.   Child as "tabula rasa" or "blank slate"

   2.   John B. Watson (1878–1958)—behaviorism

     a.   *Classical conditioning*—neutral stimulus associated with meaningful one over time leading "conditioned" response that can be elicited by neutral stimulus alone as though it were the meaningful one

     b.   *Psychological Care of the Infant and Child* (1928)

   3.   B. F. Skinner—student of Watson

     a.   Mechanistic-learning theory

     b.   *Operant or instrumental conditioning*—behavior is reinforced or extinguished by positive or negatively experienced consequences such as use of "time-out" for misbehavior

   4.   Albert Bandura and Walter Mischel—social learning theory

     a.   Influenced by both behaviorism and psychodynamic theories

    b. Behavior results from interaction of individual characteristics, the environment and the behavior itself

    c. Modeling—learning from direct observation and subsequent imitation of what is seen and done by significant others in the proximal environment

- Ethologic Theories

    1. Konrad Lorenz—*sensitive periods* as biologically-programmed periods predisposed for particular learning, e.g., *imprinting*

    2. Harry Harlow—Wisconsin primate laboratory's classic rhesus monkey experiments on separation, isolation and "terry cloth vs. wire surrogate mothers"

        a. Maternal separation and social isolation resulted in dramatic impairment of social-emotional development

        b. Physical contact and comfort as necessary for normal social and emotional development

    3. John Bowlby: *Attachment and Loss* (1969)

        a. Attachment defined as "an affectional tie the infant forms to another specific person that binds the two together in space and endures over time"

        b. Importance of early mothering and consequences of "maternal deprivation" as observed in orphanages and asylums

    4. Marshall Klaus and John Kennel—*Maternal-Infant Bonding* (1976)

        a. Seminal studies on the impact of early contact vs. separation on maternal-infant bonding

        b. Influential in advocating change in hospital policies regarding rooming-in and father participation in the delivery room

    5. Mary Ainsworth: *Patterns of Attachment: A Study of the Strange Situation* (1978)—developed laboratory paradigm "Strange Situation" to assess security or insecurity of the attachment relationship

        a. Early maternal responsiveness to infant needs promotes secure attachment

        b. Secure maternal-infant attachment provides "safe base" from which the child can begin to actively explore the environment and a source of comfort when distressed

        c. Securely attached infants show more optimal cognitive gains and later school performance, illustrating the interconnectedness of psychosocial and cognitive domains

- Humanistic Theories

    1. Abraham Maslow (1908–1970)

        a. Theory of basic needs and human potential derived from study of healthy, creative individuals; few people achieve self-actualization

    b. Hierarchy of needs

        (1) Physiologic

        (2) Safety, security and stability

        (3) Affiliation, acceptance and love

        (4) Ego, self-worth, confidence, competence and success

        (5) Self-actualization

2. Carl Rogers

    a. Client-centered approach from a phenomenologic perspective

    b. Key strategies for intervention

        (1) Unconditional positive regard, empathy and genuineness

        (2) Empathy

        (3) Congruence or the ability to be genuine

- Moral Development

  1. Lawrence Kohlberg's stages of moral development

    a. Based on his original cross-sectional study of 84 school-aged boys (10 to 16 years) recruited from two suburban Chicago schools who were later followed longitudinally

    b. Responses to hypothetic moral dilemmas

    c. Preconventional or pre-moral level

        (1) Stage 1: Punishment-obedience—child behaves to avoid punishment.

        (2) Stage 2: Instrumental-exchange—child behaves well for some gain or reward

    d. Conventional level

        (1) Stage 3: Good-boy/good-girl orientation—child behaves for approval

        (2) Stage 4: Law and order perspective—child behaves to avoid getting caught

    e. Postconventional level

        (1) Stage 5: Social contract—child/adolescent behaves in accordance with generally accepted social norms

        (2) Stage 6: Universal ethical principles—child/adolescent decides on moral standards of behavior through individual reflection and reasoning

  2. Carol Gilligan: Gender differences in moral development

    a. Male social development orients to ethic of *principles* with moral issues decided on the basis of fairness and justice

b. Female social development orients to ethic of *interpersonal relationships* with moral issues decided on the basis of compassion and caring

- Language Development: L. S. Vygotsky (1896–1934)

    1. Language as biologically-programmed but children learn language actively through direct experience and culture

    2. Zone of proximal development (ZPD): Zone between child's opportunity to observe/participate and ability to internalize the learned behavior

Transactional and Contextual Theories of Development

- Heredity-Environment Interactions

    1. Growth and developmental outcomes result from "main effects" and "interaction effects" of and between both heredity (nature) and environment (nurture)

    2. *Reaction Range*—range of phenotypes that may emerge from similar genotypes developing under varied environmental contexts

- Transactional and Resiliency as Models of Development

    1. Transaction model first described in 1975 as a "continuum of reproductive risk and caretaking casualties" by Arnold Sameroff and Michael Chandler

    2. Research based on transactional model emerged in 1980s describes risk and protective factors associated with vulnerability and resilience in the face of adversity

        a. Emmy Werner (1982)—Kauai longitudinal study from birth to adulthood to explore perinatal risk and environmental factors on subsequent developmental outcomes

        b. Michael Rutter (1979; 1987)—epidemiological studies of children of mentally ill parents to examine risk and protective factors influencing subsequent psychopathology

        c. Alan Sroufe's longitudinal study of competence as a developmental construct

    3. Examples of clinical problems with multifactorial etiology better understood through a transactional perspective include failure-to-thrive, child abuse, attention deficit hyperactivity, conduct, and eating disorders

- Ecological Model or "Development in Context"

    1. Developed and described by Urie Bronfenbrenner in 1979 publication—*Ecology of Human Development: Experiments by Nature and Design.*

    2. Person-place-process model

        a. Microsystems—immediate settings within which a child spends time during development (e.g., home, school, hospital)

        b. Mesosystem—relationship or linkages between microsystems (e.g., service coordination)

      c. Exosystem—settings that may indirectly influence development (e.g., parent's work place, school boards)

      d. Macrosystem—broad-based historical, cultural, demographic and institutional context, (e.g., managed care and welfare reform initiatives)

  3. Understanding how and why a child changes or stays the same over time requires examination not only of the child's emerging capabilities but the quality of the settings (places and processes) where children spend time, communication/linkages between these settings, influence of policy decisions, and overall social, cultural, and political context

  4. Examples of clinical interventions better understood through an ecological perspective include early intervention services, home visiting services, and care coordination/case management strategies

- Collaborative effort toward integration of scientific knowledge concerning childhood development and implications for policy and practice (Shonkoff & Phillips, 2000)

Infant Growth and Development (Birth to 2 years)

- Physical Domain: Major tasks—physiologic regulation/motor control

  1. Definitions

      a. Preterm—newborn with gestational age estimated as less than 37 weeks

      b. Low birth weight (LBW)— < 2500 g

         (1) Very low birth weight (VLBW)— < 1500 g

         (2) Extremely low birth weight (ELBW)— < 1000 g

      c. Assessment of weight for gestational age

         (1) AGA—appropriate for gestational age

         (2) LGA—large for gestational age; weight > 90th percentile; often associated with diabetic pregnancies

         (3) SGA—small for gestational age

            (a) Symmetric intrauterine growth retardation (IUGR)—weight, length and head circumference are SGA; reflects long-standing compromise and/ or intrinsic to infant

            (b) Asymmetric intrauterine growth retardation (IUGR)—underweight for length and head circumference; reflects acute compromise extrinsic to fetus such as placental insufficiency

  2. Average U.S. newborn is 20 to 21 inches (51 cm), weighs approximately 7 pounds (3.1 kg), with head circumference of 13 to 14 inches (33.0 to 35.6 cm) and with chest circumference measuring approximately 2 cm less than head circumference

  3. Initial 10% weight loss in average newborn in first 3 to 4 days of life is usually regained by 14 days

4. Weight doubles by 4 months, triples by one year and q

   a. 6 to 8 oz weight gain per week during first 6 mon

   b. 3 to 4 oz weight gain per week during 6 to 12 mon

   c. Average weight gain in second year is 8 to 9 oz (.2

5. Length usually increases by 50% by one year, doubles by
   years—increases by 1 inch per month during first 6 month   ₂ ᵢₙcn per month
   through first year

6. Head circumference increases $\frac{1}{2}$ inch per month during first 6 months then $\frac{1}{4}$ inch per month through first year

7. Serial measurements and observation over time with use of standardized growth charts—National Center for Health Statistics (NCHS)

8. Dental development

   a. Formation of teeth begins during the third fetal month and continues through adolescence

   b. Primary or deciduous teeth are first set of teeth that are later replaced by permanent teeth

   c. Eruption timing can vary greatly but eruption sequence of deciduous teeth is generally consistent—see Table 1

Table 1
Timetable: Primary Teeth Eruption

Primary Teeth	Maxillary Eruption	Mandibular Eruption
(1) Central incisors	6–8 months	5–7 months
(2) Lateral incisors	8–11 months	7–10 months
(3) Cuspids (Canines)	16–20 months	16–20 months
(4) First molars	10–16 months	10–16 months
(5) Second molars	20–30 months	20–30 months

9. Motor development

   a. Early reflexive responses—involuntary responses to stimuli that may be viewed as precursors to late motor skills

      (1) Survival reflexes

         (a) Breathing, hiccups, sneezes, spitting up as infant tries to regulate breathing, sucking and swallowing

         (b) Temperature control reflexes—cry, shivering, tucking legs close to body

         (c) Feeding reflexes—sucking, rooting, crying, and swallowing

(2) Nonsurvival reflexes—Babinski, stepping, swimming, grasping, moro or startle

b. Gross and fine motor milestones—age of attainment varies but sequence is generally consistent (see Tables 2 and 3)

Table 2
Gross Motor Milestones

Milestone	Age
Good head control	2–3 months
Rolls—front to back	4–5 months
Rolls—back to front	5–6 months
Sits alone	5–6 months
Creeps or crawls	7–8 months
Pulls to standing, cruises	9–10 months
Stands alone	11–12 months
Walks—forward	12–14 months
Walks—backwards	14–16 months
Walks—up steps with assistance	16–18 months
Walks—up and down steps alone	22–24 months
Jumps with both feet	24–28 months

Table 3
Fine Motor Milestones

Milestone	Age
Grasp and shakes rattle	2–3 months
Reaches for object or person	3–4 months
Brings hands to mid-line	4–5 months
Hand-to-hand object transfer	5–6 months
Unilateral reaching	6–7 months
Raking grasp	6–7 months
Finger feeding	7–9 months
Pincer grasp	8–10 months
Simple games—pat-a-cake	9–10 months
Makes marks on paper with pencil/crayon	10–12 months
Opens book, turns pages	12–13 months
Stacks 2 blocks	12–15 months
Uses eating utensils	15–17 months
Stacks 3 blocks	17–18 months
Simple puzzles—circles shapes first	18–20 months
Stacks 6–7 blocks	22–24 months

- Cognitive Development: Major tasks—sensorimotor and early language development

  1. Vision

     a. Presence of blink reflex and pupil constriction to light are indications of newborn vision

b. Newborns can focus on objects between 4 to 30 inches including mother's face during feeding

c. Binocular vision develops between 4 to 6 months

d. Visual acuity is difficult to measure during infancy; distance acuity has been estimated between 20/150 to 20/400 in newborns; improves to 20/70 by 2 years and 20/30 by 5 years

2. Hearing

a. Infants have greater auditory acuity for high rather than low frequency sounds

b. Responsiveness to "motherese" as high-pitched "baby talk"

3. Sensori-motor development (Piaget)

a. Reflexes (birth to 1 month)

b. Primary circular reactions (1 to 4 months)—adaptation of reflexes to the environment through coordination of 2 actions such as seeing and grasping

c. Secondary circular reactions (4 to 8 months)—increased awareness of objects, persons and expected responses

d. Coordination of means and ends (8-12 months)—object permanence introduces this substage with awareness that people and objects continue to exist when out of sight

e. Tertiary circular reactions—active exploration and trial-and-error learning (12 to 18 months)

f. Mental combinations—ability to problem-solve simple situations without trial-and-error (18 to 24 months)

4. Language development—receptive language precedes expressive abilities (see Table 4)

Table 4
Language Milestones

Milestone	Age
Responds to sounds	Birth
Smiles and coos	2–3 months
Laughs, expresses delight	4–5 months
Babbles	5–6 months
"Dada" & "mama"	8–9 months
Waves "bye-bye"	8–9 months
Understands "no"	9–10 months
2 words other than "mama/dada"	11–12 months
Jabbering	12–13 months
Begins to point to body parts	15–18 months
2-word phrases & sentences	18–22 months
30-50 word vocabulary	22–24 months

- Psychosocial Development: Major tasks—goodness of fit between temperament and environment; development of secure attachment relationship

  1. Temperament—the "how" of behavior rather than "what" or "why"

     a. New York Longitudinal Study (NYLS) defined 9 dimensions of temperament—activity, rhythmicity, approachability, adaptability, intensity, threshold of arousal, mood, distractibility, and attention

     b. Categories of temperamental profiles

        (1) Easy—rhythmic, approachable, adaptable, positive moods, and low intensity (40%)

        (2) Slow-to-warm-up—less active, more avoidant, less adaptable, more negative moods and low intensity (15%)

        (3) Difficult—arrhythmic, more avoidant, less adaptable, more negative moods and high intensity (10%)

        (4) Intermediate high and intermediate low (35%)

  2. Parent-infant interaction and the attachment relationship

     a. Synchrony—sensitive, coordinated, mutually regulated and reciprocal style of social interactions that evolve between parent and infant during the first year of life leading to a secure attachment by one year

     b. Emotional development begins with physiologic experience and expression of "comfort/discomfort" which later differentiates into more fine-tuned emotions

        (1) Social smile in response to persons begins around 6 weeks

        (2) Emergence of fears and anxiety accompanies the cognitive milestone of object permanency as the infant distinguishes "mother" from "stranger;" fear of strangers (stranger anxiety) begins around 6 months and peaks about 12 months; separation anxiety begins between 8 to 9 months and peaks around 14 months

     c. Attachment (definition)—the enduring and specific, affective bond that develops over the first year of life

        (1) Secure attachment—underlying emotion is love

        (2) Insecure-avoidant—underlying emotion is anger

        (3) Insecure-anxious—underlying emotion is anxiety/ambivalence

        (4) Insecure-disorganized—underlying process is confusion/ dysfunction

Toddler and Preschooler Growth and Development

- Physical Domain: Major tasks—locomotion and continued motor development

  1. Physical growth

a. Reduced rate of growth between 2 to 6 years resulting in fewer caloric needs and decreased appetite

b. Growth in length is approximately 3 inches (7 cm) per year and weight gain approximately 4 ½ pounds (2 kg) per year

c. Average U.S. 6 year old weighs about 46 pounds (21 kg) and is 46 inches (117 cm) tall

2. Motor development

a. CNS maturation during toddler and preschool years allows for better control and coordination of both gross motor and fine motor skills

b. Motor developmental milestones—see Table 5

Table 5
Gross and Fine Motor Milestones

Gross Motor Milestones	Mean Age
(1) Balance on each foot 2 seconds	2 ½ years
(2) Hops	3 ½ years
(3) Walks upstairs alternating feet	3 ½ years
(4) Walks on tip toes	3 ½ years
(5) Heel-to-toe walking	4 ½ years
Fine Motor Milestones	**Mean Age**
(1) Tower of 8 cubes	2 ½ years
(2) Thumb wiggle	2 ½ year
(3) Copies circle	3 to 3 ½ years
(4) Draws a person with 6 parts	4 ½ years
(5) Copies square	5 years

3. Cognitive development—symbolic thinking and increased language development

a. Pre-operational thinking (Piaget)

(1) Preconceptual (2 to 4 years)

(2) Intuitive (2 to 7 years)

b. Centration—preschoolers' tendency to focus on one idea or characteristic feature of an object or situation at one time

(1) Egocentrism—tendency to focus thinking and understanding about the world from their own perspective only

(2) Animism—everything animate or inanimate thinks and feels the way the preschooler does

c. Difficulty distinguishing fact from fantasy—normative "lying," nightmares, imaginary friends, and potential to feel responsible for bad or good things happening based on their own thoughts, feelings, or behaviors

d. Language development

    (1) Expressive language

        (a) Up to 425 word vocabulary with 75% speech understandable—2 ½ years

        (b) Increased complexity of sentences including 4 to 5 words—3 ½ years

    (2) Receptive language

        (a) Carries out 2 to 3 item commands—3 years

        (b) Understands opposite analogies—4 years

        (c) Understands "if," "because" and "when"—5 years

4. Psychosocial development: Major tasks—autonomy, impulse control/discipline and gender identity

    a. Parenting styles and discipline

      (1) Authoritarian parent—strict parenting with firm or harsh discipline and without questioning; high expectations, low support, low parent-child communication

      (2) Permissive parenting—few demands and low expectations

        (a) Democratic-indulgent—low expectations with high support and high parent-child communication

        (b) Permissive-neglectful—low expectations with low support and low parent-child communication

      (3) Authoritative parenting—firm limits but opportunity for dialogue; high expectations, high support and high parent-child communication; associated with best-child outcomes

    b. Aggression and impulse control

      (1) Instrumental aggression—common form of aggression among preschoolers focused on retrieving an object, space or special privilege; frequency decreases with increased understanding of sharing and impulse control

      (2) Hostile aggression—person-oriented aggression that is not common among preschoolers but may emerge with school entry if impulse control remains problematic

    c. Play as the major medium for early mastery of a variety of physical, cognitive and social skills has been appropriately described as the "work of children"

      (1) Infancy—solitary play as the earliest level of sensorimotor or skill mastery play; associated with little awareness of other children

(2) Toddlers

   (a) Onlooker play is common at this age with curious watching of other children playing

   (b) Parallel play—becomes predominant style of play with toddlers engaged in similar play activity but with minimal interaction

(3) Preschoolers play—more social in character including:

   (a) Associative play—some interaction and sharing of toys may occur but not organized and consistent enough to be called a game

   (b) Cooperative play—children are taking turns and actively playing together

   (c) Dramatic or pretend play—make believe play during which the children create and act out a scene such as "playing house"

   (d) Rough-and-tumble play—physical play involving gross motor activities like running, jumping, chasing and wrestling that appears aggressive but is actually playful

d. Fears

   (1) Nightmares

   (2) Night terrors—partial arousal for deep non-REM sleep with minimal recollection of screaming/thrashing

e. Gender identity—emerging sense of self as a male or female person

   (1) 2-year-olds can distinguish gender and will identify themselves as boy or girl

   (2) 3- to 4-year-olds tend to show sex-typed preferences; gender identity is usually firmly established and unlikely to change

   (3) 5- to 6-year-olds begin to express notions about how males and females should dress, behave and feel

School-Aged Development

- Physical Domain: Motor coordination and skill development

  1. Physical growth—relatively stable, smooth and uneventful

     a. Average school-aged child gains about 5 pounds and $2\frac{1}{2}$ inches per year

     b. By age 10, the average school-aged child weighs about 70 pounds and is 54 inches tall

  2. Motor development—few gender differences except for stronger forearm strength in males and increased flexibility in females

  3. Permanent teeth timing and eruption sequence—see Table 6

Table 6
Timetable: Permanent Teeth Eruption

Permanent Teeth	Maxillary Eruption	Mandibular Eruption
a. Central incisors	7–8 years	6–7 years
b. Lateral incisors	8–9 years	7–8 years
c. Cuspids (Canines)	11–12 years	9–11 years
d. First premolar (Bicuspids)	10–11 years	10–12 years
e. Second premolar (Bicuspids)	10–12 years	11–13 years
f. First molars	6–7 years	6–7 years
g. Second molars	12–13 years	12–13 years
h. Third molars	17–22 years	17–22 years

- Cognitive Development: Major task—concrete thinking and adaptation to school

    1. Concrete operational thought (Piaget)

        a. "5 to 7 shift"—transition period between preoperational and concrete operational thinking

        b. Logical operations include:

            (1) Reversibility—ability to reverse a process or action such as understanding that if $2 + 3 = 5$ then $5 - 3 = 2$

            (2) Conservation (number, mass and volume)—understanding that certain aspect or quality of an object can change in appearance without changing the object itself

            (3) Classification—ability to group objects on the basis of similar characteristics such as color or shape

            (4) Seriation—arrangement of items in a series such as by increasing size

    2. School readiness

        a. School entry is a major transition for children

        b. School refusal may reflect separation anxiety masked as vague somatic complaints

- Psychosocial Development: Major tasks—self-esteem, peers, and after school activites

    1. Self-esteem—competence to think, learn, and make decisions as well as believe that one is worthy of love and respectful treatment from others

    2. Peers and development of prosocial behavior through cooperative games, sports, and activities

    3. The need for organized after school activities has become critical with the increasing numbers of children who are regularly left unsupervised after school because of parental work schedules and variations in family structure in the U.S.

Adolescent Development

- Physical Domain: Major tasks—puberty, sexual maturation

    1. Physical growth

        a. Average U.S. female gains about 38 pounds (17 kg) and $9\frac{1}{2}$ inches (24 cm) between 10 to 14 years.

        b. Average U.S. male gains about 42 pound (19 kg) and $9\frac{1}{2}$ inches (24 cm) between 12 to 16 years.

    2. Puberty—period of rapid physical growth and sexual maturation resulting in adult size, shape and reproductive potential

        a. Sequence of puberty—individual variation in onset but sequence of somatic and physiologic changes is relatively set

            (1) Females

                (a) Puberty onset 9 to 10 years

                (b) Precocious puberty < 8 years

                (c) Delayed puberty > 13 years

                (d) First physical sign—breast buds

                (e) Peak height velocity—12.4 years

                (f) Menarche—12.5 years

                (g) Fertility—15 years

            (2) Males

                (a) Puberty onset 11 to 12 years

                (b) Precocious puberty < 9 years

                (c) Delayed puberty > 14 years

                (d) First physical sign—testicular growth

                (e) Peak height velocity—14.4 years

                (f) Spermarche—13 to 14 years

                (g) Fertility—15 years

        b. Anovulatory cycles are common during the first two years after menarche (50% of cycles vs. 20% after 5 years)

        c. Stages of genital maturity in males—takes approximately 4 years to move from stage 2 to 5 (Tanner staging)

            (1) Stage 1: Pre-adolescent testes, scrotum and penis

            (2) Stage 2: Enlargement of scrotum and testes; scrotum reddens and roughens

(3) Stage 3: Penis enlarges primarily in length

(4) Stage 4: Penis enlarges in breadth and development of glans

(5) Stage 5: Adult size and shape

d. Stages of breast development in females (Tanner staging)

(1) Stage 1: Pre-adolescent breast with nipple elevation

(2) Stage 2: Breast buds with areolar enlargement

(3) Stage 3: Breast enlargement without separate contour with nipple

(4) Stage 4: Projection of areola and nipple as secondary mound to breast

(5) Stage 5: Adult breast with areola receding and nipple projecting from breast

e. Stages of pubic hair development in males and females (Tanner staging)

(1) Stage 1: Pre-adolescent without pubic hair

(2) Stage 2: Sparse, pale, fine pubic hair

(3) Stage 3: Darker, more curled, increased amount of pubic hair

(4) Stage 4: Hair is adult in character but doesn't cover entire pubic area

(5) Stage 5: Adult distribution in quantity, quality and pattern

- Cognitive Development: Major tasks—ability to abstract and decision-making

  1. Formal operational thought—ability to abstract (Piaget)

  2. Characteristic ways of thinking

     a. Egocentrism—difficulty an adolescent may have in thinking rationally about their own personal experiences as completely unique

     b. Invincibility fable—sense of invincibility that can lead to risk-taking behaviors

     c. Personal fable—variation of adolescent egocentrism whereby adolescent feels personally gifted in some way

     d. Imaginary audience—exaggerated sense that everyone is watching and focused on the adolescent resulting in feeling self-conscious

- Psychosocial Development: Major tasks—independence, intimacy, vocation or career goals

  1. Majority of adolescents cope well with their transition to adulthood and do not experience "storm and stress" as once assumed

  2. A second phase of "separation-individuation" occurs during adolescence that requires new approaches to parenting, communication, decision-making and independence

  3. Three psychosocial periods of adolescence

     a. Early adolescence—middle school (11 to 14 years)

(1) Importance of peers and feeling "normal"

(2) Moodiness

b. Middle adolescence—high school (15 to 17 years)

(1) Body image, sexuality, dating

(2) Asserting independence

c. Late adolescence—vocation and career choices (18 to 21 years)

(1) Identity formation—achievement, moratorium, foreclosure, diffusion

(2) Vocation and career choices including college, military, and employment opportunities

(3) Intimacy in relationships

The Changing American Family as Context for Growth and Development

- Demographic Changes

  1. Increasing rates of divorce and remarriage

  2. Delays and declines in child-bearing

  3. Rise in female participation in work force—voluntary, dual earner families, female head of household, and welfare reform work requirements

  4. Increasing incidence of single parent families, childhood poverty, and homelessness

- Variations in Family Structure

  1. Decrease in "traditional" two-parent family

  2. Increase in single-parent households—divorce, births to unmarried mothers, death of spouse, adoption

  3. Remarriage, blended families, and step-parenting

  4. Extended and/or "skip generation" families with grandparents as primary caregivers and/or with several generations living together

  5. Foster families—estimated 300,000 children in foster care at any given time

  6. Group living including homeless shelters—estimated 43% of the homeless population include families with children

  7. Gay and lesbian families—estimated 5 million lesbian mothers and 3 million gay fathers caring for between 6 to 14 million children

- Family Functioning: Critical concepts

  1. Family functioning is more directly related to healthy growth and development than is family structure

  2. Components of family functioning include provision of a stable and safe physical environment as well as financial and emotional resources necessary to provide supportive and nurturing care with appropriate supervision and guidance

3. Screening and assessment tools

   a. Family Inventory of Life Events (FILE)

   b. Family Coping Strategies (F-COPES)

   c. Adolescent-Family Inventory of Life Events and Changes (A-FILE)

   d. Parenting Stress Index (PSI)

4. Family-centered care—Institute for Family-Centered Care

   a. Recognition that the family is the constant in a child's life

   b. Family-professional collaboration at all levels

   c. Respect for family diversity in structure, race, ethnicity, culture and socioeconomic status

   d. Recognition of family strengths, uniqueness and diversity in coping strategies

   e. Communication and sharing of information on an ongoing basis with families in a supportive and non-judgmental manner

   f. Support and facilitation of family-to-family support

   g. Understand and incorporate strategies supportive of growth and developmental needs of children and their families into health care settings/systems

   h. Implementation of policies and programs to support emotional and financial well-being of families

   i. Accessible health care that is flexible, culturally competent and responsive to family-centered need

5. Resources: Institute for Family-Centered Care
     http://www.familycenteredcare.org

Deviations in Physical Growth and Behavioral Development

Failure-to-Thrive (FTT)

- Definition

1. No consensus on definition

2. Descriptive rather than diagnostic term

3. Generally refers to infants and young children whose weight is below the 3rd percentile on National Center for Health Statistics (NCHS) growth standards and/or whose weight trajectory has decreased by two major growth percentiles

4. Traditional categories include organic FTT, non-organic FTT, and mixed etiology FTT

5. Newer categories include neurodevelopmental FTT and socioemotional FTT

- Etiology/Incidence
  1. Multifactorial etiology including underlying organic disease or predisposing medical condition, maladaptive parent-infant interaction, maternal depression, poverty, deficits in parenting information and skills, child abuse and neglect
  2. Accounts for between 3% to 5% of all pediatric admissions of infants less than one year with as many as 50% without underlying medical condition
  3. Males and females are equally affected
- Clinical Findings
  1. Inadequate intake—inadequate milk production, mechanical problems with suck/swallow coordination, systemic disease, errors in formula preparation, misunderstanding about infant needs and feeding practices
  2. Increased losses or decreased utilization—vomiting and/or malabsorption
  3. Increased caloric requirements--underlying disease process including cardiac, respiratory, hyperthyroid, cancer, recurrent infection
  4. Altered growth potential—prenatal insult, genetic disorder or endocrine dysfunction
- Differential Diagnosis
  1. Organic causes
     a. Gastrointestinal—gastroesophageal reflux (GER), pyloric stenosis, cleft palate, lactose intolerance, Hirschprung disease, milk-protein intolerance, hepatitis, malabsorption
     b. Cardiopulmonary—cardiac defects, bronchopulmonary dysplasia (BPD), asthma, cystic fibrosis (CF), tracheobronchial malformations
     c. Endocrine—hypothyroid, diabetes, adrenal insufficiency, pituitary disorders, growth hormone deficiency
     d. Infection—parasitic or bacterial, TB, HIV
     e. Neurologic—mental retardation, fetal alcohol syndrome, lead poisoning, prematurity, neuroregulatory difficulties
     f. Genetic—mitochondrial diseases
  2. Social-emotional and environmental causes
     a. Maternal depression, isolation, marital difficulties
     b. Poverty/inadequate resources
     c. Inadequate parenting knowledge and skills
     d. Difficult temperament
     e. Child abuse and neglect

- Diagnostic Methods/Findings

    1. History—prenatal, perinatal, neonatal; complete diet history and feeding practices; environmental, social, and family history

    2. Identification of risk factors—premature, LBW, difficult temperament, regulation problems, social stresses

    3. Height, weight, head circumference; review longitudinal growth data, corrected for gestational age as appropriate; vital signs including blood pressure if child is over 3 years

    4. Physical examination—signs of underlying organic disease; severity of malnutrition, evidence of abuse or neglect

    5. Developmental assessment and caregiver concerns

    6. Feeding observation to assess behavioral or interactional contributing factors

    7. Home visit or public health nurse referral to assess environmental factors.

    8. Laboratory assessment should be judicious based on history and clinical findings; CBC, UA if applicable; serum creatinine, total protein/albumin; electrolyte screen; other labs as indicated by history, blood lead levels, TB test; thyroid function; test for reflux/malabsorption; sweat test, stool specimen for parasites; bone age if height is poor

- Management/Treatment

    1. Importance of developing therapeutic alliance with caregiver

    2. Usually managed on an outpatient basis if possible with hospitalization indicated when there is evidence of abuse or severe neglect, severe malnutrition, medical instability or when outpatient management has failed

    3. Interdisciplinary approach is optimal utilizing health care, nutritional, mental health and social services

    4. Provide caregivers with necessary information regarding nutritional needs of child and appropriate feeding skills to promote optimal growth

    5. Close monitoring and follow-up on growth and development, social environment and interdisciplinary/interagency communication

Stuttering

- Definition: Speech dysfluency with initial onset during the preschool years that is characterized by repetitions of sounds, syllables, and/or short words as well as pauses in timing of speech.

    1. Mild or developmental stuttering—speech dysfluency most notable when a preschool-aged child is tired or excited that usually resolves spontaneously if not given excessive attention

2. Moderate or severe stuttering (sometimes referred to as acquired stuttering)—persistent speech dysfluency that is inappropriate for age and usually has a neurologic and/or psychogenic etiology

- Etiology/Incidence

   1. Multifactorial etiology with a 3:1 male to female ratio of occurrence

   2. Prevalence estimated at 1% among pre-pubertal children with decrease to 0.8% estimate post-puberty

   3. Mild developmental stuttering occurs in 4% to 5% of children between 2 to 5 years that spontaneously resolves; approximately 20% of early stuttering does not resolve without intervention

- Clinical Findings

   1. Repetition and/or prolongation of sounds, syllables or short words

   2. Pauses within words or sentences

   3. Signs of physical tension and struggling with speech such as eye blinking and trembling lips

   4. Avoidance of words that cause particular problems

   5. Child and/or parents are frustrated and/or embarrassed by stuttering posing difficulty at home, in school, or with peers

- Differential Diagnosis

   1. Normal developmental dysfluency

   2. Hearing impairment

   3. Speech-motor deficit

- Management/Treatment

   1. Assess frequency, type and duration of dysfluency

   2. Encourage parents to avoid excessive attention to dysfluency and be patient in listening to child's speech

   3. Refer to speech and language pathologist for assessment if child is showing signs of embarrassment, speech dysfluency interferes with communication and/or parent expresses significant concern regardless of severity

   4. Stuttering Foundation of America
      PO Box 11749
      Memphis, TN 38111-0749
      (800) 992-9392

Autism and Pervasive Developmental Disorder (PDD)

- Definition: Type of pervasive developmental disability characterized by a spectrum of symptoms and characteristics that may range in severity but usually manifest themselves within the first three years of life; symptoms include altered responses to sensory stimuli, impairments in communication, language, play and other social interactions; DSM-IV-TR and International Categories of Disease-10 (ICD-10) categorize PDD similarly to include:

1. Autistic disorder or autism

2. Pervasive developmental disorder, not otherwise specified (PDD-NOS) or atypical autism

3. Asperger's syndrome

4. Rett's disorder

5. Childhood disintegrative disorder

- Etiology/Incidence

1. Underlying neurological disorder caused by brain insult/injury during fetal development and not by psychosocial circumstances as previously believed

2. Associated etiological factors include genetic link (10%) as well as history of perinatal infection; no clear etiological determination for majority of children with autism

3. Rates are 4 times higher among males than females; occurrence in females tends to be severe; no racial, ethnic, or socioeconomic differences; epidemiological data indicate overall incidence rates of 2 to 5 per 10,000

- Clinical Findings

1. Normal growth and development usually reported until 2 to 2 $\frac{1}{2}$ years when parents notice delays in language, symbolic or imaginative play, and/or other social interactions; onset of such delay or abnormal behavioral pattern before 3 years of age is considered part of diagnostic criteria.

2. DSM-IV-TR (2000) diagnostic criteria require a total of six behavioral manifestations from three categories including:

   a. Qualitative impairment in social interaction—poor eye contact; lack of shared enjoyment in activities with peers or family

   b. Qualitative impairment in communication—delayed or deviant language development; lack of interest in toys, activities for symbolic or imaginative play appropriate for age

   c. Restrictive repetitive and stereotypic patterns of behavior, interests and/or activities—repetitive rituals or motor movements such as spinning or hand flapping

3. Associated problems may include other cognitive delays, problems learning, unusual responses to sensory stimuli, difficulties with sleeping and eating, differences in emotional responsiveness, and seizure activity

4. Significant variation in clusters of symptoms and characteristics ranging from mild to severely affected

- Diagnostic Tests/Findings

    1. No specific medical diagnostic test for autism

    2. EEG indicated for associated problems including seizures and language delay

    3. Laboratory studies to assess etiological factors

        a. Urine amino acids and organic acids; metabolic screen for metabolic disorders such as PKU

        b. DNA probe for fragile X on blood plasma

    4. MRI or CT scan may show structural abnormalities in cerebellum but otherwise not particularly helpful in absence of clinical signs such as asymmetries, focal tremors or paralyses

- Differential Diagnosis

    1. Mental retardation

    2. Sensory impairment (hearing or vision)

    3. Severe abuse or neglect

    4. Subtypes of pervasive developmental disorders

    5. Childhood psychosis

    6. Gifted child

    7. Tourette's syndrome

    8. Fragile X

- Management/Treatment

    1. No specific medical interventions currently available

    2. Early screening, diagnosis and referral to early intervention is critical

    3. Treatment is primarily psychoeducation requiring individualized plan

    4. Interdisciplinary team to coordinate care including parents, teachers, primary care provider, psychologist, physical therapy, speech and language and other early intervention staff as appropriate

    5. Address associated problems through specific therapies (sensory integration) counseling (family adjustment, behavioral management), medications (seizures and behavioral problems)

    6. Community education, resource identification and parent-to-parent support

        a. Autism Society of America
        7910 Woodmont Avenue, Suite 650
        Bethesda, MD 20814-3015

        b. CHAT—checklist for autism in toddlers (Baron-Cohen, Cox, Baird, Swettenham, Nightengale, Morgan, Drew, & Chaman, 1996)

Obesity

- Definition
    1. Excess accumulation of body fat relative to lean body mass that results from excessive caloric intake relative to energy expenditure
    2. Operational definitions (cut-off values) vary in the literature
- Etiology/Incidence
    1. Multifactorial etiology with interaction of genetic, environmental, developmental and behavioral factors
        a. Genetic predisposition and parental obesity
        b. Dietary patterns
        c. Inactivity (television, video games)
        d. Cultural and familial food preferences
        e. Use of food as emotional buffer
        f. Physical disorders with decreased energy expenditure (spina bifida, Down syndrome, Prader-Willi syndrome)
    2. Most prevalent nutritional problem in U.S.
    3. Childhood obesity prevalence is rising with current estimates ranging from 15% to 30% depending on definition and cut-off values
- Clinical Findings
    1. Parent and/or child concern regarding body weight
    2. Clinical observation of large size and/or excess fat on child
- Differential Diagnosis
    1. Endocrine dysfunction
    2. Congenital disorders/short stature
    3. Large frame
    4. Muscular hypertrophy
    5. Medication induced obesity (corticosteroids, psychotropic drugs)
- Diagnostic Tests/Findings
    1. History includes detailed dietary and activity level history (past and present), family history of obesity and related morbidities including hypertension, cardiovascular disease, hyperlipidemia, diabetes, depression; review of systems for associated morbidity (glucose intolerance, orthopedic difficulties); developmental milestones, psychosocial concerns about weight
    2. Physical examination, vital signs, blood pressure
    3. Anthropometric measurements

a. Weight for height ratio greater than 95th percentile on NCHS growth charts is commonly used but doesn't account for large frame or increased muscle mass

b. Percent of ideal body weight greater or equal to 120%; calculated by dividing child's actual weight by ideal body weight (50th percentile for age and sex) and multiplied by 100

c. Skin-fold thickness per calibrated caliper measurements at or above 85th percentile for age, sex, and race; tricep measurements are most common and reference charts are available

d. Body Mass Index (BMI) considered most useful index

    (1) Weight in kilograms/height in meters^2

    (2) Screening classifications using BMI in adolescents

        (a) Obesity—BMI equal or greater than 95th percentile for age and gender

        (b) At risk for obesity—between 85th and 95th percentile or with rapid weight gain of > 2 BMI units in one year

    (3) No current consensus on BMI classification of obesity among younger children

    (4) More recent reference percentiles provide age, gender and ethnic-specific distributions (Rosner, Prineas, Loggie & Daniels, 1998)

e. New NHANES III growth chart reference standards will include BMI distributions

    4. CBC, UA, thyroid function, lipid profile

- Management/Treatment

    1. Prevention in infancy through parent education regarding nutritional needs and feeding strategies

    2. Discuss moderate modification of diet and caloric content while increasing exercise program

    3. Goal for younger child is weight maintenance rather than weight reduction while linear growth catches up; goal for adolescent may include weight reduction if treated after growth spurt

    4. Behavior modification strategies directed at alternative coping measures to deal with stress, maintain motivation, and reinforce regimen

    5. Involvement of family in therapeutic program increases likelihood of success

    6. Refer to and collaborate with available community resources as appropriate

Child Abuse and Neglect

- Definition: Abuse usually refers to actual "acts of commission" and neglect refers to "acts of omission" although there remains no consensus on specific definitions

1. First described as "Battered Child Syndrome" by Dr. Henry Kempe in 1962

2. Legal definitions and reporting requirements vary from State to State but all 50 States have mandated reporting of suspected abuse or neglect by health care providers

3. Categories include physical, sexual and emotional abuse, negligent care, and Munchausen syndrome by proxy (MSP)

    a. Soft tissue injuries most common—bruises, abrasions and lacerations

    b. Head injuries less frequent but cause majority of deaths— "Shaken Baby Syndrome" (altered consciousness with or without signs of head injuries)

    c. Burns account for 10% of abuse injuries

    d. Abdominal injuries—usually blunt injuries from hitting or kicking; liver lacerations; kidney/pancreas contusions

    e. Fractures—rib, spiral and multiple fractures at same or various ages should trigger suspicion

    f. Sexual abuse—probably least reported and underdiagnosed

    g. Munchausen syndrome by proxy (MSP)—disturbed parent-child relationship with fabrication or actual harm to produce symptoms of illness requiring medical attention

- Etiology/Incidence:

    1. Etiological factors associated with abuse and neglect

        a. Perpetrator—history of being maltreated as a child; cognitive or psychiatric impairment; socially isolated; inadequate parenting knowledge and skills including unrealistic expectations of child

        b. Victim—unwanted pregnancy; difficult temperament; premature and/or disabled; no significant gender differences

        c. Social context—violence (family/community); poverty; unemployment; substance abuse

    2. An estimated 903,500 children were victims of substantiated reports to Child Protective Services (CPS) from 39 states in 2001 (U.S. Department of Health and Human Services, 2003)

        a. Neglect (52%) is most common form of maltreatment followed by physical abuse (24%), sexual abuse (12%), emotional abuse (6%), medical neglect (3%) and other forms (16%)

        b. Approximately equal numbers of males (48%) and females (51.5%) experienced documented child maltreatment in 2001

        c. African-American and Native American children had rates twice as high as national average

        d. Most (80%) perpetrators are parents

3. Child abuse/neglect is a significant cause of pediatric mortality in infants (second to SIDS) and young children (second to accidents)

   a. 1,300 deaths resulting from abuse or neglect were reported in 2001

   b. Most deaths (84.5%) were of children 6 years or younger

- Clinical Findings

  1. History is vague, inconsistent and/or incompatible with child's developmental stage and severity of injury

  2. History may change during course of interview

  3. Delay in seeking medical attention for injury

  4. History of recurrent injuries

  5. Soft tissue injuries with markings characteristic of source of abuse such as hand marks, curved mark of a belt, burn mark in shape of electric iron

  6. Bruises in various stages of healing

  7. Burn markings characteristic of immersion

  8. Undernutrition, poor hygiene

  9. Developmental delays

  10. Inappropriate parent-child interaction

- Differential Diagnosis

  1. Unintentional injury

  2. Inadequate parenting skills

  3. Underlying disease process, e.g., hemophilia, leukemia, osteogenesis imperfecta

  4. Birth marks, Mongolian spots, and/or other variations in skin pigmentation

  5. Folk-medicine and cultural practices, e.g., coin rubbing

  6. Sudden Infant Death Syndrome (SIDS)

- Diagnostic Tests/Findings

  1. History to determine and precisely document type of injury, alleged circumstances and action taken by caregiver

  2. Observation of parent and child for behavioral extremes or exaggerated responses

  3. Physical examination to assess location, type, and characteristic of any lesions or burns for characteristic pattern, shape or outline; bruises should be noted for coloring

  4. Coagulation studies for severe bruising; radiographs of long bones, ribs and/or skull series as indicated by history and physical examination; ultrasound for suspected visceral injury

- Management/Treatment

    1. Appropriate medical care for child including immediate hospitalization if indicated by severity of injuries

    2. Ensure safety of child utilizing foster care or relatives if necessary

    3. Communicate identified concerns (moderate or severe injuries or threats to child's well-being) and legal imperative to notify child protective services as a mandated reporter of suspected child maltreatment

    4. Assessment of siblings for maltreatment and assurance of safety

    5. Identify and make appropriate referrals to available community resources to facilitate interdisciplinary and interagency collaboration—child protective services, public health, parenting classes, child care/school programs

    6. Education and prevention

        a. Identify families with risk factors associated with child maltreatment and make referrals to appropriate community-based preventive resources before serious abuse occurs

        b. Close primary care supervision and acute care follow-up for at-risk families and children

        c. Early reporting of suspected abuse or neglect

        d. Support community-based child abuse prevention efforts

Attention Deficit Hyperactivity Disorder (ADHD)

- Definition

    1. A behavioral syndrome characterized by a persistent pattern of inattention, poor concentration, impulsivity and overactivity that exceeds normal developmental variation

    2. DSM-IV-TR (2000) defined sub-types

        a. Attention deficit/hyperactivity disorder—predominantly inattention type

        b. Attention deficit/hyperactivity disorder—predominantly hyperactive-impulsive type

        c. Attention deficit disorder—combined type

- Etiology/Incidence

    1. Multifactorial etiology that remains poorly understood but may be associated with:

        a. Delayed CNS maturation

        b. Genetic factors

        c. Prenatal, perinatal, or postnatal trauma or illness

        d. Dysfunction of catecholamine neurotransmitters

e. Male-to-female ratio ranges from 4:1 (general population) to 9:1 (clinic populations)

2. Controlled studies have not demonstrated evidence of additives, sugar or salicylates as associated factors

3. Approximately 3% to 5% of school-aged children meet DSM-IV criteria

- Clinical Findings: DSM-IV-TR (2000) diagnostic criteria for ADHD include:

   1. Six (or more) symptoms of inattention

      a. Poor attention to detail/careless mistakes

      b. Difficulty maintaining attention during activities

      c. Failure to listen even when directly spoken to

      d. Problems following directions and/or with completion of assignments or tasks

      e. Disorganized in activities and tasks

      f. Avoids activities that require focused mental attention

      g. Frequently loses items necessary for successful completion of task, activity or assignment

      h. Easily distracted by external stimuli

      i. Forgetful
         or

   2. Six (or more) symptoms of hyperactivity/impulsivity

      a. Fidgets and squirms

      b. Difficulty staying seated when expected or appropriate

      c. Excessive running and climbing

      d. Difficulty with quiet play activities

      e. Very high energy and activity level

      f. Excessively verbal and talkative

      g. Answers questions abruptly before question is completed

      h. Difficulty waiting for turn

      i. Frequently interrupts others and acts intrusively
         and

   3. Symptom onset prior to 7 years of age

   4. Symptoms identified as problemsome in at least two settings, e.g., home and school

   5. Negative impact of symptoms on social, academic and/or work performance

   6. Symptoms not attributed to more significant underlying psychiatric or medical disorder

- Differential Diagnosis

    1. Age appropriate for highly active child

    2. Inadequate environments (understimulating or chaotic)

    3. Learning disabilities/sensory impairment

    4. Seizures or mental retardation

    5. Situational anxiety and/or depressive reaction

    6. Oppositional behavior and/or conduct disorder

- Diagnostic Tests/Findings

    1. History—Perinatal (maternal substance abuse); past (early health problems including ear infections, lead poisoning, iron deficiency anemia, frequent injuries due to activity), present (frequency, severity and context of symptoms at home and school); social and developmental; parenting style; review of systems

    2. Physical examination, screen for "neurological soft signs;" affective behavior; laboratory data of limited value; CBC, lead screen

    3. Height, weight, blood pressure, vital signs

    4. Vision and hearing screen

    5. Sample behavioral assessment from multiple settings—(home, babysitter/child care, relatives, school) using rating scale of direct observation

        a. Connor's Abbreviated Parent-Teacher Questionnaire

        b. ADHD Comprehensive Teacher rating scale

        c. Achenbach and Edelbrach's Child Behavior Checklist

        d. Edelbrach Child Attention Problem Scale

        e. DuPaul ADHD Rating Scale for Teachers

    6. Psychological evaluation and cognitive testing

- Management/Treatment

    1. Provide structured environment—regular routine, clear and simple rules, firm limits, minimize distraction, overstimulation and fatigue

    2. Behavioral management—formal operant conditioning techniques to reward/reinforce good behaviors; punishment strategies (time-out) or extinction techniques (systematic ignoring) to decrease unacceptable behaviors

    3. Evaluate need for mental health referral

        a. Child-based therapy for depression, anxiety, low self-esteem; cognitive-behavioral training to increase self-control

        b. Parenting classes or family therapy for relationship difficulties

    4. CNS stimulant medication—(children > 5 years)

    a. Methylphenidate—effective in 75% to 80% with trial of at least 2 to 3 weeks; give 20 to 30 minutes before meals to maximize effectiveness; avoid p.m. doses to minimize insomnia

    b. Dextroamphetamine—effectiveness in 70% to 75% with rapid response

    c. Amphetamine mixture—newer drug being utilized that is a combination of dextroamphetamine and amphetamine; onset of action is slower and smoother than methylphenidate or dextroamphetamine; adequate clinical trials are still pending

    d. Magnesium pemoline—effective in 65% to 70% with trial of 2 to 3 weeks; can cause liver toxicity

    e. Desipramine and imipramine (tricyclic antidepressants)—effectiveness with 60% to 70% when other medications are ineffective or have unacceptable side-effects; may work better with children having underlying depression

5. Close follow-up assessment and monitoring of growth and response to medication and behavioral management plan every 3 to 4 months

6. Ongoing coordination and communication with family, school personnel, primary care provider and mental health resources is critical to successful management

7. Medication may be discontinued after 2 to 3 month trial if no change in behavior

8. Non-conventional treatments (no documented evidence of effectiveness in controlled studies)

    a. Megavitamins/mineral therapy

    b. Elimination of sugar, additives, coloring

    c. Neurophysiologic interventions (patterning, sensory integration, optometric training)

9. Community resources

    a. Children and Adults with Attention Deficit Disorder (CHADD)
    International non-profit parent support organization
    499 N.W. 70th Ave., Suite 109
    Plantation, Florida 33317
    (305) 587-3700

    b. National Attention Deficit Disorder Association
    (800) 487-2282
    http://www.add.org

Aggression, Defiance and Disruptive Behavioral Disorders

- Normal behavior vs. dysfunctional patterns and clinical disorders

1. Most children manifest some degree of developmentally normative aggressive, defiant and disruptive behavior during infancy and early childhood, e.g., breath-holding, temper tantrums, lying, fighting, breaking things

2. Almost half of all parents consult with primary care providers regarding difficulty managing disruptive and defiant behaviors of their preschoolers

3. Repetitive and persistent patterns of aggressive, defiant, and disruptive behaviors lasting over 6 months warrant detailed assessment and possible mental health referral

- Conduct Disorder: A repetitive and persistent dysfunctional pattern of aggressive behavior and/or violation of the law, social norms, and basic human rights

    1. Etiology/Incidence

        a. Multifactorial etiology—biological-genetic component suggested from twin/adoption studies

        b. Child onset (less than 10 years) has graver prognosis with increased risk of later substance abuse and anti-social personality disorder than adolescent-onset

        c. Incidence greater among males with estimates of 6% to 16%; female estimates of 2% to 9%

    2. Clinical Findings—DSM-IV-TR (2000) criteria include:

        a. Aggressive/threatening behavior to people or animals

        b. Deliberate, intentional destruction of property

        c. Lying, stealing

        d. Serious rule violations such as staying out all night, running away, truancy

    3. Differential Diagnosis:

        a. Adjustment disorder

        b. ADHD

        c. Oppositional-defiant disorder

        d. Manic episode

    4. Diagnostic Tests/Findings

        a. Separate interview with parent and child

        b. Assessment of parental anxiety regarding dependency/control issues; impact on family functioning

        c. Severity of behaviors with respect to intensity, frequency, duration, context, and developmental stage

        d. Identify contributing psychosocial risk factors—poverty, abuse, neglect, exposure to violence, parental mental illness and/or substance abuse

    5. Management/Treatment

        a. Identify and communicate concern for child and family well-being

        b. Refer for psychological/psychiatric evaluation and intervention

    c. Refer to social service and/or other community resources for parenting education, support, and to reduce family stress and potential for violence

- Oppositional-Defiant Disorder: A repetitive and persistent dysfunctional pattern characterized by negative, disobedient, defiant and hostile behavior directed at authority figures

  1. Etiology/Incidence

    a. Multifactorial etiology associated with difficult temperament, disruption in early caregiving environment, harsh, inconsistent and/or neglectful parenting; history of psychiatric disorder in at least one parent including maternal depression

    b. Incidence among males is greater than females until puberty after which rates become more equal; overall estimates range from 2% to 16% depending on population

  2. Clinical Findings

    a. Loses temper easily

    b. Argumentative with adult authority figures

    c. Actively defiant of rules and adult requests

    d. Deliberately annoys other people

    e. Blames others for mistakes and misbehavior

    f. Edgy and easily annoyed

    g. Frequently resentful or angry

    h. Spiteful and vindictive behavior

  3. Differential Diagnosis

    a. Within normal range of oppositional behavior for age and developmental level

    b. Conduct disorder

    c. ADHD

    d. Mental retardation

  4. Management/Treatment

    a. Early identification and monitoring of defiant, aggressive, and oppositional behaviors

    b. Parenting education, support, and effective discipline

    c. Refer for family therapy/intervention if child manifests four or more of clinical behavioral features that have persisted for longer than 6 months

Learning Disabilities (LD)

- Definition
    1. Generic term referring to a heterogeneous cluster of disorders manifested by significant difficulties in the acquisition and use of language, listening, reading (dyslexia), writing (dysgraphia), reasoning, or mathematical abilities (dyscalculia)
    2. School performance in deficit areas significantly below that expected for age, grade, and level of intelligence
- Etiology/Incidence
    1. Multifactorial etiology of genetic and environmental factors
    2. Possible abnormal function in parietal and/or occipital lobes of brain
    3. Conditions associated with LD
        a. Developmental delay
        b. Lead poisoning
        c. Fetal alcohol syndrome
        d. Fragile-X syndrome
    4. General prevalence estimated at 6% to 11% of school-age children
    5. Dyslexia—most common LD, affects 2% to 10% of general population
- Clinical Findings
    1. Specific academic skill deficits
        a. Basic reading skills, reading comprehension, spelling
        b. Mathematical calculations and reasoning
        c. Disorders of written expression and writing skills
    2. Perceptual-motor impairments
        a. Distinguishing shapes and sizes
        b. Fine motor skills, e.g., writing, coloring, cutting
        c. May make letter and number reversals
    3. Memory and thinking impairment (integrative processing)
        a. Haphazard, ineffective study habits and strategies for memorization
        b. Sequencing of data
        c. Understanding abstract concepts, e.g., time, space, parts, whole
        d. Lacking skills for effective problem-solving and task completion
    4. Speech and language deficits
        a. Language delay

    b. Difficulty with grammar (syntax), meaning (semantics) and/or social use of words (pragmatics)

5. Attention deficits—difficulty concentrating and staying on task

6. Hyperactivity—difficulty sitting still, constantly in motion

7. Impulsiveness

    a. Often acting without thinking

    b. Poor planning skills

    c. Lack of self-regulation skills

8. General deficits in coordination—clumsiness

9. Emotional problems

    a. Lability and moodiness

    b. Often isolated or rejected by peers

    c. May exhibit inappropriate attention-getting behaviors

    d. Difficulty reading nonverbal social cues

    e. May be passive learners

- Differential Diagnosis

  1. Undiagnosed sensory impairment—vision or hearing deficits

  2. Attention deficit hyperactivity disorder (ADHD)

  3. Seizure disorder

  4. Mental retardation

  5. Maladaptation to chronic disease

  6. Social and environmental factors

      a. Child abuse and neglect

      b. Situational anxiety or depressive reaction

      c. Ethnic or cultural minority

- Physical Findings

  1. Neurological soft signs commonly present

      a. Poor fine motor coordination and tactile discrimination

      b. Strabismus

      c. Poor hand-eye coordination

      d. Balance problems

  2. Phenotypic features of associated conditions—FAS, Fragile-X

  3. Other abnormal physical findings likely to be related to LD

- Diagnostic Studies/Findings: Diagnosis requires multidimensional assessment
    1. Complete medical and social history
    2. Developmental and behavioral history
    3. Educational history and school functioning
    4. Physical examination—soft neurological signs
    5. Laboratory studies—associated conditions
        a. Lead screening
        b. EEG if seizures suspected
    6. Psychoeducational testing
    7. Analysis of history, test results, and academic achievement leads to diagnosis
- Management/Treatment
    1. Developmental surveillance, early identification and referral is critical
    2. Early intervention to optimize learning and minimize emotional sequelae
    3. Thorough psychoeducational evaluation to determine skills and deficits
    4. Interdisciplinary conference to evaluate findings (M-team)
    5. Individualized education plan (IEP) developed based on multidimensional assessment
    6. Yearly re-evaluation of IEP with revisions as needed
    7. Address other associated behavioral, social and family issues through counseling and direct instruction
    8. Inform parents of legal rights under Individuals with Disabilities Education Act (IDEA) and availability of appropriate special services

Eating Disorders: Anorexia Nervosa and Bulimia Nervosa

- Definition: Chronic and often severe disturbances in eating behavior accompanied by distorted perception of body weight, size and shape
    1. Anorexia nervosa—eating disturbance associated with weight loss and refusal to maintain body weight at minimally normal level (85% of expected body weight for age and sex) with subsequent amenorrhea
    2. Bulimia nervosa—eating disturbance associated with episodic binge eating followed by compensatory efforts to prevent weight gain (self-induced vomiting, dieting, fasting, excessive exercise or misuse of laxatives, enemas and/or diuretics)
    3. Anorexia may occur with or without associated binging/purging (restricting vs. binge-eating/purging types); bulimia may occur with or without purging (purging vs. non-purging types)

- Etiology/Incidence
    1. Family enmeshment hypothesis—rigid, overprotective families with difficulty with conflict resolution; separation-individuation
    2. Fear of sexual maturation; history of sexual abuse
    3. Social pressure to be thin
    4. Ballet dancers and gymnasts at particular risk
    5. Associated with psychological profile of low self-esteem in spite of outward successfulness.
    6. Both disorders are more common among females.
    7. Anorexia affects approximately 1% of white middle/upper class females; 5% to 10% of cases are male often associated with gender identity conflict
    8. Bimodal distribution with one peak at 14 years and second at 18 years
    9. Bulimia is more common than anorexia with later age onset
    10. Suicide rates of 2% to 5% of those with chronic anorexia with overall mortality rate as high as 10%
    11. Normal to high intelligence, overachievers, perfectionists
- Clinical Findings
    1. Self-imposed weight loss
    2. Anemia, jaundice, and secondary amenorrhea
    3. Vigorous exercise regimen to increase weight loss
    4. Constipation (chronic laxatives) and reflux esophagitis (self-induced vomiting)
    5. Dry skin, brittle nails
    6. Lower body temperature, blood pressure and heart rate
    7. Lanugo
    8. Sore throat, calluses on dorsum of fingers, loss of tooth enamel (from induced vomiting)
- Differential Diagnosis
    1. General medical condition—gastrointestinal disease, diabetes, thyroid disorder, AIDS, systemic lupus erythematosus
    2. Pregnancy
    3. Depressive disorder or substance abuse
- Diagnostic Tests/Findings
    1. History—include nutritional patterns as well as effort to lose weight (dieting, exercise, vomiting); preoccupation with food and/or feeling ''fat''; past medical, family and social; review of systems (amenorrhea)

2. Weight and height percentiles—degree of malnutrition determined as percentage below ideal weight (IBW)

   a. Mild malnutrition— < 20% below IBW

   b. Moderate malnutrition—20% to 30% below IBW

   c. Severe malnutrition— > 30% below IBW

3. Physical examination—signs of malnutrition; dry skin, brittle nails, muscle weakness, flat affect, decreased blood pressure, pulse and body temperature; Tanner staging delays

4. CBC, serum albumin, glucose, electrolytes, thyroid function, ECG; others as appropriate based on history and clinical findings

- Management/Treatment

  1. Interdisciplinary treatment plan including nutritional intervention, behavior modification techniques, psychotherapy (individual, family and/or group therapy), pharmacologic management with antidepressants if appropriate

  2. Hospitalization for rehydration and refeeding if condition warrants

  3. Approximately one half of patients show varying degrees of improvement; 25% show long-term improvement; 25% do poorly regardless of intervention

  4. Refer to appropriate community resources for assessment tool, support and education:

     Eating Disorder Inventory-2
     Psychological Assessment Resources, Inc.
     PO Box 998
     Odessa, Florida 33556

     Foundation for Education about Eating Disorders
     PO Box 1637
     Baltimore, MD 21210
     (410) 467-0603

     The American Anorexia and Bulimia Association
     293 Central Park West, Suite 1R
     NY, NY 10024
     (212) 501-8351
     http://members.aol.com/amambu

     National Association of Anorexia Nervosa and Associated Disorders
     PO Box 7
     Highland Park, IL 60035
     (847) 831-3438
     http://www.anad.org

Childhood Depression

- Definition: Behavioral pattern lasting at least two weeks that is characterized by affective and behavioral symptoms including sad or tearful moods, irritability and/or social withdrawal with associated decreased interest and pleasure in developmentally appropriate activities

- Etiology/Incidence: Multifactorial etiology with associated risk factors including:

    1. History of traumatic event(s) involving significant separation(s) or loss(es) of parent, caregiver or significant other

    2. Family history of depression especially in mother; evidence of genetic component from twin and adoption studies

    3. Chronic neglect and lack of nurturance due to family disruptions or dysfunction including long-term effects of poverty and/or homelessness

    4. Substance abuse, physical or sexual abuse in household

    5. Chronic illness and/or disability may increase risk especially with familial predisposition

    6. Estimated incidence of 3% for overall pediatric population and as high as 9% for adolescents; no gender differences in early childhood depression but increases among females in adolescence with ratio of 5:1

- Clinical Findings

    1. Major depressive episode—significant distress and/or interference with normal daily functioning lasting at least 2 weeks associated with:

        a. Depressed or irritable mood and/or decreased interest and pleasure in developmentally appropriate activities and a minimum of 4 additional symptoms

        b. Appetite changes with associated weight gain or loss

        c. Insomnia or hypersomnia

        d. Difficulty concentrating; decline in school performance

        e. Feelings of worthlessness, guilt, fearfulness, isolation

        f. Social withdrawal from friends, family, school refusal and/or truancy

        g. General somatic complaints of aches and pains with non-specific etiology, e.g., fatigue, headaches, stomachaches

        h. Agitation, irritability and/or disruptive behavior

        i. Recurrent thoughts of death and/or suicidal ideation

    2. Dysthymic disorder—long-standing depressed or irritable mood lasting one year or more but symptoms of distress and interference with normal daily functioning not as pronounced as a major depressive episode

    3. Adjustment disorder with depressed mood—depressed or irritable mood, sadness, tearfulness and/or feelings of hopelessness causing some degree of impairment of

daily functioning that occurs within 3 months of a significant and identifiable stressful life event

- Differential Diagnosis

    1. Normal periods of sadness and/or mood swings

    2. Acute depressive reactions/adjustment disorder with depressed mood in response to identifiable life stress

    3. Masked depressive disorder—somatization and denial of feelings

    4. Underlying physical disorder

    5. Substance abuse

    6. Psychiatric depressive disorder with suicidal risk

- Diagnostic Tests/Findings

    1. Behavioral symptoms according to DSM-IV-TR diagnostic criteria

    2. History—developmental, family, social and school; current medications; chronic disease/disability

    3. Separate interview with child or adolescent is essential

    4. Physical examination—neurological screening

    5. Height, weight, vital signs, assess for recent weight loss or gain

    6. Laboratory tests—as indicated by history (drug screen; pregnancy test)

- Management/Treatment

    1. Early screening and identification of children and adolescents at risk for depression

        a. Center for Epidemiologic Studies Depression Scale for Children

        b. Children's Depression Rating Scale

        c. Children's Depression Inventory

        d. Child Behavior Checklist

        e. Rose Institute Adolescent Depression Scale

        f. Mood Questionnaire for Adolescents

    2. Evaluate severity of depression including suicidal risk and make appropriate referrals

    3. Psychiatric intervention is necessary for major depressive episode or dysthymic disorder

        a. Family and/or individual psychotherapy

        b. Pharmacotherapy—may be included as part of multimodal treatment plan

            (1) Selective serotonin reuptake inhibitors (SSRI)—most effective medication for major depressive episodes (fluoxetine or sertraline)

(2) Tricyclic antidepressants have limited clinical use with equivocal effectiveness demonstrated in controlled studies (monitor blood levels)

4. Supportive counseling for adjustment disorder with depressed mood

5. Resources

Depression/Awareness, Recognition, and Treatment (D/ART)
National Institutes of Mental Health
Room 10-85
5600 Fishers Lane
Rockville, Maryland 20857

Suicidal Behavior

- Definition: Passive or active thoughts/wishes about death and dying (suicidal ideation); talking and/or threatening to take one's life, or self-injury without intent to die (suicidal gesture); deliberate self-injury with the intent to die but not resulting in death (suicide attempt) and self-inflicted death (completed suicide)

- Etiology/Incidence

  1. Accounts for 10% of teenage deaths representing second leading cause of adolescent mortality

  2. 15% to 40% of completed suicides were preceded by one or more suicide gestures/attempts

  3. Females have higher rates of suicide attempts; males have higher rates of completed suicides

  4. Higher rates among Native American, Asian, and chronically ill adolescents

  5. Ingestion of medication is most common method; violent methods (hanging and shooting) are more frequently used by males than females and are more often fatal

- Clinical Findings

  1. Severe and/or chronic depression

  2. Hopelessness

  3. Previous suicidal gestures

  4. History of suicide in family

  5. Existence of specific plan

- Differential Diagnosis

  1. Unintentional injuries due to carelessness and/or adolescent sense of ''invincibility''

  2. Suicidal gesture as desperate call for help

  3. Imminent risk/acute suicidal intent

  4. Psychotic episode

- Diagnostic Tests/Findings

    1. History—past and present health, chronic depression, chronic illness or disability; school performance; family history of depression and/ or suicide; current medications; substance abuse

    2. Suicidal risk—suicidal ideation, extent of premeditation and existence of plan; likelihood of rescue; suicide notes, previous suicidal gestures

    3. Observation and/or reports of suicidal behavior by family, teachers, or peers

- Management/Treatment

    1. Refer immediately for crisis intervention resources, e.g., 24 hour hot-line

    2. Suicidal ideation and/or gestures with existence of plan requires immediate psychological evaluation

    3. Assure safe environment for child/adolescent including hospitalization if necessary

    4. Short-term hospitalization is recommended for all suicide attempts; attending to emergency treatment and/or surgical management is necessary but insufficient without additional follow-up intervention

    5. Treat underlying depression

    6. Inform child/adolescent of seriousness of concern and need to notify family and mobilize necessary community resources

        a. The Youth Suicide National Center
        1825 I Street NW
        Washington, DC 20006
        (202) 429-0190

        b. National Adolescent Suicide Hotline
        (800) 621-4000

        c. American Association of Suicidology
        2459 South Ash
        Denver, Colorado 80222
        (303) 692-0985
        http://www.cyberpsych.org/aas.htm.

Substance Abuse (Tobacco, Alcohol, and Other Drugs)

- Definition: Use of any drug or chemical for purposes of stimulation, pleasure or in a way that interferes with normal functioning and/or threatens health; includes misuse of legal 'recreational' drugs, prescribed or non-prescribed medications, as well as illegal substances; DSM-IV-TR distinguishes substance abuse from dependence (APA, 1994):

    1. Substance abuse—a maladaptive pattern of substance use associated with significant impairment or distress including inability to meet expected daily obligations, use of substance in situations/context that may be hazardous to self or others, and/or resulting in legal and/or other interpersonal conflicts

2. Substance dependence—a pattern of repeated substance abuse that results in tolerance, withdrawal, and/or compulsive use that can be psychological and/or physiologic-based

3. Categories of substances include—alcohol; marijuana (cannabis); nicotine; amphetamines; caffeine; cocaine; hallucinogens; inhalants; opioids; phencyclidine (PCP); sedatives and hypnotics; anabolic steroids

- Etiology/Incidence

1. Multifactorial etiology including some evidence of biological predisposition along with psychosocial and environmental risks such as impulsivity, non-conformity/rebellion, peer pressure, ineffective coping with stress, undiagnosed depression, family dysfunction, history of child abuse or neglect, parental substance abuse

2. Majority of adolescents will engage in some form of drug use at some point

3. More frequent use of all substances among males vs. females

4. Highest overall incidence of substance abuse among Caucasian teen-agers followed by Hispanic youth, lowest incidence among African-American teen-agers (O'Malley, Johnston, & Bachman, 1995)

5. Most recent national drug use survey reported increasing prevalence of current illicit drug use—11.4% teen-agers from 12 to 17 years of age (SAMSA, 1998)

- Clinical Findings:

1. Nicotine—decreased exercise tolerance, fatigue, muscle weakness; pallor; tachycardia; staining of teeth; tobacco odor on breath and clothes

2. Alcohol—initial euphoria and talkativeness; grogginess; impaired short-term memory; decreased reaction time; hypoglycemia

3. Marijuana (THC, pot, cannabis, joint, reefer, weed, hash, grass)—euphoria; drowsiness; slowed reaction time and motor coordination; time distortions; tachycardia and transient hypertension; blood shot eyes

4. Amphetamines—dilated pupils, tachycardia, anorexia, insomnia, weight loss, anxiety and suicidal behavior

5. Cocaine (coke, free-base, crack, nose, flake)—agitation, hyperactivity, euphoria followed by depression, confused thinking, occasional paranoid ideation; tachycardia; habitual "snorting" induced nasal septum scabbing or necrosis

6. Hallucinogens

   a. LSD—dilated pupils; visual and auditory hallucinations and flashbacks; disorganized and confused thinking; increased attention to stimuli; chronic use can lead to psychosis and major personality changes

   b. PCP—euphoria, motor incoordination, hallucinations; paranoia with aggressive/violent behavior

7. Inhalants/volatile substances (glue, hydrocarbons)—relaxation, hallucinations, light headedness, giddiness; seizures, coma, cardiac arrhythmias and sudden death

8. Anabolic steroids—used to increase muscle mass and strength (non-substantiated effect); fluid retention, mood swings, menstrual abnormalities; male gynecomastia, female hirsutism, breast atrophy

9. Opiates include naturally occurring (e.g., morphine, codeine); semisynthetic (e.g., heroine, dilaudid) and synthetic (e.g., fentanyl, meperidine, methadone); constricted pupils; respiratory depression; euphoria, analgesia; dermatologic lesions "tracks"; tattoos in unusual places to conceal track marks; chronic infections (skin, HIV, scarring and cellulitis); constipation, decrease in libido; urinary retention

- Differential Diagnosis

  1. Social recreational use of legal substances

  2. Experimentation vs. abuse

  3. Chronic depression

  4. Neurological disorder

  5. Learning disabilities

- Diagnostic Tests/Findings

  1. History—past and present, environmental, family, social, and academic history; review of systems; current medications; specific drug history including specific drugs, frequency of use, settings of use, impairment of daily functioning including suspensions or legal difficulties

  2. Interviews with and observations from child/adolescent, parents, school personnel, peers

  3. Physical examination with close assessment of skin integrity (nasal septum, skin lesions/track marks); neurological assessment; vital signs, weight, height, blood pressure

  4. Serum and urine toxicology; HIV testing; others as appropriate to specific history

- Management/Treatment

  1. Assure appropriate privacy, confidentiality and non-judgmental atmosphere

  2. Referral to appropriate substance abuse treatment resources

  3. Identify and provide appropriate referrals for management of underlying psychosocial difficulties contributing to substance abuse

  4. Educate and counsel regarding legal and physical risks of substance abuse

  5. Support community-based prevention programs

  6. Additional National Resources

National Institute on Drug Abuse (NIDA)
Hotline: (800) 662-HELP
National Institute on Drug Abuse Prevention
(800) 638-2045
National Federation of Parents for Drug-Free Youth
(800) 544-KIDS
National Clearinghouse for Alcohol and Drug Abuse Information
(800) 729-6686

Health Supervision as Ongoing Surveillance, Screening and Assessment of Physical Growth and Behavioral Development

- Definitions:

    1. Surveillance: A continuous process of periodic assessment and monitoring of growth and development overtime through a variety of methods including direct observation, health history, parent/child interviews, and physical examination

    2. Screening: Use of standardized or generally accepted methods with essentially well populations in order to identify individuals who may be at risk for physical, cognitive or psychosocial abnormality and warrant further assessment; good screening tools are simple, inexpensive, acceptable, valid and reliable

    3. Assessment: A more systematic evaluation using a standardized or generally accepted method leading to recommendations for intervention

    4. Sensitivity: Proportion of those with the abnormality who are correctly identified through screening (true positives)

    5. Specificity: Proportion of those without the abnormality who are correctly identified as negative through screening (true negatives)

    6. Positive predictive value (PPV): Proportion of those individuals correctly screened as positive of all those who actually have the abnormality

- Examples of Screening and Assessment Tests Used in Child Health Supervision

    1. Physical assessment and laboratory screening

        a. Newborn genetic screening (blood spot on filter paper)

            (1) Newborn screening for hypothyroidism and phenylketonuria (PKU) required in all States; galactosemia and hemoglobinopathies required in the majority of States

            (2) Newborn screening for additional conditions include—biotinidase deficiency, maple syrup urine disease (MSUD), congenital adrenal hyperplasia, cystic fibrosis, homocystinuria, congenital toxoplasmosis, tyrosinemia

            (3) Requirements for voluntary vs. mandatory screening vary by State

        b. Anthropometric body measurements—weight (wt), length or height (ht), head circumference (hc), skin-fold thickness

    (1) American Academy of Pediatrics (AAP) recommendations:

       (a) Birth to 2 years (wt, length, and hc) at each visit

       (b) 3 to 5 years (wt, ht) annually

       (c) 6 to 20 years (wt, ht) every other year

    (2) NCHS age and gender specific growth charts for serial measurements

    (3) Body mass index (BMI)—adolescents

    (4) Risks—growth retardation, malnutrition, obesity, eating disorders

c. Blood pressure screening

    (1) AAP recommendations:

       (a) Annually from 3 to 6 years

       (b) Every other year thereafter

    (2) Risks—hypertension

d. Cholesterol screening (serum levels)

    (1) AAP recommendations:

       (a) Universal screening not recommended

       (b) Children > 2 years with family history of hypercholesterolemia and/or premature cardiovascular disease

    (2) Risks—coronary artery disease in adulthood

e. Anemia screening (hemoglobin/hematocrit)

    (1) AAP recommendations—measure once during

       (a) Infancy (6 to 9 months)

       (b) Early childhood (1 to 5 years)

       (c) School-age (5 to 12 years)

       (d) Adolescents (14 to 20 years)

    (2) Risks—iron deficiency anemia

f. Lead screening—AAP recommends targeted screening based on well-child surveillance of risk

g. Tuberculosis (TB) screening

    (1) Methods include Mantoux (PPD) and multiple puncture (tine)

    (2) Mantoux is preferred method with better sensitivity and specificity

    (3) AAP recommends targeted screening based on degree of risk

       (a) Annual testing for high-risk children

(b) Periodic testing for low-risk children living in high prevalence environments—between 4 to 6 years and again between 11 to 16 years

h. Urine screening (urine analysis)—AAP recommendations 6 months, 2, 8, and 18 years

i. Vision screening (visual acuity)

(1) AAP recommendations—ages 3, 4, 5, 6, 8, 12, and 18 years

(2) Methods—visual acuity

(a) Preschool children—Illiterate (tumbling) E; Allen picture cards, HOTV

(b) School-age children and adolescents—Snellen letters

j. Hearing screening

(1) NIH Consensus Statement on Early Identification of Hearing Impairment in Infants and Young Children (1993)

(a) Evoked otoacoustic emissions (EOAE) to screen all newborns

(b) Auditory Brainstem Response Audiometry (ABR) for all newborns who fail EOAE

(2) AAP recommendations

(a) Low-risk children—pure-tone audiometry at 4, 5, 12, and 18 years

(b) High-risk neonates and young children— audiology screening preferably before discharge (neonates), and no later than 3 months after being identified at risk

k. Dental screening—AAP recommends first dental screening by 3 years of age

2. Developmental screening and assessment

a. Global development

(1) Newborn Behavioral Assessment Scale (NBAS)—assessment of newborn's behavioral capacities including state control, autonomic reactivity, reflexes, habituation, and responsiveness to visual and auditory stimuli

(2) Bayley Infant Neurodevelopmental Screener (BINS)— screens for basic neurological, receptive, expressive, and cognitive functions in infants between 3 to 24 months

(3) Bayley Scales of Infant Development (second edition (BSID-II)—current ''gold-standard'' for diagnosing developmental delays and recommending intervention for children birth through 42 months with separate mental, motor, and behavioral rating scales

      (4) Ages and Stages Questionnaires (ASQ)—parent-completed child monitoring system for children 4 to 48 months

      (5) Denver II—screens in personal-social, fine motor-adaptive, language and gross motor domains in children birth to 6 years

      (6) First Step—screening test for evaluating preschoolers

  b. Cognitive development-intelligence

      (1) McCarthy Scales of Children's Abilities

      (2) Weschler Preschool and Primary Scale of Intelligence Revised (WPPSIR)

      (3) Weschler Intelligence Scale for Children-WISC III

  c. Language

      (1) Early Language Milestones Scale (ELM)—(0 to 42 months)

      (2) Receptive and Expressive Emergent Language Scale (REEL)—(0 to 36 months)

      (3) Clinical Linguistic and Auditory Milestone Test (CLAMS)—(0 to 36 months)

      (4) Language Development Survey—screening tool for toddlers using vocabulary checklist for enumeration of words

      (5) The MacArthur Communicative Development Inventory—words and gestures

      (6) The MacArthur Communicative Development Inventory—words and sentences

  d. Behaviors

      (1) Achenbach's Child Behavior Checklist (ACBCL)

      (2) Connor's Abbreviated Parent-Teacher Questionnaire

  e. Temperament

      (1) Infant Temperament Questionnaire—4 to 8 months

      (2) Toddler Temperament Scale—1 to 3 years

      (3) Behavioral Style Questionnaire—3 to 7 years

      (4) Middle Childhood Temperament Questionnaire—8 to 12 years

3. Parent-child relationship and home environment

  a. Parenting Stress Index (PSI)

  b. Home Observation for Measurement of the Environment (HOME scale)—infant, preschool and elementary school versions

    c. Pediatric Review and Observation of Children's Environmental Support and Stimulation Inventory (PROCESS)

    d. Nursing Child Assessment Feeding (NCAF) and Teaching (NCAT) scales

4. Mental health screening and diagnostic classifications

    a. 0–3 Diagnostic classification of mental health and developmental disorders of infancy and early childhood (1995)

    b. DSM-PC Classification of child and adolescent mental diagnoses in primary care (1996)

    c. DSM-IV-TR Diagnostic and statistical manual of mental disorders (2000)

Questions
Select the best answer

1. Most stage-based theories of development focus primarily on:

   a. The continuity of development
   b. The discontinuity of development
   c. Persistence of inherent personality characteristics
   d. The influence of context on development

2. The common practice of using ''time-outs'' with young children is a direct application of:

   a. Operant conditioning
   b. Classical conditioning
   c. Separation-individuation
   d. Maturational reinforcement

3. Good communication between families, schools and primary care providers is an example of which ecological concept?

   a. Microsytem
   b. Mesosystem
   c. Exosystem
   d. Macrosystem

4. Which of the following findings would be most likely associated with asymmetric intrauterine growth retardation:

   a. Weight, length and head circumference ranging from 3rd to 5th percentile
   b. Heavy maternal smoking throughout pregnancy
   c. Weight at 3rd percentile and length at 25th
   d. Gestational diabetes

5. Early reflexive responses that are not related to survival include all but:

   a. Babinski
   b. Moro
   c. Swimming
   d. Rooting

6. The most likely weight of a one-year-old child whose weight at birth was $6\frac{1}{2}$ pounds would be:

   a. 19-20 pounds
   b. 13-14 pounds
   c. 25-26 pounds
   d. Impossible to estimate

7. One of the major psychosocial tasks of infancy is:

    a. Development of secure attachment
    b. Separation-individuation
    c. Symbiosis
    d. Regulation

8. Which developmental theory best explains the multifactorial etiology of failure-to-thrive?

    a. Organismic-maturational theory
    b. Social learning theory
    c. Transactional theory
    d. Psychoanalytic theory

9. Most healthy infants are able to reach, grasp and hold onto a rattle or other small toy by about:

    a. 2 months
    b. 6 months
    c. 8 months
    d. 10 months

10. The pincer grasp is a fine motor skill that involves the ability to pick up a small object such as a raisin or piece of cereal with the thumb and forefinger that usually is mastered around:

    a. 4 months
    b. 6 months
    c. 9 months
    d. 16 months

11. The majority of American infants are able to walk by about:

    a. 11 months
    b. 12 months
    c. 13 months
    d. 14 months

12. A young child should have had a first dental screening by:

    a. 2 years
    b. 3 years
    c. 4 years
    d. School entry

13. You would be concerned about the language development of a child who:

    a. Repeats simple phrases at 32 months
    b. Stutters when excited or tired at 42 months
    c. Has a vocabulary of 10 words at 12 months
    d. Pronounces words that are not understandable at 36 months

14. The most common temperamental profile is:

    a. Easy
    b. Difficult
    c. Slow-to-warm-up
    d. Intermediate

15. The underlying emotion of an insecurely attached (avoidant) relationship is:

    a. Ambivalence
    b. Deprivation
    c. Anger
    d. Conditional love

16. The stage of cognitive development that Piaget decribed as characteristic of the way preschoolers think is the:

    a. Preoperational stage
    b. Mental combinations stage
    c. Tertiary circular function stage
    d. Sensorimotor stage

17. A preschool boy whose parents have separated and are beginning divorce procedures:

    a. May think that he caused the divorce by misbehaving
    b. Should not be told of the impending divorce until the parents are sure of their decision
    c. Is likely to experience gender identity confusion
    d. Should be able to make a decision about which parent he prefers living with

18. Which behavior would you expect to decrease during the preschool years?

    a. Rough-and-tumble play
    b. Instrumental aggression
    c. Hostile aggression
    d. Cooperative play

19. A preschool child who says that the sky is blue because it is his favorite color is illustrating the concept of:

    a. Symbolic thinking
    b. Egocentrism
    c. Centration
    d. Imaginary audience

20. Which of the following strategies would not be appropriate to include as part of your management of a 9 year old boy who is obese?

    a. Referral to nutritionist for weight reduction plan
    b. Increase physical exercise

c. Behavior modification strategies to deal with stress and/or reinforce treatment plan
d. Involve family in management program

21. Which of the following issues or concepts is relevant to the school-aged child?

   a. Operational thinking
   b. Initiative
   c. Concrete operations
   d. Separation-individuation

22. The first physical sign indicating the onset of female puberty is:

   a. Sparsely distributed fine, pale pubic hairs.
   b. Breast buds
   c. Menarche
   d. Peak height velocity

23. Which of the following findings would be helpful in distinguishing obesity vs. large body frame in an adolescent who is concerned with her weight?

   a. Tricep skinfold measurement
   b. Weight-for-height ratio
   c. Body mass index
   d. Percent of ideal body weight

24. The most common form of child abuse seen in pediatric primary care is:

   a. Burns
   b. Fractures
   c. Soft tissue injuries
   d. Shaken baby syndrome

25. A differential diagnosis for child abuse would include all of the following except:

   a. Birth marks
   b. Unintentional injury
   c. Inadequate parenting
   d. Prader-Willi syndrome

26. Which of the following symptoms are not typical of a child with ADHD?

   a. Easily distracted
   b. Difficulty playing quietly
   c. Doesn't follow directions
   d. Frequently angry and resentful

27. Which of the following clinical findings would not suggest an eating disorder with a purging component?

   a. Sore throat

   b. Brittle nails

   c. Constipation

   d. Finger calluses

28. Which of the following situations does not necessarily warrant immediate mental health assessment and/or referral?

   a. 13 year old girl who has been "down" for the last month with varied somatic complaints

   b. 9 year old boy whose parents recently separated and filed for a divorce and seems to be doing well

   c. 16 year old girl who has a history of long-standing depression but seems to be doing well in school

   d. 15 year old boy who expresses suicidal thoughts

29. Which of the following is not a test for visual acuity?

   a. HOTV

   b. Allen figures

   c. Snellen chart

   d. ELM

30. The preferred method for tuberculosis screening is:

   a. Mantoux

   b. MPT

   c. HOTV

   d. DASE

31. Which adolescent would be at greatest risk for developing anorexia nervosa?

   a. 12 year old female who just had her first period

   b. 14 year old gymnist

   c. 16 year old male runner

   d. 18 year old female college student

32. Which of the following substances is associated with pupillary constriction?

   a. Amphetamines

   b. LSD

   c. Heroin

   d. Nicotine

33. A newborn infant who was recently tested and failed the evoked otoacoustic emissions audiometry (EOAE) prior to discharge should be referred for:

   a. Pure tone audiometry

   b. Complete diagnostic evaluation

   c. Auditory brainstem response

   d. Repeat EOAE within 3 months

34. A risk factor that is common to many psychosocial pediatric problems including failure to thrive, conduct or oppositional disorders, and childhood depression is:

    a. Maternal depression or other psychiatric disorder
    b. Substance abuse
    c. Prematurity
    d. History of sexual abuse

35. Which of the following diagnoses is not more common among males?

    a. ADHD
    b. Conduct Disorders
    c. Suicide
    d. FTT

36. Newborn genetic screening is required in all or most states for all of the following disorders except:

    a. Hypothyroidism
    b. PKU
    c. Galactosemia
    d. Cystic Fibrosis

37. The diagnostic criteria for Autistic disorders includes which of the following?

    a. Speech delay, ataxia, mental retardation
    b. Impairments in social interactions, interpersonal communication and staring spells
    c. Mental retardation, impairments in social interactions and stereotypical restricted pattern of interests and activities
    d. Impairments in social interactions, in interpersonal communication and stereotypical restricted pattern of interests and activities

38. In addition to specific academic skill deficits, learning disabilities are commonly associated with which of the following characteristics?

    a. Perceptual-motor impairments, normal motor function
    b. Perceptual motor impairment, impulsiveness
    c. Perceptual motor impairments, Down syndrome
    d. Lack of impulsiveness, perceptual motor impairment

Answers

1. b	14. a	27. b
2. a	15. c	28. b
3. b	16. a	29. d
4. c	17. a	30. a
5. d	18. b	31. b
6. a	19. b	32. c
7. a	20. a	33. c
8. c	21. c	34. a
9. b	22. b	35. d
10. c	23. c	36. d
11. d	24. c	37. d
12. b	25. d	38. b
13. d	26. d	

Bibliography

American Academy of Pediatrics (1996). *The classification of child and adolescent mental diagnoses in primary care.* Elk Grove, IL: Author

American Academy of Pediatrics (2000). Clinical practice guidelines: Diagnosis and evaluation of the child with attention-deficit/hyperactivity disorder. *Pediatrics, 105*(5), 1158-1170.

American Psychiatric Association. (2000). *Diagnostic and statistical manual of mental disorders—text revision* (4th ed.). Washington, DC: American Psychiatric Association.

Avery, M. E., & First, L. R. (1994). *Pediatric medicine* (2nd ed.). Baltimore: Williams & Wilkins.

Baron-Cohen, S., Cox, A., Swettenham, J., Nightengale, N., Morgan, K., Drew, A., & Charman, T. (1996). Psychological markers in the detection of autism in infancy. *British Journal of Psychiatry, 168*(2), 158-163.

Behrman, R. E., Kliegman, R. M., & Jenson, H. B. (2002). *Nelson textbook of pediatrics* (17th ed.). Philadelphia: W. B. Saunders Company.

Berger, K. S., & Straub, R. (2000). *The developing person through the life span.* NY: Worth Publishers.

Burns, C. E., Brady, M. A., Dunn, A. M., & Starr, N. (2000). *Pediatric primary care: A handbook for nurse practitioners* (2nd ed.). Philadelphia: W. B. Saunders Company.

Dixon, S. D., & Stein, M. T. (2000). *Encounters with children: Pediatric behavior and development* (3rd ed.). St. Louis: Mosby Year Book, Inc.

Green, M. (2000). *Bright futures: Guidelines for health supervision of infants, children and adolescents* (2nd ed.) Arlington, VA: National Center for Education in Maternal and Child Health.

Hanson, S. M. H., & Boyde, S. T. (2001). *Family health care nursing: Theory, practice and research.* Philadelphia: R. A. Davis.

Hoekelman, R. A., Adam, H. M., Nelson, N. M., Weitzman, M. L., & Wilson, M. H. (2001). *Primary pediatric care* (4th ed.). St. Louis: Mosby Year Book, Inc.

Hofmann, A., & Greydanus, D. (1997). *Adolescent Medicine.* (3rd ed.) Stamford, Conn.: Appletone & Lange.

Johnson, B. H., Jeppson, E. S., & Redburn, L. (1992). *Caring for children and families: Guidelines for hospitals.* Bethesda, MD: Association for the Care of Children's Health.

Lemley, K. B., O'Grady, E. T., Rauckhorst, L., Russell, D. D., & Small, N. (1994). Baseline data on the delivery of clinical preventive services provided by nurse practitioners. *The Nurse Practitioner: The American Journal of Primary Health Care, 19*(5), 57-63.

Levine, M., Carey, W., & Crocker, A. (1999). *Developmental-behavioral pediatrics* (3rd ed.). Philadelphia: W. B. Saunders.

McMillan, J. (1999). *Oski's pediatrics. Principles and practice.* Philadelphia: Lippincott, Williams & Wilkins.

Mercugliano, M., Powers, T., & Blum, N. (1999). *The clinician's practical guide to attention-deficit/hyperactivity disorder.* Baltimore: Paul H. Brooks Publishing.

Meisels, S. J., & Fenichel, E. (1996). *New visions for the developmental assessment of infants and young children.* Washington, DC: Zero to Three.

O'Malley, P. M., Johnston, L. D., & Bachman, J. G. (1995). Adolescent substance use: Epidemiology and implications for public policy. *The Pediatric Clinics of North America, 42*(2), 241-260.

Rosner, B., Prineas, R., Loggie, J., & Daniels, S. R. (1998). Percentiles for body mass index in U.S. children 5 to 17 years of age. *J. Pediatrics, 132*(2), 211-222.

Rudolph, A. M., Hoffman, J. I., & Rudolph, C. D. (1996). *Rudolph's pediatrics* (20th ed.). Stanford, CT: Appleton & Lange.

Shonkoff, J. P., & Phillips, D. A. (2000). *From neurons to neighborhoods: The science of early childhood development.* Washington, D. C.: National Academy Press.

Substance abuse and mental health services administration (S.A.M.S.A.) (1998). Preliminary results from the 1997 National Household Survey on Drug Abuse, Substance Abuse and Mental Health Services Administration. http://wwwsamsa.gov/press/98082/ohtm

Tanner, J. M. (1978). *Fetus into man: Physical growth from conception to maturity.* Cambridge, MA: Harvard University Press.

U.S. Department of Health and Human Services. (1998). *Clinician's handbook of preventive services* (2nd ed.). Washington, DC: U.S. Government Printing Office.

U.S. Department of Health and Human Services. (1996). *Healthy people 2000: Midcourse review and 1995 revisions.* Washington, DC: U.S. Government Printing Office.

U.S. Department of Health and Human Services. (2001). *Child maltreatment 2001: Reports from the states to the national child abuse and neglect data system.* Washington, DC: U.S. Government Printing Office.

Valadian, I., & Porter, D. (1977). *Physical growth and development.* Boston: Little, Brown & Co.

Zero to Three. (1995). *Diagnostic classification: 0-3: Diagnostic classification of mental health and developmental disorders of infancy and early childhood.* Washington, DC: Zero to Three.

Health Promotion and Well Child Care for Infants, Children and Adolescence

Bernadette Mazurek Melnyk
Leigh Small

Overview: Health Maintenance and Health Promotion

Pediatric nurse practitioners (PNPs) have long been on the forefront of promoting and maintaining optimal physical and mental health for children and their families. Because of their understanding of the multiple factors that may influence the overall health and development of children and adolescents, PNPs are able to implement evidence-based, individualized as well as group interventions and appropriately involve all family members to enhance health outcomes.

One strategy for enhancing health and developmental outcomes in children, teens and their families is the implementation of routine child health supervision. Health supervision is comprised of those measures that promote health, prevent morbidity and mortality, and facilitate optimal development and maturation within the context of the family and community. It involves routine well child visits which include health promotion strategies, anticipatory guidance, as well as specific screening procedures at regular, timed intervals throughout childhood and adolescence.

Child Health Supervision

- Components

  1. The parent/child interview

  2. Developmental and educational surveillance

  3. Observation of parent/child interaction

  4. Physical examination

  5. Screening

  6. Assessment of strengths and vulnerabilities (concerns, problems and stressors affecting the child and family)

  7. Evidence-based individualized interventions, including health promotion strategies and anticipatory guidance

- General Interviewing Approaches

  1. Determine who will be present for interview

  2. Provide privacy and empathetic environment

  3. Maintain good eye contact and relaxed facial expressions

  4. State you will be taking notes during interview to enhance accuracy of recorded data

  5. Obtain history with child clothed

  6. Begin with open ended questions, e.g., "Tell me what concerns you today," or "tell me why you are here today"

  7. Use direct questions to obtain specific information, e.g., "How old is Bobby?"

8. Avoid leading questions, e.g., "Your child doesn't have behavioral problems, does he?"

9. Use language parents and child understand

10. Provide undivided attention; listen carefully

11. Build self-esteem and confidence throughout interview

12. Conduct interview with cultural sensitivity

- Communication with Parents (same as general approaches, plus)

   1. Obtain parent's perception of any concerns or problems; if both parents present, obtain each parent's view of concerns or problems

   2. Restate parental concerns to ensure accuracy and understanding

   3. Be supportive, not judgmental, e.g., "Why didn't you bring your child in earlier?"

- Communication with Young Children (less than six years of age)

   1. Talk to child at his/her eye level

   2. Use play to enhance comfort

   3. Use projective techniques to elicit information about how child is feeling, e.g., "Tell me how your bear is feeling today."

   4. Use nonthreatening words, e.g., tube instead of needle; opening instead of cut, since young children engage in magical thinking

   5. Allow adequate time for responses

   6. Remember that young children have difficulty giving detailed information

- Communication with Younger School-age Children

   1. Communicate with parent first if child is initially shy

   2. Ask questions and give explanations using concrete terminology

   3. Use simple diagrams when asking child to describe location of symptoms

   4. Allow time for responses

   5. Give permission to express fears and concerns

- Communication with Older School-age Children and Adolescents

   1. If parent is present, conduct part of interview (questions dealing with personal or sensitive information) when alone with the older child or adolescent

   2. Interview while fully clothed

   3. Start interview with nonthreatening questions

   4. Inform older child/adolescent that all questions you are asking have to do with his/her health; that you ask all older children/adolescents these questions

5. Acknowledge that, although all of your questions are necessary, some may feel uncomfortable to answer

6. Inform older child/adolescent that information shared is confidential unless he/she tells you about wanting to hurt him/herself or someone else has hurt him/her

7. Encourage expression of feelings and concerns

8. Enhance self-esteem and provide positive feedback during interview

- Confidentiality Issues and Informed Consent

    1. Health care providers are required by law to keep the information gathered in the course of a child's care confidential; in 2003, national standards to protect the privacy of personal health information were established as part of the Health Insurance Portability and Accountability Act (HIPAA) of 1996 (DHHS, 2003)

    2. Privileged information may only be shared among health care professionals involved in the care of a child when parental consents are signed or in medical emergencies when release of information is in the best interest of the child and absolutely necessary for the provision of care

    3. Many States mandate reporting by health care professionals of special circumstances (reasonable cause to suspect child physical or sexual abuse or neglect; suicidal intent; gunshot and stab wounds)

    4. Some States require reporting of births, deaths, certain diseases, and other vital statistics.

    5. Consents should be signed by child's parent or legal guardian before information concerning child is released; emancipated minor (under the age of 18 years and married; parent of his or her own child; or self-sufficiently living away from home with parental consent) also may sign consents

    6. Minor's informed consent laws vary across States by status (emancipated) and conditions

        a. Most states have statutes allowing access to contraceptives, pregnancy testing/prenatal care as well as the diagnosis, treatment and prevention of sexually transmitted diseases per consent of minor

        b. Approximately half of the States have statutes allowing HIV testing and treatment per consent of minor

The Pediatric History

During the examination of a pediatric patient, the history is critical in the early detection of problems and prevention of long-term negative outcomes. Approximately 80% of the information used to arrive at a diagnosis is derived from the history.

- New Patient History

    1. Identifying data—demographic data; name and reliability of person providing the history as well as his/her relationship to child

2. Chief complaint (C.C.)—purpose of visit

3. Interim health—health since child was last seen by their primary care provider

4. Current health

    a. Nutrition

    b. Elimination

    c. Sleep

    d. Development—including school performance; daily activities; recreation and hobbies; social adjustment; behavior; and temperament

    e. Discipline

    f. Safety

    g. Immunizations and screening

    h. Allergies—including type of response

    i. Medications

    j. Substance use—alcohol, drug, cigarette, tobacco, caffeine use

    k. Reproductive/sexual if applicable (e.g., character and frequency of menses with associated symptoms [headaches, backaches]; last menses; last intercourse; presence of abdominal pain or vaginal discharge; current contraception)

5. Past medical history

    a. Birth—obtain if child is less than 3 years of age or if child is older than 3 years and having developmental or neurological problems

        (1) Prenatal

            (a) Planned or unplanned pregnancy

            (b) Onset of prenatal care

            (c) Medications, drugs, alcohol use during pregnancy

            (d) Medical problems during pregnancy—e.g., bleeding; infections; toxemia

        (2) Perinatal

            (a) Length of labor and delivery

            (b) Type of delivery

            (c) Medications or anesthesia

            (d) Complications

            (e) Birth weight

            (f) Gestation at birth; Apgar scores

(g) If multiple births, birth order

   (3) Postnatal

      (a) Maternal and infant problems

      (b) Age and weight at discharge

  b. Illnesses and injuries

  c. Hospitalizations and surgeries

  d. Growth and development

    (1) Physical growth

    (2) Developmental milestones

    (3) Mental health/social-emotional development—e.g., temperament, relationships, mood state, coping abilities

    (4) School—e.g., performance; attendance; problems; early intervention or Head Start

6. Family history

  a. Family profile and medical history (use pedigree chart)—include serious chronic, inherited and congenital problems in immediate family (blood relatives); drug and alcohol abuse; mental health problems; and age of first myocardial infarction if applicable

  b. Family social history—members of household and their relationship to the child; physical environment; employment/financial situation of parents or legal guardian; health care coverage; child care; family stressors (e.g., marital separation; illness); exposure to conflict or violence; presence of social support

7. Review of systems—does this child now or has this child ever had problems with any of the following systems?

  a. General

  b. Head/eyes/ears/nose/throat (HEENT)

  c. Lymph

  d. Respiratory

  e. Cardiac

  f. Gastrointestinal

  g. Genitourinary

  h. Musculoskeletal

  i. Skin

  j. Hematological

  k. Neurological

l. Psychological/mental health

m. Sexual/reproductive

- Interval History

    1. Chief complaint (C.C.)

    2. Interim health—since last visit

    3. Current health—e.g., nutrition; elimination; sleep; development; allergies; immunizations

    4. Update any changes in history since last visit

    5. Review of systems since last history

- History of Present Illness (H.P.I.) or Problem

    1. Description of present illness or problem

        a. Onset

        b. Location; character

        c. Temporal aspects

        d. Precipitating/aggravating factors; relieving factors

        e. Past treatment

        f. Associated symptoms

        g. Course

        h. Effect on daily activities

        i. Similar symptoms in family members or friends

        j. Pertinent negatives

        k. Other current illnesses/health problems

        l. Allergies

- Telephone History (telephone triage)

    1. Requires triage decision

        a. Telephone management

        b. Office visit

        c. Refer to emergency department or other health care provider

    2. Telephone protocol books are helpful in assessment and management of common illnesses and problems encountered by phone

    3. Critical elements

        a. Identify yourself

        b. Identify caller, his or her relationship to child, and caller's telephone number

    c. Obtain child's name, age and approximate weight

    d. Ascertain thorough history of present illness or problem

    e. If not medically necessary to see child, explain rationale and evaluate comfort of caller in home management

    f. Tell caller when to call back which includes advising on signs of worsening status

    g. Ask caller to telephone again to give progress report if there are any concerns about the child; if caller does not telephone as requested, IT IS CRITICAL TO MAKE THE FOLLOW-UP CALL

    h. Ask caller to write down information that has been given or at least to repeat the information

    i. Offer simple, understandable explanations

    j. Advise caller to contact you again with any questions

    k. Convey warmth, empathy and support

    l. Document all telephone conversations, including history, diagnosis, and management plan

- Sexual/Reproductive History

  1. Inform child that these questions are asked of all older school-age children and adolescents

  2. Reenforce that, although these questions are very personal or sensitive, they are necessary to gain a complete picture of that child or adolescent's health

  3. Reassure child or adolescent that the information he or she shares is confidential unless information about harm to self or others is revealed

  4. Progress from least to most sensitive questions

  5. It is best to phrase questions—"When was the first time you had intercourse?" instead of "Have you ever had intercourse?"

  6. Make sure older child or adolescent understands meaning of terms used

  7. Essential elements of sexual/reproductive history

      a. Date of menarche (first menses)

      b. Frequency, length and quantity of menses with associated symptoms, e.g., cramping, headache or backache

      c. Date of last menses

      d. Use of tampons or pads

      e. Age of first intercourse; date of last intercourse

      f. Sexual preference, e.g., males, females, or both; same sex exploration is common in teenagers; number of sexual partners

g. Types of sexual practices, e.g., male, female; oral sex, intercourse

h. Reasons for sexual activity, e.g., increases self-esteem; enjoyment; peer pressure

i. Pregnancies and outcomes

j. Current contraception

k. History of any sexually transmitted diseases (STD), naming each disease, e.g., gonorrhea, chlamydia, etc.

l. Vaginal or penile discharge

m. Date of last pelvic examination

n. Contraceptive history; current contraception; use of condoms

o. Knowledge of STDs, AIDS, pregnancy, and prevention measures

p. Date of prior test or desire for HIV testing

q. Performance of self-breast or testicular exam

r. History of sexual abuse

The Pediatric Physical Examination

- General Information

    1. Examination should be comprehensive and systematic

    2. Observation is first critical component of the examination beginning as soon as the child is seen

    3. Use examination to teach child about his or her body

- Age-related Issues (Infants)

    1. Developmental considerations

        a. Stage of trust versus mistrust

        b. Stranger anxiety develops at 6 to 7 months

        c. Separation anxiety develops at 8 to 9 months

        d. Major fears—separation from parents and pain

    2. Approaches to physical examination

        a. Approach slowly

        b. Conduct as much of examination with infant on parent's lap

        c. Provide infant with security objects, e.g., special blanket or toy

        d. Use distraction and engaging facial expressions during the examination

        e. Conduct examination using noninvasive to invasive sequence, e.g., auscultate heart and lung sounds first; examine ears and throat last

      f.   Allow for brief break if infant is hungry or stressed

- Age-related Issues (Toddlers)

   1. Developmental considerations

      a.   Stage of autonomy versus shame/doubt

      b.   Striving for independence

      c.   Negativism and temper tantrums (common)

      d.   Beginning of magical thinking

      e.   Major fears—separation from parents; intrusion of body orifices; loss of control; pain

   2. Approaches to physical examination

      a.   Use of distraction is helpful

      b.   Allow child to touch and hold equipment before examination

      c.   Demonstrate examination on doll, toy, or parent before conducting examination on child

      d.   Give child choices when possible

      e.   When necessary, tell child what you are going to do instead of gaining permission, e.g., "I am going to check your tummy" versus "Is it OK with you if I check your tummy?"

      f.   Conduct as much of examination as possible on parent's lap

      g.   Conduct examination using noninvasive to an invasive sequence

- Age-Related Issues (Preschool Children)

   1. Developmental considerations

      a.   Stage of initiative versus guilt

      b.   Magical thinking

      c.   Egocentrism

      d.   Major fears—separation from parents; loss of control; body mutilation; pain

   2. Approaches to physical examination

      a.   Inform child what you are going to do and what he/she can do to help

      b.   Role play with equipment, e.g., let child examine ears of doll first

      c.   Head to toe examination sequence can usually be implemented

      d.   Choose words carefully due to magical thinking

      e.   Allow choices whenever possible

      f.   Teach child about his/her body during course of examination

  g. Praise child for helping and attempting to cooperate

- Age-Related Issues (School-age Children)
    1. Developmental considerations
        a. Industry versus inferiority
        b. Concrete thinking
        c. Desires to act brave
        d. Enjoys gathering scientific information
        e. Modesty emerges with older school-age child
        f. Major fears—separation from peers; loss of control; pain; death, beginning at age 9 years
    2. Approaches to physical examination
        a. Head to toe sequence
        b. Scientific terminology with concrete explanations
        c. Answer questions factually with age-appropriate vocabulary
        d. Explain use of equipment, e.g., otoscope
- Age-Related Issues (Adolescents)
    1. Developmental considerations
        a. Stage of identity versus role diffusion
        b. Striving for independence and control
        c. Formal operational thinking
        d. Bodily concerns
        e. Concerns about being different
        f. Major fears—change in body image; separation from peers; loss of control; death
    2. Approaches to physical examination
        a. Assure privacy
        b. Examine without parent unless adolescent prefers parent remain in room
        c. Inform adolescent of each step of examination
        d. Give choices whenever possible
        e. Cover parts of body not currently being examined
        f. Assure privacy
        g. Teach adolescent about his/her body during course of examination
        h. Provide reassurance of ''normalcy'' during course of examination

      i. Recognize and discuss apprehension about breast, pelvic and testicular examinations

- Measurement of Vital Signs
  1. Temperature
     a. Rectal temperature—most accurate method, but proper technique must be used to avoid injury
     b. Tympanic membrane temperature—quick and noninvasive measurement, reliability is a problem
     c. Temperature of 100.4° F (38° C) and above is considered a fever
  2. Pulse
     a. Norms

	Beats/minute
(1) Newborn	120–170
(2) 1 year	80–160
(3) 3 years	80–120
(4) 6 years	75–115
(5) 10 years	70–110
(6) 17 years	60–100

     b. Conditions that commonly elevate pulse

       (1) Temperature—for every 1 degree of temperature elevation in fahrenheit, pulse increases by 10 beats per minute

       (2) Anxiety/stress; excitement

       (3) Exercise

       (4) Severe anemia

       (5) Hyperthyroidism

       (6) Hypoxia

       (7) Heart disease

  3. Respirations

     a. Norms

	Breaths per minute
(1) Newborn	30–80
(2) 1 year	20–40
(3) 3 years	20–30
(4) 6 years	16–20

    (5) 10 years   16–20

    (6) 17 years   12–20

  b. Conditions that commonly elevate respirations

    (1) Temperature—for every 1 degree of temperature elevation in fahrenheit, respirations increase by 4 breaths per minute

    (2) Anxiety/stress; excitement

    (3) Pain

    (4) Respiratory conditions, e.g., pneumonia

    (5) Heart disease

4. Blood Pressure

  a. Appropriate cuff size required for accurate reading

    (1) Bladder width should not be more than $\frac{2}{3}$ the length of upper arm

    (2) Bladder length should cover $\frac{3}{4}$ of the arm circumference

  b. Use Korotkoff sound IV (muffling sound) as diastolic blood pressure in children under 13 years of age; use Korotkoff sound V (disappearance of sound) as the diastolic blood pressure in children 13 years of age and older

  c. Plot blood pressure on standard blood pressure graphs for boys or girls

  d. Begin to measure blood pressure at well-child visits, starting at 3 years of age

  e. A single elevated blood pressure measurement in an apparently healthy child does not necessarily reflect disease

  f. Hypertension—average systolic and/or diastolic blood pressure $\geq$ 95th percentile for age and sex on at least 3 separate occasions using the same arm, same cuff, and same position

Age	Systolic (mm Hg)	Diastolic (mm Hg)
Infant	$\geq$ 112	$\geq$ 74
3–5 years	$\geq$ 116	$\geq$ 76
6–9 years	$\geq$ 122	$\geq$ 78
10–12 years	$\geq$ 126	$\geq$ 82
13–15 years	$\geq$ 136	$\geq$ 86
16–18 years	$\geq$ 142	$\geq$ 92

  g. Taller, heavier children have higher blood pressure than smaller children of same age

  h. Pulse pressure—difference between systolic and diastolic blood pressures (normal is 20 to 50 mm Hg)

(1) Wide pulse pressure from high systolic pressure is usually due to fever, exercise, or excitement

(2) Wide pulse pressure from low diastolic pressure is usually due to patent ductus arteriosus, aortic regurgitation, or other serious heart disease

Specific Normal Findings and Common Variations

- Head and Neck

    1. History indicating possible abnormalities

        a. Difficult birth; use of forceps

        b. Unusual head shape or preferred position at rest

        c. Poor head control for age

        d. Lack of neonatal screening for hypothyroidism

    2. Selected physical examination findings

        a. Head circumference is approximately 2 cm larger than chest during first year of life; head and chest circumferences should be equal at 1 year of age; during childhood, chest is usually 5 to 7 cm larger than head

        b. Fontanels—best to assess while infant is sitting up and not crying

            (1) Posterior fontanel rarely palpable at birth; closes by 2 months of age

            (2) Size of anterior fontanel should be no larger than 4 to 5 cm in diameter

            (3) Anterior fontanel closes between 9 to 18 months of age

                (a) Early closure usually leads to synostosis

                (b) Late closure is commonly seen with increased intracranial pressure, hypothyroidism, rickets; syphilis, Down syndrome, osteogenesis imperfecta

            (4) Large anterior fontanel may indicate:

                (a) Chronically increased intracranial pressure

                (b) Subdural hematoma

                (c) Rickets

                (d) Hypothyroidism

                (e) Osteogenesis imperfecta

            (5) Bulging anterior fontanel is usually seen with conditions that cause increased intracranial pressure, e.g., meningitis/encephalitis, fluid overload

            (6) Sunken anterior fontanel is usually seen with severe dehydration (more than 10%)

        c. Unusual head size or shape

(1) Hydrocephalus—excessively large head at birth or head that grows abnormally rapid; usually associated with distended scalp veins, widely separated cranial sutures, large and tense anterior fontanel, and "sunset eyes"

(2) Microcephaly—head circumference > 2 standard deviations below the mean for age, sex and gestation; reflects an abnormally small brain; common causes are intrauterine infections (e.g., herpes, rubella, syphilis); genetic defects; drug usage during pregnancy (especially alcohol)

(3) Macrocephaly—head circumference > 2 standard deviations above the mean for age, sex and gestation; common causes are hydrocephalus, masses, increased intracranial pressure; skeletal dysplasias (osteogenesis imperfecta)

(4) Head tilt—common causes include strabismus, CNS lesions, or short sternocleidomastoid muscle

(5) Caput succedaneum—diffuse edema of the soft tissue of the scalp which usually crosses suture lines; may be seen with bruising due to traumatic vaginal birth; seen at birth; no specific treatment necessary; usually resolves in 2 to 3 days

(6) Cephalohematoma—subperiosteal collection of blood which does not cross suture lines; often does not appear until several hours after birth and may increase over 24 hours; no specific treatment indicated; resolves over a few weeks to months; observe for hyperbilirubinemia

(7) Premature or irregular closure of suture lines can cause unusual head shape (craniosynostosis)

(8) Bossing (bulging) of frontal area is associated with rickets and prematurity

d. Head Control

(1) By 4 months of age, head should be held erect and in midline

(2) By 6 months of age, there should be no head lag when infant is pulled from supine to sitting position—if present, may indicate neuromuscular disorder; may be the *first sign* of cerebral palsy

e. Neck

(1) Pain and resistance to flexion may indicate meningeal irritation

(2) Torticollis (restriction of motion)—can result from birth trauma (e.g., injury to the sternocleidomastoid muscle with bleeding into the muscle); muscle spasm, viral infection, or drug ingestion

(3) Webbed neck—common in Turner's syndrome, a chromosomal abnormality, occurring 99% of the time in females, which results in webbed neck, widespread nipples, abnormal ears, micrognathia and lymphedema of hands and feet

    (4) Unusual position of trachea could indicate serious lung problem

    (5) Mass in the neck

       (a) Thyroglossal duct cyst—usually seen near midline of neck; cyst moves up and down with protrusion of tongue; may become infected and present as an abscess; surgical excision recommended

       (b) Brachial cleft cyst—can appear as swelling anterior to sternocleidomastoid (SCM) muscle or as opening along anterior border of SCM, may drain and become infected

       (c) Hematoma (of sternocleidomastoid muscle)—more common in breech deliveries

       (d) Enlarged thyroid—due to hyperthyroidism or hypothyroidism; visible thyroid gland is almost always enlarged

       (e) Enlarged lymph node—most frequent cause of lateral neck mass

- Face

  1. History indicating possible abnormalities

    a. Difficult delivery; use of forceps

    b. Asymmetry of face when crying or speaking

    c. Facial features which are unusual or do not match family characteristics

    d. Drug or alcohol use during pregnancy

  2. Selected physical examination findings

    a. Asymmetry of nasolabial folds or drooping mouth indicates facial nerve impairment or Bell's palsy

    b. Child who demonstrates open mouth breathing and facial contortions may have allergic rhinitis

    c. Dysmorphic facial features are hallmark of numerous syndromes (e.g. fetal alcohol syndrome) and diagnosis should be pursued

- Eyes

  1. History indicating possible abnormalities

    a. Premature infant who required resuscitation; needed ventilator or oxygen support; had retinopathy of prematurity

    b. Infant who does not track faces or objects; absent blink in response to bright lights or sudden movements

    c. Children less than 6 years of age who:

      (1) Rub eyes excessively, squint, have photophobia

      (2) Have difficulty reaching for or picking up small objects

      (3) Engage in head tilting

(4) Hold objects close to face

d. School-age children (same as young children, plus) who:

    (1) Sit close to blackboard or TV in order to see

    (2) Are making poor progress in school not explained by intellectual deficit or learning disability

e. Any age child who:

    (1) Demonstrates white area in pupil visible in photographs (retinoblastoma)

    (2) Complains of headaches not present upon awakening, but progress during the day (accommodative errors)

    (3) Has problems with excessive tearing—allergies, (accommodative errors)

    (4) Has an eye which turns in or out (strabismus)

2. Selected physical examination findings

a. Position and placement—inner canthal distance averages 2.5 cm; epicanthal folds present in Asian children; palpebral fissures lie horizontally

    (1) Hypertelorism (wide set eyes)—present in Down syndrome

    (2) Epicanthal folds can be frequently seen in Down syndrome, renal agenesis, or glycogen storage disease

    (3) Ptosis could be normal or may indicate paralysis of oculomotor nerve

    (4) Exophthalmos (protruding eyeballs)—can be seen with hyperthyroidism

b. Eyelids normally same color as surrounding skin

    (1) "Stork Bite" mark—telangiectatic nevi disappear by 12 months

    (2) Blocked tear duct (dacryostenosis)—may lead to infection of lacrimal sac evidenced by swelling, redness, and purulent discharge (dacryocystitis)

    (3) Periorbital edema—soft swelling that may be associated with renal or cardiac problems or sinusitis; acute onset of unilateral eyelid edema with erythema, induration and tenderness indicates periorbital cellulitis

c. "Allergic shiners"—bluish discoloration and soft edema below eyes usually indicates allergies

d. Sclera and conjunctiva

    (1) Sclera is shiny, clear and white

    (2) Bulbar conjunctiva (covers sclera) is moist and transparent and palpebral conjunctiva (lines the eyelids) is pink and moist

    (3) Spots of brown melanin may be seen in dark skinned races

    (4) Yellow sclera indicates jaundice

(5) Redness may indicate bacterial or viral infection, allergy or irritation, e.g., chemicals

(6) Excessive pallor of the palpebral conjunctiva indicates anemia

(7) Cobblestone appearance of palpebral conjunctiva (lining the eyelids) can indicate severe allergy or contact lens irritation

e. Pupils and iris

(1) Unequal pupils (anisocoria)—usually congenital and normal, but can indicate increased intracranial pressure from head trauma or other intracranial disease processes, e.g., meningitis

(2) Dilated, fixed pupils—usually indicate severe brain damage

(3) Dilated pupils—may result from use of anticholinergic drugs (e.g., atropine) and substance abuse (e.g., amphetamines)

(4) Abnormally small pupils—may result from brain damage, use of morphine, or substance abuse (e.g., cocaine)

f. By 3 to 4 months, infants should have binocular vision (ability to fixate on one visual field with both eyes simultaneously)

(1) Assessment techniques to elicit phoria (movement of eye when covered) or tropia (obvious turning in or out of eye without coverage) (e.g., strabismus)

(a) Cover-uncover test (when eye is covered, it may deviate in (esophoria) or out (exophoria) and return to midline when uncovered

(b) Corneal light reflex (Hirschberg's test)—with light held 12 to 14 inches from eyes, reflection of light should be the same on both corneas; if unequal, it is suggestive of phoria or tropia

(2) Intermittent alternating convergent strabismus—normal from 0 to 6 months of age

3. Ophthalmoscopic examination—red reflex should be elicited in every newborn and at each well-child visit

a. Absence of red reflex or an opacity of the lens may indicate cataracts in the newborn

b. Presence of white instead of red reflex may indicate retinoblastoma

- Ears

1. History indicating possible abnormalities

a. Prenatal exposure to maternal infection, irradiation, or drug abuse

b. Birth weight less than 1500 g

c. Anoxia in neonatal period

d. Ototoxic antibiotic usage (e.g., gentamycin)

e. Cleft palate

f. Infections

g. Meningitis

h. Encephalitis

i. Recurrent or chronic otitis media

2. Behaviors suggestive of hearing loss

    a. No reaction to loud or strange noises

    b. No babbling in infant after 6 months

    c. No communicative speech; reliance on gestures after 15 months of age

    d. Language delays

3. Selected physical examination findings

    a. Position and placement—low or obliquely set ears may indicate genitourinary or chromosomal abnormality or a multisystem syndrome

    b. Pain

        (1) Pain produced by manipulation of auricle or pressure on tragus may indicate otitis externa

        (2) Pain and tenderness over mastoid process may indicate mastoiditis

    c. Examination of tympanic membrane (TM)

        (1) For best visualization of TM—pull auricle down and back in children under 3 years of age; pull auricle up and back for children over 3 years of age

        (2) Crying produces erythema of TM bilaterally; landmarks are still visible with succinct light reflexes and +4 TM mobility

        (3) Pneumatic otoscopy is critical for assessment of fluid in middle ear

            (a) Decreased TM mobility—indicates fluid in middle ear

            (b) In child with pressure equalization (PE) tubes, decreased mobility of TM indicates obstruction or dysfunction of tubes

- Nose and Sinuses

1. History indicating possible abnormalities

    a. Inability to move air through both nares

    b. Discharge

    c. Nasal flaring or narrowing on inspection

    d. Hypernasal voice—snoring, hypertrophied adenoids

2. Selected physical examination findings

a. Flattened nasal bridge (in other than Asian or African-American children) may indicate congenital anomalies

b. Boggy nasal mucous membranes (bluish, pale, edematous) with serous drainage indicates allergic rhinitis

c. Persistent copious or purulent discharge is indicative of sinusitis

d. Unilateral purulent discharge suggests foreign body

- Throat/Mouth

    1. History indicating possible abnormalities

        a. Lack of, or excessive fluoride supplementation or fluoridated water

        b. Infant or toddler who goes to sleep with bottle of milk or juice

        c. Thumbsucking or pacifier use beyond 2 years of age

        d. Unusual sequence of tooth eruption

    2. Selected physical examination findings

        a. Lips

            (1) Cherry red color indicates acidosis

            (2) Drooping of one side of lips indicates facial nerve impairment

            (3) Fissures at corners of mouth may indicate riboflavin or niacin deficiency

        b. Teeth

            (1) Mottling may indicate excessive fluoride intake

            (2) Green or black staining can result from oral iron intake

        c. Palate—decay of maxillary incisors may result from baby bottle caries syndrome

            (1) Palpation of palate is important in newborns to detect submucosal cleft

            (2) Uvula rises and remains in midline when saying ''ah''; deviation or absence of movement indicates involvement of glossopharyngeal or vagus nerves

            (3) Bifed uvula is suggestive of a submucosal cleft palate

        d. Tonsils

            (1) During childhood, tonsillar hypertrophy is a normal immunological response; largest in size between 8 and 9 years of age and decreases in size after puberty

            (2) Asymmetrically enlarged tonsil without infection may suggest tonsillar lymphoma

        e. Voice

(1) Nasal quality indicates enlarged adenoids

(2) Hoarse cry may indicate croup, cretinism or tetany

(3) Chronic hoarseness may indicate vocal cord polyps

(4) Shrill, high-pitched cry may indicate increased intracranial pressure

f. Temporomandibular joint (TMJ)

(1) Findings indicative of TMJ dysfunction—pain upon palpation of TMJ; decrease in mandibular movement; TMJ sounds (popping and clicking); malocclusion; and abnormal morphology of mandible (micrognathia)

(2) Inability to open jaw (trismus) associated with fever and sore throat is suggestive of peritonsillar abscess

- Heart

1. History indicating possible abnormalities

   a. Infant

   (1) Increased respirations, especially during sleep

   (2) Prolonged feeding time; tires during feedings

   (3) Cyanosis of mucous membranes of mouth

   (4) Eyelid edema

   b. Child

   (1) Increased respirations, especially during sleep

   (2) Squatting or sleeping in knee chest position

   (3) Eyelid edema

   (4) Cyanosis of mucous membranes of mouth

   (5) Exercise intolerance

2. Selected physical examination findings

   a. Heart sounds and area of clearest auscultation

   (1) S_1 (closure of mitral and tricuspid valves)—heard best at apex

   (2) S_2 (closure of aortic and pulmonic valves)—heard best at aortic and pulmonic areas

   (3) Physiological splitting of S_2 during inspiration is normal; if fixed (heard upon inspiration and expiration), may indicate atrial septal defect or pulmonic stenosis

   (4) S_3—heard best at apex (sounds like Kentucky); due to blood rushing through mitral valve and hitting an empty ventricle; normal in almost all children; if loud in character, may indicate high diastolic pressure in involved ventricle as found in acute ventricular failure

(5) S$_4$—heard best at apex (sounds like Tennessee); almost never normal; indicates high pressure in either ventricle as found in pulmonic and aortic stenosis and systemic hypertension

b. Normal variations in heart rhythm—in sinus arrythmia, heart rate increases with inspiration and decreases with expiration; disappears with exercise or holding breath

c. Innocent (functional) murmurs—present in approximately 50% of children

    (1) Characteristics

        (a) Usually systolic in timing

        (b) Usually soft; never more than Grade III

        (c) Rarely transmitted

        (d) Low pitched, vibratory, musical, or twangy

        (e) Short duration

        (f) Usually loudest at left lower sternal border or at the second or third intercostal space

        (g) Varies in loudness and presence from time to time

        (h) Heard loudest in the recumbent position, during expiration, and after exercise

        (i) Diminishes with change in positioning from recumbent to sitting

        (j) No cyanosis

        (k) Normal pulses, respiratory rate and BP

        (l) Normal growth and development

        (m) Absence of a thrill (vibratory sensation felt over murmur with palm of hand)

    (2) Types of innocent heart murmurs in children

        (a) *Pulmonary ejection murmur* (heard at the pulmonic area)—early to mid systole; distinct gap between first heart sound and murmur and end of murmur and second heart sound

        (b) *Vibratory or Still's murmur*—musical or vibratory murmur; heard best at the lower left sternal border

        (c) *Venous hum*—heard best above or below clavicles, second or third interspaces; more coarse quality; very dependent upon position; disappears when child lies down or turns neck which decreases blood velocity through internal jugular veins

    (3) Conditions that increase intensity of innocent heart murmurs—exercise, fever, and anemia due to increased cardiac output

    (4) Innocent murmurs in the newborn

(a) Transition from fetal to adult circulation may take up to 48 hours

(b) Usually grade I or II

(c) Systolic

(d) Not associated with other signs and symptoms

(5) Point of Maximal Impulse (PMI)

(a) Children less than 8 years of age—4th intercostal space, mid-clavicular line

(b) Children more than 8 years of age—5th intercostal space, slightly right of mid-clavicular line

(c) Displacement of PMI with cardiac enlargement

(d) Increased pulsation of PMI indicates conditions which increase cardiac output, e.g., anemia, anxiety, fever, fluid overload

(6) Peripheral pulses—normally palpable, equal in intensity and rhythm; weak or absent femoral pulses may indicate coarctation of the aorta

- Lungs
  1. History indicating possible abnormalities
     a. Family history of tuberculosis, cystic fibrosis, allergy, asthma, atopic dermatitis
     b. Infants and young children
        (1) Premature infant with any respiratory complications
        (2) Sudden onset of coughing or difficulty breathing
        (3) Difficulty feeding
        (4) Apnea episodes
     c. Older children and adolescents
        (1) Smoking
        (2) Cocaine use
        (3) Recurrent or chronic cough
        (4) Exercise intolerance
  2. Selected physical examination findings
     a. Normal breath sounds—breath sounds are best heard by having child breath through mouth
        (1) Vesicular—low pitch, soft intensity; inspiration is more than expiration with a ratio of 5:2; heard over peripheral lung fields
        (2) Bronchovesicular—medium pitch, moderate intensity; inspiration equals expiration with a ratio of 1:1; heard over main bronchus

(3) Bronchial/tracheal—high pitch, loud intensity; inspiration less than expiration with a ratio of 1:2

 b. Abnormal breath sounds

  (1) Rhonchi—course sounds heard on expiration that are indicative of secretions in the large airways; usually present in bronchitis; clear with coughing; associated with rhonchal fremitus (course vibrations felt with hand on chest as air passes through exudate in bronchi)

  (2) Transmitted rhonchi—course sounds that result from the transmission of sound from congested nasal passages to the chest; can be avoided by having child breathe through mouth

  (3) Wheezing—high pitched musical or whistling sounds produced as air passes through narrowed airways; heard in bronchiolitis, asthma; cystic fibrosis; foreign body aspiration (unilateral wheezing)

  (4) Crackles—fine crackling sounds heard upon inspiration indicative of air passing through moisture in alveoli; usually suggests pneumonia or congestive heart failure

  (5) Pleural friction rub—creaking or grating sound caused by inflamed parietal and visceral pleural linings rubbing together; usually inspiratory and expiratory; subsides when child holds breath

 c. Chest movement

  (1) Children under 7 years of age are diaphragmatic (abdominal) breathers

  (2) Girls over 7 years of age become thoracic breathers; boys continue as abdominal breathers

  (3) Chest structural abnormalities may compromise lung function

   (a) Pectus carinatum—protuberant sternum

   (b) Pectus excavatum—depressed sternum

- Breasts (see Endocrine Disorders chapter)

 1. History indicating possible abnormalities

  a. Prepubertal breast enlargement in girls

  b. Gynecomastia in boys at any age

  c. Breast mass

  d. Galactorrhea not associated with childbearing

 2. Selected physical examination findings

  a. Neonate may have gynecomastia and milky discharge which disappears within 2 weeks (or, at least, 3 months)

  b. Gynecomastia can be normal variant in males due to temporary estrogen/testosterone imbalance (usually begins at Tanner Stage II to III and can last for 1 to

2 years); most commonly felt as small, tender, oval subareolar mass measuring up to 2 to 3 cm in diameter

c. Gynecomastia also may be indicative of

    (1) Obesity or increased muscle (pseudo-gynecomastia)

    (2) Testicular tumor (testes must be palpated in any male with gynecomastia)

    (3) Medication usage—estrogen, steroids, tricyclic antidepressants (e.g., imipramine), respiridol, mellaril, amphetamines, digoxin, cimetidine

    (4) Klinefelter's syndrome (47XXY)—associated with small penis and testes, scoliosis, aspermia, decreased testosterone levels, and height greater than 6 feet

d. Asymmetric breast development is normal in the adolescent female

e. Galactorrhea may be indicative of:

    (1) Pregnancy

    (2) Recent abortion

    (3) Pituitary tumor—associated with increased prolactin level; increased headaches; amenorrhea; peripheral vision loss

    (4) Drug use—marijuana; opiates (codeine, heroin, morphine); amphetamines; hormones (oral contraceptives); digoxin; valium; cimetidine; phenothiazines (thorazine, mellaril); haloperidol; tricyclic antidepressants; respiridol

    (5) Hypothyroidism

d. Breast masses in adolescents

    (1) Benign breast masses (obtain ultrasound versus mammogram due to dense breast tissue in adolescents)

        (a) Fibroadenoma—most common breast mass in adolescents; increased incidence in African-Americans

            (i) Characteristics—single, unilateral mass; round or discoid in shape; firm and smooth in consistency; no retraction; mobile; nontender

            (ii) No variation with menstrual cycle

        (b) Fibrocystic breasts—usually result of hormonal imbalance

            (i) Characteristics—breast pain with or without lumps; symptoms worsen a few days before menses and resolve with completion of menses

            (ii) Mobile cysts or areas are more dense and fibrous; usually resolve in 1 to 3 months

(2) Neoplastic breast masses (very rare)—firm; nonmobile; painless; overlying skin changes; nipple discharge

- Abdomen
  1. History indicating possible abnormalities
     a. Birth weight under 1500 g places infant at high risk for necrotizing enterocolitis
     b. Failure to pass first meconium stool within 24 hours
     c. Jaundice
     d. Failure to grow or unexplained weight loss
     e. Projectile vomiting or blood in emesis
     f. Chronic diarrhea or constipation
     g. Enlargement of the abdomen with or without pain
     h. Abdominal or pelvic pain
  2. Selected physical examination findings—flexion of knees and hips facilitates examination
     a. Prominent abdomen (pot-belly)—normal in early childhood in sitting and supine positions due to poorly developed musculature; children up to 13 years of age may have prominent abdomen in standing position
     b. Liver edge—may be palpable 1 to 2 cm below right costal margin, especially with deep inspiration
     c. Spleen tip—may be palpable 1 to 2 cm below left costal margin, especially with deep inspiration
     d. Diastasis recti—separation of rectus abdominis muscles several cm wide from xiphoid bone to umbilicus; may extend to symphysis pubis; normal as long as not associated with hernia
     e. Bowel sounds
        (1) Active bowel sounds—heard every 5 to 15 seconds; range of 4 to 12 sounds per minute
        (2) Hypoactive bowel sounds—heard at more than 15 second intervals or less than 4 sounds per minute
        (3) Hyperactive bowel sounds—heard less than every 5 seconds or more than 12 sounds per minute
     f. Palpation of fecal mass in LLQ common with constipation
- Reproductive System
  1. History indicating possible abnormalities
     a. Discharge or bleeding from vagina or penis

    b. History or suspicion of sexual abuse

    c. Sexual intercourse without use of contraceptives

    d. Scrotal swelling with crying or bowel movement

    e. "Empty" scrotum versus retractable testes

    f. Unusual voiding pattern

2. Selected physical examination findings (see Human Growth and Development Infancy through Adolescence chapter for Tanner stages and sequence of pubertal development)

    a. Signs and symptoms of possible sexual abuse

        (1) Evidence of general physical abuse or neglect

        (2) Evidence of trauma or scarring in genital, anal or perianal areas

        (3) Changes in skin color or pigmentation in genital or anal area

        (4) Any sexually transmitted disease

        (5) Anorectal itching, bleeding, pain or poor sphincter tone

        (6) Rashes, sores or discharge in genital area

        (7) Dysuria, frequency of urination, enuresis

        (8) Behavioral or emotional changes

        (9) Deterioration in school performance

      (10) Inappropriate sexual behavior for developmental level

    b. Labial adhesions

        (1) Rule out ambiguous genitalia

        (2) Adhesions of labia minora most common in young infants

    c. Male genitalia

        (1) Phimosis—foreskin that cannot be easily retracted over the glans penis before 5 years of age

        (2) Undescended testes (cryptorchidism)—if testicle can be "milked" down into scrotum, consider it descended; refer undescended testicle after 1 year of age

        (3) Hypospadias or epispadias should be referred

        (4) Large scrotum—hydrocele; spermatocele; varicocele

            (a) Testicular tumor (common in adolescents and young men)

            (b) Indirect inguinal hernia

- Musculoskeletal System (see Musculoskeletal Disorders: Infancy through Adolescence chapter)

1. History indicating possible abnormalities

   a. Birth history—large for gestational age; abnormal presentation; anoxia in perinatal period

   b. Delay in motor developmental milestones

   c. Unusual style of movement—dragging of legs while crawling

   d. Hand dominance in an infant—may indicate weakness of other hand

   e. Leg pain/limp

2. Selected physical examination findings

   a. Barlow and Ortolani tests to detect hip dislocation or subluxation in infants—more common in females and breech deliveries

      (1) Barlow's test—hip is flexed and thigh is adducted which causes displacement of femoral head from acetabulum with a palpable "clunk"

      (2) Ortolani's test—hip is flexed at 90 degree angle and abducted with examiner's finger over the greater trochanter which reduces dislocated hip; a "clunk" is heard and felt

   b. Allis sign to detect hip dislocation or shortened femur—unequal leg length is abnormal

   c. Trendelenburg test to detect hip dislocation—child stands and raises one leg off the ground; lowering of iliac crest on side opposite weight-bearing leg indicates defect in weight bearing hip

   d. Gower's sign shows generalized muscle weakness; often indicative of muscular dystrophy—use of hands on legs to push self to standing position is abnormal

   e. Scoliosis (lateral curvature of the spine)

      (1) Functional—child can voluntarily straighten spine; disappears when child is recumbent

      (2) Structural—persistent curvature; unequal height of shoulders and iliac crests when standing erect; presence of rib hump when leaning forward

   f. Developmental differences

      (1) Longitudinal arch of foot can be obscured by fat pad until 3 years of age; child appears "flat footed"

      (2) Bowlegs (genu varum) and wide-based gait—common in toddlers

      (3) Knock knees (genu valgum)—common in preschool children

   g. "Turned-in" foot may have different causes

      (1) Femoral anteversion—most common between 3 and 8 years; 99% resolve by 8 years of age

Table 1
Infant Reflexes

Reflex	Appearance	Disappearance
Palmar grasp	birth	2–3 months
Plantar grasp	birth	10–12 months
Moro	birth	4–6 months
Stepping	birth	3–4 months
Tonic neck	birth to 6 weeks	4–6 months
		3–4 months, except during sleep up to 12
Rooting	birth	months

(2) Tibial torsion—most common between 1 and 3 years of age; growth alone will correct 99% of cases

(3) Metatarsus adductus

h. Hip should always be examined in child complaining of knee pain

- Neurologic System

1. History indicating possible abnormalities

   a. Delay or regression in developmental milestones; unusual behavior for age; learning or school difficulties

   b. Headaches/seizures

   c. Clumsiness or progressive weakness; irritability or lethargy

2. Selected physical examination findings

   a. Infant reflexes (automatisms)—see Table 1

   b. Absence of infantile automatisms or persistence beyond expected time of disappearance may indicate severe CNS dysfunction

   c. Spasticity—may be early sign of cerebral palsy

   d. Use of Denver II or other general developmental screening tool yields much data regarding age appropriate skills

   e. Babinski sign—normal up to 2 years of age

   f. Age of disappearance of individual "soft signs" is typically 8 years

- Dermatologic System (see Dermatologic Conditions: Infancy through Adolescence chapter)

1. History indicating possible abnormalities

   a. Family history of atopic dermatitis, allergic skin disorders, familial hair loss, or unusual pigmentation patterns

   b. Chronic or repeated acute episodes of skin lesions

   c. Frequent scratching or rubbing of body area

2. Selected physical examination findings

a. Birthmarks (nevi)

   (1) Salmon patch (stork-bite)—common on eyelids, nasolabial region or nape of neck; disappears by 12 months

   (2) Nevus flammeus (port-wine stain)—enlarges as child grows

   (3) Strawberry nevus (raised hemangioma)

      (a) Begins as circumscribed grayish white area; later becomes red and raised; not always present at birth

      (b) Majority resolve spontaneously by 10 years of age

   (4) Mongolian spot (hyperpigmented nevi)

      (a) Usually in sacral or gluteal areas

      (b) Generally seen in newborns of African-American, Asian or Latin descent

   (5) Café-au-lait spots (light brown, flat patches)—6 or more may be associated with neurofibromatosis

b. Common color changes in newborns

   (1) Acrocyanosis—cyanosis of hands and feet due to vascular instability

   (2) Cutis marmorata—transient mottling when infant is exposed to decreased temperature

   (3) Erythema toxicum—transient, benign, pink papular rash with vesicles on thorax, back, buttocks and abdomen

   (4) Harlequin color change—as infant lies on side, dependent portion of body becomes pink and upper portion is pale

   (5) Jaundice (see Hematological/Oncological/Immunologic Disorders: Infancy through Adolescence chapter)—skin blanches yellow with pressure instead of white as with carotinemia

      (a) Jaundice appears first on head and then progresses down body

      (b) Approximate level of hyperbilirubinemia by cephalocaudal distribution—nose (3 mg/dL); face (5 mg/dL); chest (7 mg/dL); abdomen (10 mg/dL); legs (12 mg/dL); palms (20 mg/dL)

      (c) Physiological jaundice—appears 2 to 3 days after birth

      (d) Appearance of jaundice in first 24 hours indicates hemolytic disease or infection

      (e) Breast feeding infants who develop jaundice in the second to third week may have breast milk jaundice

      (f) First appearance of jaundice at 2 to 3 weeks of age—must suspect biliary atresia (indirect bilirubin is elevated and AST and ALT also may be elevated)

(g) Factors contributing to development of hyperbilirubinemia—metabolic acidosis, lowered albumin levels, free fatty acids, drugs (maternal or fetal), other conditions (e.g., fetal distress, hypoxia, hypothermia, hypoglycemia, infant bruising, maternal or fetal infection

c. Degree of dehydration can be estimated by length of time skin retains "tenting" after it is pinched

  (1) < 2 seconds = < 5% loss of body weight

  (2) 2 to 3 seconds = 5% to 8% loss of body weight

  (3) 3 to 4 seconds = 9% to 10% loss of body weight

  (4) > 4 seconds = > 10% loss of body weight

- Lymph Nodes

  1. History indicating possible abnormalities

     a. Recurrent infections—tonsillitis, adenoiditis, bacterial infections, oral candidiasis, chronic diarrhea

     b. Poor growth; failure to thrive

     c. Maternal HIV infection

     d. IV drug use

     e. Multiple and indiscriminate sexual contacts

  2. Selected physical examination findings

     a. Normal size is up to 1 cm in inguinal area; 2 cm in cervical area; in other areas, up to 3 mm is normal

     b. Nodes enlarged due to infection are firm, or fluctuant, warm, tender, mobile, and may be accompanied by redness of overlying skin

     c. "Shotty" nodes (e.g., under 0.5 cm in diameter, firm, mobile and non-tender) can be present at any time in childhood and usually indicate past infection

     d. Suspect malignancy or tuberculosis if supraclavicular nodes are palpated

Selected Laboratory Tests and Values

- General Considerations

  1. Cost, pain, and invasiveness versus need for data to make accurate diagnosis

  2. Anesthetic cream used topically can ease venipuncture, especially in highly anxious children

  3. Laboratory values should be referenced against specified norms of laboratory conducting the testing since normal values may vary from laboratory to laboratory

- Hematology—CBC with differential

Table 2
Normal Range of Values
CBC

	Newborn	1 month	1 year	2–6 yrs	6–12 yrs	12–18 yrs
Hgb (g/dL)	14–24	11–17	11–15	11–15	11.5–15	12–16 (Males) 11.5–16 (Females)
Hct (%)	42–60	33–55	33–41	34–42	34–43	37–50 (Males) 36–44 (Females)
RBC (mill/mm³)	4.1–7.5	4.2–5.2	4.1–5.1	3.9–5.3	4. 0–5.2	4.5–5.3 (Males) 4.1–5.1 (Females)
WBC × 1000/mm³	9–30	5–19.5	6–17	5–15.5	4.5–13.5	4.5–13.5
Neutrophils (Segs%)	33–60	32–60	31–60	33–60	33–60	33–60
Bands (%) (Immature neutrophils)	0–5	0–5	0–5	0–5	0–5	0–5
Lymphocytes (%)	25–33	31–57	31–61	31–59	31–57	20–45
Monocytes (%)	3–7	3–7	3–7	3–7	3–7	3–10
Eosinophils (%)	1–4	1–4	1–4	1–4	1–4	1– 7
Basophils (%)	0–.75	0–.75	0–.75	0–.75	0–.75	0–.75
Platelets (10³/mm³)	84–478	150–400	150–400	150–400	150–400	150–400
Reticulocyte count (%)	3–7	.2–2	.2–2.8	.5–4	.5–4	.5–1.5
MCV (Mean Cell Volume+; μm³)	95–120	70–95	70–95	70–95	70–95	78–100
MCHC (Mean Cell Hemoglobin Concentration*)	31–37	31–37	31–37	31–37	31–37	31–37

+ Mean cell volume—average size of red cells
* Mean cell hemoglobin concentration—ratio of hemoglobin weight to hematocrit; helps to distinguish between normal colored cells (normochromic cells) and paler (hypochromic) cells

1. Normal range of values for complete blood count (CBC) with differential (see Table 2)

2. Common causes of variation in CBC with differential

   a. Hemoglobin variations

      (1) Increased—may indicate polycythemia (an overproduction of RBCs as a result of hypoxia); dehydration, or intravascular hemolysis

      (2) Decreased—may indicate anemia, hemodilution, sickle cell anemia, thalassemia; hemorrhage, or hyperthyroidism

   b. Hematocrit variations

      (1) Increased—may indicate polycythemia, dehydration or erythrocytosis

      (2) Decreased—may indicate anemia, hemorrhage; hyperthyroidism; leukemia, or cirrhosis

   c. Red blood cell variations

      (1) Increased—may indicate dehydration; hemorrhage; severe diarrhea; acute poisoning

      (2) Decreased—may indicate blood loss, low iron intake, lead poisoning, leukemia, rheumatic fever; systemic lupus erythematosis, or subacute bacterial endocarditis

d. White blood cell variations

    (1) Increased—first week of life; may signal bacterial infection (e.g., tonsillitis, sepsis, meningitis, appendicitis), or indicate acute hemorrhage, serum sickness, steroid use; hemolysis or leukemia

    (2) Decreased—indicates bone marrow depression which may result from viral infection; rickettsial infection; hypersplenia; leukemia; certain drugs (e.g., antiseizure medications, antibiotics, antihistamines, diuretics, analgesics, tricyclic antidepressants)

e. Neutrophils variations

    (1) Increased—may indicate bacterial infection; ischemic necrosis from burn injuries; metabolic disorders (e.g., diabetic ketoacidosis); stress response, emotional distress; inflammatory diseases (e.g. rheumatic arthritis), or hemolysis

    (2) Decreased (neutropenia)—viral infections (e.g., hepatitis, mononucleosis); chemotherapy or radiation; immune deficiencies; malignancies

f. Band cell or stab (immature neutrophil) variations—increased (known as a shift to the left); usually indicates severe bacterial infection (e.g., sepsis, pneumonia)

g. Lymphocytes variations

    (1) Increased—may indicate a viral infection; lymphocytic leukemia; ulcerative colitis; immune diseases

    (2) Decreased—indicates severe debilitating illnesses (e.g., congestive heart or renal failure, advanced TB); immunosuppressive therapy; Hodgkin's disease; after burns or trauma; Cushing syndrome; corticosteroid usage; HIV infection

    (3) Atypical lymphocytes—common in premature and healthy newborn infants; may indicate viral infection (e.g., mononucleosis, hepatitis); lymphocytic leukemia; ulcerative colitis; immune diseases

h. Monocyte variations

    (1) Increased—may indicate recovery from acute infection; SBE; leukemia; Hodgkin's disease; rickettsial infection; SLE; rheumatoid arthritis; hepatitis

    (2) Decreased—may indicate rheumatoid arthritis; HIV infection; prednisone usage

i. Eosinophil variations

    (1) Increased—may indicate allergic disorders (e.g., asthma, allergic rhinitis, atopic dermatitis) or parasite infection

    (2) Decreased—stress responses due to trauma, shock, burns, and emotional stress; Cushing syndrome

    j. Basophil variations

        (1) Increased—may indicate certain leukemias, Hodgkin's disease, inflammatory conditions (e.g. ulcerative colitis); polycythemia, chronic hemolytic anemia; infections such as TB, varicella, influenza

        (2) Decreased—may indicate hyperthyroidism, pregnancy, stress, prolonged use of steroids, allergic reaction

    k. Platelet variations

        (1) Increased—may indicate acute infection; malignancy; post-splenectomy; trauma; rheumatoid arthritis; Kawasaki disease

        (2) Decreased (thrombocytopenia)—may indicate leukemia; idiopathic thrombocytopenic purpura (ITP); autoimmune disorders; drugs (e.g., penicillin, ampicillin, cephalothin); hemolytic uremic syndrome; DIC; viral infection; HIV infection

    l. Reticulocyte count variations

        (1) Increased—may indicate hemorrhage/blood loss; increased destruction of RBCs; response to initiation of iron therapy

        (2) Decreased—may indicate iron deficiency anemia; chronic infection; radiation; aplastic anemia

    m. MCV variations

        (1) Increased—may indicate macrocytic anemia due to folic acid or vitamin B_{12} deficiency

        (2) Decreased—may indicate microcytic anemias caused by iron deficiency and thalassemia; anemia of chronic disease or lead poisoning

    n. MCHC variations

        (1) Increased—may indicate spherocytosis

        (2) Decreased—suggests hypochromic anemia caused by iron deficiency; chronic blood loss or thalassemia

- Chemistry

    1. Sodium chloride (mEq/L)

        a. Newborn—134 to 144

        b. Child—135 to 145

        c. Increased—dehydration; vomiting or diarrhea; diabetes insipidus; Cushing syndrome

        d. Decreased—vomiting; diarrhea; burns; diabetic ketoacidosis; Addison's disease; acute or chronic renal failure; syndrome of inappropriate antidiuretic hormone (SIADH)

    2. Potassium (mEq/L)

    a. Newborn—3.7 to 5.9

    b. Child—3.5 to 5.0

    c. Increased—may indicate acidosis or renal failure

    d. Decreased—may indicate diarrhea, vomiting, dehydration, malabsorption, use of diuretics or anti-inflammatory drugs

3. Blood urea nitrogen (BUN)

    a. Normal range—5 to 20 mg/dL

    b. Increased—may indicate a high protein diet; renal or urinary obstruction or disease; GI hemorrhage; malignancies; dehydration; shock

    c. Decreased—hemodilution; pregnancy; nephrotic syndrome; liver failure

4. Creatinine (more sensitive indicator of renal function than BUN)

    a. Normal value—0.3 to 1 mg/dL

    b. Increased—may indicate renal dysfunction; urinary tract obstruction, dehydration, muscle disease

5. Bilirubin (mg/dL)

    a. Birth—1.5

    b. Three to four days postnatal

        (1) Breastfed—7.3

        (2) Bottlefed—5.7

    c. Older infant and child

        (1) Total—less than 1.5

        (2) Direct (conjugated)—0.2 to 0.4 (higher levels require investigation for pathology)

        (3) Indirect (unconjugated) bilirubin—0.4 to 0.8 (levels greater than 20 mg/dL may be neurotoxic to brain)

6. Cholesterol (mg/100 mL)

    a. Full-term newborn—45 to 167

    b. Infant—70 to 190

    c. Child and adolescent—less than 170

7. Lead—normal value (less than 10 μg/dL)

- Urine

1. pH

    a. Newborn—5.0 to 7.0

    b. Older infant and child—4.8 to 7.8

    c. Increased (alkaline)—may indicate urinary tract infection; salicylate intoxication

    d. Decreased (acidic)—may indicate acidosis; renal failure; diarrhea or dehydration

2. Specific gravity

    a. Newborn—1.001 to 1.020

    b. Older infant and child—1.001 to 1.030

    c. Increased—may indicate dehydration, nephrosis, glomerulonephritis

    d. Decreased—may indicate diabetes insipidus; severe renal damage

3. Glucose (should be negative)—presence of sugar may indicate diabetes mellitus or other metabolic disorders; liver disease or renal tubular disorders

4. Protein (should be negative)—presence of protein may indicate renal disease (e.g., nephritis, nephrosis); exercise; SLE; orthostatic proteinuria; asymptomatic proteinuria

5. Ketones (should be negative)—presence of ketones may indicate fever, dehydration, anorexia, diarrhea, fasting, prolonged vomiting or anorexia

6. Nitrites (should be negative)—presence of nitrites strongly suggests urinary tract infection

7. WBC

    a. Normal range—0 to 4 WBC/HPF

    b. Increased—may indicate urinary tract infection; fever; pyelonephritis; TB; nephrosis

8. RBC

    a. Normal range 1 to 2 RBCs/HPF

    b. Increased—may indicate urinary tract infection; pyelonephritis; SLE; renal stones; trauma; TB; hemophilia; ployarteritis nodosa; malignant hypertension

9. Bacteria (should be negative)—100,000 colonies/mL or more of a single pathogen on urine culture by clean catch method confirms a urinary tract infection; repeat urine culture should be obtained for a result of 10,000 to 100,000 colonies/mL

- Cerebrospinal fluid (CSF)

1. Pressure—70 to 180 mm H_2O; higher indicates increased intracranial pressure which may be the result of a tumor; cerebral hemorrhage; meningitis; obstructed shunt

2. Appearance—Clear

    a. Bloody—may indicate traumatic tap; cerebral hemorrhage

    b. Yellow—may indicate hyperbilirubinemia or metastatic melanoma

    c. Cloudy—suggests increased WBC as found in bacterial meningitis

3. Glucose—60 to 80 mg/dL

   a. Increased—diabetes

   b. Decreased—may indicate bacterial meningitis, TB meningitis; hypoglycemia; leukemia with metastasis

4. Protein—15 to 45 mg/dL; increased in encephalitis; bacterial meningitis; TB meningitis; acoustic neuroma

5. Cell count

   a. Infant—0 to 20 WBC/mm^3

   b. Child and adolescent—0 to 10 WBC/mm^3

   c. Increased—bacterial meningitis; early viral meningitis; cerebral abscess

Selected Screening Tests

- Newborn Screening

  1. Screening should be conducted according to State law

  2. Most States require testing for:

     a. Hypothyroidism

     b. Phenylketonuria (PKU)

     c. Galactosemia

     d. Hemoglobinopathies (e.g., sickle cell disease)

  3. Other tests may include screening for:

     a. Maple syrup urine disease

     b. Homocystinuria

     c. Biotinidase deficiency

     d. Tyrosinemia

     e. Congenital adrenal hyperplasia

     f. Cystic fibrosis

     g. Toxoplasmosis

  4. Initial specimens should be obtained at least 24 hours after birth, but not more than 7 days of age

  5. Most States recommend a second metabolic screening in the first week of life for those infants tested before the first 36 to 48 hours of life

- Vision Screening

  1. Identify risk factors

     a. Prenatal infections

   b. Congenital cyanotic heart disease

   c. Structural malformation

   d. Family history of eye or vision problems

   e. Excessive oxygenation in neonatal period

   f. Hearing problems

   g. Parent concern about the child's visual functioning

   h. Deterioration in school performance

  2. Conduct age appropriate screening measures

   a. Young infant

    (1) Assess pupillary response to light

    (2) Illicit blink reflex

    (3) Determine ability to fix on and follow an object

    (4) Assess red reflex

   b. Older infant and toddler

    (1) Determine ability to fix on and follow an object

    (2) Perform corneal light reflex test (Hirschberg)

    (3) Perform cover/uncover test

    (4) Assess red reflex

   c. Preschool child (same as toddler, plus)

    (1) Conduct visual acuity tests (Allen figures, HOTV, Sjogren hand, illiterate E)—refer for further evaluation with visual acuity of 20/50 or worse or a two-line difference or more in scores between eyes

    (2) Use Ishihara for color perception

   d. School-age child and adolescent (preschool child, plus)

    (1) Far vision—Snellen chart

    (2) Near vision—Rosenbaum or Jaeger card

    (3) Refer children for further evaluation with:

     (a) Abnormal or asymmetric red reflex

     (b) Asymmetric corneal light reflex

     (c) Abnormal cover/uncover test

     (d) Structural abnormality

     (e) Failure to follow object equally when covering each eye

     (f) Visual acuity of 20/30 or worse at 7 years of age

(g) Two line difference or more in scores between eyes

- Hearing Screening
    1. Identify infants and children at risk for hearing problems
        a. Neonatal risk criteria
            (1) Affected family member
            (2) Bilirubin > 20 mg/dL
            (3) Congenital CMV, herpes, rubella
            (4) Defects in ENT structure
            (5) Birth weight < 1500 g
            (6) Bacterial meningitis
            (7) Use of ototoxic medications for more than 5 days
            (8) Mechanical ventilation for cardiopulmonary disease for more than 48 hours
            (9) Intracranial hemorrhage
        b. Risk criteria for children less than 2 years of age (neonatal risk factors, plus)
            (1) Parental concerns regarding hearing or language development
            (2) Head trauma with temporal bone fracture
            (3) Infections known to cause sensorineural hearing loss (e.g., measles, mumps)
            (4) Recurrent otitis media or middle ear effusion
    2. Conduct age-appropriate screening measures
        a. Newborn
            (1) Healthy infants—observe responses to voices, loud noises
            (2) High-risk infants—auditory brainstem response (ABR) or evoked otoacoustic emissions (EOAE)
            (3) AAP goal of early identification of infants with hearing loss before 3 months with intervention implemented prior to 6 months of age (AAP, 1995)
        b. Four to 24 months (same as newborn, plus)
            (1) Observe orientation to sound
            (2) Assess language development
        c. Two to 3 years (same as above, plus)—play audiometry
        d. Older than 3 years

(1) Examine ears using an otoscope with pneumatic otoscopy before conducting audiometry

(2) Conduct pure tone audiometry—test each ear at 500, 1000, 2000 and 4000 Hz (hand-held audiometers have not proven effective in screening children)

(3) Use tympanometry to further assess middle ear air pressure and tympanic membrane compliance if pneumatic otoscopy was abnormal

3. Refer children to an audiologist for further evaluation if hearing threshold levels are greater than 20 dB at any of the above frequencies; if the reliability of a test with an individual child is uncertain, repeat screening before referral

- Tuberculosis screening

1. Mantoux test should be used for testing; uses .1 cc of purified protein derivative (PPD) which contains 5 tuberculin units; administer via intradermal injection on the volar aspect of the forearm to produce a 6 to 10 mm wheal; multiple-puncture tests do not have adequate specificity and sensitivity

2. Test should be read 48 to 72 hours following injection by a measurement of the area of *INDURATION,* not redness

3. BCG vaccination is NOT a contraindication to TB skin testing

4. Positive skin tests include children who have reaction of:

   a. At least 15 mm *INDURATION* with no risk factors

   b. At least 10 mm *INDURATION* who are less than 4 years of age or those with medical risk factors (e.g., born in, or whose parents were born, in areas of prevalent TB [Asia, Middle East, Africa, or Latin America] or exposed to adults who are HIV positive, homeless, illicit drug users, nursing home residents, incarcerated or institutionalized persons, or migrant farm workers)

   c. At least 5 mm *INDURATION* who are household contacts of active or previously active TB cases as well as children with immunosuppressive conditions, including HIV infection

5. Current recommendations for TB testing are based on degree of risk rather than routine, universal screening

6. Immediate TB testing should be conducted on children who are contacts of individuals with confirmed or suspected infectious TBI; have been in contact with persons who have been incarcerated in the last five years; are immigrating from or with a history of travel to endemic countries, and those with clinical or radiologic findings of TB.

7. Annual TB testing should be conducted for children at high risk, beginning as early as 3 months of age

   a. HIV positive or living with an HIV infected person

   b. Institutionalized and/or incarcerated children and adolescents

8. Testing every two to three years

   a. Children exposed to the homeless, HIV-infected individuals, nursing home residents, institutionalized or incarcerated adolescents, illicit drug users, and migrant farm workers

9. Periodic TB testing between 4 to 6 years and again between 11 and 16 years for children living in high prevalence areas or with uncertain history of risk factors

10. See most recent AAP *Red Book* for specific updated guidelines

- Lead Screening

  1. The Centers for Disease Control (CDC) no longer recommend universal screening; targeted screening should be based on surveillance of risk (see Hematological/Oncological/Immunologic Disorders chapter)

  2. Risk factors include children who: live in poverty; have poorly maintained housing or an inner city residence; had a house painted before 1950; live in a home or child care near heavily traveled highways; live in a home built before 1978 that is being remodeled; are of minority race; have pica

  3. Most children with lead poisoning are between the ages of 1 and 5 years

  4. The blood lead level is more specific and sensitive than the erythrocyte protoporphyrin (EP) level (only 50% of children with a blood lead level of 32 μg/dL have elevated EP leads)

  5. Venous blood samples are more reliable than capillary samples

  6. The CDC defines lead poisoning as a blood lead level of ≥ 10 μg/dL as elevated; all children with blood lead levels equal to or more than 20 μg/dL should be screened for iron deficiency and receive treatment as recommended by CDC

  7. Children who have blood lead levels of 10 to 14 μg/dL need periodic testing, but no treatment

  8. Children who have blood lead levels between 15 to 19 μg/dL need education and dietary advice coupled with re-testing

- Cholesterol Screening

  1. Universal screening for all children not recommended

  2. Children more than 2 years of age who have a parent with a total cholesterol level of 240 mg/dL or greater should receive a total cholesterol screen

  3. Children more than 2 years of age with a family history of premature cardiovascular disease (e.g., a parent or grandparent with a myocardial infarction, sudden cardiac death, angina pectoris, coronary arteriography for diagnostic purposes, or cardiac bypass surgery at the age of 55 years or younger) should be screened with a serum lipid profile

  4. Children receiving total cholesterol screening may eat a normal diet before the test

5. Children receiving a serum lipid profile should fast for 12 hours (except for water) before their blood is drawn

6. An acceptable total cholesterol level in children and teens is less than 170 mg/dL; an acceptable LDL cholesterol level is less than 130 mg/dL.

7. A high total cholesterol level in children and teens is greater than or equal to 200 mg/dL; a high LDL cholesterol level is greater than or equal to 130 mg/dL

- Urine Screening

   1. Routine screening should be performed at 6 months and again at 2, 8, and 18 years of age

   2. Positive results of bacteriuria from a bagged urine specimen on an infant should be confirmed by catheterization or suprapubic aspiration

   3. "Clean catch" mid-stream urine specimens in children and adolescents are best for reliable results

- Sexually Transmitted Diseases/HIV

   1. All sexually active adolescents should be screened for gonorrhea and chlamydia as well as have a Pap smear performed as a screening for Human Papillomavirus (HPV)

   2. High-risk adolescents should be screened for syphilis and offered HIV testing (e.g., those with multiple sexual partners, who reside in areas with a high prevalence of STD/HIV infection, who have been sexually abused by or have had sexual contact with individuals with documented STD/HIV infection or parenteral drug use)

Special Examinations

- The Newborn Examination

   1. Immediately after birth, obtain APGAR scores at 1 and 5 minutes; composite scores range from 0 to 10 based on 5 criteria

Criteria	0	1	2
Heart rate	Absent	Slow (< 100)	> 100
Respiratory rate	Absent	Slow, irregular	Good strong cry
Muscle tone	Limp	Some flexion of extremities	Active motion
Reflex irritability	No response	Grimace	Cough or sneeze
Color	Blue, pale	Body pink, extremities blue	Completely pink

2. Obtain length, weight, head circumference percentiles, and vital signs

3. Assess vision and hearing

4. Assess gestational age (Ballard, Dubowitz)

5. HEENT

    a. Palpate anterior and posterior fontanels—note presence of molding, craniosynostosis, cephalohematomas, asymmetry

    b. Assess presence of red reflex

    c. Note size, shape and position of ears and characteristics of TM

    d. Assess for patency of nares, intact palate, and any unusual findings in the mouth

6. Assess neck for webbing; palpate for masses

7. Auscultate lungs and assess thorax for shape, symmetry, and character of respirations

8. Perform cardiac evaluation, including auscultation for murmurs and assessment of brachial and femoral pulses

9. Conduct abdominal examination, including the number of blood vessels in cord (two umbilical arteries and one umbilical vein), cord appearance, and condition of stump

10. Assess genitourinary system, including prominence of labia; number of testicles and position; position of urethra; circumcision prior to discharge

11. Conduct musculoskeletal examination, including hips; feet; range of motion; presence of crepitus; Ortolani and Barlow maneuvers

12. Perform neurological examination, including assessment of head lag and muscle tone; illicit the following reflexes

    a. Root/suck

    b. Gag reflex

    c. Moro

    d. Plantar/palmar

    e. Stepping

    f. Tonic neck

13. Assess skin for cyanosis, jaundice, meconium staining, rashes, lesions and birthmarks

- The Sports Evaluation

    1. Purpose

        a. Identify risk factors associated with morbidity and mortality

        b. Identify conditions that place the child at risk for injury

        c. Identify conditions which could worsen with sports participation

        d. Determine appropriate sports activities for child's abilities

2. Most important history-taking question—has the child ever fainted or lost consciousness during exercise?

3. The physical examination should be comprehensive with emphasis on:

   a. Cardiac examination, including blood pressure

     (1) Presence of a systolic murmur that increases on sitting or with valsalva maneuver requires an echocardiogram

     (2) An arrythmia that does not subside with exercise requires referral to a cardiologist

   b. Musculoskeletal examination

     (1) Perform scoliosis screen

     (2) Have child perform the "duck walk" (squat on heels, walk 4 steps, and stand up)

     (3) Assess shoulder flexion and rotation

   c. Genitalia exam

     (1) Tanner stage

     (2) Presence of hernias

     (3) Presence of both testicles in males

4. Excluding conditions for contact collision sports include:

   a. Atlantoaxial instability (as found in Down syndrome)

   b. Carditis

   c. Absence of a paired organ (e.g., kidneys)

   d. Hepatosplenomegaly

   e. Poorly controlled seizure disorder

   f. Ventriculoperitoneal (VP) shunt

- Breast and Pelvic Examinations

1. Breast

   a. Although breast disease is rare in adolescent females, assessment of the breasts should be performed routinely as part of the well child physical examination from the start of puberty (as soon as breast budding occurs)

   b. In addition to detection of disease, the breast examination is a wonderful opportunity to teach adolescents about breast development and self-breast examination as well as provide reassurance about the "normalcy" of their breasts

2. Pelvic

a. Recognize the pelvic examination produces much fear and anxiety for adolescents, especially those who are experiencing it for the first time, have had a prior difficult experience, and have been sexually abused

b. Prepare the adolescent for the examination by showing her illustrations of the reproductive system and explaining the procedure

c. Provide concrete objective information about sensations the adolescent will feel during course of the examination which will help her cope better with the experience

d. Suggest ways to maintain control and decrease anxiety during examination (e.g., relaxation techniques)

e. Use largest speculum that will fit comfortably within vagina (usually small plastic or Pederson speculum work best for this age group)

f. Warm speculum before insertion

g. Inform adolescent of what you are doing throughout the examination

h. Encourage the adolescent to become involved with the examination if she desires (e.g., a mirror can be positioned to see the area being examined)

i. Verbal or visual modes of distraction are helpful (e.g., interesting posters on the ceiling or wall)

j. Use examination to teach adolescent about her body and to reassure her of "normalcy"

k. Provide as much privacy as possible, e.g., while dressing

l. Give positive feedback to the adolescent for her cooperation or assistance

m. Recognize that cervical ectopy is a normal finding during the examination, especially in adolescents taking hormonal contraceptives

Problem-Oriented Health Record

- Organized system for recording health visits to allow for thorough, concise data, easy retrieval of data, enhanced communication between health professionals; documentation of problem assessment/management, and decreased risk of liability

- Components of the problem-oriented health record

    1. Data base—medical history, physical examination, growth charts, developmental flow sheets, screening and laboratory tests, and problem-specific progress notes

    2. Problem list—conditions that require diagnostic work-up or ongoing management

    3. Management plan—includes information related to the diagnosis, management, education and follow-up for specific health problem

    4. Progress notes—includes documentation of each patient visit and is usually recorded in SOAP format

        a. S—subjective information provided by child and parent or caregiver

      b. **O**—objective information which consists of observations, physical examination, and laboratory findings

      c. **A**—assessment (diagnosis)

      d. **P**—plan

          (1) Medications

          (2) Treatments (e.g., warm compresses)

          (3) Further laboratory studies

          (4) Consultations or referrals

          (5) Diet or activity modifications

          (6) Teaching

          (7) Follow-up schedule (visit or telephone contact)

Child Health Supervision Schedule of Visits with Key Issues (Nutrition, Development, Screening, Immunizations, Anticipatory Guidance and Health Education)

- Prenatal Visit

    1. General Considerations

      a. Major purposes—ensure the health of the fetus, child, family; establish relationship with family; answer questions; provide anticipatory guidance and plan of care

      b. Timing—between 30 to 35 weeks gestation

      c. Include both parents and/or grandparents if single parent

    2. Family history—parents and siblings' ages; health of parents, siblings, and blood relatives, including chronic illnesses such as asthma, cystic fibrosis, and heart disease as well as mental disorders

    3. Obstetrical history—current gestational age; beginning of prenatal care; ultrasound or amniocentesis results; name of obstetrician; medications, drugs, cigarettes or alcohol usage during this pregnancy; prior pregnancies and outcomes

    4. Preparation for childbirth and infant

      a. Readiness for parenthood

      b. Planned or unplanned pregnancy

      c. Prenatal classes, childbirth preparation

      d. Sibling preparation, if applicable

      e. Choice of infant feeding (breast/bottle)—this visit is an excellent time to encourage breastfeeding, clarify misperceptions, and answer questions

      f. Circumcision, if applicable

      g. Genetic testing, if applicable

     h. Arrangements for child care

     i. Special concerns of prospective parents

     j. Current life stressors

5. Social history

     a. Family type—single parent, nuclear

     b. Number and types of pets

     c. Perceived social support

     d. Health care practices/religion

     e. Financial information, including insurance

     f. Cultural issues

6. Plan of care and anticipatory guidance

     a. Timing of health supervision visits

     b. Immunizations

     c. Organization of practice, e.g., team approach with nurse practitioners and physicians

     d. How and where to access care when needed; available hours

     e. Fees/medical coverage

     f. Need for transportation

     g. General infant care and supplies needed

     h. Safety information, e.g., car seats; pets

     i. Psychological adjustment of parents and siblings

- Newborn Visit

1. Purposes—obtain complete history; physical examination; anticipatory guidance and plan of care

2. Initial history—from chart review and parent/s

     a. General health of mother

         (1) Mother's age and gestation at first prenatal visit; regularity of visits

         (2) History of maternal infection and prenatal complications

         (3) Substance abuse, tobacco use

         (4) History of chronic disease

         (5) Medications during pregnancy

         (6) Weight gain; nutritional status

         (7) Number of weeks of gestation

(8)   Number of living children

b.   Labor and delivery

(1)   Length of labor

(2)   Medications used—anesthesia

(3)   Type of facility—birthing center, hospital, other

(4)   Type of delivery—spontaneous, C-section (explanation needed if yes)

(5)   Blood type, including Rh factor

c.   Infant's status at delivery

(1)   Identification verified

(2)   Term, preterm (number of weeks)

(3)   Determination of gestational age (Ballard/Dubowitz)

(4)   Apgar scores

(5)   Complications

(6)   Oxygen or any other treatment(s) required

(7)   Blood, type, Rh Factor; other values

(8)   Length, weight, head and chest circumference (including percentiles)

(9)   Physical examination results—note any abnormal findings

(10)   Correct date of birth

d.   Nursery course—presence of jaundice; type of treatments; medications, immunizations; length of stay; circumcision/cord condition

e.   Family history—maternal/paternal

(1)   Review of systems (ROS)—includes physical and mental health problems

(2)   Home environment—members of household; pets; smokers; infant supplies and sleeping arrangements

f.   Common parental concerns

(1)   Initial weight loss, appearance of infant (cephalohematoma, molding); normalcy of infant

(2)   Rashes, skin markings—telangiectasis, cafe-au-lait, hemangiomas

(3)   Infant's habits—feeding, stooling, sleeping, development, normal crying

(4)   Female infant—breast engorgement, vaginal discharge

g.   Objective data

(1)   Verify identification of mother, infant

(2) Parent/infant interaction—eye contact; holding; response to crying, vocalization

(3) Behavioral—consolability, self-quieting

(4) Physical examination (see Newborn Examination under Special Examinations in this chapter)

h. Plan of care

(1) Reinforce infant care; cord care; circumcision care; instructions on when to seek medical advice

(2) Emphasize individual variability of infant temperament noting positive aspects and challenges

(3) Breast-feeding mothers

    (a) Quiet alert state optimal time for nursing

    (b) Initial feedings 3 to 5 minutes/each breast every $1\frac{1}{2}$ to 2 hours; increase time as tolerated

    (c) Supplemental formula unnecessary

    (d) Colostrum present first 2 to 4 days

    (e) Increase maternal fluid intake especially at 6 weeks and 3 months during infant growth spurts

    (f) Adequate infant intake indicated by 6 or more voids/day

    (g) Vitamins unnecessary unless at risk for nutritional deficiencies, e.g. inadequate sunlight as vitamin D source

(4) Bottle-feeding mothers

    (a) Alleviate guilt if it exists for not breast-feeding

    (b) Amount and frequency varies

        (1) 0 to 1 month—2 to 4 oz. every 3 to 4 hours

        (2) 2 to 4 months—5 to 7 oz. every 4 to 5 hours

    (c) Inform them that iron-fortified formulas are best

    (d) Suggest partial hydrolysate formula if infant at risk for atopic disease, e.g., strong family history of atopic disease

(5) Crying—infant's first way of communicating needs

    (a) Less than 2 hours/day during first month; peaks at 6 weeks

    (b) Decreases as infant learns other ways to communicate

(6) Colic—excessive crying in otherwise healthy infants beginning at 2 to 3 weeks; may last 3 to 4 months

    (a) Rule out physical problems

      (b)   Assess for over/under feeding

      (c)   Acknowledge stressful situation; encourage breaks from infant if possible; reassure that it usually subsides by 3 to 4 months

      (d)   Avoid sudden and overstimulation of infant

      (e)   If nursing, eliminate possible offending sources from maternal diet, e.g., coffee, spices, chocolate, milk, gas-forming foods

      (f)   Soothing techniques—rocking, walking, background "white noise," car rides

      (g)   Antiflatulent if indicated by history and examination

  (7) Sleep patterns

      (a)   Usually sleeps 8 hours by 3 months

      (b)   Early introduction of solids—doesn't cause infants to sleep through the night

      (c)   Position on side or supine as SIDS preventive measure unless medically contraindicated

  (8) Bowel movements

      (a)   Usually after feeding (especially if breast fed); normal variation may be up to one/week

      (b)   Avoid laxatives; use stool softener if constipated

  (9) Reminder to schedule office visit for 2 weeks-of-age

- Interim Visits—2 Weeks to 1 Year (2 weeks; 2, 4, 6, 9 & 12 months)

  1. Subjective information

    a. Feeding—type, amounts, time at breast, name of formula

    b. Elimination—frequency, color, consistency of stools; number of saturated diapers per day

    c. Sleep

    d. Development, including behavior and temperament

    e. Concerns of parent, caregiver

    f. Interval history—health since last visit; emergency care; illnesses, medications used

  2. Objective data

    a. Age, height, weight, head circumference percentiles; vital signs

    b. Caregiver/infant interaction

    c. Vision and hearing screening

    d. Physical examination

e. Developmental screening—Denver II or equivalent and results

f. Laboratory

(1) Bilirubin, if indicated

(2) Urinalysis at 6 months unless indicated otherwise

(3) Hematocrit between 6 and 9 months or if indicated otherwise

(4) Blood lead level between 9 to 12 months or sooner if indicated

3. Plan of care, including health promotion strategies and anticipatory guidance

a. Administer immunizations as indicated after obtaining consent and assessing response to previous immunizations—contact Centers for Disease Control and Prevention and the American Academy of Pediatrics for updated recommended childhood and adolescent schedules

(1) Inform parents of common side effects of immunizations; there is a website designed and maintained by the Center for Disease Control (CDC) regarding the National Immunization Program (NIP) that has the most up to date information about immunization and possible side effects (Http:/www.cdc.gov/nip)

(2) The National Childhood Vaccine Injury Act of 1986 requires all health providers who administer vaccines to report occurrences of certain adverse events stipulated in the Act—the Vaccine Adverse Event Reporting System (VAERS) website has the most up-to-date listing of reportable events and the associated time intervals from vaccine administration (http://www.vaers.org/reportable.htm). Additionally, providers may report adverse effects online using this website

b. Inform parents of any medications prescribed, including name, rationale, dosage, frequency, course and potential side effects

c. Implement health promotion strategies and anticipatory guidance appropriate for age and developmental level (ideally should be done before or at the very beginning of a developmental stage or problem); best to focus on one or two per visit with input from the parent or caregiver

4. Anticipatory guidance—nutrition and feeding

a. Nutritional requirements are 110 to 120 calories/kg/day

b. Consumption of more than 32 oz of formula per day usually indicative of need for solids once an infant is at least 4 months of age

c. Formula recommended up to 1 year of age; whole milk until two years of age

d. Judicious use of juices—some fortified with vitamin C; best to place in cup versus bottle

e. Best to avoid giving infants a bottle in bed, especially containing formula or juice (leads to dental caries)

f. Introduction of solids

(1) Usually best to delay introduction of solids until 6 months of age—earlier introduction may lead to overfeeding and allergies

(2) Cereal usually first food added to diet followed by vegetables, fruits and meats

(3) Add only 1 new food every 3 to 5 days

(4) Do not give common allergenic foods until one year of age, e.g. cow's milk, egg whites, wheat, citrus fruits

(5) Avoid the following until 3 years of age to prevent choking—nuts, potato chips, popcorn, raw celery and carrots; hotdogs; fish with bones; tough meat; small, hard candies

g. Introduction of cup—when infant loses interest in bottle (7 to 10 months); spout cup may be used initially

h. Weaning (breast or bottle)—gradually decrease number of feedings over several weeks; night feeding usually last to be eliminated

5. Anticipatory guidance—sleep

a. 2 to 4 month old infant—8 to 12 hours at night; 2 to 3 naps

b. 6 to 12 month old infant—11 to 12 hours at night; 2 to 3 naps

c. Side-lying or supine sleep position through 6 months

d. Strategies for parents

(1) Put infant in crib when drowsy rather than asleep

(2) Quiet, non-stimulating night feedings

(3) Night waking once night feedings stop—briefly stroke infant lightly; don't pick infant up

(4) Avoid pattern of placing infant in parent's bed

6. Anticipatory guidance—infant stimulation

a. Provide variety of age-appropriate stimulation

b. Formal infant stimulation programs for infants at risk for developmental delays

7. Anticipatory guidance—teeth

a. Eruption typically begins at approximately 6 months of age

b. Signs and symptoms—local sensitivity and inflammation; increased drooling, biting, irritability

c. No evidence that teething causes fever, diarrhea, or other systemic illnesses

d. Comfort measures—hard rubber teething toy, chilled teething ring; wet wash cloth; avoid liquid filled teething rings

8. Stranger/anxiety—emerging awareness and preference for mother/ primary caregiver; early indicator of healthy attachment process emerging around 6 months

9. Separation anxiety—emerging awareness that infant is an individual distinct from primary attachment figure/caregiver

    a. Develops around 9 months; peaks at around 18 months

    b. Suggestions for parents

        (1) Recognize that bedtime, going to daycare, having a babysitter at home are all separations

        (2) Gradually introduce child to new situations and caretakers

        (3) The child learns to accept separation through multiple, brief separations and reunions

        (4) Games such as "peek-a-boo" and "hide-and-seek" may be helpful

10. Safety—prevention of ingestion/aspiration of foreign objects

    a. Keep pins, buttons, and other small objects off the floor and out of reach

    b. Do not feed infants hard foods (e.g., nuts, hard candies)

    c. Discard broken or cracked rattles with beads

    d. Do not give infant balloons

    e. Do not prop infant's bottle

    f. Select pacifier with shield too large to enter infant's mouth

    g. Learn emergency procedure for dealing effectively with choking

11. Injury prevention

    a. Keep electrical wires out of reach; outlets covered; cabinet safety locks; medicines, poisons out of reach

    b. Install smoke detectors in household

    c. Keep syrup of ipecac readily available in case of accidental poisoning; Poison Control telephone number available, other emergency phone numbers

    d. Use car seat appropriate for infant's weight and age

    e. Avoid walkers and stairs; use gate to barricade doorways and unsafe areas, e.g., kitchen and bathroom

    f. Do not place necklaces or pacifier cords around infant's neck

    g. Discourage infant jewelry

    h. Position crib or playpen away from window blind or curtain cords

    i. Use a crib with side rails spaced no more than $2\frac{3}{8}$ inches apart

    j. Secure infant with belt on changing table

      k. Lower crib mattress when infant begins to stand

12. Water safety—prevention of drowning and burns

      a. Set hot water heater temperature at 120° F or less

      b. Do not leave infant unattended in bathtub

      c. Do not allow child to play in water unattended, e.g., toilet bowls, sinks, buckets of water

      d. Use of safety devices around swimming pools, lakes and in boats, e.g., life jackets

      e. Lock fences around swimming pools

      f. Continuous supervision around water

      g. Do not leave other children in charge of infants around any body of water

13. Sun safety and sunburn protection—use lotion with sun protective factor (SPF) of at least 15; avoid use around eyes; use caps with sun visors or bonnets to protect eyes; keep infants in shaded areas, even with sunscreen; sun avoidance for infants < 6 months

14. Alternative child care arrangements—babysitters and day care; appropriate supervision and stimulation/activities (language, visual and motor)

15. Emphasize positive qualities of the infant and the parent-child relationship and mutually agree upon a plan with the parent to strengthen needed areas

16. Make referrals to other nurse practitioners, physicians, clinics and community resources as needed

17. Schedule for next visit

- Interim Visits—Toddler (1 to 3 years) (12, 15, 18, & 24 months)

1. Subjective data—nutrition/appetite; elimination; sleep; development; parental concerns; health since last visit

2. Objective Data

      a. Assess parent-child interaction and parenting style

      b. Height, weight; head circumference (up to 2 years)

      c. Vision and hearing screening

      d. Physical examination

      e. Developmental screening—Denver II or equivalent and results

      f. Laboratory

          (1) Hematocrit at 2 years or if otherwise indicated

          (2) Urinalysis at 2 years of age or if otherwise indicated

(3) Lead screening by 2 years of age as appropriate based on well-child surveillance of risk (CDC) (See Hematological/Oncological/Immunologic Disorders: Infancy through Adolescence chapter)

- Management

   a. Update immunizations—contact Centers for Disease Control and Prevention and the American Academy of Pediatrics for updated recommended childhood and adolescent schedules; inform parents of common side-effects of immunizations

   b. Advise parents of any medications prescribed, including vitamins and fluoride, e.g., name, rationale, dosage, frequency, course and potential side effects

   c. Nutrition appropriate for age

      (1) Nutritional requirements are 102 cal/kg

      (2) Provide foods from the five major food groups in realistic amounts; $\frac{1}{4}$ to $\frac{1}{3}$ of adult portion or one measuring tablespoon for each year of the child's age

      (3) Physiological anorexia is common between 15 and 18 months of age

      (4) Parental concerns regarding nutrition—decreased appetite; food jags; rituals; variable intake; definite likes and dislikes

      (5) Potential nutritional problems—iron deficiency anemia (especially if toddler is drinking more than 32 oz of milk per day); low intake of calcium, vitamin A, zinc, ascorbic acid; obesity

      (6) Provide regular meals and snacks

      (7) Avoid food battles

   d. Toilet Training

      (1) Most children are psychologically and physiologically ready between 18 to 30 months

      (2) Majority of children achieve daytime bowel and bladder training simultaneously; average age is 28 months

      (3) Nighttime control generally occurs about 1 year after daytime control is achieved

      (4) Toilet training should not be started when family is unduly stressed (e.g., new baby, moving, holidays, divorce)

      (5) Suggestions for parents—praise all efforts; expect accidents to happen; don't punish; if child is resistant, try again in a few weeks; follow usual pattern of elimination; limit time on potty to 5 to 10 minutes

   e. Sleep

      (1) One to 3 year olds usually sleep 10 to 12 hours at night and take 1 to 2 naps

(2) Toddlers need rituals and consistency at bedtime as well as security objects, e.g., blanket, special toy

(3) Nightmares start at approximately 3 years; child generally wakens and remembers dream

(4) Night terrors generally occur between 2 to 4 years; child does not waken

(5) Tips for parents—quietly reassure child; let child fall asleep in own bed

f. Negativism

   (1) Normal behaviors in toddlers as they strive to develop sense of autonomy

   (2) Expressed as "no," temper tantrums, breathholding

   (3) Tips for parents

      (a) Give child as much control as possible (e.g, offer choice of two acceptable objects or actions); allow independence when possible

      (b) Ignore temper tantrums, however expect a "response burst" initially when ignored

g. Sibling rivalry

   (1) Can occur throughout childhood; is often most troublesome just after birth of new baby if older sibling is under 2 years

   (2) Tips for parents

      (a) Involve children in preparation for new baby

      (b) Praise "big-kid" behaviors; ignore regression

      (c) Provide special time for each child every day

      (d) Stay out of minor sibling conflicts, but discipline if aggression occurs

      (e) Foster individual interests of each child and avoid comparing children

h. Thumb Sucking—peaks between 18 to 21 months; ignore before age 4 unless child is not thriving

i. Safety—apply recommendations given earlier that are appropriate for toddlers, plus

   (1) Emphasize street safety—begin teaching the basic rules of pedestrian and traffic safety

   (2) Avoid strangers; teach child methods to avoid encounters with strangers which can be harmful

   (3) Continued use of car seats according to weight—all toddlers should ride

forward-facing and upright (studies show safest place for the child is middle of back seat)

    (4) Keep medicine and poisons out of reach in locked cabinets—highest incidence of poisoning occurs in 2-year-olds

    (5) Use of helmets with any type of bicycle use, either as a passenger or alone

    (6) Enroll child in swimming lessons and always supervise when in or around water

j. Dental care—use of toothbrush; first dental visit recommended at approximately 3 years of age

k. Parenting and Discipline

    (1) Use limit setting and time-out for inappropriate behavior—1 minute of time-out for each year of age

    (2) Praise good behavior

    (3) Emphasize consistency especially between parents

    (4) Spend time with child; read to child on a daily basis

    (5) Parents set example as role models

    (6) Assign chores appropriate for age, e.g., put toys away

    (7) Begin socialization with other children

l. Television

    (1) Limit television viewing to appropriate children's programs

    (2) Limit time spent watching TV

    (3) Strong correlation between viewing aggression-type programs and child's level of aggressive play

    (4) TV fosters negative outcomes—rapid paced, superficial problem-solving; obesity

    (5) Watch TV with child and provide reality base; opportunity to discuss values, and stereotypes

    (6) Set good example through parenteral TV habits

m. Child care arrangements—day care; head start programs; nursery school; preschool programs; babysitters

n. Emphasize positive qualities of the child and the parent-child relationship and mutually agree upon a plan with the parent to strengthen needed areas

o. Make referrals to other nurse practitioners, physicians, clinics and community resources as needed

p. Schedule for next visit

- Interim Visits For Preschool Child (Ages 3, 4 & 5 years)

    1. Subjective information—nutrition/appetite; elimination; sleep; development, including behavior and temperament; caregiver concerns; interim health since last visit including stressful life changes, e.g., move, divorce

    2. Objective Data

        a. Assess parent-child interaction and parenting style

        b. Height, weight and blood pressure (starting at age 3 years)

        c. Vision and hearing screening

        d. Physical examination

        e. Developmental screening—Denver II or equivalent and results

        f. Laboratory

            (1) Mantoux test for TB screening between 4 and 6 years of age if at risk

            (2) Cholesterol screening if indicated

    3. Management

        a. Immunizations—contact Centers for Disease Control and Prevention and the American Academy of Pediatrics for updated recommended childhood and adolescent schedules; review status and update as indicated; inform parents of common side-effects of immunizations

        b. Advise parents of any medications prescribed, including vitamins and fluoride, e.g., name, rationale, dosage frequency and potential side effects

        c. Nutrition appropriate for age

            (1) Nutritional requirements are 90 cal/kg

            (2) Provide foods from the five major food groups in realistic amounts

            (3) Provide nutritious snacks during television viewing (e.g., fruits, vegetables) instead of high-fat foods (e.g., potato chips, cookies)

            (4) Potential nutritional problems (same as in the toddler years)

        d. Elimination—expect occasional night-time accidents until 4 years of age; do not punish or embarrass child

        e. Sleep

            (1) The 3 to 5-year-old child usually sleeps 8 to 12 hours per night and gradually eliminates naps

            (2) Prepare parents for an increase in nightmares

        f. Development

(1) Discuss the change from the pleasing 3-year-old to the sometimes aggressive, frustrating behavior of the 4-year-old; provide reassurance that "calmness" usually begins at age 5 years

(2) Emphasize the "magical thinking" of the preschool child and how it places the child at risk for accidental injury and an increase in fears

(3) Discuss the child's rigid superego and how children this age feel guilty for negative events

(4) Inform parents that they can expect "tall tales," the use of "toilet talk" and the construction of imaginary playmates

(5) Discuss need for peer companionship and school readiness

g. Sex education—begins in infancy and toddlerhood when parents label the genitals and accept genital exploration and masturbation as normal activities

(1) Preschool children are curious about gender differences and "how babies are made," their questions should be answered briefly and accurately

(2) Explore parents' feelings about masturbation and prepare for a possible increase in this behavior

(3) Talk with child about "good touch" and "bad touch"; encourage parents to re-enforce prevention

h. Dental care

(1) Brush teeth after each meal if possible and at bedtime

(2) Recommend first dental visit if not previously done

(3) If thumbsucking is persistent at age 4, have dental evaluation to rule out malocclusion; speech evaluation if tongue thrust is suspected

i. Safety—apply recommendations given earlier that are appropriate for preschool children, plus

(1) Reinforce pedestrian safety—children ages 3 to 7 years are more frequently involved in pedestrian-related motor vehicle accidents

(2) Teach guidelines for bicycle safety; avoid busy streets

(3) Devise fire escape plan and teach the child; conduct routine fire drills

(4) Teach child to roll and to smother clothing if it catches on fire

(5) Teach safety—the danger of matches, open flames

(6) Always supervise child when swimming or near any water

(7) Frequently check playground equipment for stability, loose nuts and bolts, and suitable landing surface

(8) Keep child away from power equipment, including lawn mowers

(9) Never clean or handle a gun in the presence of the child

(10) Discard old refrigerators and other large appliances or remove all doors during storage to avoid entrapment during play or exploration

(11) Do not allow chewing gum or eating while running or jumping

j. Exercise—encourage frequent periods of outdoor activities and limit television viewing

k. Emphasize positive qualities of the child and the parent-child relationship and mutually agree upon a plan with the parent to strengthen needed areas

l. Make referrals to other nurse practitioners, physicians, clinics and community resources as needed

m. Schedule for next visit

● Interim Visits: School-age Children—annual visit (6 to 12 years)

1. Subjective Data

a. Nutrition/appetite

b. Elimination—especially constipation and enuresis

c. Sleep

d. Development—include school, activities, exercise, friends, behavior and family relationships

e. Allergies and reactions

f. Medications

g. Drug, alcohol, cigarette and caffeine usage (for older school-age child)

h. Concerns of child and caregiver; current/recent stressors, e.g., move, divorce

i. Interim health since last visit (include review of systems); for older school-age children, obtain sexual/reproductive history as indicated

2. Objective

a. Assess parent-child interaction and child behavior

b. Height and weight, including percentiles

c. Vital signs, including blood pressure

d. Vision and hearing screening

e. Physical examination, including assessment for scoliosis and Tanner staging

f. Laboratory

(1) Mantoux test for TB screening of high-risk child if not performed in the pre-school period

(2) Hematocrit at 8 years of age

(3) Urinalysis at 8 years of age; cholesterol, if indicated

        (4)   Cholesterol if indicated

3. Management

   a.   Immunizations—review status and update as indicated—contact Centers for Disease Control and Prevention and the American Academy of Pediatrics for updated recommended childhood and adolescent schedules; inform parents of common side-effects

   b.   Advise parents of any medications prescribed, including vitamins and fluoride, e.g., on name, rationale, dosage, frequency and potential side effects

   c.   Nutrition

        (1)   Nutritional requirements are approximately 70 cal/kg

        (2)   Most behavioral problems with food resolved

        (3)   Potential nutritional problems—obesity, iron deficiency

        (4)   Encourage good nutritional practices (e.g., balanced meals, nutritious snacks, no meal skipping)

   d.   Development characteristics and behaviors

        (1)   Ages 6 to 7—nervous mannerisms; restless activity; egocentric thinking; rigid superego

        (2)   Ages 8 to 10—takes on idols and heros; friends serve as allies against adults; less rigid superego

        (3)   Ages 10 to 12—increased self-awareness and self-consciousness; body image concerns; mood swings, stormy behavior; need for independence

        (4)   Inform parents that use of dirty words may occur

        (5)   Prepare for pubertal changes and menstruation in girls

        (6)   Discuss with parents the importance of and strategies for bolstering the child's self-esteem

   e.   Good health habits—assist child and parents to establish early patterns of behavior, e.g., regular exercise, sufficient sleep, regular dental care, avoidance of drugs, alcohol, tobacco

   f.   Communication—encourage parents to assist child in developing good communication skills, problem-solving strategies and stress management

   g.   Drugs, smoking and alcohol—encourage parent/child discussions

   h.   Sex education—anatomy and physiology; sexual activity; values clarification; decision making; contraception; prevention of STDs and AIDS

   i   Parenting strategies

        (1)   Although the child is maturing, quality time, attention and affection from parents is important (evidence exists supporting "connectedness" to parents and/or another adult decreases risk-taking behaviors)

    (2)   Encourage independence and decision-making

    (3)   Promote responsibility and accountability by assigning appropriate chores

    (4)   Maintain adequate supervision

    (5)   Discuss methods of discipline; use positive re-enforcement and appropriate consequences for inappropriate behavior

    (6)   Establish fair rules

    (7)   Respect the child's need for privacy

    (8)   Set example by being a good role model

    (9)   Provide child with an allowance

    (10)   Select movies and TV programming and video games that are appropriate for child's developmental level

    (11)   Praise child for achievements

    (12)   Encourage school attendance

    (13)   Refer parents to resources that can assist them in building assets and preventing psychosocial morbidities (see Melnyk et al., 2003, for KySS (Keep yourself/your children Safe and Secure) Campaign Strategic Plan, a national effort by the National Association of Pediatric Nurse Practitioners (NAPNAP to decrease emotional and behavioral problems in children and adolescents).

  j. Safety

    (1)   Bicycle, skateboarding, rollerblading; use of helmets and protection padding

    (2)   Seat belt use

    (3)   Prevention of sexual abuse, e.g., inappropriate touching; what to do if it occurs

    (4)   Water safety; swimming

    (5)   Fire prevention safety; home fire drill; proper use of appliances

    (6)   Sunburn prevention

    (7)   Prevention of violence in home; lock up guns, ammunition; teach child gun safety

    (8)   Pedestrian safety

  k. Lying and cheating (common in school-age children)

    (1)   School-age children lie to avoid trouble or gain an advantage

(2) Appropriate response—confront child in a positive way; try to understand reason for lie; follow through with age-appropriate discipline when needed

(3) Adults should model honesty

l. Sports

(1) For 6 to 8-year-olds, sports participation should be noncompetitive and focused on learning rules, teamwork and having fun

(2) Older school-aged children and teenagers should have a pre-participation physical examination

m. Emphasize positive qualities of the child and the parent-child relationship and mutually agree upon a plan with the parent to strengthen needed areas

n. Make referrals as needed

o. Schedule for next visit

- Interim Visits: Adolescent—annual visit (13 to 18 Years)

1. Subjective information—gather "sensitive" information when alone with the adolescent

a. Nutrition—especially appetite; meal-skipping

b. Elimination—especially use of aids such as laxatives, diuretics

c. Sleep practices

d. Development—special emphasis on assessment of mental and emotional health (including school performance and attendance; self-esteem, friends and relationships; family functioning and "connectedness"; hobbies; activities; work; stress and anger management; coping skills; risk-taking behaviors, such as driving while drinking and use of weapons; violent or aggressive behavior; ideations about hurting self or others)

e. Allergies

f. Medications

g. Drug, alcohol, cigarette, and caffeine consumption

h. Sexual activities, reproductive issues

i. Concerns/worries; current and recent stressors

j. Interim health since last visit—include review of systems, with special emphasis on gathering psychological and sexual/reproductive data

k. Specific questions when alone with parent

(1) Family communication patterns and relationship with the adolescent

(2) Parent's description of the adolescent's strong and weak points, attitudes, and behaviors

      (3) Discipline practices and response

      (4) Specific concerns and worries about the adolescent

2. Objective data

    a. Observation of parent-adolescent interaction (e.g., parental support of adolescent; does the parent allow the adolescent to answer questions)

    b. Height and weight; percentiles

    c. Vital signs, including blood pressure

    d. Vision and hearing screening

    e. Physical examination—including scoliosis screen, Tanner stage, and breast examination; pelvic examination if adolescent female is sexually active, having irregular menses, or is more than 16 years of age

    f. Laboratory

      (1) Urinalysis

      (2) Hematocrit

      (3) VDRL, GC, Chlamydia and HIV if sexually active or history of sexual abuse

      (4) Pap smear if pelvic examination performed

      (5) Liver function tests (if history of drug usage); cholesterol, if indicated

3. Management

    a. Update immunizations—contact Centers for Disease Control and Prevention and the American Academy of Pediatrics for updated recommended childhood and adolescent schedules; Hepatitis B vaccine series should be encouraged for all adolescents who may not have received the immunization in their earlier childhood years, especially sexually active adolescents or those who are using IV drugs; provide information on common side effects

    b. Advise regarding any medications prescribed, e.g., include name, rationale, dosage, frequency, course and potential side effects

    c. Nutrition appropriate for age

      (1) The adolescent diet should be similar to an active adult with extra calories during rapid growth periods; prudent consumption of high fat foods, e.g., red meats, butter, and eggs

      (2) Nutritional issues—irregular meals, chaotic lifestyle; increase in meals eaten away from home; increase in snacks; skipping of meals; fad diets; vegetarianism

      (3) Potential nutritional problems—increased need for calcium, iron, zinc; eating disorders; obesity

      (4) Encourage well-balanced meals and nutritious snacks

    (5)   Discuss adolescent's perception of his/her weight

    (6)   Encourage healthy weight loss strategies if indicated, e.g., decreasing fat intake; increasing exercise

d. Safety—same as school age child, plus

    (1)   Emphasize the possible consequences of drinking and use of drugs while driving

    (2)   Discourage being a passenger when the driver has been drinking or using drugs

    (3)   Discuss typical high-risk situations and how to avoid them; role play healthy behaviors to use in high-risk situations

    (4)   Encourage safe swimming and diving practices

    (5)   Discuss proper use of safe sports equipment and maintenance

    (6)   Instruct adolescent in proper training and warm-up exercises for sports and physical activities

    (7)   Educate regarding safe and proper use of firearms and other potentially dangerous objects such as firecrackers

    (8)   Discuss use and misuse of over-the-counter medications

e. Developmental Issues

    (1)   Discuss dating and peer pressure

    (2)   Encourage open communication with parents, peers, and school personnel

    (3)   Teach stress reduction techniques and coping skills

    (4)   Educate regarding healthy outlets for anger

    (5)   Discuss plans for the future—further education; work; recreation; hobbies; marriage; parenthood

    (6)   Educate regarding acne—e.g., cause, myths and proper skin care

f. Discuss issues related to sexuality—decision making; mature relationships; assertiveness; safe sex/prevention of STDs, including HIV; pregnancy and contraception; implications of potential parenthood; ''normalcy'' of occasional masturbation

g. Encourage good health habits—e.g., regular exercise; sufficient sleep, regular dental care

h. Continue education regarding use of drugs, alcohol, cigarettes, and caffeine

i. Inform parents of major developmental characteristics of adolescents

    (1)   Increased self-awareness, self-consciousness and self-appraisal

    (2)   Body image concerns

  (3) Mood swings and stormy behavior

  (4) Need for independence

  (5) Using peer values as criteria with which to judge own values, but still needing family to provide acceptance and feeling of self-worth

  (6) Interest in opposite sex

 j. Parenting strategies with adolescents

  (1) Fairness in rules and reasonable limit setting

  (2) Allow decision making

  (3) Respect adolescent's privacy

  (4) Expect periods of estrangement (be available; adolescent needs supportive family)

  (5) Praise achievements at home, school, extracurricular activities

  (6) Bolster self-esteem

  (7) Supervision as needed

  (8) Encourage independence, new experiences, after-school activities, including part-time job

  (9) Promote family communication

  (10) Serve as role model—practice good health habits, e.g., parents should not smoke if they do not want child to imitate their behavior

  (11) Recognize signs of probable substance abuse—drop in school performance; personality change; mood swings; sleepiness or fatigue; depression

 k. Emphasize positive qualities of the adolescent and the parent-adolescent relationship and mutually agree upon a plan to strengthen needed areas

 l. Make referrals as needed

 m. Refer parents to resources that can assist them in building their teen's assets as well as with their parenting skills (Melnyk et al., in press)

 n. Schedule for next visit

Questions
Select the best answer

1. Sixteen-year-old Sarah makes the following statements to you during a health visit. Which of the following pieces of information should not be kept confidential?

   a. "I have been sexually active with three of my boyfriends."
   b. "I sometimes smoke marijuana."
   c. "I want to get pregnant."
   d. "Sometimes I feel like ending my life."

2. In performing a physical examination on a nine-month-old infant, which of the following developmental fears would not be appropriate for you to consider?

   a. Stranger anxiety
   b. Pain
   c. Separation from parents
   d. Bodily harm

3. When performing a physical examination on a toddler, which of the following body parts would you examine last?

   a. Heart and lungs
   b. Abdomen and genitals
   c. Ears and throat
   d. Hips and extremities

4. Role play with equipment during the course of a physical examination would be most beneficial with which of the following age groups?

   a. Toddlers
   b. Preschoolers
   c. Young school-age children
   d. Older school-age children

5. Providing reassurance of "normalcy" during the course of an examination would be most important for:

   a. Preschool children
   b. Young school-age children
   c. Older school-age children
   d. Adolescents

6. Which of the following would not elevate the pulse of a child?

   a. Fever
   b. Anemia
   c. Hypothyroidism
   d. Exercise

7. Which of the following sounds should be considered the diastolic blood pressure in children under 13 years of age?

   a. The muffling sound (Korotkoff IV)
   b. The disappearance of sound (Korotkoff V)
   c. Korotkoff sound I
   d. Korotkoff sound II

8. Blood pressure should be measured at well child visits, beginning at age:

   a. 2 years
   b. 3 years
   c. 4 years
   d. 5 years

9. A wide pulse pressure that results from a high systolic blood pressure is usually not due to which of the following?

   a. Fever
   b. Exercise
   c. Excitement
   d. A patent ductus arteriosus

10. Head and chest circumferences should be equal at:

   a. 6 months of age
   b. 1 year of age
   c. 2 years of age
   d. 3 years of age

11. The anterior fontanel usually closes by:

   a. 2 months of age
   b. 6 months of age
   c. 18 months of age
   d. 24 months of age

12. Diffuse edema of the soft tissue of the scalp which usually crosses suture lines in the newborn is:

   a. Bossing
   b. Caput succedaneum
   c. Cephalohematoma
   d. Macrocephaly

13. An infant should no longer have a head lag when pulled from the supine to sitting position at what age?

   a. 2 months
   b. 4 months

c. 6 months

d. 9 months

14. "Boggy" nasal mucous membranes with serous drainage upon examination usually suggests:

    a. Sinusitis

    b. Polyps

    c. URI

    d. Allergic rhinitis

15. A white instead of red reflex upon eye examination of a 1-year-old child would suggest:

    a. An accommodative error

    b. Retinoblastoma

    c. Papilledema

    d. Retinal detachment

16. A cobblestone appearance of the palpebral conjunctiva usually indicates:

    a. Bacterial infection

    b. Chemical irritation

    c. Viral infection

    d. Severe allergy

17. An eye that deviates in when covered but returns to midline when uncovered is an:

    a. Esophoria

    b. Exophoria

    c. Esotropia

    d. Exotropia

18. Pain produced by manipulation of the auricle or pressure on the tragus suggests:

    a. Acute otitis media

    b. Otitis externa

    c. Otitis media with effusion

    d. Mastoiditis

19. A hypernasal voice and snoring in a child is suggestive of:

    a. Polyps of the larynx

    b. Nasopharyngeal tumor

    c. Hypertrophied adenoids

    d. Cleft palate

20. Physiological splitting of the second heart sound during inspiration in a child:

    a. Is normal

    b. Should be evaluated with an EKG

    c. Suggests an ASD

    d. Should be referred to a cardiologist

21. Which of the following is not characteristics of innocent heart murmurs in children?

    a. Systolic in timing

    b. Varies in loudness with positioning

    c. Usually transmitted to the neck

    d. Usually loudest at lower left sternal border or at second or third intercostal space

22. A Grade II musical or vibratory murmur heard best at the lower left sternal border that changes with positioning is suggestive of a:

    a. Pulmonary ejection murmur

    b. Ventricular septal defect

    c. Venous hum

    d. Vibratory or Still's murmur

23. Wheezing in a child may not be found in which of the following conditions?

    a. Asthma

    b. Bronchiolitis

    c. Pleural friction rub

    d. Cystic fibrosis

24. Gynecomastia in a male may not be a finding in which of the following?

    a. Normal pubertal development

    b. Steroid usage

    c. Hyperthyroidism

    d. Testicular tumor

25. Which of the following would usually not be considered a sign of a pituitary tumor in an adolescent female?

    a. Dysfunctional uterine bleeding

    b. Galactorrhea

    c. Loss of peripheral vision

    d. Increase in headaches

26. Which of the following is not a specific examination test for a dislocated hip?

    a. Barlow's test

    b. Ortolani's test

    c. Trendelenburg test

    d. Gower's test

27. In addition to the knee, which of the following should be examined in a child complaining of knee pain?

    a. Foot
    b. Ankle
    c. Hip
    d. Spine

28. Which of the following infant reflexes should not disappear by 6 months of age?

    a. Moro
    b. Rooting
    c. Tonic neck
    d. Plantar grasp

29. Spasticity in an infant may be an early sign of:

    a. Neurofibromatosis
    b. Hydrocephalus
    c. Cerebral palsy
    d. Muscular dystrophy

30. A shift to the left is present when which of the following are elevated?

    a. Neutrophils
    b. Bands or stabs
    c. Lymphocytes
    d. Eosinophils

31. Which of the following is usually elevated with viral infections?

    a. Neutrophils
    b. Eosinophils
    c. Lymphocytes
    d. Basophils

32. Decreased platelets may not be found in which of the following?

    a. Leukemia
    b. Anemia
    c. ITP
    d. Medication usage (e.g., ampicillin, cephalothin)

33. Which of the following does not suggest a urinary tract infection?

    a. Increased protein
    b. Increased WBCs
    c. Increased RBCs
    d. Increased nitrites

34. A Mantoux test in a child with no risk factors is considered positive with a reaction of:

    a. At least 5 mm induration
    b. At least 8 mm induration
    c. At least 10 mm induration
    d. At least 15 mm induration

35. Children should receive TB testing at which of the following ages if low risk but is living in a high prevalence neighborhood?

    a. 4 and 14 years of age
    b. 1, 2, 4, and 10 years of age
    c. 1, 4, 10 and 18 years of age
    d. 4, 10 and 14 years of age

36. Cholesterol screening should be done:

    a. Once for all children at 3 years of age
    b. Once for all children at 6 years of age
    c. Once for children whose parents have a total cholesterol level of 200mg/ dL or greater
    d. Only for children with a family history of premature cardiovascular disease

37. For which of the following screening tests should children fast for 12 hours before the test is done?

    a. Total cholesterol
    b. Serum chemistry profile
    c. Serum lipid profile
    d. Hematocrit

38. Which of the following is the most important history-taking question for a sports evaluation?

    a. Has the child ever had a head injury?
    b. Has the child ever fainted or lost consciousness during exercise?
    c. Does the child ever get short of breath with exercise?
    d. Has the child ever had prior surgeries?

39. Which of the following conditions would not exclude a child from participating in contact collision sports?

    a. Hepatosplenomegaly
    b. Absence of a paired organ
    c. Atlantoaxial instability
    d. Prior head injury

40. Which of the following topics would not be appropriate to include when providing anticipatory guidance to the parent of a 4-month-old infant?

    a. Introduction of solid foods
    b. Teething

    c. Negativism

    d. Introduction of a cup

41. Which is the correct order for introduction of solid foods to an infant?

    a. Fruits, cereal, vegetables, and meats

    b. Cereal, meats, vegetables, and fruits

    c. Fruits, cereal, meats, and vegetables

    d. Cereal, vegetables, fruits, and meats

42. Which of the following topics is not appropriate to include when providing anticipatory guidance to the parent of an 18-month-old?

    a. Temper tantrums

    b. Toilet training

    c. Dental care

    d. Stranger anxiety

43. Appropriate anticipatory guidance for the parents of an 8-year-old girl should not include:

    a. Preparation for an increase in nervous mannerisms and restless activity

    b. Preparation for pubertal changes

    c. Information that friends begin to serve as allies against adults

    d. Information that their daughter will take on idols and heroes

44. Which of the following children could routinely receive the MMR vaccine?

    a. A child who has had an anaphylactic reaction to the ingestion of eggs

    b. A child whose mother is pregnant

    c. A child who is receiving chemotherapy

    d. A child with mild diarrhea

45. A pelvic examination should not be performed on which of the following adolescents?

    a. A 14-year-old who is sexually active

    b. A 15-year-old who has just started menarche

    c. A 17-year-old who is having irregular menses

    d. An 18-year-old healthy female

Answers

1. d	16. d	31. c
2. d	17. a	32. b
3. c	18. b	33. a
4. b	19. c	34. d
5. d	20. a	35. a
6. c	21. c	36. d
7. a	22. d	37. c
8. b	23. c	38. b
9. d	24. c	39. d
10. b	25. a	40. c
11. c	26. d	41. d
12. b	27. c	42. d
13. c	28. d	43. a
14. d	29. c	44. d
15. b	30. b	45. b

Bibliography

American Academy of Pediatrics (AAP) (2003). Report of the committee on infectious diseases. AAP: Committee on Infectious Diseases.

Department of Health and Human Services (DHHS) (2003). Retrieved December 29, 2003, from http://www.hhs.gov/ocr/hipaa/.

Department of Health and Human Services Center for Disease Control National Immunization Program (2003) Retrieved December 29, 2003, from http://www.cdc.gov/nip/.

Colyar, M. R. (2003). *Well-child assessment for primary care providers.* Philadelphia: F.A. Davis Company.

Fox, J. A. (Ed.) (2002). *Primary health care of infants, children, & adolescents* (2nd edition). St. Louis: Mosby.

Green, M., & Cark, E. M. (Eds.) (2001). *Bright futures: Guidelines for health supervision of infants, children and adolescents.* Georgetown University: National Center for Education in Maternal and Child Health.

Gunn, V. L., & Nechyba, C. (2002). *The Harriet Lane handbook* (16th edition). Philadelphia: Mosby.

Hoekelman, R. A. (Ed.). (2001). *Primary pediatric care.* (4th Ed.). St. Louis: Mosby-Year Book, Inc.

Jellinek, M., Patel, B. P., & Froehle, M. C. (2002). *Bright futures in practice: Mental Health.* Georgetown University: National Center for Education in Maternal and Child Health.

Melnyk, B. M., Brown, H. E., Jones, D. C., Kreipe, R., & Novak, J. (2003). Improving the mental/psychosocial health of U.S. children and adolescents: Outcomes and implementation strategies from the national KySS summit. *Journal of Pediatric Health Care* (Supplement), 17 (6), S1-S24.

Story, M., Holt, K., & Sofka, D. (2002). *Bright futures in practice: Nutrition* (2nd edition). Georgetown University: National Center for Education in Maternal and Child Health.

Vaccine Adverse Event Reporting System (2003) Retrieved December 29, 2003, from http://www.vaers.org/.

Head, Eye, Ear, Nose, Mouth and Throat Disorders

Connie Paczkowski

Head

Microcephaly

- Definition: Head circumference (HC) 2 to 3 SD or more below the mean for age and sex or HC percentiles that drop with increasing age

- Etiology/Incidence (2.5% of total population)

  1. Primary variety of dysmorphic syndromes produced by genetic/chromosomal disorders

  2. Acquired from multiple causes including

     a. Intrauterine infections, e.g., TORCH—toxoplasmosis, other agents [HIV, listeria, syphilis, gonococcus, group β streptococcus, varicella-zoster, malaria], rubella, cytomegalovirus inclusion disease, herpes simplex

     b. Fetal exposure to toxic substances including alcohol, phenylketones (maternal PKU)

     c. Fetal exposure to radiation in first and/or second trimesters

     d. Placental insufficiency, prenatal hypoxia, trauma, maternal hypoglycemia, degenerative diseases, e.g., Tay Sachs

     e. Extremely poor nutrition during the first six months of life

     f. Significant risk for isolated microcephaly—alcohol use, inadequate weight gain during pregnancy, inadequate prenatal care, African-American and low educational level (Krauss, 2003)

- Signs and Symptoms

  1. In full term birth and up to six months of age, chest circumference surpasses head circumference (unless child is very obese)

  2. Delayed developmental milestones; neurological problems, mental retardation

  3. Family history of microcephaly

- Differential Diagnosis

  1. Craniosynostosis

  2. Endocrine disorders, e.g., hypopituitary function, hypothyroidism

  3. Severe malnutrition

- Physical Findings

  1. Early closure of fontanel; prominent cranial sutures

  2. Marked downward sloped forehead with narrowed temporal diameter and occipital flattening (familial microcephaly)

  3. Skull asymmetries, high arched palate and dysplastic teeth (dysmorphic and chromosomal disorders)

- Diagnostic Tests/Findings
    1. Karyotyping for chromosomal disorders, e.g., Fragile X syndrome
    2. Antibody titers for TORCH infections
    3. Test infant serum and urine for amino and organic acids
    4. CT or MRI to detect calcification, malformations or atrophy
- Management/Treatment
    1. Complete history and physical findings crucial to finding treatable disorders, e.g., hypopituitarism, severe protein-calorie malnutrition
    2. Premature closure of sutures may be surgically corrected
    3. Most disorders are untreatable; accurate diagnosis is essential for appropriate genetic and family counseling (Behrman, 2000)
    4. Management is supportive

Macrocephaly

- Definition: Head circumference greater than 2 to 3 SD from the mean for age, sex and gestation or one that increases too rapidly
- Etiology/Incidence
    1. Most likely causes of excessive head growth include hydrocephalus, extra-axial fluid collections, metabolic/genetic disorders and neoplasms
    2. Normal head growth with large heads include:
        a. Familial macrocephaly (benign)
        b. Megalencephaly (large brain) found with neurofibromatosis
- Signs and Symptoms
    1. Excessive head growth
    2. Dependent on cause, e.g., hydrocephalus
- Differential Diagnosis
    1. Benign macrocephaly—familial or catch up growth in thriving premature infant
    2. Pathological macrocephaly
- Physical Findings
    1. Progressive excessive head growth greater than 2 to 3 SD above the mean for age/sex as delineated on growth chart
    2. Transillumination of skull may reveal chronic subdural effusions, hydrocephaly or large cystic defects
    3. May have extensive findings depending on underlying cause

- Diagnostic Tests/Findings: CT, MRI or ultrasonography of anterior fontanel (if not closed) can:

  1. Define structural cause; determine if operable disorder

  2. If benign, provide more accurate diagnosis, prognosis, guide to management and genetic counseling

  3. Provide basis of comparison if future study is necessary

- Management/Treatment

  1. CT, MRI or ultrasound of head if any signs/symptoms of increased intracranial pressure

  2. Surgical correction of premature closure of sutures

  3. Genetic counseling

Caput Succedaneum

- Definition: Diffuse swelling of soft tissue of the scalp which usually crosses suture lines with possible bruising

- Etiology/Incidence: Trauma to scalp while baby descends through birth canal causing edema of scalp, skin and muscles; associated with molding

- Signs and symptoms: Swelling of scalp with some ecchymosis involving the presenting portion of occiput during vertex delivery

- Differential Diagnosis: Cephalohematoma

- Physical Findings: Swelling and bruising of parietal region of the scalp; edema crosses suture line

- Diagnostic Tests/Findings: None

- Management/Treatment

  1. Usually unnecessary with spontaneous resolution within a few days

  2. If extensive ecchymosis, may require phototherapy for hyperbilirubinemia

Cephalohematoma

- Definition: Subperiosteal collection of blood bound by suture lines

- Etiology/Incidence

  1. Slow subperiosteal bleed from trauma due to difficult delivery

  2. Coagulopathy or intracranial hemorrhage

  3. 25% overlie linear skull fracture—not depressed

- Signs and Symptoms

  1. Presents hours to days after delivery; limited to periosteum at suture margins

  2. Occasionally prolongs neonatal jaundice

- Differential Diagnosis
  1. Caput succedaneum
  2. Cranial meningocele
- Physical Findings: Nonecchymotic swelling of parietal area that does not cross suture lines
- Diagnostic Tests: None
- Management/Treatment
  1. Usually unnecessary with resolution within a few weeks/months
  2. Calcification of hematoma possible; may be felt as bony prominence
  3. Observance for hyperbilirubinemia

Hydrocephalus

- Definition: Increased production, impaired absorption or obstruction in flow of cerebrospinal fluid (CSF), leading to dilatation of cerebral ventricles
- Etiology/Incidence
  1. Obstruction of CSF flow anywhere along its route
  2. Origin may be:
     a. Congenital, due to primary cerebral malformation
     b. Acquired postnatally, secondary to tumor, hemorrhage or infection
  3. Obstructive or noncommunicating hydrocephalus
     a. Major cause of hydrocephalus
     b. Obstruction of CSF within ventricular system before CSF reaches subarachnoid space
     c. Sites include aqueduct of Sylvius and obstruction of fourth ventricle (Arnold-Chiari and Dandy-Walker)
  4. Nonobstructive or communicating hydrocephalus
     a. Impairment of CSF within subarachnoid space
     b. Impairment of absorption
     c. Usually caused by scarring due to subarachnoid hemorrhage or meningitis
     d. Most commonly occurs over convexities
  5. Choroid plexus papilloma
     a. Overproduction of CSF
     b. Rare cause of hydrocephalus

- Signs and Symptoms: Presentation is variable depending on age and etiology

    1. Birth to 12 months—apparent large head, sluggish feeding, vomiting, piercing cry and irritability

    2. 12 months through adolescence—signs of increased intracranial pressure (ICP), headache following sleep, lethargy or irritability; confusion, personality changes; possible decline in academic performance; signs and symptoms related to specific focal lesion or tumor; possible sixth nerve palsies; chronic papilledema

- Differential Diagnosis

    1. Macrocephaly

    2. Megalencephaly

    3. Benign large head

    4. Macrocrania

    5. Meningitis

    6. Sepsis

    7. Tumor

- Physical Findings

    1. Infancy—bulging anterior fontanel, scalp vein distention, bossing, "setting sun sign", separated skull sutures, slow PERRL, hypertonia, hyper-reflexia, spasticity

    2. Childhood—strabismus, extrapyramidal tract signs (ataxia), papilledema, optic atrophy, growth failure from endocrine dysfunction

- Diagnostic Tests/Findings

    1. Cranial radiograph—separated sutures

    2. CT scan/ultrasound—impaired CSF circulation causing ventricular enlargement

    3. Ventriculography—obstruction detection

- Management/Treatment

    1. Most cases require extracranial shunts, particularly ventriculoperitoneal types (Behrman, 2000)

    2. Treatment of underlying cause, e.g., mass or lesion, inflammation, infection, vasogenic edema

    3. Anticipatory guidance for families and caregivers throughout child's life

        a. Referral to support groups

        b. Teaching signs and symptoms of ICP

        c. Daily head circumference measurements

        d. Management of psychomotor challenges

EYE

Conjunctivitis of the Newborn (Ophthalmia Neonatrum)

- Definition: Infection and/or inflammation of conjunctiva in first month of life
- Etiology/Incidence
    1. Chemical—irritation from use of silver nitrate or other ophthalmic preparations (occurs in 10% of newborns); erythromycin ophthalmic ointment commonly used in place of silver nitrate with less irritation
    2. Gonococcal—perinatal transmission of *Neisseria gonorrhoeae;* prophylactic treatment with erythromycin ophthalmic ointment 0.5%, topical silver nitrate 1%, tetracycline 1%, or povidone-iodine 2.5% (AAP, 2003)
    3. Inclusion—perinatal transmission of *Chlamydia trachomatis* during vaginal birth; occurs in 50% of infants born to infected mothers (AAP, 2003)
    4. Other pathogens after first week of life include *Haemophilus influenzae, Staphylococcus aureus,* enterococci Group B Streptococcus and herpes simplex virus (HSV)
- Signs and Symptoms
    1. Chemical—mild injection of conjunctiva, presents several hours following ophthalmic drop/ointment instillation lasting no longer than 3 to 4 days
    2. Gonococcal—acute purulent discharge 2 to 4 days after birth
    3. Chlamydia—usually presents with mild mucopurulent discharge a few days to several weeks after birth
    4. Other bacteria—purulent discharge normally seen on 5th day
    5. Virus—serous discharge
- Differential Diagnosis
    1. Dacryostenosis
    2. Foreign body
    3. Corneal abrasion
- Physical Findings
    1. Chemical—conjunctival hyperemia, minimal lid edema, scanty discharge
    2. Gonococcal—chemosis, significant lid edema; purulent discharge
    3. Chlamydia—minimal lid edema, conjunctival hyperemia, chemosis, concomitant pneumonia (afebrile, repetitive staccato cough, tachypnea and rales)
    4. Other bacteria—lid edema and chemosis
    5. Herpes simplex—possible serous discharge

- Diagnostic Tests/Findings

  1. Gram and Giemsa stain—gonococci revealed as intracellular gram negative diplococci; chlamydia is revealed as basophilic intracytoplasmic inclusions in the conjunctival epithelial cells

  2. Cultures—positive for specific organism

  3. Direct fluroscent antibody staining or enzyme immunoassay—detection of HSV antigens

  4. Immune fluorescent antibody testing for chlamydia organisms

- Management/Treatment

  1. Chemical—no treatment necessary; resolves spontaneously without sequelae; decreased incidence with use of erythromycin ophthalmic ointment in place of silver nitrate

  2. Gonococcal—hospitalization is necessary; eye should be irrigated initially with normal saline every 10 to 30 minutes gradually decreasing to every 2 hour intervals until purulent discharge is cleared; ceftriaxone 25 to 50 mg/kg/day, IV or IM not to exceed 125 mg given as a single dose; cefotaxime 100 mg/kg/day, IV or IM given as a single dose is an alternative; topical treatment alone is inadequate and unnecessary when systemic therapy is given (AAP, 2003)

  3. Chlamydia conjunctivitis and pneumonia—oral erythromycin 50 mg/kg/day in four divided doses for 10 to 14 days; oral sulfonamides may be used after immediate neonatal period for infants intolerant to erythromycin; topical treatment ineffective and unnecessary; efficacy of erythromycin therapy is 80%, second course sometimes required (AAP, 2003)

  4. Other bacteria—organism dependent; erythromycin ointment every six hours for gram positive organisms; gentamicin ophthalmic solution every six hours for gram negative organisms; moist compresses

  5. Stress thorough hand washing, no sharing of wash cloths or towels

  6. Herpes simplex—treat with 0.1% idoxuridine, 1-2% trifluridine, or 3% vidarabine topical ophthalmic preparations in addition to parenteral antiviral therapy, under ophthalmologists direction (AAP, 2003)

  7. Mothers and sexual partner(s) should also be treated appropriately

Conjunctivitis of Childhood

- Definition: Inflammation and/or infection of palpabral (lining of eye lids) and bulbar (layer of tissue over the sclera) conjunctiva in children one month or older

- Etiology/Incidence

  1. Most frequent ocular disorder in children; may be associated with otitis media indicating bacterial infection with beta-lactamase resistant organism

  2. Very contagious especially in day care and school age children

3. Bacterial conjunctivitis—most common pathogens include *Staphylococcus aureus, Haemophilus influenzae* and *Streptococcus pneumoniae* (Finberg & Kleinman, 2002; Behrman, 2000)

4. Viral conjunctivitis primarily due to adenovirus 3, 4 and 7; also caused by herpes simplex and varicella zoster

5. Allergic and vernal (chronic allergic) conjunctivitis—often with unidentified cause; commonly associated with seasonal allergens

- Signs and Symptoms
    1. Pruritus, foreign body sensation, tearing
    2. Headache
    3. Possible sensitivity to light
    4. Discharge
        a. Viral, allergic—watery or thick/stringy mucoid
        b. Bacterial—purulent

- Differential Diagnosis
    1. Nasolacrimal duct obstruction
    2. Blepharitis in older children
    3. Keratitis (can be seen with herpes simplex conjunctivitis)
    4. Systemic infection presenting with conjunctivitis, e.g. rubella, rubeola, Kawasaki
    5. Periorbital cellulitis

- Physical Findings
    1. Discharge, rhinitis
    2. Eyelid edema
    3. Moderate to severe erythema of conjunctiva; chemosis
    4. Preauricular adenopathy commonly seen with viral pathogens
    5. Malaise, pharyngitis and fever may be present
    6. Cobblestone-like papillary hypertrophy along inner aspect of upper lid (vernal conjunctivitis)

- Diagnostic Tests/Findings
    1. Cultures and sensitivities usually unnecessary unless pseudomonas, neisseria or other virulent organism suspected (Finberg & Kleinman, 2002)
    2. Rule out corneal infiltration with fluorescein stain

- Management/Treatment
    1. Bacterial—most respond readily to topical ophthalmic antibiotics, e.g., tobramycin,

erythromycin (used if gram negative bacteria suspected), sulfacetamide, polymyxin B sulfate-trimethoprim, or fluoroquinolone drops or ointment; if concomitant otitis media, also treat with oral antimicrobials

2. Viral—artificial tears for lubrication, topical steroids (only by ophthalmologist) if keratitis present

3. Herpes—initial infection self limited, virus remains latent; can recur in children with recurrent keratitis, ophthalmologist referral necessary; **any child with a history of a herpes ocular infection who presents with red eye, lid vesicles or corneal staining with fluorescein should be referred immediately;** treatment includes topical and systemic antivirals

4. Allergic—avoidance of known allergens, cold compresses, systemic or topical antihistamines, nonsteroidal anti-inflammatories or topical mast cell stabilizers (e.g., cromolyn sodium), refer to ophthalmologist for chronic conjunctivitis

5. Good hand washing and hygiene; stress control of cross contamination, avoid shared linen; cleanse eye lashes with warm sterile water wiping from inner canthus outward

6. Ophthalmologist referral needed:

   a. If conjunctivitis is unresponsive to treatment within 2 to 3 days

   b. If associated with loss of vision, pain, photophobia

   c. If severe conjunctivitis or with corneal/orbital cellulitis involvement

Dacryostenosis

- Definition: Unilateral or bilateral obstruction of the nasolacrimal duct, usually at nasal punctal opening

- Etiology/Incidence

  1. Due to failure of duct canalization during gestation

  2. May also occur secondary to trauma or infection

  3. 90% spontaneous resolution by 12 months

  4. Most common lacrimal disorder in infants

- Signs and Symptoms: Continuous or intermittent tearing (wet look in the eye) with crusting of lashes

- Differential Diagnosis

  1. Ophthalmia neonatorum, conjunctivitis

  2. Dacryocystitis—inflammation/infection of obstructed nasolacrimal duct

  3. Glaucoma

  4. Intraocular inflammation

  5. External irritation

- Physical Findings
  1. Tearing
  2. Expression of thin mucopurulent exudate from lacrimal sac
  3. Inflammation/infection of conjunctiva
  4. Signs of dacryocystitis—fever, erythema and edema of lid and/or over lacrimal sac or duct, excoriation of surrounding tissue

- Management/Treatment
  1. Gently massage lacrimal sac and nasolacrimal duct by frequently stroking skin from brow area along lateral aspect of nose
  2. For conjunctivitis or purulent discharge, administration of sodium sulfacetamide or erythromycin ointment
  3. Referral to ophthalmologist by six months of age or earlier for evaluation and treatment if no improvement with antibiotics and massage
  4. Persistent obstruction and recurrent purulent drainage beyond six to twelve months, may require surgical probing of duct, and/or silicone tube intubation; For older children balloon catheter dilation is more effective than simple probing due to stenosis of distal nasal lacrimal duct (Lueder, 2002)
  5. Severe dacryocystitis requires referral to ophthalmologist and systemic antibiotics
  6. Newborns with lacrimal sac mucoceles can experience respiratory distress and need probing with nasal endoscopy (Wagner, 2001)

Chalazion

- Definition: Obstruction of meibomian glands lining posterior margins of upper or lower lids; usually involves midportion of tarsus resulting in an inflammatory lipogranuloma
- Etiology/Incidence: Unknown cause
- Signs and Symptoms
  1. Progressive swelling of lid
  2. Slight discomfort
  3. Minimal redness
- Differential Diagnosis
  1. Blepharitis
  2. Hordeolum
  3. Sebaceous cell carcinoma (rare)
- Physical Findings
  1. Firm, nontender, nonmovable nodule often on palpebral surface of lid
  2. Large chalazions may cause chronic pressure on cornea leading to astigmatism

- Diagnostic Tests/Findings: None indicated
- Management/Treatment
  1. Small chalazions may resolve without treatment
  2. Warm compresses 2 to 3 times a day for 20 minutes for 2 to 3 days
  3. Treat large, recurrent or infected lesions with local antibacterial drops or ointments (sulfacetamide sodium 10%) q.i.d. for one week
  4. If unresponsive to treatment, refer to opthalmologist for surgical excision, curettage or corticosteroid injections

Blepharitis (Granulation of Eyelids)

- Definition:
  1. Common acute or chronic inflammation of eyelash follicles and meibomian glands of eyelid margins
  2. Types
     a. Seborrheic, ulcerated or combination of both
     b. Bacterial infection of lash follicles
- Etiology/Incidence
  1. Seborrheic blepharitis may be associated with seborrheic dermatitis, psoriasis, eczema or allergies; chemicals, smoke, air pollution and cosmetics can aggravate condition
  2. *Staphylococcus aureus* is primary causative pathogen
  3. Common in early childhood; associated with Down Syndrome; eczema
- Signs and Symptoms
  1. Irritation, burning
  2. Sensation of foreign body
  3. Erythema of eyelid margins
  4. Pruritus
  5. Loss of eye lashes
- Differential Diagnosis
  1. Chalazion, conjunctivitis, superficial keratitis
  2. Hordeolum
  3. Seborrhea, pediculosis of eyelashes
- Physical Findings
  1. Seborrheic form—hypertrophy and desquamation of epidermis adjacent to eye lid margin

2. Loss of eye lashes

3. Translucent, easily removable scales

4. Ulcerative form—purulent inflammation with ulcer formation on lid margins with erythema and bleeding; if condition progresses, leads to eyelid margin distortion and possible ectropion

5. May be associated with conjunctivitis and superficial keratitis

- Diagnostic Tests/Findings: None indicated

- Management/Treatment: Similar for both forms

  1. Warm moist compresses to lid margins several times/day

  2. Daily mechanical scrubbing and cleansing of lid margins with cotton tipped applicator or soft cloth, dipped in dilute baby shampoo

  3. Application of topical antibiotic ointment massaged into lid margins (sulfacetamide sodium 10% or polymyxin B-bacitracin)

  4. When seborrheic dermatitis of the scalp is present, frequent shampooing with selenium sulfide recommended

  5. Continue treatment for several weeks if necessary; recurrences are common

Hordeolum (Stye)

- Definition: An acute localized inflammation of one or more sebaceous glands (meibomian or zeisian) of eyelids

- Etiology/Incidence: Most common infectious pathogen is *Staphylococcus aureus;* highest incidence in children/adolescence

- Signs and Symptoms

  1. Sudden onset of tenderness, redness and swelling of affected lid

  2. Foreign body sensation

- Differential Diagnosis

  1. Chalazion

  2. Blepharitis

  3. Inclusion cyst

- Physical Findings

  1. Painful erythematous swelling on either skin (external stye) or conjunctival (internal stye) surface

  2. May suppurate and drain spontaneously

- Diagnostic Tests/Findings: Culture not necessary

- Management/Treatment
    1. Warm moist compresses for 15 minutes three to four times a day
    2. Sulfacetamide sodium 10% or polymyxin B-bacitracin drops or ointment
    3. Cleanse eye lids with baby shampoo once a day
    4. Refer for incision and drainage if unresponsive to treatment
    5. Dispose of old eye makeup; discourage use of eye makeup until hordeolum is resolved; stress good hand and eye hygiene

Orbital/Periorbital Cellulitis

- Definition
    1. Orbital—inflammation of the orbital contents posterior to orbital septum
    2. Periorbital—inflammation/infection of the skin and subcutaneous tissue surrounding eye; often associated with trauma, septicemia, sinusitis and bacteremia or local infection near the eye

- Etiology/Incidence
    1. Orbit or preseptal areas are infected from local trauma or spread from proximate structures or body parts
    2. Most common causes of bacterial orbital cellulitis in children are paranasal sinusitis and ethmoiditis
    3. Other causes include insect stings or bites, impetigo, foreign body
    4. Most common organisms are *Staphylococcus aureus*, *Streptococcus pneumoniae*, *Haemophilus influenzae*
    5. Periorbital cellulitis much more common than orbital cellulitis

- Signs and Symptoms
    1. Orbital cellulitis
        a. Insidious onset
        b. Orbital pain, headache
        c. Decreased vision
        d. Fever
        e. Potentially devastating consequences
    2. Periorbital cellulitis
        a. Acute onset of unilateral eyelid swelling
        b. Warmth, swelling and tenderness of overlying skin
        c. Eye itself and vision are usually normal
    3. Rhinorrhea, fever (102° to 104° F)

- Differential Diagnosis
    1. Differentiate between orbital (within true orbit), periorbital or preseptal (surrounding orbital septum) cellulitis
    2. Edema secondary to trauma
    3. Allergic periorbital edema
    4. Insect bite
- Physical Findings
    1. Orbital cellulitis
        a. Lid edema
        b. Chemosis
        c. Proptosis
        d. Decreased ocular mobility
        e. Decreased visual acuity
        f. Ophthalmoplegia (paralysis of eye muscles) and proptosis (protrusion of eyeball)—classic findings and distinguish orbital from periorbital cellulitis
    2. Periorbital cellulitis
        a. Unilateral eyelid edema
        b. Erythema
        c. Tenderness of overlying skin
        d. Visual acuity usually normal
- Diagnostic Tests/Findings
    1. Visual acuity exam—decreased vision with orbital cellulitis only
    2. Sinus roentgenograms or CT scan—determine sinus involvement
    3. Orbital sonography—determine orbit involvement
    4. CBC with differential—leukocytosis
    5. Blood and/or eye cultures—determine pathogen
    6. Lumbar punctures with infants—rule out sepsis
- Management/Treatment
    1. **Prompt assessment, treatment and referral**
    2. Systemic antibiotic therapy, primarily IV
    3. Moderate to severe cases or children under 1 year old may need hospitalization
    4. Complications may include loss of vision, subperiosteal or orbital abscess, meningitis, epidural and subdural abscess, thrombosis in the retina or sinus

5. Hib vaccine introduction—sharp decline in annual case rate of periorbital and orbital cellulitis (Ambati, 2001)

Cataracts

- Definition: Partial or complete opacity of the lens
- Etiology/Incidence: May be congenital or acquired during childhood; unilateral or bilateral; can result in significant amblyopia
  1. Congenital—results from genetic anomalies, prematurity and/or drug exposure, hypocalcemia, or maternal rubella during first trimester; incidence 2/10,000 births (Bhatti, 2003)
  2. Acquired cataracts due to:
     a. Trauma to the orbit
     b. Systemic disease—diabetes mellitus, Trisomy 21, hypoparathyroidism, galactosemia, atopic dermatitis, hypocalcemia, Marfan's syndrome
     c. Ingestion of poisons found in moth balls/crystals, insecticides
     d. Long term use of systemic corticosteroids or ocular corticosteroid drops
     e. Complications from other ocular abnormalities, e.g., glaucoma, uveitis, strabismus, pendibular nystagmus with severe amblyopia
- Signs and Symptoms: Severity of visual acuity deficits depends on location and degree of opacity; no pain
- Differential Diagnosis
  1. Retinoblastoma
  2. Glaucoma
- Physical Findings
  1. Strabismus—may be initial sign of cataract in child
  2. Absent red reflex, black dot(s) surrounded by red reflex, or white plaque-like opacities
  3. Signs of other systemic diseases and ocular abnormalities as noted in etiology
- Management/Treatment
  1. Prompt referral to ophthalmologist for diagnosis/treatment
  2. Surgical measures indicated if vision unable to develop due to extent of cataract; visual correction
  3. Determine etiology; any positive family history of congenital cataracts; question if an isolated disorder or part of systemic disorder

Glaucoma

- Definition: Increased intraocular pressure from disruption of aqueous fluid circulation involving one or both eyes resulting in optic nerve damage with loss of visual acuity and eventual blindness

- Etiology/Incidence

  1. Congenital—present at birth and up to 3 years of age

  2. Primary—isolated anomaly of drainage apparatus; 50% of infantile glaucoma is primary; occurs in only 0.03% (Behrman, 2000)

  3. Secondary or juvenile (3 to 30 year olds) from various causes, e.g., trauma, intraocular hemorrhage, intraocular tumor

  4. Possible complication of corticosteroid therapy, ocular injury or disease

  5. May be associated with other developmental anomalies, e.g., Marfan's, neurofibromatosis, congenital rubella syndrome, Pierre Robins syndrome

- Signs and Symptoms

  1. Classic triad ($\frac{1}{3}$ of infants demonstrate these)—photophobia, abnormal overflow of tears (epiphora), blepharospasm (eyelid spasm) (Behrman, 2000)

  2. Decreased vision (peripheral first) leading to tunnel vision

  3. Persistent, extreme pain (occasionally)

- Differential Diagnosis: Cataracts

- Physical Findings

  1. Corneal and ocular enlargement demonstrated as linear white opacities; corneal haziness and edema; firm to pressure

  2. Stretching of corneal and scleral tissues (in primary); thin, bluish sclera with pupillary dilation

  3. Deep cupping of optic disc

  4. Moderate injection or erythema (frequently unilateral) usually bulbar near limbus

- Diagnostic Tests/Findings: Glaucoma pressure test will show increased pressure

- Management/Treatment

  1. Immediate referral to ophthalmologist to confirm diagnosis and initiate therapy

  2. Topical beta blockers and carbonic anhydrase inhibitors; surgery indicated to relieve intraocular pressure (75% success rate)

  3. Enucleation may be necessary

  4. Glaucoma progresses slowly; blindness is highly probable without treatment

Strabismus

- Definition: Ocular misalignment; eyes may deviate outward (exotropia), inward (esotropia), downward (hypotropia) or upward (hypertropia)
- Etiology/Incidence
    1. Constant strabismus is termed "tropia"
    2. Intermittent alternating esotropia or exotropia normal in first four to six months of life
    3. Historical risk factors include prematurity, family history, cerebral palsy, most chromosomal and other major genetic anomalies, prenatal drug exposure, fetal alcohol syndrome, major head trauma, major congenital or acquired structural ocular defects (Ticho, 2003)
    4. Suppression is an adaptation to diplopia; without correction permanent loss of vision is probable
    5. Acquired strabismus occurring after 6 months of age usually from cataracts, retinoblastoma, anisometropia or high refractive errors
    6. Strabismus occurs in 4% of children under 6 years; esotropia is most common (Behrman, 2000)
    7. Patients with congenital vision loss are more likely to develop esotropia; and those with acquired vision loss are more likely to develop exotropia (Havertape, 2001)
    8. Pseudostrabismus—eyes appear to be crossed due to epicanthal folds on either side of bridge of nose; no ocular deviation
- Signs and Symptoms
    1. Varies with age
    2. Squinting
    3. Decreased vision
    4. School problems
    5. Head tilting
    6. Face turning
    7. Over pointing
    8. Awkwardness
- Differential Diagnosis
    1. Cataracts
    2. Retinoblastoma
    3. Anisometropia
    4. High refractive errors

5. Amblyopia

6. Head trauma

7. Other congenital eye muscle syndromes

- Physical Findings

    1. Misalignment of eye(s)

    2. Intermittent, alternating or continuous esotropia, exotropia, hypertropia or hypotropia

- Diagnostic Tests/Findings

    1. Abnormal Hirschberg (corneal light reflex unequal) and/or cover/uncover test (movement of covered eye)

    2. Vision screen—may reveal refractive errors, amblyopia or anisometropia

- Management/Treatment

    1. Establish period of onset, progression frequency and amplitude (constant versus intermittent), presence or absence of fixation preference, family history of strabismus or amblyopia, evidence of any associated neurologic or other disorders (Ticho, 2003)

    2. Referral to ophthalmologist

        a. Any children over 6 months with fixed or continuous strabismus; constant exotropia under 3 months of age

        b. Earlier if other developmental delays are present or deviations are continuous or fixed

        c. Signs of differential diagnosis present

        d. Suspicious history

        e. Immediate if hypotropia or hypertropia is present at any age

    3. Acquired—appropriate treatment depending on pathology and/or refractive errors

    4. Patching of fixing eye forces use of deviating eye; orthoptic exercises, corrective lenses may or may not be indicated; surgical alignment may be considered

Nystagmus

- Definition: Involuntary, horizontal, vertical, rotary, or mixed rhythmic movement of eyes

- Etiology/Incidence

    1. Caused by abnormality in one of three basic mechanisms—fixation, conjugate gaze or vestibular mechanisms (Behrman, 2000)

    2. May be familial

    3. Associated with albinism, refractive errors, central nervous system (CNS) abnormalities and various diseases of inner ear and retina

    4. Classified according to direction of movement

- Signs and Symptoms
    1. Irregular eye movements
    2. Abnormal head movements; may be rhythmic
- Differential Diagnosis: Underlying cause
- Physical Findings
    1. Involuntary rhythmic eye movements
    2. Vision screen may be abnormal
- Diagnostic Tests/Findings: Abnormal visual acuity test
- Management/Treatment
    1. Refer to ophthalmologist and neurologist (as necessary)
    2. Treat underlying cause
    3. Monitor child closely

Retinoblastoma

- Definition: Congenital malignancy of retina
    1. Most common malignant intraocular tumor of childhood
    2. See discussion in chapter on Hematologic/Oncologic/Immunologic Disorders

Refractive Errors

Hyperopia (Farsightedness)

- Definition: Alteration in refractive power when visual image is focused behind the retina; ability to see objects clearly at a distance, but not at close range
- Etiology/Incidence
    1. Axial length of eye too short and/or due to insufficient convexity of the refracting surfaces of the eye especially the cornea
    2. Familial pattern common
- Signs and Symptoms
    1. Often asymptomatic due to children's ability to easily accommodate for hyperopia
    2. Headache and eye strain during prolonged periods of close work in older children
    3. Strabismus often seen with severe hyperopia
- Differential Diagnosis
    1. Astigmatism
    2. Myopia
    3. Anisometropia

    4. Amblyopia

- Physical Findings: Abnormal vision screen
- Diagnostic Tests/Findings
    1. Vision screen shows hyperopia
    2. Passing vision screen is 20/40 (age 3 to 4 years), 20/30 (older children)
    3. A difference of two lines between the 2 eyes is significant
- Management/Treatment
    1. Refer to ophthalmologist or optometrist
    2. If strabismus present, see previous section for management
    3. Annual eye examinations

Myopia (Nearsightedness)

- Definition: Alteration in refractive power when visual image is focused in front of retina; ability to see objects clearly at close range, but not at a distance
- Etiology/Incidence
    1. Axial length of eye too long and/or increased curvature of the refracting surfaces of the eye, especially the cornea
    2. Familial pattern common; frequently associated with prematurity
    3. Myopia may be present at birth; usually appears around 8 to 10 years of age
- Signs and Symptoms
    1. Distant objects blurred
    2. Squinting forms physiologic pinhole to improve acuity
    3. Difficulty reading blackboard
- Differential Diagnosis
    1. Hyperopia
    2. Astigmatism
    3. Anisometropia
    4. Amblyopia
- Physical Findings: Abnormal vision screen
- Diagnostic Tests/Findings: Abnormal vision screen (see hyperopia)
- Management/Treatment
    1. Refer to ophthalmologist or optometrist
    2. Importance of annual eye examinations

Astigmatism

- Definition: Refractive error due to an irregular curvature of the cornea or changes in the lens causing light rays to bend in different directions
- Etiology/Incidence
    1. Familial developmental variations in the curvature of the cornea
    2. Depending on severity of curvature variation, retina can not focus regardless of distance
    3. Increased risk secondary to injury, periorbital or eyelid hemangiomas or ptosis (Behrman, 2000)
- Signs and Symptoms
    1. Commonly found in conjunction with other refractive errors
    2. Pain in and around eyes, headache, fatigue, reading problems, frowning
- Differential Diagnosis
    1. Myopia
    2. Hyperopia
    3. Amblyopia
    4. Anisometropia
- Physical Findings: Possible abnormal vision screen
- Diagnostic Tests/Findings: Vision screen with possible abnormality
- Management/Treatment
    1. Refer to ophthalmologist or optometrist
    2. Corrective lenses or contacts may be prescribed; patching may be recommended

Blindness (Amaurosis)

- Definition
    1. Varies from inability to distinguish light from darkness to partial vision
    2. Best corrected visual acuity between 20/70 to 20/200
    3. Legal blindness is distant acuity 20/200 in better eye or visual field; includes an angle of no greater than 20 degrees
    4. Primary blindness—present at birth
- Etiology/Incidence
    1. $\frac{1}{3}$ of blindness in children from trauma
    2. Variety of pathological causes—cataracts, glaucoma, retinopathy of prematurity (ROP) (most common cause of severe visual impairment); retinoblastoma, trauma,

detached retina, cranial nerve II problems, infection, hydrocephalus, genetic problems

- Signs and Symptoms: Varies with age and mode of onset, abilities of child, laterality and severity of deficit

    1. Developmental delays, e.g., gross motor, walking often delayed to 18 to 24 months

    2. Social skills—increased passivity, increased anxiety around strangers

    3. Decreased social communication and school performance

    4. Increased self-stimulating behavior, e.g., hand flapping, rocking, rubbing eyes

    5. Language delay; cognitive delays, understanding of object permanence; cause/effect

    6. Delay in development of conversational skills

    7. Photophobia, chronic tearing, wandering eyes

    8. Lack of smiling response to visual stimuli

- Differential Diagnosis: If primary or from birth

    1. Developmental malformations

    2. Damage consequent to gestational/perinatal infection

    3. Anoxia, hypoxia, perinatal trauma

    4. Genetically determined diseases

- Physical Findings: In primary blindness

    1. Nystagmus (may be first clue)

    2. Enlarged or cloudy cornea; abnormal or absent red reflex

    3. Lack of pupillary reflex; optic disc pallor; pigmentary deposits

    4. Fixed or intermittent strabismus beyond 6 months of age

    5. History of prematurity with retinopathy of prematurity (ROP)

    6. Possible neurological disorder

- Diagnostic Tests/Findings

    1. Ophthalmologic examination—abnormal as described above

    2. Developmental testing—delays as outlined

    3. CT or MRI—rule out physiological abnormalities

- Management/Treatment

    1. Obtain complete family genetic visual impairment history

    2. Address family issues; social and emotional needs of child

    3. General medical and developmental history

4. Metabolic and genetic studies

5. Prompt referral to ophthalmologist, neurologist and developmental specialist

Amblyopia (Lazy Eye)

- Definition: Decreased visual acuity in one or both eyes with no apparent abnormality on physical examination, despite correction of any refractive error; suppression of retinal image in affected eye to avoid diplopia

- Etiology/Incidence

    1. Organic—trauma, organic lesion, cataract, diseases of the eye or visual pathways, ptosis

    2. Nonorganic—sensory stimulation deprivation or disuse; abnormal binocular interaction during infancy and early childhood (greatest risk between 2 to 3 years of age but can continue until 9 years of age); large difference in refractive errors between both eyes (anisometropia)

    3. Rarely bilateral; associated with strabismus

    4. Occurs in 2% to 5% of general population

    5. Five types—deprivation (ptosis, opacities), strabismic, anisometropic, occlusion (patching good eye too much), ametropic (both eyes large refractive errors, typically hyperopic and/or astigmatism)

- Signs and Symptoms: Wandering eye

- Differential Diagnosis

    1. Cataracts

    2. Blindness

    3. Ptosis

- Physical Examination

    1. Negative red reflex

    2. Ptosis

    3. Strabismus

- Diagnostics Tests/Findings

    1. Abnormal vision and/or ophthalmic examination—abnormal red reflex, positive cover/uncover test, unequal corneal light reflex

    2. Abnormal ocular movements

- Management/Treatment

    1. Early detection, prompt intervention, referral to ophthalmologist

    2. Effective vision screening before 3 years of age

    3. Corrective lenses

4. Occlusion therapy forcing stimulation of amblyopic eye (patching good eye)

5. Close monitoring of occlusion therapy

6. Reassurance and support throughout treatment

Eye Injuries

General information regarding corneal abrasion, foreign body, hyphema, ecchymosis and chemical injuries

- Definition/Incidence/Etiology
    1. $\frac{1}{3}$ of blindness in children < ten years of age is due to trauma
    2. Sports and activities in which ocular trauma is common include BB guns (most common), archery, darts, motorcycling, bicycling, racquet sports, boxing, basketball and baseball

- Physical Examination
    1. Steps in proper evaluation include:
        a. Recognizing life threatening nonocular conditions, e.g., chemical injuries
        b. Taking adequate history to assess potential risk of injury
        c. Examining in detail (visual acuity, external ocular motility unless ruptured globe suspected), pupil, anterior segment and fundus
        d. Referral for signs and symptons or history of severe ocular injury
    2. Use caution—severe intraocular injury may be concealed behind minimal external trauma
    3. Examine lids, lacrimal system, adnexa, sclera and conjunctiva for lacerations, foreign body or perforation
    4. Palpate orbital rim for crepitus; CT scan when orbital fracture suspected; can be associated with significant intracranial and ocular injuries
    5. A dislocated lens presents with a quivering iris
    6. Topical anesthetic recommended for examination only; slows healing of cornea

- Management/Treatment
    1. Ocular injuries requiring immediate referral include:
        a. Chemical injuries
        b. Globe lacerations, severe lacerations of lid
        c. Hyphemas
        d. Penetrating intraocular injury
    2. Avoid pressure to globe by placing a protective shield over injured eye

3. Nonaccidental trauma or child abuse should be considered with presence of lid ecchymosis, conjunctival hemorrhages, hyphema or retinal hemorrhages; ideally injuries should be photographed when possible

4. Acetaminophen for pain, no acetylsalicylic acid (ASA)

5. Injury prevention (e.g., protective eyewear) will reduce ocular trauma by 90%

6. Date of last tetanus vaccine

7. Rabies prophylaxis if trauma from animal bite

8. Refer to ophthalmologist for further assessment

Corneal Abrasion

- Definition: Loss of epithelial lining from corneal surface of one or both eyes
- Etiology/Incidence—abrasion, trauma or foreign bodies in upper lid leading to corneal injury, e.g., paper, brushes, toys or fingernails, contact lenses, ultraviolet light exposure; most common ocular injury in children
- Signs and Symptoms
    1. Possible evidence of foreign body
    2. Severe pain and tearing
    3. Blepharospasm
    4. Injection of sclera
    5. Photophobia
- Physical Findings: Epithelial injury visible with use of fluorescein stain and Wood's lamp
- Management/Treatment
    1. Topical anesthetic for evaluation only
    2. Remove foreign body via irrigation with normal saline
    3. Broad spectrum antibiotic ointment with a short acting cycloplegic agent for pain if necessary, plus daily follow-up until abrasion is healed; patching is not recommended (Forbes, 2001)
    4. Refer to ophthalmologist if abrasion is not healed within 3 days
    5. Acetaminophen for discomfort

Foreign Body Eye Injury

- Definition: Foreign body in the eye
- Etiology/Incidence
    1. Surface—nonadherent/loosely adherent to cornea or conjunctival epithelium (most likely sources dirt, sand, grass)

    2. Penetrating—into but not through cornea or sclera

    3. Perforating—through cornea or sclera and into globe

- Signs and Symptoms
    1. Foreign body sensation
    2. Pain
    3. Sensitivity to light
    4. Tearing
    5. Eye rubbing

- Differential Diagnosis
    1. Corneal abrasion
    2. Chemical injury

- Physical Findings
    1. Foreign body may be visualized
    2. Positive fluorescein examination if corneal abrasion present
    3. Epiphora
    4. Possible visual acuity abnormality

- Diagnostic Tests/Findings
    1. Visual acuity—to determine any deviation from normal
    2. Fluorescein test—to determine presence of corneal abrasion
    3. Possible radiographs to visualize foreign body

- Management/Treatment
    1. All intraocular foreign bodies require referral to ophthalmologist
    2. Topical ophthalmic anesthetic drops for examination unless perforating wound suspected
    3. If persistent corneal abrasion after 24 hours with treatment, penetrating or perforation wound, refer to ophthalmologist
    4. Thoroughly examine lashes, lids, cornea and conjunctival surfaces
    5. Remove foreign body via irrigation with normal saline
    6. After removal, examine for corneal abrasion, treat appropriately

Hyphema

- Definition: Accumulation of blood in anterior chamber
- Etiology/Incidence

1. Due to blunt or perforating trauma (e.g., balls, fists and sticks) leading to rupture of iris or ciliary body blood vessels; increased risk of rebleeding in first 5 days and glaucoma with traumatic hyphema (Behrman, 2000)

2. May also occur with bleeding disorders, e.g., sickle cell disease

3. Usually lasts 5 to 6 days

- Signs and Symptoms

    1. History of ocular injury

    2. Drowsiness

    3. Pain

    4. Light sensitivity

- Physical Findings

    1. Blood in anterior chamber

    2. Visual acuity changes

- Management/Treatment

    1. Refer to ophthalmologist

    2. Reduce activity for several days, bed rest in supine position with head of bed elevated 30 to 40 degrees to promote reabsorption of blood; hospitalization often necessary; eye patch for 5 days on injured eye; no aspirin or reading

    3. Surgery may be necessary to remove blood

Ecchymoses ("Black Eye")

- Definition: Bruising of periorbital region

- Etiology/Incidence: Blunt contusion injury; due to isolated periorbital injury or other orbital/ocular injury

- Signs and Symptoms

    1. Pain

    2. Visual impairment due to occlusion from edematous eyelid

- Differential Diagnosis: Other orbital/ocular injury (e.g., lens dislocation, globe rupture, retinal detachment)

- Physical Findings

    1. Edema

    2. Ecchymosis

- Diagnostic Tests/Findings

    1. Ophthalmic examination—determine other orbital/ocular injuries

    2. Visual acuity

- Management/Treatment
    1. Uncomplicated—cold compresses for 24 to 48 hours; then warm compresses until swelling resolves; elevate head; inform parents/patient that ecchymosis and edema may spread
    2. Refer to ophthalmologist—closed head injury, damage to skull, facial bone fracture

Chemical Injuries

- Definition: Burns of the eye lids, conjunctiva and/or cornea
- Etiology/Incidence
    1. Steam, intense heat and common household agents
    2. Severe alkali injuries characterized by corneal opacification
    3. Amount of damage directly related to duration of exposure
- Management/Treatment
    1. **Acute ocular emergency**
    2. Copious irrigation with normal saline for 20 to 30 minutes—patch and refer to ophthalmologist immediately to rule out corneal or other ocular trauma
    3. Severe chemical injury to eye(s) requires hospitalization
    4. Topical anesthetic may reduce pain from injury and irrigation
    5. Pseudomonal contamination common with any burn possibly leading to corneal ulceration; prevention—antibiotic preparation containing polymyxin B, gentamicin, tobramycin or colistin should be instilled into the injured eye(s) 3 to 4 times a day

Ear

External Otitis Media (EOM)

- Definition: Acute infection and/or inflammation of external auditory canal; "swimmer's ear"
- Etiology/Incidence
    1. More common in summer months due to excessive wetness (swimming, bathing or increased environmental humidity) which changes the acidic environment and promotes bacterial/fungal growth due to abnormal neutral or basic environment
    2. Common organisms are *Pseudomonas aeruginosa* (most common), *Staphylococcus aureus, Streptococcus pyogenes, Enterobacter aerogenes, Proteus mirabilis, Klebsiella pneumoniae, Staphylococcus epidermis,* and fungi, e.g., candida, aspergillus, trichophyton (Ecker, 2003)
    3. Loss of protective cerumen or chronic irritation
    4. Trauma disrupting lining of auditory canal, e.g., foreign body, digital irritation

5. Excessive dryness (eczema, psoriasis); contact dermatitis, e.g., poison ivy, medications, hair spray, perfumes

- Signs and Symptoms

    1. Itching of ear canal (early symptom)

    2. Acute and possibly severe ear pain upon manipulation of pinna/tragus, or performance of otoscopic examination; mastoid pain

    3. Pressure/fullness in ear, possible hearing loss (conductive or sensorineural) (Ecker, 2003)

- Differential Diagnosis

    1. Acute otitis media with perforation

    2. Dental infection

    3. Mastoiditis, furunculosis

    4. Foreign body

    5. Eczema

- Physical Findings

    1. May be difficult to visualize tympanic membrane (TM), however usually normal

    2. Edematous/erythematous external canal

    3. Black spots on TM indicative of fungal infection

    4. Furuncle may be noted with localized infection

    5. Otorrhea (rare), occasional regional lymphadenopathy

    6. Observe for signs of mastoiditis or cellulitis beyond external canal

- Diagnostic Tests/Findings: Culture of discharge unnecessary unless unresponsive to treatment

- Management/Treatment

    1. Withdraw any foreign bodies or debris from external canal by gentle irrigation with warm water or normal saline

    2. Topical antibiotic otic drops containing combinations of neomycin, polymyxin, propylene glycol and corticosteroids, 3 to 4 drops, 3 to 4 times/day for 7 to 10 days

    3. If significant swelling, insert cotton wick saturated with antibiotic solution for first 24 to 48 hours

    4. Systemic analgesic often required for severe pain

    5. Re-examine 1 to 2 weeks for evaluation of TM and removal of any debris

    6. Prevention—instillation of white vinegar and rubbing alcohol (50/ 50) in both ear canals after swimming; avoid water in canals, vigorous cleaning, scratching or prolonged use of cerumenolytic agents

7. Incision and drainage (I + D) of furuncle if present

8. Fungal infection treated with 5% boric acid in ethanol solution for 5 to 7 days

Acute Otitis Media (AOM)

- Definition: Inflammation of the middle ear with fluid and associated signs and symptoms of ear infection (suppurative otitis media)

- Etiology/Incidence

  1. Fluid/pathogen accumulation in middle ear due to eustachian tube malfunction secondary to obstruction caused by allergies, viral infections, decreased patency and/or other mechanical factors

  2. Common pathogenic agents

     a. *Streptococcus pneumoniae* (most common, 40%)

     b. *Haemophilus influenzae* (25% to 30%)

     c. *Moraxella catarrhalis* (10% to 20%)

     d. Less common pathogens—*Staphylococcus aureus,* group A beta hemolytic streptococcus and *Pseudomonas aeruginosa,* (more common in chronic otitis media)

     e. Viruses—Influenza, RSV (most common), adenovirus, parainfluenza and coronavirus

     f. Prevalence of β-lactamase producing strains highest in past 15 years

     g. Increase in drug resistant bacteria, especially in children younger than 24 months; those who recently were treated with β-lactamase antibiotics and children exposed to large numbers of children

     h. No growth found in 16% of AOM

  3. Predisposing factors

     a. Physiological considerations—eustachian tube of child under 6 years of age is short, wide, and horizontal allowing access of pathogens from nasopharynx to reach middle ear

     b. Possible hereditary factors

     c. Common occurrence with/following upper respiratory infection

     d. Bottle feeding in supine position and/or no breast feeding

     e. Craniofacial abnormalities, e.g., cleft palate

     f. Allergic rhinitis

     g. Tobacco smoke exposure

     h. Children in group day care centers at higher risk than those in home care

4. One of the most common pediatric diagnoses—highest prevalence between 6 to 36 months

5. Highest incidence in winter/spring; males, Caucasians, American Indians, Eskimos and lower socioeconomic groups

6. Children who develop OM early in life are prone to recurrent OM and chronic otitis media with effusion (OME); recurrent OM rose from 18.7% in 1981 to 26% in 1988 with greatest increase among infants in day care

7. Natural history of untreated otitis media—70% to 90% spontaneous resolution

- Signs and Symptoms

  1. Fever in $\frac{1}{3}$ to $\frac{1}{2}$ of cases

  2. Complaints of ear fullness, pain or discomfort 50% of the time

  3. Poor appetite/feeding, irritable with sleep disturbances (especially in infants)

  4. Nausea/vomiting

  5. Runny nose

  6. Tugging on ears

- Differential Diagnosis

  1. Crying child with normal erythematous tympanic membranes

  2. Damage to TM

  3. Tympanosclerosis

  4. Cholesteatoma

  5. Otitis externa

  6. Rare complications—mastoiditis; sepsis in young infant; hearing loss, developmental/speech delay

- Physical Findings: Diagnosis is determined by changes in color, contour, vascularity and mobility of TM

  1. Color is erythematous or yellow and opaque

  2. Contour may be dull or bulging; light reflexes usually distorted

  3. Distinct vascularity

  4. Mobility decreased or absent via tympanometry or pneumatic otoscopy

  5. Conductive hearing loss

- Diagnostic Tests/Findings: Use depends on age of child, and stage of middle ear disease

  1. Pneumatic otoscopy—visualize degree of mobility impairment

  2. Tympanometry using electroacoustic impedance bridge to measure compliance of the TM—identifies middle ear effusion, perforation, patent ventilation tubes, or excessive hard packed cerumen

Table 1
Antibiotic Therapy for Management of Otitis Media

Drug Category
First line therapy Amoxicillin
Second line therapy 1. Amoxicillin-clavulanate 2. Cefuroxime 3. Clindamycin 4. Ceftriaxone 5. Cefprozil 6. Ceftibuten 7. Azithromycin 8. Clarithromycin 9. Loracarbef 10. Cefpodoxime
Prophylactic therapy 1. Amoxicillin 2. Sulfisoxazole

3. Audiometric tests—to rule out conductive hearing loss, especially for otitis media with effusion in children 3 months and older

4. Language screen—assess degree of possible speech delay

- Management/Treatment

1. Judicious use of antimicrobials due to increased bacterial resistance; consider no antibiotic use during the first 24 to 48 hours; if no better an antibiotic should be given

2. Select appropriate antibiotic—see Table 1

    a. Children considered high risk include less than 24 months, attend day care, antibiotic use in the last 30 days, anatomic abnormalities, an immature immune system and siblings with history of recurrent AOM; first line treatment high dose of amoxicillin

    b. Children considered low risk, first line treatment lower dose of amoxicillin

3. Maintain realistic expectations—90% to 95% symptom relief within 48 to 72 hours; if no better, change antibiotic to 2nd line therapy

4. Children older than 24 months with uncomplicated AOM can be treated with a five day regimen of antibiotics; children less than 24 months with chronic or recurrent AOM or a perforated tympanic membrane, give a 10-day course of antibiotics (Ecker, 2003)

5. Use tympanocentesis sparingly; only used for retreatment failures with severe symptoms

6. Monitor residual OME—may last for several months; persistent OME for 6 to 8 weeks, consider treatment with second line antibiotics (see Table 1)

7. Pain and fever control

   a. Analgesics—acetaminophen, ibuprofen

   b. Local anesthetic otic drops (contraindicated in acute/chronic perforations and ventilation tubes)

8. Decongestant use is controversial; usefulness unproven

9. Recheck AOM after 10 to 21 days

10. Prevention

    a. Proper feeding techniques for infants

    b. Encourage breast feeding—shown to be protective against otitis media

    c. Eliminate exposure to tobacco smoke

    d. Antibiotic prophylaxis—see Table 1; only used for control of chronic AOM, e.g., 3 or more episodes in 6 months or 4 episodes in 12 months (AAP, 2003)

    e. Immunization with pneumococcal and influenza vaccines

11. Referral to otolaryngologist

    a. Persistent AOM resistant to treatment over 1 to 2 months

    b. Frequent recurrent OM—3 in 6 months, 4 to 5 episodes in one year, 6 episodes by 6 years of age

    c. Persistent/chronic OME > 3 months

    d. Evidence of hearing deficit and/or language delay

    e. Determine need for tympanostomy tube placement

Otitis Media with Effusion (OME)

- Definition: Inflammation/fluid accumulation in middle ear with decreased TM mobility on pneumatic otoscopy but without signs and symptoms of ear infection; also referred to as serous, secretory, mucoid, and allergic otitis media or "glue ear"

- Etiology/Incidence

  1. Caused by eustachian tube malfunction as frequent sequelae of acute otitis media; negative pressure in middle ear results in fluid accumulation by effusion

  2. OME accounts for 25% to 35% of all cases of OM

  3. 30% to 40% have OME associated with allergic rhinitis

  4. Majority (50% to 80%) clear within 2 to 3 months

  5. Mild to moderate hearing loss with concomitant language delays may occur with OME contributing to subsequent behavioral difficulties including poor attention and school performance

- Signs and Symptoms
  1. Sometimes none or mild discomfort
  2. Behavioral changes, e.g., hearing loss, decreased attention span
- Differential Diagnosis: Same as AOM
- Physical Findings
  1. Color—opaque or translucent TM; possible presence of air, fluid levels or bubbles
  2. Contour—appears retracted due to negative pressure in middle ear
  3. Vascularity—none visible
  4. Mobility—decreased, tympanometry reveals high negative pressure
- Diagnostic Tests/Findings: Same as AOM
- Management/Treatment:
  1. Most cases resolve without antibiotics
  2. Limit use of antibiotic prophylaxis due to marginal benefit
  3. Limit passive smoking exposure, treat other infections, control allergies
  4. Audiogram after 3 months; referral to otolaryngologist
  5. Consider surgery for chronic OME accompanied by pain, recurrent AOM; speech or hearing problems (Ecker, 2003)
  6. Decongestants and antihistamines not recommended
  7. Follow up every 3 to 4 weeks
  8. Prevention, education and referral recommendations, same as AOM

Tympanostomy Tubes
- Definition
  1. Surgical incision of ear drum (myringotomy with placement of ventilation tube) to relieve pressure and drain pus/fluid from middle ear
  2. Two types
     a. Short term—intended to remain in TM 8 to 15 months
     b. Long term—intended for more than 15 months
- Etiology/Incidence
  1. One million tubes inserted annually
  2. Indicated for children with failed antibiotic prophylaxis of 4 months or longer; those allergic to penicillin or sulfonamides; those with associated hearing loss of 20 dB or other complications

3. With increasing number of resistant bacteria, possibility of more frequent use of tubes

- Management/Treatment

    1. Fitted ear plugs with swimming

    2. If drainage occurs from tubes, treat with antibiotic otic suspension, e.g., fluoroquinolone otic drops (first line therapy) polymyxin B with neomycin and hydrocortisone

Chronic/Acute Perforations

- Definition: Spontaneous perforation of tympanic membrane during episode of AOM
- Etiology/Incidence

    1. Chronic—perforation lasts longer than one month

    2. Chronic suppurative O.M.—associated with discharge

    3. Chronic sites of perforation

        a. Central—relatively safe from cholesteatoma formation

        b. Peripheral—especially in pars flaccida, increased risk of cholesteatoma

- Signs and Symptoms: Painless ear discharge if infection present
- Differential Diagnosis

    1. Cholesteatoma

    2. Mastoiditis

    3. Extradural, subdural or brain abscess

    4. Meningitis

    5. Labrynthitis

    6. Lateral sinus thrombophlebitis

- Physical Findings

    1. Thickened, inflamed middle ear mucosa

    2. May contain granulation tissue or polyps

    3. Conductive hearing loss dependent on size of perforation

    4. Site of perforation important to note

- Diagnostic Tests/Findings

    1. Culture discharge—*Pseudomonas aeruginosa* and *Staphylococcus aureus* most often seen

    2. PPD—rule out tuberculosis

    3. CT scan of mastoid—rule out mastoiditis

- Management/Treatment

    1. Oral antibiotics (see Table 1) for 14 days plus antibiotic ear drops (3 to 4 drops four times a day, for 7 days); if not responsive, suspect mastoiditis or cholesteatoma

    2. Patients with central nervous system sequelae, refer immediately

    3. Hospitalization may be necessary

    4. Follow up every week to 3 months; most heal within 2 weeks

    5. Refer to otolaryngologist

        a. Unresolved perforation after 1 year duration

        b. Surgical repair delayed until 9 to 12 years of age

- Prevention of recurrent infection

    1. Cotton plugs with petroleum jelly (on outer surface) when bathing and hair washing

    2. Discourage swimming (use fitted earplugs if unavoidable)

    3. Diving, jumping into water, and underwater swimming forbidden

    4. Exposure to air is helpful

Mastoiditis

- Definition: Infection of the mastoid antrum and air cells with potential destruction of the mastoid airspaces, a suppurative complication of otitis media

- Etiology/Incidence

    1. Uncommon, due to successful antibiotics for AOM

    2. Develops secondary to OM leading to periostitis and osteitis with abscess formation

    3. Unusual before two years of age

    4. Common pathogens

        a. Most common—*Streptococcus pneumoniae, Streptococcus pyogenes, Staphylococcus aureus*

        b. Less common—*Haemophilus influenzae*

        c. Other agents—Pseudomonas (chronic mastoiditis), *Mycobacterium tuberculosis* (rare), *Moraxella catarrhalis,* enteropathic gram negative rods

- Signs and Symptoms

    1. Pain, tenderness behind ear

    2. Fever or irritability

- Differential Diagnosis

    1. Meningitis

2. Extradural abscess

3. Subdural empyema

4. Focal otic encephalitis

- Physical Findings

    1. Severe tenderness over mastoid bone

    2. Mastoid area often edematous with erythema

    3. Presence of AOM

    4. Pinna displaced downward and outward (late finding)

    5. Narrowing of ear canal in posterior superior wall due to pressure from mastoid abscess

    6. Purulent drainage and debris may be present in ear canal

- Diagnostic Tests/Findings

    1. CBC—elevated WBC

    2. Blood culture—rule out sepsis

    3. PPD—rule out exposure to tuberculosis

    4. Radiography or CT scan of mastoid(s)—diffuse clouding of mastoid cells; later in disease, bony destruction and resorption of the mastoid air cells; CT also done if brain abscess is suspected

    5. Tympanocentesis—identify pathogen

    6. Lumbar puncture—rule out meningitis

- Management/Treatment

    1. Prompt referral to ENT and hospitalization

    2. Incision and drainage of abscess; systemic intravenous antibiotics

    3. Complications—meningitis, brain abscess, cavernous sinus thrombosis, acute suppurative labrynthitis, facial palsy

    4. Oral systemic antibiotics for 4 to 6 weeks after discharge

Cholesteatoma

- Definition: Cyst like mass with lining of stratified squamous epithelium filled with desquamated debris; most common in middle ear and mastoid area

- Etiology/Incidence

    1. Congenital or acquired

    2. Varied theories explaining formation, e.g., inflammatory process; perforation or failure of desquamated tissue to clear from middle ear

    3. Incidence unknown

4. If surgery delayed, it can invade and destroy other structures of the temporal bone and possibly spread to intracranial cavity

5. If untreated, may lead to facial nerve paralysis, intracranial infection

-   Signs and Symptoms

    1. Dizziness

    2. Hearing loss

-   Differential Diagnosis: Aural polyps

-   Physical Findings

    1. Pearly white, shiny, greasy lesion on or behind tympanic membrane

    2. History of chronic OM with foul smelling purulent otorrhea

-   Diagnostic Tests/Findings: Audiogram to rule out hearing deficit

-   Management/Treatment

    1. Referral to ENT for surgical excision

    2. Complications

        a. Irreversible structural damage

        b. Permanent bone damage

        c. Facial nerve palsy

        d. Hearing loss

        e. Intracranial infection

Hearing Loss

-   Definition: A deficit in hearing process; classified as conductive, sensorineural or mixed; can range from mild to severe; may be congenital or acquired; quantified by measured hearing threshhold

    1. Conductive loss—normal bone conduction and reduced air conduction due to obstruction of transmission of sound waves through external auditory canal and middle ear to the inner ear; usual range of 15 to 40 dB loss

    2. Sensorineural loss—cochlea hair cells and/or auditory nerve damage; may range from mild to profound

    3. Mixed—components of conductive and sensorineural hearing loss present

    4. Hearing loss criteria in children differs from adults since children are in the process of speech and language development (Behrman, 2000)

        a. Mild—15 to 30 dB

        b. Moderate—30 to 50 dB

        c. Severe—50 to 70 dB

        d. Profound—70 dB and above

- Etiology/Incidence
    1. Hearing loss can be classified in five ways
        a. Age of onset
        b. Type—conductive, sensorineural, mixed or central
        c. Degree—ranging from mild to profound
        d. Configuration—decibel (dB) loss
        e. Hearing status of parent(s)
    2. Congenital
        a. Sensorineural—moderate to profound loss; 1–2:1000 live births (Behrman, 2000)
            (1) Genetic—autosomal dominant (80%), autosomal recessive (20%)
            (2) In utero infections—TORCH, CMV and rubella most common causes in newborn
            (3) Erythroblastosis fetalis
            (4) Anoxia
            (5) Birth trauma
            (6) Birth weight < 1500 g
            (7) Exposure to ototoxic drugs
            (8) Prolonged mechanical ventilation
        b. Conductive—congenital atresia, deformities or stenosis of ossicles
    3. Acquired
        a. Sensorineural
            (1) Meningitis
            (2) Mumps, measles
            (3) Labyrinthitis, ototoxic drug exposure
            (4) Severe head trauma
            (5) Noise induced hearing loss (NIHL) from loud music, firecrackers, firearms, toy cap pistols, squeaking toys, recreational vehicles, farm equipment, lawn mowers, inappropriate hearing aids
        b. Conductive
            (1) Otitis media with middle effusion—75% of children have one episode of AOM with conductive hearing loss
            (2) Cerumen impaction; foreign bodies in external canal

(3) Perforated/damaged tympanic membrane; severe head trauma

(4) Cholesteatoma, otosclerosis

- Signs and Symptoms
  1. Infants
     a. Failure to elicit startle or blink reflex to loud sound
     b. Failure to be awakened by loud sounds
     c. General indifference to sound
     d. Lack of babbling by 7 months
  2. Children
     a. Substitution of gestures for words, especially after 15 months
     b. Failure to develop intelligible speech by 24 months
     c. Asking to have statements repeated
     d. Inappropriate response to questions
     e. Markedly inattentive

- Differential Diagnosis
  1. Mental retardation
  2. Profound deprivation
  3. Communication disorder—articulation disorders, expressive language delay, global language disorder, autism

- Physical Findings
  1. Careful evaluation of TM, e.g., decreased mobility, bulging, opacity
  2. Congenital abnormalities—external canal abnormalities, craniofacial malformations, structural abnormalities of external ear

- Diagnostic Test/Findings
  1. Audiogram appropriate for age to rule out hearing loss
  2. CT Scan—rule out physiologic abnormalities
  3. Weber and Rinne tests—abnormal response

- Management/Treatment
  1. History screening at two week old visit—family history of hearing loss, perinatal infections (TORCH), anatomic malformations involving head or neck, birth weight < 1500 g, hyperbilirubinemia, bacterial meningitis, asphyxia
  2. Detect hearing loss as young as possible; take parental suspicions seriously; many tests available for all age groups including newborn (otoacoustic emissions-OAE, auditory brainstem response-ABR)

3. Referral for full audiological testing and language evaluation as soon as deficit is strongly suspected

4. Psychosocial considerations—rehabilitation, hearing aids, educational programs

5. Prevention

   a. Early identification and intervention; periodic hearing and language screening; (birth to 4 months—responds appropriately to loud noises; 4 to 24 months—responds to noise out of field of vision; older children—pure tone audiometry)

   b. Appropriate management and treatment of auditory canal obstruction and middle ear disease

   c. Avoid repeated exposure to loud noises to prevent NIHL

   d. Control erythroblastosis with use of RhoGAM; hyperbilirubinemia with photo-therapy and exchange transfusions

   e. Prevent mumps and measles with immunization

   f. Avoid ototoxic medications

Nose

Allergic Rhinitis

- Definition: IgE mediated response to inhaled allergens or irritants producing nasal mucosa inflammation

- Etiology/Incidence

  1. Types—seasonal or perennial depending on exposure/sensitization to allergen

     a. Seasonal—inhaled pollens, e.g., trees, grasses; more common after age 6

     b. Perennial—house dust mites, mold spores, animal dander; may occur in children under age of 6, rarely seen under 24 months

  2. Most common pediatric atopic disease; commonly associated with conjunctivitis, sinusitis, OME and/or atopic dermatitis

  3. Strong genetic predisposition

- Signs and Symptoms

  1. Chronic, clear nasal discharge

  2. Episodes of sneezing with itching of eyes, ears, nose, palate, pharynx

  3. Open mouth facies, snoring with sleep

  4. Excessive tearing

  5. Purulent secretions indicate secondary infection (e.g., sinusitis, foreign body)

  6. Symptoms year-round with perennial rhinitis

- Differential Diagnosis

    1. Bacterial or viral upper respiratory infection, e.g., strep pharyngitis, influenza, OM, sinusitis

    2. Vasomotor rhinitis

    3. Congenital or anatomical abnormalities leading to obstruction, e.g., nasal polyps, foreign body

- Physical findings

    1. Allergic "shiners" and "salute" with nasal crease

    2. Hypertrophied turbinates; halitosis

    3. Nasal mucosa pale blue, boggy, and edematous with watery or mucoid secretions

- Diagnostic Tests/Findings

    1. Nasal smear for eosinophils—10% considered confirmatory

    2. RAST and skin testing—elevations or reactions to specific allergens

    3. CBC differential—elevated eosinophils and total IgE

- Management/Treatment: Referral to allergist may be necessary

    1. First line of therapy—identify and avoid allergen(s)

    2. Environmental controls—removal of carpets, drapes, and stuffed animals; plastic covers for mattresses and pillows; decrease humidity with air conditioner, use of air purifiers, and avoidance of tobacco smoke

    3. Drug therapy—antihistamine H_1 receptor antagonists

        a. Fexofenadine hydrochloide—(> 12 years) 60 mg every 12 hours; nonsedating

        b. Loratadine—(> 6 years and 30 kg) 10 mg daily; nonsedating

        c. Cetirizine—5 mg daily; 10 mg if 12 years of age or older

        d. Montelukast, 4 mg, 5 mg or 10 mg tablets daily

        e. Diphenhydramine—(5 mg/kg/day) every 6 hours; sedating

        f. Oral sympathomimetic (e.g., pseudoephedrine) for short term relief by producing vasoconstriction of respiratory tract mucosa

        g. Mast cell stabilizer nasal spray to prevent allergic response— cromolyn sodium (> 2 years) one spray intranasally 4 times/day

        h. Topical nasal corticosteroids to decrease immediate and late phase allergic reactions with reduction of influx of inflammatory cells; start about 1 to 2 weeks before allergy season

            (1) Beclomethasone—(> 6 years) by nasal inhalation

            (2) Flunisolide—(> 6 years) by nasal inhalation

    4. Referrals if symptoms not responsive to avoidance and/or medication

Head, Eye, Ear, Nose, Mouth and Throat Disorders ——— 197

a. Allergist for skin testing for possible long-term immunotherapy

b. Immunotherapy effective in relieving symptoms due to dust mites, animal dander, pollens, molds, insect stings and drug sensitivities

c. HEENT specialist for consultation and possible surgical interventions, e.g., myringotomy tubes

Chronic Rhinitis

- Definition: Chronic nasal discharge with or without acute exacerbations
- Etiology/Incidence

    a. May reflect underlying disorder e.g., nasal polyps, chronic sinusitis, chronically infected tonsils, cystic fibrosis, allergy, foreign body, deviated septum, congenital malformation, syphilis

    b. May result from prolonged topical nasal decongestant use

- Signs and Symptoms: Variable

    1. Foul smelling, nasal discharge

    2. Possible bloody discharge, e.g., with foreign body, syphilis

    3. Disturbances in taste and smell

    4. Fever with superimposed infection

- Differential Diagnosis: Allergic rhinitis
- Physical Findings

    1. Excoriation of anterior nares and upper lip

    2. Nasal discharge—usually clear

- Management/Treatment: Directed at underlying cause

    1. Antibiotic for bacterial infection

    2. Environmental controls to minimize exposure to allergens

    3. Special attention to nutritional status, rest and prevention of exposure to new infections

Foreign Body in Nose

- Definition: Foreign body in either nostril
- Etiology/Incidence: Common items include food, crayons, small toys, erasers, paper wads, beads, beans and stones, alkaline button batteries
- Signs and Symptoms

    1. Initial—sneezing, mild discomfort, rarely pain; can increase with time

    2. Infection usually follows—unilateral purulent, malodorous or bloody discharge is always suggestive of a foreign body

- Differential Diagnosis
    1. Nasal polyps, nasal tumors
    2. Purulent rhinitis, sinusitis
- Physical Findings
    1. Unilateral foul smelling nasal discharge
    2. Visualization of foreign body
- Diagnostics Tests/Findings: None usually; head mirror or light will provide visualization of object
- Management/Treatment
    1. Remove promptly with forceps or nasal suction
    2. Generally infection resolves after removal
    3. Referral to otolaryngologist if unable to remove

Epistaxis

- Definition: Bleeding from the nose
- Etiology/Incidence
    1. Most cases are benign and frequent in childhood due to increased vascularity of nasal mucosa
    2. Trauma and inflammation of mucosal lining (sudden onset) most common cause—nose picking, foreign body insertion, direct blunt trauma, violent sneezing
    3. Nasal mucosal drying (intermittent bleeding) from poorly humidified air, e.g., heating systems
    4. Chronic infection of nasal tissue—viral or bacterial
    5. Substance abuse, e.g., cocaine, cannabis
    6. Systemic diseases—consider with bleeding that is severe, prolonged or recurrent
        a. Hypertension—exacerbates problem
        b. Clotting abnormalities, e.g., hemophilia, aplastic anemia, leukemia, idiopathic thrombocytopenia, platelet dysfunction
        c. ASA and NSAID overuse, neoplasms (gradual onset), cancer treatments, hormonal influences, e.g., menses, birth control pills (BCP), pregnancy
- Signs and Symptoms
    1. Bleeding from nares—usually unilateral
    2. Tarry stools—occasionally with frequent bleeds
- Differential Diagnosis
    1. Foreign bodies

2. Infection

3. Substance abuse

4. Allergies

5. Chronic rhinitis

6. Chronic nasal spray use

- Physical Findings

  1. Determine location of bleeding

     a. Anterior bleed—most common site (90%) Kesselbach's plexus

     b. Posterior bleed—can see only if nose is normal, no inflammation and with special instruments; may see posterior oropharynx blood flow

     c. High nasal bleed—may represent nasoethmoid or orbit fracture

     d. Recurrent—consider bleeding disorder or chronic irritation

- Diagnostic Tests/Findings

  1. Stool for occult blood—determine if child is swallowing blood

  2. Roentgenograms, CBC with differential, platelets, PT, PTT; coagulation profile (if bleeding disorder is suspected)

- Management/Treatment

  1. Complete history including—recurrent or acute; unilateral or bilateral; duration; recent URI, allergic rhinitis; ASA or NSAID use; signs of underlying disease

  2. Monitor vital signs, especially blood pressure

  3. Apply pressure to anterior nasal septum with patient sitting in upright position with head tilted forward, (most stop within 10 to 15 minutes); application of ice; increase humidity of home; avoid nose blowing

  4. Antibiotics (topical and oral) may be indicated if infection is suggested

  5. Topical nasal vasoconstrictor drops (phenylephrine $\frac{1}{4}$% to $\frac{1}{2}$%) and packing may be needed

  6. Recurrent or severe cases—refer to otolaryngologist

Sinusitis

- Definition: Acute, subacute or chronic inflammation of mucosal lining in one or more of paranasal sinuses

- Etiology/Incidence

  1. Common pathogens (also commonly found in AOM)

     a. Predominately in acute sinusitis—*Streptococcus pneumoniae, Haemophilus influenzae* and *Moraxella catarrhalis*

b. Prevalent in chronic sinusitis are anaerobes (e.g., Group A beta hemolytic streptococcus and *Staphylococcus aureus*) due to low oxygen content and low pH of fluid

c. Viruses—less common

2. 5% to 10% of URIs in children develop into sinusitis

3. May be secondary to allergies, adenoidal hypertrophy, anatomical abnormalities, dental abscess, diving and swimming

4. Higher incidence in boys affecting maxillary and ethmoid sinuses

5. Maxillary and ethmoid sinuses most frequently involved

6. Acute sinusitis—persistent symptoms > 10 days and < one month

7. Chronic sinusitis—> 30 days

- Signs and Symptoms: Children have less specific complaints; adolescents usually present with classical symptoms

1. Persistent URI (beyond 7 to 10 days) with purulent or watery drainage

2. Cough, low grade fever

3. Facial pain, toothache, headache or tenderness over involved sinus

4. Postnasal drip, bad breath, sore throat

5. Increased pain with cough, bending over or abrupt head movement

6. Fatigue, malaise, anorexia

7. Periorbital swelling in morning

- Differential Diagnosis

1. Dental infections, cleft palate, foreign bodies, tumors and polyps, nasal trauma, malformations

2. Allergic and purulent rhinitis, common cold

3. Cystic fibrosis, immunodeficiency states, allergy, or asthma

- Physical Findings

1. Clear or mucopurulent rhinorrhea and/or postnasal drainage

2. Erythema of nasal mucosa and/or throat

3. Pain on percussion with possible erythema/edema in area of affected sinus

4. OME common finding—especially in younger child

- Diagnostic Tests/Findings

1. Nasal scrapings—eosinophils present with allergy

2. Roentgenography—rule out cysts, polyps, abscess

3. CT scan—used in complicated sinusitis, intraorbital and intracranial involvement, abscess and sinonasal neoplasms

- Management/Treatment
    1. Antibiotic therapy—same as used in AOM (see Table 1)
        a. To penetrate sinuses, need 14 to 21 days of treatment; up to 6 weeks in chronic cases
        b. Trimethoprim/sulfamethoxazole should not be used if group A streptococci is suspected
    2. Decongestants/antihistamines not proven effective except with concomitant allergic manifestations
    3. Comfort measures—analgesics, increased humidity, increase oral fluids
    4. Inflammation control with topical steroid nasal spray, e.g., beclomethasone
    5. Diving/swimming in moderation; consider elimination of activity with chronic cases
    6. Complications
        a. Intracranial complications—subdural empyema, brain abscess, sinus thrombosis
        b. Orbital cellulitis secondary to ethmoiditis (medical emergency)
    7. Refer to otolaryngologist and/or allergist for chronic sinusitis and allergy control

Nasal Polyps

- Definition: Benign pedunculated tumors
- Etiology/Incidence
    1. Originate from edematous, chronically inflamed nasal mucosa in ethmoid sinus
    2. Common in children with cystic fibrosis; 25% develop nasal polyps
- Signs and Symptoms
    1. Nasal obstruction
    2. Mouth breathing
- Differential Diagnosis
    1. Chronic sinusitis
    2. Cystic fibrosis
    3. Chronic allergic rhinitis
    4. Asthma
- Physical Findings
    1. Hyponasal obstruction

2. Profuse mucoid/mucopurulent rhinorrhea

3. Shiny grey, grape like mass(es) between nasal turbinates and septum

- Diagnostic Tests/Findings: Sweat test to rule out cystic fibrosis on every child with polyps

- Management/Treatment

    1. Care in distinguishing swollen turbinates from polyps

    2. Antihistamines if allergy related

    3. Local/systemic decongestants/corticosteroids not helpful

    4. Refer for surgical removal in those with complete obstruction or uncontrolled deformity

Mouth

Oral Candidiasis (Thrush)

- Definition: Common fungal infection of oral cavity

- Etiology/Incidence

    1. *Candida albicans* (monilial)

    2. More common in neonate and infant than in other age groups; (transmission during vaginal delivery)

    3. Predisposing factors

        a. Steroid therapy

        b. Antibiotic therapy

        c. Compromised immune system

    4. 50%–60% incidence (AAP, 2003)

- Signs and Symptoms: White patches in mouth

- Physical Findings

    1. Characteristic white, curd like adherent plaques that are not easily removed; found on the buccal mucosa, tongue, pharynx and/or tonsils

    2. Bleeding occurs with attempts to remove plaques

- Diagnostic Tests/Findings: Systemic/immune status evaluation if persistent or resistant to treatment

- Management/Treatment

    1. Antifungal therapy—nystatin oral suspension applied to oral mucosa 4 times/day for 10 days; if not responding, consider gentian violet application or fluconazole systemically in severe cases (AAP, 2003)

2. If breast feeding consider examining and treating mother for candidiasis of breast (cross-infection)

3. Check diaper area for concurrent diaper rash

4. Sterilize nipples, pacifiers if bottle fed; apply nystatin to nipples if breast feeding; if recurrent, look for other causes, e.g., H.I.V.

Cleft Lip/Palate

- Definition:
    1. Cleft lip—failure of embryonic structures surrounding oral cavity to join
    2. Cleft palate—failure of palatal shelves to fuse
    3. Occurs in various degrees

- Etiology/Incidence
    1. Genetic influence with cleft lip more than palate
    2. Both can occur sporadically
    3. More common to have combination of both than one without the other
    4. Cleft lip with or without palate—1:800 births
    5. Cleft palate alone—1:1,750 births
    6. More common in males, Asians and with maternal drug exposure
    7. Lower incidence in African-Americans
    8. Increase in middle ear/nasopharyngeal/sinus infections with associated hearing loss
    9. Recurrent otitis media is common

- Signs and Symptoms: Separation of lip and/or palate

- Differential Diagnosis: None

- Physical Findings
    1. Degree of cleft varies from small notch to complete separation
    2. Unilateral or bilateral
    3. Involves soft and/or hard palate
    4. Bifid uvula indicates submucosal cleft palate

- Diagnostic Test/Findings: Audiogram to rule out hearing deficit

- Management/Treatment
    1. Surgical repair; timing individualized—lip usually by 2 months, palate by 9 to 12 months
    2. Teach feeding techniques (breast or bottle) before and after repair
    3. Referral for dental restoration if needed

4. Referrals to otolaryngologist, plastic surgeon, pediatric dentist, prosthodontist, orthodontist, speech therapist, psychiatrist, social worker and genetic counselors

5. Support family adjustment and management

Dental Caries

- Definition: Demineralization of tooth surface secondary to production of organic acids by bacterial fermentation of dietary carbohydrates (Behrman, 2000)
- Etiology/Incidence
    1. Mutans streptococci are primary etiological organism responsible for human dental caries
    2. Rate of formation depends on frequency of acid environment in mouth; availability of fluoride for remineralization; oral hygiene
    3. Nursing bottle tooth decay (nursing caries)
        a. Tooth decay resulting from repeated/prolonged contact with milk, formula, or juice
        b. Children put to bed with bottle or sleep at the breast or use either the breast/bottle as pacifier are at increased risk
    4. Most pediatric dental caries occur on the occlusal surfaces of posterior and lingual aspect of the maxillary incisors, molars and cuspids
    5. New teeth are at greater risk for caries than established teeth
    6. Fluoride is critical in the process of remineralization
- Signs and Symptoms
    1. Sensitive or painful tooth
    2. Severe decay—pain, edema and infection
    3. Weight loss
    4. Feeding problems
- Physical Findings: Initial decalcification of enamel appears as opaque white spots that turn light brown progressing to dark brown with destruction of tooth
- Management/Treatment
    1. Prevention of dental caries/periodontal disease
        a. Well balanced diet with appropriate feeding practices; low sugar and complex carbohydrate consumption
        b. Wean from bottle, pacifier and breast at one year of age
        c. Brush/clean/wipe teeth as soon as they appear
        d. Daily brushing and flossing of teeth; for children under 8 years, parental involvement needed

      e. Fluoride supplement, dental sealants to occlusal surfaces of the posterior teeth

      f. Early dental visits—American Academy of Pediatric Dentists recommend starting dental visits at 12 to 18 months of age for initial discussion of oral hygiene, weaning and fluoride supplementation; routine dental checkups starting at 3 years

   2. Dental referral for identified caries

Aphthous Ulcers (Canker Sores)

- Definition: Shallow, painful mouth ulceration
- Etiology/Incidence
  1. Usually affects oral mucosa on ventral surface of tongue, soft palate, buccal mucosa or floor of mouth; occasionally may affect other body tissues
  2. Idiopathic
  3. Precipitated by trauma, stress, sun, allergies, endocrine or hematologic disorders
  4. Onset often in adolescence (20%) and recurrent
  5. "Minor"—1 to 5 lesions, 1 cm, lasting 7 to 14 days
  6. "Major"—10% of cases greater than 1 cm, lasting 6 weeks
- Signs and Symptoms
  1. Burning or tingling before appearance of lesion
  2. Pain at lesion site
  3. Afebrile
- Differential Diagnosis
  1. Herpetic lesions (simplex zoster)
  2. Herpangina (coxsackievirus A)
  3. Trauma
  4. Chemical burns
  5. Hand, foot and mouth disease (coxsackievirus A5, A10, A16)
- Physical Findings
  1. Single or multiple, small, oval, indurated papules with erythematous halo, develops pale center that erodes into ulcers
  2. No systemic symptoms
- Diagnostic Test/Findings: None
- Management/Treatment
  1. Oral analgesics, e.g., 6 to 12 years use chloraseptic spray; greater than 12 years use viscous xylocaine solution

2. Antibacterial (tetracycline) rinses may shorten disease course in children > 9 years of age

3. Referral pediatric dentist if condition lasts more than 14 days

Herpes Labialis (Cold Sore, Fever Blister) and Herpes Simplex Stomatitis

- Definition
  1. Ulceration and inflammation of oral mucosa
  2. Acute primary herpetic gingivostomatitis (APHGS) occurs in previously unexposed children

- Etiology/Incidence
  1. Virus acquired from individual who has mouth sore or herpetic whitlow on a finger or toe; caused by Herpes Simplex Virus 1 (HSV1)
  2. Illness starts 5 to 10 day after exposure
  3. Spontaneous recovery in 7 to 10 days
  4. 50% develop subsequent cold sore episodes after primary acute episode
  5. Oral recurrence—one to several lesions with local pain for 3 to 7 days

- Signs and Symptoms
  1. May be asymptomatic especially cold sores/fever blisters
  2. Initial symptoms include fever, chills, irritability, tender submandibular adenopathy, ulcerative exanthem of the gingiva and mucous membranes of the mouth (AAP, 2003)
  3. Sore throat, burning in mouth and throat
  4. Anorexia from pain; could lead to dehydration

- Differential Diagnosis
  1. Aphthous ulcers
  2. Hand, foot and mouth syndrome
  3. Herpangina

- Physical Findings
  1. Cold sores—grouped vesicles on erythematous base; commonly found on mucocutaneous border of lips
  2. Primary gingivostomatitis—vesicles on oral mucosa, gingiva, tongue, and lips; ulcer formation following vesicle stage
  3. Cervical adenopathy with gingivostomatitis
  4. May spread to perioral skin

- Diagnostic Tests/Findings: None
- Management/Treatment
    1. "Over the counter" (OTC) cold sore treatment
    2. Pain management—acetaminophen or ibuprofen; topical relief with occlusive gels, e.g., infant oral anesthetic agents; 1:1 mixture of diphenhydramine combined with antacid preparations consisting of magnesium and aluminum hydroxide *or* anti-diarrheal preparations to provide a protective coating for the oral mucosa (severe cases add 2% viscous lidocaine sparingly)
    3. Spontaneous recovery

Hand, Foot, and Mouth Disease

- Definition: Acute viral illness presenting with vesicular enanthem on tongue, gums, palate, oral mucosa; papulovesicular exanthem on hands, feet, legs and occasionally the buttocks
- Etiology/Incidence
    1. Coxsackievirus A16 (most common), A5 and A10
    2. Enterovirus 71—severe illness (aseptic meningitis, encephalitis, paralytic disease common)
    3. Seasonal, predominant in summer and fall
    4. Incubation 4 to 6 days
    5. Spontaneous resolution in one week
- Signs and Symptoms
    1. Fever
    2. Anorexia
    3. Dysphagia
    4. Vomiting
- Differential Diagnosis
    1. Acute primary herpetic gingivostomatitis
    2. Aphthous stomatitis, herpangina
    3. Trauma, burns
- Physical Findings
    1. Small vesicles erode to ulcers on buccal mucosa, hard palate, tonsils, and tongue
    2. Vesicular lesions appear as blanching red lesions on arms, legs, palms, soles and occasionally buttocks

- Diagnostic Tests/Findings: Unnecessary
- Management/Treatment: See Herpangina

Herpangina

- Definition: Acute viral illness presenting with ulceration and inflammation of oral mucosa
- Etiology/Incidence
    1. Coxsackievirus, group A (most common)
    2. Coxsackie B viruses and echoviruses (less common)
    3. Seasonal in U.S.—predominant in summer months
    4. Resolves spontaneously in 3 to 5 days
- Signs and Symptoms
    1. Fever in moderate range
    2. Headache, myalgia, malaise
    3. Dysphagia, vomiting (25%), anorexia, significant oral discomfort, drooling
- Differential Diagnosis
    1. Acute primary herpetic gingivostomatitis
    2. Aphthous stomatitis
    3. Trauma or burns
    4. Hand, foot and mouth disease
- Physical Findings: Small vesicles or punched-out ulcers, especially on soft palate and tonsillar pillars
- Diagnostic Tests/Findings: Unnecessary
- Management/Treatment
    1. Fever and/or pain control—acetaminophen, ibuprofen
    2. Topical relief with 1:1 mixture of diphenhydramine combined with antacid preparations consisting of magnesium and aluminum hydroxide *or* anti-diarrheal preparations to provide a protective coating for the oral mucosa (severe cases add 2% viscous lidocaine; use sparingly)
    3. Encourage fluids to ensure adequate hydration

Throat

Pharyngitis and Tonsillitis

- Definition: Acute inflammation and infection of the throat; when tonsils are main focus of inflammation, tonsillitis is more appropriate term to use

- Etiology/Incidence

  1. Causes vary by geographic location, season, age, and amount/time of exposure; most common in 5 to 15-year-olds

  2. Viruses

     a. Virus is probable cause in conjunction with nasal congestion and rhinorrhea

     b. Adenovirus (12 types) account for 23% of cases

     c. Epstein-Barr virus

     d. Influenza A and B, RSV, parainfluenza virus, cytomegalovirus, rotavirus

     e. Enteroviruses (e.g., coxsackievirus A and echovirus) seen in summer and fall

  3. Bacteria

     a. Group A beta hemolytic streptococcus (GABHS) account for 10 to 15% of all pharyngitis cases; typically occurs in winter and spring

     b. *Haemophilus influenzae*—less common with use of HIB vaccine

     c. *Neisseria gonorrhoeae*—in sexually active adolescents or sexually abused children

     d. *Corynebacterium haemolyticum* and *Corynebacterium diphtheriae*—characteristic presence of grey pseudomembranous exudate on pharynx and tonsils which bleeds with attempts at removal; quite rare in U.S.; still seen in undeveloped countries

  4. Other causes

     a. *Mycoplasma pneumoniae*—5% of cases in school age children

     b. Fungal—*Candida albicans*

     c. Parasites

     d. Streptococcal toxin postulated as cause of Kawasaki

  5. Noninfectious causes (nearly 50% of cases)

     a. Trauma from tobacco smoke, heat, alcohol

     b. Allergic rhinitis or postnasal drainage

  6. Transmission—through exposure to infected respiratory secretions, shared silverware and occasionally household pets

  7. Complications

     a. Peritonsillar or retropharyngeal abscess or cellulitis

     b. Cervical adenitis, AOM, sinusitis, pneumonia

     c. Acute rheumatic fever in untreated group A beta hemolytic streptococcal pharyngitis—prevented if treatment started within 9 days of initial complaints of sore throat

d. Glomerulonephritis—host/immune response to nonrenal infection with GABHS; not all strains are nephritogenic; manifests in 1 to 3 weeks after pharyngeal or skin infection of GABHS; unrelated to treatment

- Signs and Symptoms: Common symptomatology with some variability by causative organism

    1. Sudden or gradual onset of symptoms

    2. Sore throat

    3. Fever, variable

    4. Headache, anorexia, occasional nausea, vomiting, abdominal pain and malaise

    5. Viral pharyngitis—hoarseness, conjunctivis, runny nose, cough, cold symptoms

    6. GABHS pharyngitis—usually seen at 2 years of age and older, sudden onset of fever with complaints of headache, abdominal pain and vomiting; rash, "strawberry tongue" may be present

- Differential Diagnosis

    1. Stomatitis

    2. Peritonsillar or retropharyngeal abscess, epiglottitis

    3. Allergic rhinitis, postnasal drainage

- Physical Findings

    1. Erythema of pharynx, petechial lesions with or without ulcer formation; petechial lesions on uvula and soft palate common with GABHS

    2. Enlarged tonsils with exudate (occurs in $\frac{1}{3}$ of those with GABHS)

    3. Erythema of nasal mucosa with coryza

    4. Cervical nodes usually enlarged with possible tenderness

- Diagnostic Tests/Findings

    1. Rapid strep test to determine presence of GABHS

        a. 70% to 85% sensitivity; 95% specificity

        b. Treat if positive; throat culture to confirm negative test

    2. CBC—WBC elevated with bacterial infection; decreased with viral agent

    3. Consider other studies—dependent on history, age and clinical presentation, e.g., mono spot, EBV, culture for gonorrhoeae, diphtheria culture

- Management/Treatment

    1. Viral pharyngitis/tonsillitis—symptomatic/supportive care

        a. Saline gargles, throat lozenges

        b. Analgesics for fever/pain (acetaminophen, ibuprofen)

    c. Encourage fluids for maintaining hydration

  2. Bacterial pharyngitis/tonsillitis

    a. GABHS—penicillin drug of choice, 125 to 250 mg every eight hours for 10 days or IM Penicillin G Benzathine (600,00 U for less than 60 pounds, 1.2 million U for greater than 60 pounds); erythromycin or first generation cephlosporin for those with penicillin allergy; communicability is eliminated after 24 hours of antibiotic therapy

    b. Second line therapy include macrolides, cephalosprins, or clindamycin

    c. Gonococcal pharyngitis—one IM injection of ceftriaxone

    d. Diphtheria—hospitalization and treatment with erythromycin or penicillin G

    e. *Mycoplasma pneumoniae*—erythromycin for 10 days

Acute Nasopharyngitis (Common Cold)

- Definition: Acute viral infection of upper respiratory tract with potential involvement of nasal passages, sinuses, eustachian tubes, middle ears, conjunctiva and nasopharynx

- Etiology/Incidence

  1. Causative pathogens

    a. Over 100 infectious pathogens—respiratory syncytial virus (RSV) most common

    b. Other common pathogens include parainfluenza viruses, corona viruses, adeno-viruses, enterovirus, influenza viruses, *Mycoplasma pneumoniae (Behrman, 2000)*

  2. Pathogen shed in large amounts through nasal secretions and easily spread through self-inoculation from fingers and hands to objects (clothing, environmental surfaces)

  3. Universal susceptibility; children average 5 to 8 infections/year with a peak incidence during first 2 years

  4. Increased susceptability associated with active/passive smoke exposure

  5. More frequent in crowded situations

  6. Occurrence in cooler months in temperate climates—peaks in early fall, late January and early April

- Signs and Symptoms: Generally last one week; dry cough with mild runny nose, may persist up to 3 weeks

  1. Infants

    a. Irritability, restlessness, fever (100° to 102° F)

    b. Rhinorrhea

    c. Occasional diarrhea

    d. Changes in feeding and sleep patterns

2. Older children
    a. Afebrile or low grade fever, stuffy nose, watery nasal discharge
    b. Sore throat, sneezing, cough, chills
    c. Occasional headache, malaise

- Differential Diagnosis
    1. Underlying secondary bacterial infection—sinusitis, O.M., pharyngitis, lower respiratory tract disease
    2. Allergic rhinitis
    3. Foreign body
    4. Substance abuse in older children and adolescents, or overuse of medicated nasal spray

- Physical Findings
    1. Coryza
    2. Inflamed, moist nasal mucosa and oropharynx
    3. Chest clear

- Diagnostic Tests/Findings
    1. Viral cultures expensive; generally unnecessary
    2. If suspicious of differential diagnosis, consider throat and nose culture, drug screen

- Management/Treatment: Symptomatic/supportive care
    1. Analgesics for sore throat, muscle aches and fever > 101° F
    2. Relief of nasal congestion
        a. Saline nose drops ($\frac{1}{4}$ tsp. table salt with 6 oz water); 3 drops each nostril, wait several minutes, gentle aspiration with nasal bulb syringe
        b. Cool mist humidification
        c. Antibiotics, antihistamines and decongestants not recommended in the young child and infant
        d. Older children and adolescents receive symptomatic relief with decongestant and antihistamine use
    3. If symptoms persistent beyond 7 to 10 days, consider secondary infection
    4. Maintain hydration; also helps to liquefy secretions
    5. Prevention
        a. Good hygiene and cleaning of clothes, toys and play areas
        b. Limited exposure to crowded situations

Retropharyngeal Abscess

- Definition: Inflammation of posterior aspect of pharynx with suppurative retropharyngeal lymph nodes
- Etiology
    1. Causative pathogens—GABHS (most common), anaerobic organisms; *Staphylococcus aureus*
    2. In older children—usually superinfection from penetrating injury to posterior wall of oropharynx
    3. Possible complication of bacterial pharyngitis
    4. Relatively rare infection; most common in children under 4 years of age secondary to untreated pyogenic adenitis
- Signs and Symptoms
    1. Acute onset of high fever with persistent severe throat pain
    2. Drooling due to difficulty in swallowing
    3. Tachypnea, dyspnea, stridor
    4. Neck and head hyperextension
- Differential Diagnosis
    1. Epiglottitis
    2. Peritonsillar abscess
    3. Laryngotracheobronchitis (croup)
    4. Acute infectious mononucleosis
    5. Acute pharyngitis
    6. Bacterial tracheitis
    7. Meningitis
- Physical findings
    1. Toxic appearing child; neck and head in hyperextension
    2. Noisy, gurgling respiration
    3. Drooling, meningismus
    4. Stridor, airway obstruction
    5. Prominent swelling of posterior pharyngeal wall—confirms diagnosis
- Diagnostic Tests/Findings
    1. Lateral neck radiography—retropharyngeal space wider than C4 vertebral body
    2. CBC—elevated WBC

3. Computed tomography (CT) scan to visualize abscess

- Management/Treatment

  1. **Immediate and emergency referral to ENT**

  2. Emergency hospitalization necessary

     a. Admission to pediatric ICU for continuous monitoring for airway obstruction and possible respiratory arrest

     b. Surgical incision and drainage necessary

     c. Intravenous (IV) antibiotics—penicillin, clindamycin

Peritonsillar Abscess

- Definition: Infection of tonsils spreading to tonsillar fossa and surrounding tissues (peritonsillar cellulitis); if left untreated, tonsillar abscess forms

- Etiology/Incidence

  1. GABHS (most common)

  2. *Staphylococcus aureus,* anaerobic microorganisms

  3. Can occur at any age; more common in preadolescent or adolescent age groups

  4. Complication of untreated peritonsillar abscess—lateral pharyngeal abscess leading to possible airway obstruction; aggressive early treatment will prevent suppuration

- Signs and Symptoms

  1. Severe sore throat with high fever

  2. Toxic appearance, muffled voice, spasms of jaw muscles

  3. Difficulty swallowing and drooling in severe cases

  4. Bad breath

- Differential Diagnosis

  1. Retropharyngeal abscess

  2. Epiglottitis

- Physical Findings

  1. Unilateral enlargement of tonsil(s), bulging medially with anterior pillar prominence (most common)

  2. Soft palate and uvula edematous, erythematous, displaced towards unaffected side

  3. Extreme tonsillar tenderness on palpation

- Diagnostic Tests

  1. CBC—increased WBC

  2. Rapid strep test to rule out GABHS

- Management/Treatment
    1. **Immediate referral to ENT**
    2. Surgical incision and drainage often necessary
    3. Possible need for hospitalization
    4. Antibiotics (Penicillin), IM, IV or by mouth
    5. If not hospitalized, daily follow up visits until stable

Cervical Lymphadenitis

- Definition: Inflammation affecting one or more cervical lymph nodes
- Etiology/Incidence
    1. Pathogens
        a. *Streptococcus pyogenes* and *Staphylococcus aureus* account for approximately 80% of cases
        b. *Mycobacterium tuberculosis*
        c. Other organisms (e.g., viral, fungal or parasitic)
    2. Secondary to local infections of the ear, nose and throat (most common)
    3. Prevalent among preschool children
- Signs and Symptoms
    1. Complaints of swollen neck or face
    2. Fever
    3. Stridor, hoarseness, drooling if adenopathy impinges on airway
- Differential Diagnosis
    1. Bilateral cervical adenitis—mononucleosis, tularemia, diphtheria
    2. Subacute or chronic adenitis—cat scratch fever, nonspecific viral infections
    3. Atypical mycobacterium—tuberculosis
    4. Cervical node tumors, e.g., leukemia, neurofibromatosis
    5. Mumps, cyst, hematoma
- Physical Findings
    1. Large unilateral cervical mass, greater than 2 to 6 cm
    2. Erythema may be present
    3. Extreme tenderness on palpation
- Diagnostic Tests/Findings
    1. CBC—moderate to marked WBC

2. Mantoux test—rule out tuberculosis

3. Mono spot—rule out mononucleosis

4. Throat culture—rule out GABHS

5. Serology tests if not resolving (e.g., EBV, toxoplasmosis, CMV, histoplasmosis)

6. Aspiration of node if fluctuant—aerobic/anaerobic culture

- Management/Treatment

    1. With no evidence of sepsis, treat empirically with oral antibiotics— dicloxacillin, amoxicillin clavulanate, or cephalexin for a minimum of 10 days and no less than 5 days after resolution of symptoms

    2. Measure and follow size of node

    3. Analgesics for fever and pain; application of cold compresses

    4. Re-evaluation after 36 to 48 hours; if no improvement, possible hospitalization for IV antibiotics, especially with infants and young children

    5. Referral to otolaryngologist if not improving

    6. Surgical aspiration may be necessary

    7. Persistent unexplained, symptomatic node, increasing in size despite treatment, refer for biopsy

Epiglottitis (Supraglottitis)

- Definition: Severe, rapidly developing inflammation and swelling of the supraglottic structures leading to life threatening upper airway obstruction

- Etiology/Incidence

    1. Pathogens—group A beta-hemolytic streptococci, pneumococci, *Haemophilus influenzae*

    2. Can occur at any age, highest incidence 2 to 7 years of age

    3. Decreasing incidence from *Haemophilus influenzae* with use of HIB vaccine by 99% in children under 5 years (AAP, 2003)

- Signs and Symptoms

    1. Acute, sudden onset of high fever, severe sore throat, muffled voice, drooling, poor color, labored breathing in a previously well child

    2. Choking sensation, refuses to speak

    3. Restless, irritable, anxious, apprehensive, frightened

    4. Hyperextension of neck, leaning forward and chin thrust out, prostration; ''sniffing dog'' or tripod position—provides best possible airway

- Differential Diagnosis

    1. Acute laryngeal edema, croup syndrome, foreign body aspiration

2. Pertussis, diphtheria, Kawasaki syndrome

3. Bacterial tracheitis, retropharyngeal abscess

- Physical Findings

  1. Rapidly progressive respiratory distress—suprasternal and subcostal, soft inspiratory stridor, nasal flaring leading to possible respiratory arrest

  2. Toxic, distressed appearance

  3. Beefy erythematous epiglottis

  4. If epiglottitis suspected, do not attempt to visualize

- Diagnostic Tests/Findings: Often deferred to minimize distress

  1. CBC—WBC (greater than 18,800); laboratory examination is low priority in child with severe respiratory distress

  2. Cultures of blood, tracheal or epiglottis secretions—50% of cases, positive for *Haemophilus influenzae* type b

  3. Radiograph—lateral neck shows a thickened/swollen epiglottis ("thumb sign"); may elect not to perform radiograph due to possibility of airway obstruction and respiratory arrest; airway can be safely visualized in surgery

- Management/Treatment

  1. **Requires prompt recognition and treatment; represents a true medical emergency; death can occur within hours**

  2. While waiting for emergency transport, provide oxygen, keep child calm, be prepared for emergency cardiopulmonary resuscitation

  3. Following diagnosis, airway must be established by nasotracheal or endotracheal intubation or elective tracheotomy immediately; usually extubated within 24 to 48 hours after reducing epiglottis and afebrile

  4. IV antibiotic therapy for 2 to 3 days

     a. Third generation cephalosporins until initial pathogen identified

     b. In areas with penicillin and cephalosporin resistant pneumococci, vancomycin is drug of choice

  5. Oral antibiotic to follow IV to complete 10 day course

  6. Coricosteroid therapy to reduce swelling

  7. Prevention—*Haemophilus influenzae type b* vaccine at 2, 4, 6 or 12 and 15 months of age; no vaccines against other pathogens

Questions
Select the best answer

1. Which of the following would not alert you to microcephaly?

   a. Prominent sutures
   b. Early closure of anterior fontanel
   c. Normocephalic skull
   d. Severe malnutrition

2. When diagnosing an infant with microcephaly, an inappropriate differential diagnosis may be:

   a. Craniosynostosis
   b. Hyperthyroidism
   c. Hypopituitarism
   d. Severe malnutrition

3. At the 6 month well-child visit, you note another increase of 2 SD on the head circumference growth chart which is similar to the increase at the 4 month visit. Which of the following would not be considered a possible cause?

   a. Hydrocephalus
   b. Metabolic/genetic disorder
   c. Benign familial macrocephaly
   d. Hypothyroidism

4. Appropriate treatment of this 6-month-old would not consider:

   a. Waiting until 9 month visit to see if intervention is needed
   b. Ultrasound through anterior fontanel
   c. Referral to neurologist
   d. Referral for genetic counseling

5. A newborn presents with swelling of soft tissue of the scalp which crosses the suture lines with bruising. You suspect:

   a. Cephalohematoma
   b. Child abuse
   c. Caput succedaneum
   d. Hydrocephalus

6. In treating this infant you will need to order:

   a. Nothing, as it will resolve spontaneously
   b. Phototherapy to prevent hyperbilirubinemia
   c. Referral for drainage of lesion
   d. Skull radiographs to rule out fracture

7. Which of the following would not be included in management of cephalohematoma?

    a. No intervention needed
    b. Explain to parents, the hematoma may calcify but will eventually resolve
    c. Observe for hyperbilirubinemia
    d. May need to tap and drain hematoma

8. Which of the following would not be included in the management of hydrocephalus on an infant with macrocephaly, bulging anterior fontanel and separated suture lines?

    a. Complete history with referral for surgical treatment ASAP
    b. Treatment of underlying cause
    c. Order ultrasound of head
    d. Monitor head circumference every day for 1 to 2 weeks, then consider referral if needed

9. The appropriate time to refer an infant for intermittent esotropia would be:

    a. At four weeks
    b. At six months or just over
    c. Not until nine months
    d. Not until twelve months

10. Which of the following would not be included in treatment of a hordeolum?

    a. Warm moist compresses for 15 minutes throughout the day
    b. Incision and drainage
    c. Topical antibiotic eye drops
    d. Diphenhydramine for 72 hours

11. Joey (30-months-old) presents with headache, rhinorrhea, fever of 103.8° F, erythema, edema of the right eye lid, conjunctival chemosis, proptosis and decreased ocular movements. You would suspect:

    a. Periorbital cellulitis
    b. Orbital cellulitis
    c. Insect bite or trauma
    d. Acute bacterial conjunctivitis

12. Astigmatism is defined as:

    a. Nearsightedness
    b. Each eye has different refractive errors
    c. Curvature variation of the optical system
    d. Decreased vision in an eye from disuse

13. Which of the following eye disorders would not need a referral to an ophthalmologist?

    a. Pseudostrabismus
    b. Nystagmus in a 9-month-old infant

c. Nasal lacrimal duct stenosis in a 6-month-old

d. Cataracts

14. Signs and symptoms of bacterial conjunctivitis would not include:

a. Mucopurulent discharge

b. Foreign body sensation

c. Cobblestone appearing conjunctiva

d. "Fire red" palpebral conjunctiva

15. Absence of the red reflex usually indicates:

a. Cataract

b. Glaucoma

c. Astigmatism

d. Iritis

16. The cover/uncover test is used for detecting:

a. Nystagmus

b. Cataracts

c. Strabismus

d. Astigmatism

17. Which of the following ocular injuries would not need immediate referral?

a. Chemical burns

b. Corneal abrasions

c. Hyphema

d. Perforation wound to orbit

18. The drug of choice for the treatment of chlamydial conjunctivitis in the newborn is:

a. Systemic penicillin G 50,000 U/kg/day for 10 days

b. Ceftriaxone 25 to 50 mg/kg/day given once

c. Sodium sulfacetamide 10% ophthalmic solution 4 times a day for 21 days

d. Erythromycin 50 mg/kg/day 4 times a day for 14 days

19. Unilateral or bilateral purulent discharge and erythema of conjunctiva is most likely indicative of:

a. Chemical conjunctivitis

b. Bacterial conjunctivitis

c. Herpes simplex keratoconjunctivitis

d. Vernal conjunctivitis

20. A 10-year-old child presents with a non-tender, irritating mass in the left upper eye lid. This best describes a:

a. Hordeolum

b. Chalazion
c. Foreign body
d. Corneal abrasion

21. Which of the following is not included in this child's treatment?

a. Immediate referral for surgical removal
b. Warm compresses 2 to 3 times a day for 3 days
c. Local antibiotic eye drops
d. Corticosteroid injections

22. The most effective way to prevent spread of conjunctivitis among children and staff in day care settings is to:

a. Cleanse eye secretions with sterile cotton balls
b. Disinfect toys
c. Isolate the infected child until antibiotic therapy is completed
d. Use good hand washing technique

23. When performing the corneal light reflex assessment in a 12-month-old, the light reflected in the left eye is at 2 o'clock; light in right eye is at 12 o'clock. You would not:

a. Consider this a normal finding
b. Refer for further evaluation
c. Perform the cover/uncover test
d. Document this as an abnormal finding

24. The refractive error that occurs when light is focused in front of the retina is known as:

a. Astigmatism
b. Hyperopia
c. Myopia
d. Anisometropia

25. Which of the following clinical findings would not be seen in children with strabismus?

a. Head tilting
b. Face turning
c. School problems
d. Rhythmic eye movements

26. The following statement is false about glaucoma:

a. Anomaly of ocular drainage system
b. May follow eye disease
c. Occurs bilaterally in 25% of cases
d. Associated with congenital rubella

27. Which of following are not included in the classic triad of symptoms in glaucoma?

    a. Photophobia
    b. Epiphora
    c. Blepharospasm
    d. Persistent pain (most of the time)

28. Which of the following would not be included in the primary management of glaucoma?

    a. Instillation of anti-glaucoma drops
    b. Warn parents that blindness is inevitable
    c. Immediate referral to an ophthalmologist for diagnosis and treatment
    d. Enucleation

29. The first clue a child may have primary blindness would be the presence of:

    a. A history of prematurity
    b. Strabismus beyond 6 months
    c. Nystagmus
    d. Pigmented deposits on pupil

30. Based on your knowledge of amoxicillin oral suspension which is supplied in 400 mg/5 ml concentration with recommended dose being 40 mg/kg/day divided 2 times a day, you would order the following for Jeremy (45 pounds)?

    a. 1 tsp. orally b.i.d. for 10 days
    b. 1-$\frac{1}{4}$ tsp. orally b.i.d. for 10 days
    c. 1-$\frac{3}{4}$ tsp. orally b.i.d. for 10 days
    d. 2 tsp. orally b.i.d. for 10 days

31. Why are infants and young children predisposed to development of otitis media?

    a. Immaturity of immune mechanisms and eustachian tube is short and horizontal
    b. Eustachian tubes are long, narrow and curved
    c. The cartilage lining of the ear is undeveloped making the eustachian tube less expandable
    d. The lack of lymphoid tissue in pharynx increases vulnerability to infection

32. Sarah, age 6 years, weighing 50 pounds, presents with a history of URI and is complaining of pain in the left ear. On exam, the left ear reveals thickened bulging erythematous TM, absent light reflex, and poor mobility with pneumatic otoscopy. She has a history of penicillin allergy. Your first line antibiotic would be:

    a. Azithromycin
    b. Amoxicillin
    c. Amoxicillin/clavulanate
    d. No antibiotic is indicated with these findings

33. A tympanogram provides direct information on:

    a. Conductive hearing function

b. Tympanic membrane mobility
c. Semicircular canals fluid levels
d. Pressure in the inner ear

34. Which of the following is not a characteristic of "swimmer's ear"?

   a. Erythema and exudate of the ear canal
   b. Pruritus of ear canal
   c. Pain upon movement of the tragus
   d. Decreased hearing secondary to TM perforation

35. Your management of external otitis media would be:

   a. Neomycin/polymyxin/corticosteroid otic suspension
   b. Amoxicillin 40 mg/kg/day b.i.d. for 10 days
   c. Nothing at this time; recheck in 2 to 4 weeks
   d. Vinegar and alcohol (1:1) solution, 3 to 4 drops before and after swimming until the infection is resolved

36. The most common bacteria found with otitis media is:

   a. *Haemophilus influenza*
   b. *Streptococcus pneumoniae*
   c. *Moraxella catarrhalis*
   d. *Streptococcus pyogenes*

37. Which of the following should not be taught as preventive ear hygiene?

   a. Encouragement of supine positioning during feedings
   b. Encouragement of breast feeding
   c. Weaning off bedtime bottles
   d. Cessation of smoking around children

38. Which of the following ear disorders does not need an otolaryngologist referral?

   a. Cholesteatoma
   b. Persistent/acute O.M. unresponsive to treatment over 1 to 2 months
   c. Persistent chronic O.M.E. for 8 weeks
   d. Evidence of hearing loss and/or language delay

39. A language delay is noted in a 5-year-old child who has had repeated episodes of middle ear effusion. Among the following, the most likely cause of the delay is:

   a. Attention deficit hyperactivity disorder
   b. Conductive hearing loss
   c. Mental retardation
   d. Sensorineural hearing loss

40. Which of the following would not be associated with acquired conductive hearing loss?

    a. Perforated T.M.
    b. Otitis media with effusion
    c. Impacted cerumen
    d. Meningitis

41. Which of the following is not a common complication of acute nasopharyngitis?

    a. Otitis media
    b. Sinusitis
    c. Nasal polyps
    d. Allergic rhinitis

42. A 4-year-old presents with seasonal symptoms of allergic rhinitis. Which of the following is likely to be among the most common allergens for this child?

    a. Dust mite
    b. Mold
    c. Inhaled pollens
    d. Animal dander

43. Which of the following is not a common physical finding with this 4-year-old with allergic rhinitis?

    a. Allergic ''shiner's''
    b. Hypertrophy of gingival mucosa
    c. Purulent nasal discharge
    d. Edema of nasal mucosa

44. The most common cause of epistaxis is:

    a. Trauma
    b. Mucosal irritation (e.g. nose picking)
    c. Mucosal drying
    d. Foreign body

45. Which of the following is not a common cause of sinusitis?

    a. *Haemophilus influenzae*
    b. Adenovirus
    c. *Streptococcus pneumoniae*
    d. *Staphylococcus aureus*

46. A 15-year-old presents with rhinorrhea for 14 days, headache, halitosis, cough, fever and some facial pain. You suspect:

    a. Acute nasopharyngitis
    b. Sinusitis

    c. Seasonal allergies

    d. Cocaine use

47. Which of the following would not be included in the care of the adolescent with chronic sinusitis?

    a. Nasal cultures

    b. Local steroid nasal spray

    c. Referral to allergist and/or otolaryngologist

    d. Prophylactic antibiotic for 1 to 2 months after infection is resolved

48. Which of the following would not support the diagnosis of herpangina?

    a. Vesicles and/or ulcers present on the posterior oral cavity

    b. Fever

    c. Blisters on the lips

    d. Headache and backache

49. A common opportunistic fungal infection of the oral cavity is known as:

    a. Oral candidiasis

    b. Herpangina

    c. Hand, foot and mouth disease

    d. Herpes labialis

50. Which of the following disorders of the mouth does not present with vesicles?

    a. Herpangina

    b. Hand, foot and mouth disease

    c. Oral candidiasis

    d. Herpes labialis

51. Destruction of tooth enamel occurs from:

    a. Acid demineralization

    b. Alkaline demineralization

    c. Fluoride treatments

    d. Hypercalcification

52. In counseling a new mother about her infant with a cleft lip, which of the following choices would not be included?

    a. Surgical repair by 9 to 12 months

    b. Feeding techniques

    c. Referral to otolaryngologist

    d. Referral to pediatric dentist

53. Which statement is true about cleft lip and palate?

    a. Genetics has no influence on either condition

b. It is more common to have both than one without the other

c. They are more common in females

d. There is a higher incidence in African-Americans

54. Shallow, painful ulcers in the mouth that can be brought on by stress and/or trauma and considered idiopathic are:

a. Herpetic lesions

b. Aphthous ulcers

c. Herpangina

d. Coxsackievirus

55. The most common cause of pharyngitis in the young child is:

a. Influenza virus, serotypes A + B

b. Epstein-Barr virus

c. Adenovirus

d. Enterovirus

56. Group A beta hemolytic streptococcus accounts for _____ of all pharyngitis cases.

a. 75%

b. 50%

c. 10 to 15%

d. 5%

57. A 7-year-old male presents with an abrupt onset of high fever, stridor, drooling and hyperextension of the neck. Which of the following would you not suspect:

a. Epiglottitis

b. GABHS pharyngitis

c. Peritonsillar abscess

d. Retropharyngeal abscess

58. With examination of the throat, one tonsil is much larger than the other with marked erythema and displaced uvula. You suspect:

a. Epiglottitis

b. Peritonsillar abscess

c. Retropharyngeal abscess

d. Sinus abscess

59. Which of the following would not be included in the differential diagnosis for cervical lymphadenitis?

a. Infectious mononucleosis

b. Cat scratch fever

c. Mumps

d. Measles

60. One of the most common organisms found in cervical adenitis is:

    a. *Haemophilus influenzae*
    b. *Staphylococcus aureus*
    c. *Mycobacterium tuberculosis*
    d. Anaerobic organisms

61. To avoid the complications of GABHS including rheumatic fever and glomerulonephritis, the antibiotic of choice is:

    a. Penicillin
    b. Cephalosporins
    c. Cyclosporins
    d. Sulfatrim

62. Which of the following would not be appropriate management of epistaxis?

    a. Local compression of nares, position in upright position with head held forward
    b. Local compression of nares, position in supine position
    c. Local nasal phenylephrine HCL
    d. Referral to otolaryngologist for persistent profuse bleeding

Answers

1. c	21. a	42. c	
2. b	22. d	43. c	
3. d	23. a	44. b	
4. a	24. c	45. b	
5. c	25. d	46. b	
6. a	26. c	47. d	
7. d	27. d	48. c	
8. d	28. b	49. a	
9. b	29. c	50. c	
10. d	30. a	51. a	
11. b	31. a	52. a	
12. c	32. a	53. b	
13. a	33. b	54. b	
14. c	34. d	55. c	
15. a	35. a	56. c	
16. c	36. b	57. b	
17. b	37. a	58. b	
18. d	38. c	59. d	
19. b	39. b	60. b	
20. b	40. d	61. a	
	41. c	62. b	

Bibliography

Altemeier, W. (2001). The importance of adenoviral infections in pediatrics. *Pediatric Annals*, 30(8), 439–440.

Ambati, B. K., Ambati, J., Azar, N., Stratton, L., & Schmidt, E. V. (2001). Periorbital and orbital cellulitis before and after the advent of Haemophilus influenza type b vaccination. *Ophthalmology*, 8(9), 1514–1515.

American Academy of Pediatrics. In L. K. Pickering (Ed.). *Red Book 2003: Report of the committee on infectious diseases* (26th ed.). Elk Grove Village, IL.

Bhatti, T. R., Dott, M., Yoon, P. W., Moore, C. A., Gambrell, D., & Rasmussen, S. A. (2003). Descriptive epidemiology of infantile cataracts in metropolitan Atlanta, GA 1968-1998. *Arch Pediatric Adolescent Med*, 157(4), 341–347.

Clarke, M. P., Wright, C. M., Hrisos, S., Anderson, J.D., Henderson, J., & Richardson, S. R. (2003). Randomized controlled trial of treatment of unilateral visual impairment detected at preshool vision screening. *BMJ*, Nov 29, Volume 327, 1-5.

Dornhoffer, J., Dohar, J., Konas, D., Spektor, Z., & White, J. (2003). Managing otitis media with tubes. *Contemporary Pediatrics*, October suppplement.

Dutton, G., & Cleary, M. (2003). Should we be screening for and treating amblyopia? *BMJ*, Nov 29, Volume 327, 1242–1243.

Ecker, K., Wilson, A., & Ryan, M. (2003). Managing early childhood ear infections. *The Clinical Advisor*, 6(9), 17–24.

Finberg, L., & Kleinman, R. (Eds.). (2003). *Saunders manual of pediatric practice* (2nd ed.). Philadelphia: W. B. Saunders.

Forbes, B. (2001). Management of corneal abrasions and ocular trauma in children. *Pediatric Annals*, 30(8), 465–472.

Gasper, I., & Leilani, S. A. (2003). Are antibiotics effective for OM with effusion? *The Journal of Family Practice*, 52(4), 321–323.

Havertape, S., Cruz, O., & Chu, F. (2001). Sensory strabismus—eso or exo? *Journal of Pediatric Ophthalmology & Strabismus*, 38(6), 327–330.

Hoberman, A., & Paradise, J. (2000). Acute otitis media: Diagnosis and management in the year 2000. *Pediatric Annals*, 29(10), 609–619.

Krauss, M. J., Morrissey, A. E., Winn, H. N., Amon, E., & Leet, T.L. (2003). Microcephaly: An epidemiologic analysis. *Am Journal Obstetrics/Gynecology*, 188(6), 1484–9.

Lueder, G. T. (2002). Balloon catheter dilation for treatment of older children with nasolacrimal duct obstruction. *Arch Ophthalmology*, 120(12), 1685–8.

McConaghy, J. (2001). The evaluation and treatment of children with acute otitis media. *The Journal of Family Practice*, 50(5), 457–465.

Medves, J. (2002). Three infant care interventions: Reconsidering the evidence, *JOGNN*, 31(5), 563–569.

Minter, K., Roberts, J., Hooper, S., Burchinal, M., & Zeisel, S. (2001). Early childhood otitis media in relation to children's attention related behavior in the first six years of life, *Pediatrics*, 107(5), 1037–1042.

Mustafa, T. A., & Oriafage, I. H. (2001). Three methods of treatment of chalazia in children, *Saudi Med Journal*, Nov, 22 (11), 968–972.

Pichichero, M. (2000). Acute otitis media: Part I. *American Family Physician*, 61(7), 2051–2056.

Pichichero, M. (2000). Acute otitis media: Part II. *American Family Physician*, 61(8), 2110–2115.

Roddey, O., & Hoover, H. (2000). Otitis media with effusion in children: A pediatric office perspective. *Pediatric Annals*, 29(10), 623–628.

Rubin, S. (2001). Management of strabismus in the first year of life. *Pediatric Annals*, 30(8), 474–488.

Ruttum, M., & Alcorn, D. (2001). Case presentation of 5 year old boy presenting with congenital nystagmus. *Journal of Pediatric Ophthalmology & Strabismus*, 38(1), 36–38.

Teoh, D., & Reynolds, S. (2003). Diagnosis and management of pediatric conjunctivitis. *Pediatric Emergency Care*, 19(1), 48–55.

Ticho, B. (2003). Strabismus. *Pediatric Clinics of North America*, (50), 173–188.

Wagner, R. (2001). Management of congenital nasolacrimal duct obstruction. *Pediatric Annals*, 30(8), 481–488.

Cardiovascular Disorders

Karen Uzark

Congenital Heart Disease/Defects

- Definition: Cardiovascular malformations that result from abnormal structural development of the heart and/or vessels; most heart defects occur within first 8 weeks of gestation

- Etiology/Incidence

  1. Etiology of most defects unknown

  2. Probably genetic predisposition interacting with environmental trigger

  3. Chromosomal abnormalities account for nearly 10% of cardiac malformations (Down syndrome, Turner's syndrome, DiGeorge syndrome, others)

  4. Environmental or adverse maternal conditions account for 2% to 4%

     a. Maternal diabetes mellitus, phenylketonuria, systemic lupus erythematosus, rubella or other viruses

     b. Maternal ingestion of thalidomide, alcohol, lithium, anticonvulsant agents, other drugs

  5. Approximately 8 per 1000 live births; about 32,000 new cases of congenital heart disease per year in the U.S.

  6. Ventricular septal defect (VSD) is most common (25% to 30% of all lesions)

- Signs and Symptoms

  1. Cyanosis—usually apparent at oxygen saturation of 85% or less

     a. Central (arterial desaturation)—generalized, mucous membranes

     b. Peripheral

     c. "Spells" characteristic of tetralogy of fallot

        (1) Often in the morning with crying

        (2) Acute increase in cyanosis with hyperpnea

        (3) May be followed by limpness, loss of consciousness, rarely convulsions

  2. Increased respiratory rate and/or effort at rest or with activity

  3. Poor feeding; fatigue during feeding

  4. Excessive sweating in infant, unrelated to the environment, especially while feeding

  5. Recurrent respiratory infections

  6. Decreased exercise tolerance

  7. Squatting with fatigue (rare)

  8. Chest pain (uncommon, usually noncardiac origin)—most common with severe aortic stenosis

  9. Syncope (uncommon)

- Differential Diagnosis
    1. Pulmonary disease
    2. Arrhythmias
    3. Myocardial diseases
    4. Rheumatic fever
    5. Sepsis
    6. Hypoglycemia, anemia, polycythemia, especially in neonates
    7. Central nervous system disorders
- Physical Findings
    1. Cyanosis (central or peripheral); pallor
    2. Clubbing of the fingers or toes (with long-standing arterial desaturation)
    3. Poor growth/weight gain
    4. Abnormal respiratory patterns
        a. Tachypnea
        b. Hyperpnea
        c. Dyspnea
    5. Tachycardia
    6. Hepatic enlargement with some defects
    7. Precordial prominence or increased precordial activity, palpable thrill
    8. Abnormal heart sounds
        a. Increased intensity
        b. Abnormal splitting
        c. Ejection clicks
        d. Fourth heart sound (gallop)
        e. Murmurs (may be absent or soft in spite of serious heart defect)
    9. Abnormal peripheral pulses
        a. Decreased
        b. Bounding
        c. Unequal (decreased lower extremity pulses suggest coarctation of the aorta)
    10. Abnormal blood pressure
        a. Hypotension
        b. Upper extremity blood pressure higher than lower extremity blood pressure suggestive of coarctation of aorta

11. Peripheral edema, uncommon in infants

- Diagnostic Tests/Findings

    1. Chest radiograph to evaluate heart size and pulmonary vascular markings

    2. Electrocardiogram to evaluate rhythm, chamber enlargement or hypertrophy

    3. Arterial blood gas and hemoglobin in infant with cyanosis—if decreased PO_2 in room air, repeat arterial blood gas after 10 to 15 minutes in 100% inspired oxygen (oxygen challenge) to help differentiate between cardiac and pulmonary cyanosis; if minimal increase in PO_2, cardiac etiology suggested

    4. Echocardiogram for diagnosis of specific congenital heart defect

- Management/Treatment

    1. Referral to pediatric cardiologist

        a. Prompt referral of symptomatic neonate

        b. Prompt referral of infant with cyanotic spells

Table 1

Cyanotic Heart Defects

Defect	Anatomy	Surgical Management
Transposition of the great arteries	The aorta arises from right ventricle; pulmonary artery from the left ventricle	Arterial switch (Jatene) operation in neonatal period or intra-atrial baffle (Mustard or Senning procedure) later in infancy
Tetralogy of Fallot	Combination of four defects: (1) pulmonary stenosis, (2) ventricular septal defect, (3) overriding aorta, and (4) right ventricular hypertrophy	*Palliative:* Blalock-Taussig or other aortopulmonary shunts in infancy *Repair:* patch closure of VSD and resection of infundibular pulmonary stenosis ± pulmonary valvulotomy if necessary
Tricuspid atresia	Complete agenesis of tricuspid valve with no direct communication between right atrium and a hypoplastic right ventricle	*Palliative:* shunt (or pulmonary artery banding if increased pulmonary blood flow via a ventricular septal defect) *Repair:* pulmonary artery connected to right atrium/vena cavae (Fontan procedure)
Total anomalous pulmonary venous connection	Pulmonary veins do not enter left atrium but are connected either directly or indirectly to right atrium	*Repair:* pulmonary venous trunk connected to left atrium in infancy
Truncus arteriosus	Single arterial trunk forms aorta and pulmonary artery, overriding ventricles and receiving blood from them through a ventricular septal defect	*Repair:* closure of ventricular septal defect, removing origin of the pulmonary arteries from trunk, and connecting pulmonary arteries to right ventricle with a conduit in infancy
Pulmonary atresia with intact ventricular septum	Complete atresia of pulmonary valve and varying degrees of hypoplasia of right ventricle	*Palliative:* Blalock-Taussig shunt ± pulmonary valvulotomy *Repair:* right ventricular outflow tract reconstruction or Fontan procedure
Ebstein's anomaly of the tricuspid valve	Redundant tricuspid valve tissue with the septal and posterior leaflets displaced downward into right ventricle for a variable distance	*Repair:* tricuspid valve replacement or modified tricuspid annuloplasty (patients with less severe forms do not require surgery)

Note. From "Alterations in cardiac function" by K. Uzark. In W. Votroubek (Ed.), (1997) *Pediatric Home Care* (2nd ed., p. 135). Frederick, MD: Aspen Publishers. Copyright 1997 by Aspen Publishers. Reprinted with permission.

2. Monitoring and counseling to promote optimal growth and development

3. Primary care, immunizations

4. Endocarditis prophylaxis with dental or surgical procedures

5. Psychosocial support of child and family

6. Surgical management/treatment of most significant congenital heart defects—see Table 1

Congestive Heart Failure (CHF)

- Definition: Clinical syndrome that reflects the inability of the heart to meet metabolic requirements of the body

- Etiology/Incidence

  1. Congenital heart defects with volume or pressure overload (most common cause in pediatric age group)—see Table 2

     a. Hypoplastic left heart syndrome

     b. Coarctation of the aorta

     c. Ventricular septal defect

     d. Atrioventricular septal defect

     e. Patent ductus arteriosus

  2. Acquired heart disease (less common cause)

     a. Myocarditis

     b. Metabolic abnormalities

     c. Endocardial fibroelastosis

     d. Rheumatic heart disease

     e. Cardiomyopathy (idiopathic, doxorubicin toxicity, muscular dystrophy)

  3. Other causes

     a. Tachyarrhythmias, complete heart block in infancy

     b. Severe anemia, hydrops fetalis

     c. Acute hypertension

     d. Bronchopulmonary dysplasia

     e. Acute cor pulmonale

     f. Arteriovenous malformations

  4. Incidence unknown

- Signs and Symptoms

  1. Increased respiratory rate and/or effort at rest or with activity

Table 2

Acyanotic Heart Defects Commonly Causing Congestive Heart Failure In Infancy

Defect	Description
Hypoplastic left heart syndrome	Aortic atresia and underdevelopment of the left ventricle, mitral valve, hypoplastic aortic arch, and/or coarctation
Coarctation of the aorta	Constriction of the aorta usually located slightly distal to origin of left subclavian artery
Ventricular septal defect	Abnormal opening between right and left ventricle that may result in congestive heart failure if left-to-right shunt is large
Atrioventricular septal defect (endocardial cushion defect)	Defect in lower part of atrial septum (ostium primum) and membranous ventricular septum and a single common atrioventricular valve
Patent ductus arteriosus	Connection between pulmonary artery and aorta that fails to close after birth, allowing increased blood flow to lungs

  2. Poor feeding

  3. Excessive sweating, especially with feeding in infants

  4. Decreased exercise tolerance

  5. Poor weight gain

  6. Orthopnea in older child, chronic cough

- Differential Diagnosis

  1. Pulmonary diseases

  2. Cardiac diseases (see etiology)

- Physical Findings

  1. Tachycardia (common)

  2. Tachypnea (common)

  3. Hepatomegaly

  4. Puffy eyelids common in infants, peripheral edema less common in children

  5. Wheezing, pulmonary rales may be present

  6. Pallor, mottling of extremities

  7. Weakly palpable peripheral pulses; cool extremities

  8. Gallop rhythm with myocardial failure

  9. Cyanosis with alveolar edema

- Diagnostic Tests/Findings

  1. Chest radiograph—cardiomegaly almost always present; pulmonary vascular congestion dependent on etiology

  2. Echocardiogram to assess ventricular function, chamber enlargement, anatomy

  3. Electrocardiogram not diagnostic, may help assess etiology

- Management/Treatment

  1. Referral to cardiologist to determine etiology if heart disease suspected

  2. Drug therapy

     a. Inotropic agents—usually digoxin

     b. Diuretics

     c. Afterload-reducing agents

  3. Other measures

     a. Semi-Fowler position (infant seat, pillows)

     b. Prostaglandin E_1 if systemic perfusion dependent on patency of ductus arteriosus

     c. Caloric supplementation of formula, breast milk fortifier (low sodium formulas not recommended)

     d. Frequent rest periods

  4. Treatment of underlying condition if specific therapy available

  5. Possible referral for cardiac transplantation if refractory, end-stage heart failure

Murmurs (innocent)

- Definition:

  1. Innocent murmurs are murmurs not associated with any anatomic abnormality

  2. Result from turbulence of blood flow, usually at origin of great arteries

  3. Also referred to as functional, normal, benign, or insignificant

  4. Common innocent murmurs

     a. *Still's murmur*—vibratory, groaning, or musical systolic murmur heard best between lower left sternal border and apex, attributed to turbulence in left ventricular outflow tract

     b. *Pulmonary systolic ejection murmur* or *pulmonary flow murmur*—slightly harsh systolic ejection murmur heard best at second to third left intercostal space; attributed to turbulent flow in right ventricular outflow tract

     c. *Supraclavicular arterial bruit*—early systolic murmur heard above clavicles, attributed to turbulence at site of branching of brachiocephalic arteries

     d. *Physiologic peripheral pulmonary stenosis*—low intensity systolic ejection murmur heard best at upper left sternal border, axillae, and back bilaterally in neonates until 3 to 6 months of age, attributed to relative hypoplasia of branch pulmonary arteries at birth

     e. *Venous hum*—humming continuous murmur usually heard best at upper right sternal border in sitting position with marked decrease or disappearance of murmur in supine position

- Etiology/Incidence
  1. Heard in more than 50 percent of normal children from infancy through adolescence
  2. Still's murmur most common; heard most frequently from 3 to 7 years of age
  3. Increased intensity (incidence) associated with increased cardiac output state (fever, acute illness, anemia, anxiety, exercise)
- Signs and Symptoms: Asymptomatic
- Differential Diagnosis
  1. Congenital heart disease
  2. Conditions associated with high cardiac output
- Physical Findings
  1. No cyanosis or other cardiovascular abnormalities
  2. Normal blood pressure, peripheral pulses in upper and lower extremities
  3. Normal heart sounds, including normal splitting (not fixed) of second heart sound
  4. No clicks
  5. Characteristics
     a. Usually systolic with exception of venous hum; never diastolic alone
     b. Usually low intensity (grade 1 to 3); never associated with precordial thrill
     c. Usually short duration, not holosystolic
     d. Well-localized, poorly transmitted except neonatal peripheral pulmonary stenosis
     e. Intensity may vary with position change
- Diagnostic Tests/Findings
  1. Testing not routine
  2. May be indicated to rule out congenital heart defect
     a. Chest radiograph normal
     b. Echocardiogram if recommended by cardiologist
- Management/Treatment
  1. Inform parents of murmur
  2. Provide reassurance that child's heart is normal
  3. Referral to cardiologist if:
     a. Symptomatic
     b. Cardiovascular abnormalities on physical examination

c. Uncertainty regarding innocence of murmur

d. Persistent parental concern

Hypertension

- Definition: "Average systolic and/or average diastolic blood pressure greater than or equal to the 95th percentile for age and sex with measurements obtained on at least three occasions" (Task Force on Blood Pressure Control in Children)—see Table 3

- Etiology/Incidence

    1. Primary hypertension

        a. No known underlying disease present to cause hypertension

        b. May be related to factors such as heredity, salt intake, stress and obesity

        c. More commonly recognized in adolescents

    2. Secondary hypertension

        a. Etiology varies with age

            (1) Newborn infants—renal artery thrombosis, renal artery stenosis, congenital renal malformations, coarctation of the aorta, bronchopulmonary dysplasia

Table 3

Classification of Hypertension by Age Group

Age Group	Significant Hypertension (mm Hg)	Severe Hypertension (mm Hg)
Newborn		
7 d	Systolic BP ≥96	Systolic BP ≥106
8–30 d	Systolic BP ≥104	Systolic BP ≥110
Infant (<2 yr)	Systolic BP ≥112	Systolic BP ≥118
	Diastolic BP ≥74	Diastolic BP ≥82
Children (3–5 yr)	Systolic BP ≥116	Systolic BP ≥124
	Diastolic BP ≥76	Diastolic BP ≥84
Children (6–9 yr)	Systolic BP ≥122	Systolic BP ≥130
	Diastolic BP ≥78	Diastolic BP ≥86
Children (10–12 yr)	Systolic BP ≥126	Systolic BP ≥134
	Diastolic BP ≥82	Diastolic BP ≥90
Children (13–15 yr)	Systolic BP ≥136	Systolic BP ≥144
	Diastolic BP ≥86	Diastolic BP ≥92
Children (16–18 yr)	Systolic BP ≥142	Systolic BP ≥150
	Diastolic BP ≥92	Diastolic BP ≥98

Note. From "Task Force on Blood Pressure Control in Children" by Report of the second task force on blood pressure control in children (1987), *Pediatrics,* 79(1) p. 7. Copyright 1987 by American Academy of Pediatrics. Reproduced by permission.

        (2)   Infancy to 6 years—renal parenchymal diseases, coarctation of the aorta, renal artery stenosis

        (3)   6 to 10 year olds—renal artery stenosis, renal parenchymal disease

    b.   Other causes—endocrine disorders, neurogenic tumors, drugs or toxins, increased intracranial pressure

    c.   More common in infants and children

   3.   Prevalence of hypertension in childhood is low (1% to 3%)

- Signs and Symptoms

   1.   Primary hypertension—usually no symptoms

   2.   Severe hypertension—may complain of headaches, dizziness, visual disturbances, epistaxis

   3.   Secondary hypertension—symptoms related to underlying disease and may include:

    a.   Congestive heart failure

    b.   Respiratory distress (infants)

    c.   Failure to thrive

    d.   Irritability

    e.   Convulsions

    f.   Feeding problems

- Differential Diagnosis: Causes of secondary hypertension (see etiology)

- Physical Findings

   1.   Elevated blood pressure on at least three occasions (without acute illness)

   2.   Related to underlying disease if secondary hypertension—may include edema, pallor, increased sweating, absent or delayed femoral pulses, signs of specific syndrome

- Diagnostic Tests/Findings

   1.   Based on history, age, other clinical findings

   2.   Complete blood count (to evaluate anemia)

   3.   Urinalysis

   4.   BUN, creatinine (to evaluate renal function)

   5.   Lipid profile

   6.   Echocardiogram if hypertension severe or drug therapy considered

   7.   Additional tests based on suspected cause

- Management/Treatment

   1.   Depends on cause and degree of elevation

2. General counseling regarding cardiovascular risk factors such as family history, obesity, lack of exercise, smoking

3. Nonpharmacologic therapy

   a. Weight reduction if indicated

   b. Regular aerobic exercise programs (especially in adolescents)

   c. Dietary modification—sodium reduction

4. Antihypertensive drugs if significant diastolic hypertension; evidence of target organ injury, or if symptoms related to elevated blood pressure

   a. Thiazide-type diuretic

   b. Adrenergic inhibitor/beta blocking drugs

   c. Vasodilator or angiotensin—converting enzyme inhibitor if blood pressure control not achieved with drugs previously cited

5. If secondary hypertension, therapy for underlying disease

6. Long-term follow-up, referral to subspecialist (cardiologist, nephrologist) if poor blood pressure control

Rheumatic Fever/Heart Disease

- Definition: A post-infectious inflammatory disease, based on standardized clinical (Jones) criteria, which can result in rheumatic valvular heart disease

- Etiology/Incidence

   1. Follows a group A streptococcal infection of the upper respiratory tract

   2. Probably involves abnormal immune response of certain individuals with genetic predisposition to this complication

   3. Incidence of acute rheumatic fever (ARF) approximately 3% of individuals with untreated or inadequately treated group A streptococcal tonsillopharyngitis (greater risk of recurrence)

   4. Most common in children between 6 and 15 years of age; rarely seen before 5 years

   5. Seasonal incidence follows that of streptococcal pharyngitis; peak incidence in spring

   6. Greater frequency of rheumatic heart disease in patients who had severe cardiac involvement during initial attack or recurrence of ARF

      a. Mitral valve regurgitation most common lesion

      b. Tricuspid and pulmonary valve involvement rare

- Signs and Symptoms
    1. Diagnosis of the initial attack of acute rheumatic fever based on evidence of preceding group A streptococcal infection **PLUS** two major or one major and two minor manifestations of the following:
    2. *Major Manifestations*
        a. Cardititis (approximately 50% of patients)
            (1) Valvulitis usually, as evidenced by development of new murmur, especially apical systolic murmur of mitral regurgitation
            (2) Myocarditis in absence of valvulitis rare—evidenced by tachycardia; other signs of congestive heart failure
            (3) Pericarditis rare in absence of valvulitis—evidenced by distant heart sounds, friction rub, chest pain
        b. Polyarthritis (approximately 70% of patients)
            (1) Almost always migratory
            (2) Most frequently larger joints—knees, ankles, elbows, wrists
        c. Chorea (Sydenham's chorea)
            (1) Purposeless, involuntary, rapid movements of trunk and/or extremities
            (2) Often associated with muscle weakness and emotional lability
        d. Erythema marginatum
            (1) Macular, nonpruritic rash with serpiginous erythematous border surrounding normal looking skin
            (2) Lesions most commonly located on trunk and proximal limbs; never on face
        e. Subcutaneous nodules (rare)—firm, painless nodules over the extensor surfaces of certain joints, particularly elbows, knuckles, knees, and ankles
    3. *Minor Manifestations*
        a. Arthralgia without objective evidence of inflammation
        b. Fever usually at least 39° C (102.2° F)
        c. Elevated acute phase reactants
        d. Prolonged PR interval on electrocardiogram
        e. Other clinical features—abdominal pain, malaise, epistaxis
- Differential Diagnosis
    1. Juvenile rheumatoid arthritis
    2. Other connective tissue diseases
    3. Infective endocarditis

4. Septic arthritis

5. Viral myocarditis and pericarditis

6. Reactions to drugs or foreign serum

- Physical Findings: No single specific finding; see manifestations

- Diagnostic Tests/Findings

    1. No specific diagnostic test

    2. Elevated acute phase reactants

        a. Erythrocyte sedimentation rate

        b. C-reactive protein

    3. Elevated streptococcal antibody titer (ASO)

    4. Electrocardiogram may indicate prolonged PR interval, rarely 2nd or 3rd degree heart block

    5. Echocardiogram may show valvular regurgitation

- Management/Treatment

    1. Referral to pediatrician/cardiologist if suspected

    2. Antibiotic treatment of group A streptococcal infection

    3. Anti-inflammatory agents for treatment of arthritis or carditis

        a. Salicylates or nonsteroidal agents

        b. Possible steroids if carditis severe

    4. Bedrest for period of acute carditis

    5. Treatment of congestive heart failure, if present

    6. Prevention of streptococcal infection and recurrence of rheumatic fever

        a. Prompt and adequate treatment of streptococcal pharyngitis

        b. Administration of monthly injections of long-acting benzathine penicillin (most reliable) or daily oral antibiotic regimen

        c. Antibiotics for endocarditis prophylaxis prior to dental work or surgical procedures in patients with rheumatic heart disease

Disturbances Of Rate And Rhythm

- Definition:

    1. A heart rate below the lower limits of normal for age (bradycardia)

    2. A heart rate above the upper limits of normal for age (tachycardia)

    3. An irregularity of heart rhythm, usually related to premature contraction

- Etiology/Incidence
  1. May be congenital or acquired
     a. Congenital complete heart block (CHB); 1 in 25,000 live births, can be associated with maternal systemic lupus erythematosus or other connective tissue diseases
     b. Acquired CHB caused by damage to conduction system during cardiac surgery, severe myocarditis, acute rheumatic fever, mumps, tumors in conduction system, endocrine/metabolic disorders
  2. Other causes
     a. Drugs (theophylline, cocaine, others)
     b. Electrolyte imbalance
     c. Acidosis/hypoxia
     d. Increased intracranial pressure
     e. Cardiomyopathy, long QT syndrome, structural heart disease or surgery
  3. Supraventricular tachycardia (SVT)
     a. Most common symptomatic tachycardia in first year of life
     b. May be associated with Wolff-Parkinson-White syndrome (10% to 20%)
  4. Premature atrial contractions (PAC) and premature ventricular contractions (PVC) common in healthy children
- Signs and Symptoms
  1. Children usually asymptomatic
  2. Symptoms of low cardiac output or congestive heart failure if bradycardia or tachycardia is severe and/or prolonged
  3. Irritability, pallor, poor feeding in infants
  4. Palpitations, syncope, dizziness
  5. Seizures
  6. Rare sudden death (with ventricular tachycardia and fibrillation)
- Differential Diagnosis
  1. Normal sinus arrhythmia (phasic acceleration and deceleration of heart rate with respiration)
  2. Sinus tachycardia and associated causes
  3. Sinus bradycardia and associated causes (normal in athletes)
  4. Conditions associated with heart rate disturbances (see etiology)

- Physical Findings
    1. Bradycardia, tachycardia, or irregular rhythm
    2. Tachypnea, hepatomegaly, poor perfusion especially in infants if rate disturbance severe and/or prolonged
- Diagnostic Tests/Findings
    1. Electrocardiogram
    2. Other tests based on clinical findings and symptoms
- Management/Treatment
    1. Referral to cardiologist for evaluation and treatment if:
        a. Symptomatic
        b. Sustained arrhythmia, or
        c. Recurrent arrhythmia
    2. Treatment of underlying condition if noncardiac cause

Myocarditis

- Definition: Focal or diffuse inflammation of the myocardium in association with myocellular necrosis
- Etiology/Incidence
    1. Precise etiology usually unknown
    2. May be caused by virtually any bacterial, viral, rickettsial, fungal, or parasitic organism—viral infections the most common etiology, especially coxsackie B virus (> 50%) and adenovirus
    3. Other causes include autoimmune or collagen-vascular diseases, or hypersensitivity drug reactions (rare)
    4. Possible genetic predisposition with viral trigger
    5. Incidence unknown, as many mild cases may go undetected
    6. In patients who present with severe congestive heart failure or shock (20% to 30%), approximately one-third will die or require transplantation
- Signs and Symptoms
    1. Great variability—from no distress to severe congestive heart failure or shock
    2. Often fever or history of antecedent "flu-like" viral illness
    3. Suspect if onset of congestive heart failure with no obvious structural or functional etiology
        a. Persistent tachycardia (out of proportion to fever if present)
        b. Tachypnea, dyspnea

    c. Easy fatigue, poor feeding in infant

    d. Gallop rhythm, usually no murmur

    e. Hepatomegaly

    f. Poor perfusion

  4. Can also present as new onset arrhythmias, syncope, or sudden death

- Differential Diagnosis

  1. Carnitine deficiency

  2. Idiopathic dilated cardiomyopathy

  3. Pericarditis

  4. Endocardial fibroelastosis

  5. Hereditary mitochondrial defects

  6. Anomalies of the coronary arteries

  7. Metabolic or endocrine disorders (hyperthyroidism)

- Physical Findings: See section on congestive heart failure

- Diagnostic Tests/Findings

  1. Erythrocyte sedimentation rate and heart enzymes (CPK, LDH) elevated

  2. Viral cultures, antibody titers, and polymeraze chain reaction (PCR) may suggest viral etiology

  3. Laboratory studies to rule out metabolic causes of cardiomyopathy

  4. Echocardiography to assess ventricular function and rule out other cardiac anomalies

  5. Chest radiograph to assess cardiac enlargement which is variable

  6. Electrocardiogram may show ST segment and T wave abnormalities, possible reduced QRS voltage, or arrhythmias

  7. Endomyocardial biopsy for possible confirmation of diagnosis

- Management/Treatment

  1. Immediate referral to pediatrician and/or pediatric cardiologist if suspected

  2. Supportive measures for congestive heart failure

    a. Inotropic agents, including digoxin, at reduced dosage (may be arrythmogenic)

    b. Diuretics, afterload reduction

    c. Bedrest

  3. Treatment of arrythmias

  4. Use of immunosuppressive medication controversial

5. Possible administration of intravenous immunoglobulin—effectiveness not proven; risk of anaphylaxis

6. Psychosocial support of child and/or family—usually sudden onset of illness in previously healthy child

7. Outcome varies from complete resolution and recovery to development of chronic cardiomyopathy or death without cardiac transplantation

Hypercholesterolemia

- Definition: Elevated serum cholesterol level
    1. Total cholesterol of 200 mg/dL or above
    2. Total cholesterol of 170 to 199 mg/dL considered "borderline high"
    3. Low density lipoprotein (LDL) cholesterol of 130 mg/dL or above
- Etiology/Incidence
    1. High tracking correlations for total and LDL cholesterol levels from childhood to adulthood
    2. Potential increased risk for developing atherosclerotic or coronary heart disease as adults, especially in association with other risk factors
        a. Positive family history of premature coronary heart disease (before 55 years of age), peripheral vascular disease, or hypercholesterolemia (above 240 mg/dL)
        b. Diabetes
        c. Hypertension
        d. Obesity
        e. Smoking
        f. Physical inactivity
    3. Among children aged 2 to 11 years in U.S., about 25% with cholesterol levels in borderline high or high range
    4. Familial hypercholesterolemia (autosomal dominant) prevalence rate of heterozygous form 1 in 500, homozygous form 1 in 1,000,000
    5. Secondary causes of hypercholesterolemia
        a. Obesity
        b. Endocrine and metabolic conditions
        c. Obstructive liver disease
        d. Nephrotic syndrome
        e. Anorexia nervosa
        f. Collagen disease

g. Drugs

  (1) Corticosteroids

  (2) Isotretinoin

  (3) Thiazide diuretics

  (4) Some beta blockers

  (5) Some oral contraceptives

- Signs and Symptoms: Asymptomatic during childhood

- Differential Diagnosis: Causes of secondary hypercholesterolemia (see etiology)

- Physical Findings

  1. Rare xanthomas with familial hypercholesterolemia and very high cholesterol levels

  2. Signs of risk factors (hypertension, obesity)

- Diagnostic Tests/Findings

  1. Measurement of total cholesterol in children over 2 years of age with a positive family history or other risk factors (U.S. Department of Health and Human Services, 1991)

     a. If total cholesterol level acceptable (< 170 mg/dL), repeat measurement within 5 years

     b. If total cholesterol level borderline (170 to 199 mg/dL), repeat measurement, and if average is borderline or high, do lipoprotein analysis

     c. If total cholesterol level high (above 200 mg/dL), do lipoprotein analysis

  2. Additional studies to evaluate causes of secondary hypercholesterolemia, as indicated

- Management/Treatment

  1. Nutrition assessment/diet therapy in children over 2 years of age

     a. If LDL cholesterol ≥ 110 mg/dL, step 1 diet—no more than 30% of total calories from fat, less than 10% of total calories as saturated fat, and less than 300 mg of cholesterol per day; adequate calories to reach or maintain desirable body weight

     b. If LDL cholesterol > 130 mg/dL after 3 months of step 1 diet, step 2 diet is prescribed—saturated fatty acid intake reduced to less than 7% of calories and cholesterol intake to less than 200 mg per day; adequate amounts of nutrients, vitamins, and minerals provided

  2. Drug therapy in children aged 10 years and older if after an adequate trial of diet therapy (6 months to 1 year), LDL cholesterol ≥ 190 mg/dL or LDL cholesterol ≥ 160 mg/dL plus positive family history of premature cardiovascular disease or 2 or more other cardiovascular risk factors are present; bile acid sequestrants recommended

3. Increase exercise

4. Prevention—anticipatory guidance during all well-child maintenance visits to maintain well-balanced diet, encourage daily exercise, and avoid known risk factors

Kawasaki Disease (Mucocutaneous Lymph Node Syndrome)

- Definition: Acute febrile syndrome associated with generalized vasculitis and the leading cause of acquired coronary artery disease in children

- Etiology/Incidence

  1. Etiology uncertain

     a. Epidemiology and clinical presentation highly suggestive of infectious etiology

     b. May be associated with exposure to house dust mites or recently shampooed carpets

  2. Most frequently (80%) affects infants and children under 5 years of age; most less than 2 years

  3. Male to female ratio 1.5:1

  4. All racial backgrounds affected; highest incidence in children of Asian ancestry

  5. Approximately 20% risk of developing coronary artery abnormalities with decreased risk if intravenous gamma globulin therapy instituted before 10th day of illness

- Signs and Symptoms

  1. Vary in severity and over course of illness

  2. Early (acute phase)

     a. Preceding or concurrent respiratory symptoms—runny nose, cough, ear infection

     b. Diarrhea, vomiting, or abdominal pain (common)

     c. Irritability

     d. Persistent fever > 5 days

     e. Reddened eyes

     f. Red tongue and throat

     g. Redness and/or swelling of hands and feet

     h. Rash

     i. Swollen nodes

     j. Fast and/or irregular pulse

     k. Irritability

  3. Mid-course (sub-acute phase)

      a.   Dry, peeling skin on lips, fingers and toes

      b.   Joint pain

   4.   Late (convalescent phase)—resolution of symptoms

- Differential Diagnosis

  1. Measles

  2. Scarlet fever

  3. Drug reactions

  4. Stevens-Johnson syndrome

  5. Other febrile viral exanthems

  6. Rocky mountain spotted fever

  7. Staphylococcal scalded skin syndrome

  8. Toxic shock syndrome

  9. Juvenile rheumatoid arthritis

  10. Leptospirosis

  11. Mercury poisoning

- Physical Findings

  1. Diagnostic criteria includes presence of at least 5 of following clinical features:

     a. Persistent fever of at least 5 days

     b. Bilateral, painless bulbar conjunctival injection without exudate

     c. Lips/oral cavity—erythema and cracking of lips, strawberry tongue, erythema of oropharyngeal mucosa

     d. Peripheral extremities—acute erythema and/or edema of hands/ feet; membranous desquamation of fingertips during sub-acute and convalescent phases (1 to 3 weeks after onset of fever)

     e. Polymorphous exanthem of trunk extremeties within 4 days of fever onset

     f. Cervical nonfluctuant lymphadenopathy; at least one lymph node more than 1.5 cm in diameter; usually unilateral

  2. Coronary artery abnormalities (usually beyond 10 days of illness onset) with fever and fewer than 5 clinical features is diagnostic

  3. Other physical findings

     a. Arthritis or arthralgia

     b. Tachycardia out of proportion to degree of fever; gallop rhythm (signs of myocarditis); new murmur (less common)

     c. Sterile pyuria

     d. Aneurysm of peripheral arteries (less common)

- Diagnostic Tests/Findings
    1. No specific diagnostic test
    2. Thrombocytosis, may be marked; frequently seen after first week of illness
    3. Leukocytosis with left shift
    4. Erythrocyte sedimentation rate elevated
    5. C-reactive protein positive
    6. Mild anemia in acute phase
    7. Hypoalbuminemia
    8. Electrocardiogram abnormal in $\frac{1}{3}$ of children
        a. ST-T wave changes
        b. Decreased R wave voltage
        c. Prolonged PR or QT intervals
        d. Atrial or ventricular arrhythmias
    9. Echocardiogram—coronary artery aneurysms or ectasia; occasional pericardial effusion or decreased contractility

- Management/Treatment
    1. Immediate referral to pediatrician and/or subspecialist (immunologist, pediatric cardiologist) if suspected
    2. Management goals
        a. Reducing inflammation, particularly in the coronary arterial wall and myocardium
        b. Preventing coronary thrombosis
    3. Therapy during acute phase
        a. Intravenous gamma globulin within 10 days of onset of illness, *PLUS*
        b. High-dose aspirin (80 to 100 mg/kg/day) until patient is afebrile, then reduced to 3 to 5 mg/kg/day for 6 to 8 weeks
    4. If coronary arterial abnormalities detected
        a. Low-dose aspirin continued indefinitely
        b. Dipyridamole considered if high risk for myocardial infarction
        c. Long-term follow-up by pediatric cardiologist
    5. Administration of live virus vaccines delayed at least 5 months after intravenous gamma globulin treatment unless risk of exposure is high

6. Administration of influenza vaccine in patients on long-term aspirin therapy

7. Activity restrictions beyond initial 6 to 8 weeks based on risk for severity of coronary artery involvement

Questions
Select the best answer

1. The most common congenital heart defect in children is:

   a. Tricuspid atresia
   b. Ventricular septal defect
   c. Aortic stenosis
   d. Pulmonary atresia

2. The mother of a 4-month-old infant reports that he turned "blue" and seemed to have fast, labored breathing after vigorous crying soon after awakening. He "fell asleep" and his color and breathing seemed to improve. On physical examination, the mucous membranes of the lips and mouth appear mildly cyanotic. A systolic murmur is heard best at the mid- to upper left sternal border. Vital signs are normal with normal peripheral pulses. There is no hepatomegaly. A likely diagnosis is:

   a. Congestive heart failure
   b. Apnea
   c. Coarctation of the aorta
   d. Cyanotic spell related to Tetralogy of Fallot

3. Management of the infant with suspected heart disease and a reported cyanotic spell should include:

   a. Prompt referral to a cardiologist
   b. An apnea monitor
   c. Instructing the parent to keep a diary of these episodes
   d. Continous administration of oxygen

4. Chest pain in young children is usually:

   a. A symptom of congenital heart disease
   b. Noncardiac in origin
   c. A sign of hypercholesterolemia
   d. A symptom of congestive heart failure

5. A common cause of congestive heart failure in the first year of life is:

   a. Pulmonary stenosis
   b. Ventricular septal defect
   c. Rheumatic fever
   d. Complete heart block

6. The least likely physical finding in a 2-month-old with congestive heart failure is:

   a. Tachypnea
   b. Tachycardia
   c. Hepatomegaly
   d. Pedal edema

7. A vibratory systolic murmur is heard between the lower left sternal and the apex in a healthy 4-year-old at her preschool physical. The cardiovascular exam is otherwise normal. A likely diagnosis is:

    a. Venous hum
    b. Still's murmur
    c. Transposition of the great arteries
    d. Rheumatic heart disease

8. Characteristics of a venous hum include:

    a. A systolic murmur
    b. Radiation over precordium
    c. Marked decrease or disappearance of murmur when child is supine
    d. Heard best at lower left sternal border

9. Which of the following is true regarding innocent mumurs?

    a. The murmur is often holosystolic
    b. Prompt referral to a cardiologist is indicated
    c. A precordial thrill is present
    d. The murmur is low intensity, grade 1–3

10. Primary hypertension with no known underlying disease is most common in:

    a. Infants
    b. Children 3–5 years old
    c. Children 6–9 years old
    d. Adolescents

11. A 12-year-old girl seen at a routine visit has a blood pressure of 140/90. She denies any symptoms. The initial management would include:

    a. Intravenous pyelogram
    b. Return for two repeat blood pressure measurements
    c. No follow-up needed—blood pressure probably related to anxiety
    d. Diuretic therapy

12. A 9-year-old boy presents with a fever of 102° F and complaints of leg pains. His mother reports that he had an upper respiratory infection with a sore throat approximately two weeks ago which subsided without therapy. On physical examination, he has tender, swollen knees bilaterally. His heart rate is 120/min and a blowing systolic murmur is heard at the apex. No murmur was noted at a previous well child visit. The most likely diagnosis is:

    a. Kawasaki disease
    b. Rheumatic fever
    c. Sickle cell anemia
    d. Viral illness

13. The most useful test for evaluation of suspected acute rheumatic fever is:

    a. Antistreptolysin-O titer
    b. Electrocardiogram
    c. Hemoglobin electrophoresis
    d. Urinalysis

14. The initial attack of acute rheumatic fever is preceded by:

    a. A viral illness
    b. A group A streptococcal infection
    c. Exposure to mites
    d. Exposure to chicken pox

15. A 3-week-old infant has a one day history of irritability, pallor, and poor feeding. He is afebrile. On physical examination, his heart rate is 240/min while asleep. The most likely diagnosis is:

    a. Supraventricular tachycardia
    b. Premature ventricular contractions
    c. Sinus tachycardia
    d. Cyanotic heart defect

16. Congenital complete heart block may be associated with:

    a. Maternal lupus erythematosus
    b. Wolff-Parkinson-White syndrome
    c. Maternal myocardial infarction
    d. Kawasaki disease

17. The most common cause of myocarditis is:

    a. Bacterial
    b. Viral
    c. Drug reaction
    d. Radiation therapy

18. Which of the following is not an expected finding in a child with myocarditis?

    a. Persistent tachycardia
    b. History of antecedent "flu-like" illness
    c. A gallop rhythm
    d. A significant heart murmur

19. Hypercholesterolemia in children over 2-years-old is defined as a total cholesterol at or above:

    a. 100 mg/dL
    b. 130 mg/dL
    c. 160 mg/dL
    d. 200 mg/dL

20. A potential childhood risk factor for development of atherosclerotic or coronary heart disease as adults is:

    a. Obesity
    b. Tachycardia
    c. Heart murmur
    d. Aerobic exercise

21. Which of the following is not likely to cause secondary hypercholesterolemia?

    a. Nephrotic syndrome
    b. Hypertension
    c. Corticosteroids
    d. Obstructive liver disease

22. Which of the following is a common cause of acquired coronary artery disease during childhood?

    a. Rheumatic fever
    b. Hypertension
    c. Systemic lupus erythematosus
    d. Kawasaki disease

23. Kawasaki disease is most common in:

    a. Neonates
    b. Children less than 5 years of age
    c. Children over 6 years of age
    d. Females

24. A principal clinical feature of Kawasaki disease includes:

    a. Low grade fever for 24 hours and a pruritic rash
    b. Conjunctivitis with exudate and facial rash
    c. Arthritis and chorea
    d. Fever persisting at least five days and acute erythema and/or edema of hands and feet

25. An essential test in the evaluation of a 2-year-old with suspected Kawasaki disease is:

    a. An echocardiogram
    b. Electrolytes
    c. Cholesterol
    d. Streptococcal antibody titer

Answers

1. b	10. d	18. d
2. d	11. b	19. d
3. a	12. b	20. a
4. b	13. a	21. b
5. b	14. b	22. d
6. d	15. a	23. b
7. b	16. a	24. d
8. c	17. b	25. a
9. d		

Bibliography

Allen, H. D., Clark, E. B., Gutgesell, H. P., & Driscoll, D. J. (Eds.). (2001). *Moss and Adams' heart disease in infants, children and adolescents (including the fetus and young adult)*. Baltimore: Lippincott, Williams & Wilkins.

American Academy of Pediatrics, Committee on Nutrition. (1998). Cholesterol in childhood. *Pediatrics, 101,* 141–147.

American Heart Association, Special Writing Group from the Task Force on Children and Youth. (1994). Cardiovascular health and disease in children: Current status. *Circulation, 89,* 923–930.

American Heart Association, Special Writing Group of the Committee on Rheumatic Fever, Endocarditis, and Kawasaki Disease. (1993). Guidelines for the diagnosis of rheumatic fever: Jones criteria, updated 1992. *Circulation, 87,* 302–307.

American Heart Association, Committee on Rheumatic Fever, Endocarditis, and Kawasaki Disease. (1993). Diagnosis and therapy of Kawasaki disease in children. *Circulation, 87,* 1776–1780.

American Heart Association, Committee on Rheumatic Fever, Endocarditis, and Kawasaki Disease. (1994). Guidelines for long-term management of patients with Kawasaki disease. *Circulation, 89,* 916–922.

Behrman, R. E., Kliegman, R. M., & Jenson, H. B. (Eds.). (2000). *Nelson textbook of pediatrics* (16th ed.). Philadelphia: W. B. Saunders.

Tyler, D. C. (Ed.). (1992). *Nadas' pediatric cardiology*. Philadelphia: Hanley & Belfus, Inc.

National Cholesterol Education Program. (1992). Report of the expert panel on blood cholesterol in children and adolescents. *Pediatrics. 89,* 525–584.

Park, N. (1996). *Pediatric cardiology for practitioners* (3rd ed.). Chicago: Yearbook Medical Publishers.

Task Force on Blood Pressure Control in Children. (1987). Report of the second task force on blood pressure control in children. *Pediatrics. 79,* 1–25.

U.S. Department of Health and Services. (1991). *Report of the expert panel on blood cholesterol levels in children and adolscents* (NIH Publication No. 91-2732). Washington, DC: Author.

Lower Respiratory Disorders

Janet Johnston

Croup (Laryngotracheobronchitis)

- Definition: An acute upper airway obstruction typically caused by a viral infection of the larynx
- Etiology/Incidence
  1. Parainfluenza viruses and respiratory syncytial virus (RSV) most common organisms; influenza A and B, common organisms; bacterial causes very rare
  2. Most common in children 6 months to 5 years of age; peak incidence 2 years
  3. Males more often affected than females
  4. Peak incidence during autumn
- Signs and Symptoms
  1. Rhinitis for 3 to 4 days, low grade fever, sore throat
  2. Rapid onset of "barky" cough, inspiratory stridor, hoarseness
  3. Symptoms worse at night
  4. Often rapid improvement with exposure to cool night air or increased ambient humidity
- Differential Diagnosis
  1. Bacterial infections of the upper respiratory tract, e.g., epiglottitis, tracheitis etc.
  2. Laryngotracheomalacia
  3. Foreign body aspiration
  4. Extrinsic compression of airway from trauma, tumor, abscess, or congenital malformations
  5. Acute laryngeal edema (anaphylaxis, angioneurotic edema)
  6. Severe asthma
- Physical Findings
  1. Inspiratory stridor
  2. Brassy, barky cough
  3. Dyspnea, expiratory stridor if severe
  4. Chest sounds are usually clear
  5. Low-grade fever, high-grade fever and toxic appearance suggest bacterial etiology
- Diagnostic Tests/Findings
  1. Pulse oximetry—hypoxia indicates severe disease
  2. Radiographic image of airway—classic tapering of the subglottic trachea ("steeple sign")

3. Viral cultures of nasopharyngeal secretions—rapid identification with immunofluorescent assay

4. White blood cell count—normal or elevated (not usually done)

- Management/Treatment

    1. Mild disease—no dyspnea, hypoxia or dehydration

        a. Outpatient care—adequate oral hydration, antipyretics, calm nonintrusive care

        b. Family education regarding worsening respiratory distress

    2. Moderate to severe disease—stridor at rest, dyspnea, hypoxemia, or dehydration

        a. Hospitalize for supportive care, oxygen supplementation, medications, and intravenous fluids if indicated

        b. Fewer than 1% of patients require intubation

    3. Medications

        a. Nebulized racemic or L-epinephrine—observe for 3 hours after a dose for rebound respiratory distress

        b. Parenteral dexamethasone in doses greater than 0.3 mg/kg, oral dexamethasone (0.15–0.6 mg/kg), and nebulized corticosteroids will lessen the severity and duration of symptoms in moderate to severe disease; oral dexamethasone doses of 0.15 mg/kg are effective for mild disease; budesonide may also be effective (AAP, 2003)

        c. Antibiotics are not indicated unless a bacterial infection is present

    4. Isolation—contact precautions during hospitalization

    5. Prevention—hand washing and avoid touching face to prevent spread

Foreign Body Aspiration

- Definition: Inhalation of a foreign body that lodges in the upper trachea or lower airways, resulting in total or partial airway obstruction with local injury and inflammation

- Etiology/Incidence

    1. Food or objects with pliable, slick, or cylindrical surface; peanuts, other nuts or seeds, hot dogs, candy, grapes and latex balloons most common

    2. 80% are < 3 years of age

    3. Two-thirds of cases are males

- Signs and Symptoms

    1. Sudden, violent cough with gagging, choking, and subsequent stridor, wheezing and possible cyanosis

    2. May be asymptomatic if object is not obstructing or irritating airway

- Differential Diagnosis
  1. Acute phase—laryngotracheitis, epiglottitis, laryngeal edema, pertussis, status asthmaticus, croup, retropharyngeal abscess
  2. Chronic phase—asthma, pneumonia, bronchitis, tuberculosis, and tracheal stenosis
- Physical Findings
  1. Presentation dependent on substance aspirated as well as size and location of foreign body
  2. Rarely (6%) still coughing during examination
  3. Unilateral wheezing and decreased breath sounds on side of aspiration; may also be bilateral
  4. Voice changes, stridor, dyspnea, sputum production, and emesis possible
  5. If foreign body persists, bronchiectasis and abscess formation is likely; may present with recurrent pneumonia and/or hemoptysis
- Diagnostic Tests/Findings
  1. Pulse oximetry—decreased O_2 saturations with significant obstruction
  2. Chest radiograph—only 10% of aspirated objects are radiopaque; unilateral changes in aeration from obstruction
  3. Expiratory chest films (cooperative patients), lateral soft tissue neck films (younger patients), decubitus, or fluoroscopy (imaging throughout the complete respiratory cycle)—obstructive emphysema (failure to deflate) or atelectasis typical; right main stem bronchus main site for foreign bodies
  4. If high index of suspicion (witnessed choking ± abnormal films), rigid bronchoscopy is indicated for diagnostic and therapeutic purposes; if diagnosis uncertain, flexible bronchoscopy may aid diagnosis, but rigid bronchoscopy will still be needed if foreign body found
- Management/Treatment
  1. Institute cardiopulmonary resuscitation if needed
  2. Immediate transport to hospital for evaluation and removal
  3. Use of pulmonary clearance (chest physiotherapy) may be contraindicated if suspicion of foreign body is high—may cause object to migrate to large airways and cause severe obstruction
  4. Refer to an expert pediatric endoscopy team for rigid bronchoscopy evaluation and removal (if convincing history of foreign body aspiration, regardless of radiographic findings)
  5. Humidification, bronchodilators and anti-inflammatory medications may be useful after removal
  6. Antibiotics if evidence of pneumonia or bronchitis

7. Chest radiograph in six to eight weeks to evaluate resolution of previous findings, or sooner if child is not improving

8. Prevention

   a. Remove small items from environment of small child

   b. Sit while eating and provide adult supervision

   c. Cut food in small pieces for young children

   d. Avoid commonly aspirated foods and objects (no latex balloons etc.) in children under three years of age

Bronchitis

- Definition

  1. Acute bronchitis is transient inflammation of the larger lower airways

  2. Chronic bronchitis symptoms persist for more than two weeks; chronic bronchitis is rarely an isolated entity in children, but rather a symptom of some other condition

- Etiology/Incidence

  1. Most commonly viral—adenovirus, influenza A and B, parainfluenza type 3, RSV and rhinovirus

  2. Bacterial causes—*Mycoplasma pneumoniae, Bordetella pertussis, Chlamydia pneumoniae,* and *Corynebacterium diphtheriae*

  3. Acute bronchitis occurs most frequently in the winter and early spring; rates are higher among males

- Signs and Symptoms

  1. Initial phase includes symptoms of an upper respiratory illness

  2. Cough is the hallmark symptom; is initially dry and brassy but may become productive as illness progresses

  3. May have retrosternal pain with cough

- Differential Diagnosis

  1. Asthma

  2. Allergic disease/posterior nasal drainage

  3. Gastroesophageal reflux and/or aspiration

  4. Inhalation of irritants such as cigarette smoke

  5. Cystic fibrosis

  6. Immune deficiency

  7. Chronic sinusitis

  8. Immotile cilia syndrome

9. Foreign body aspiration

10. Airway deformity

- Physical Findings

    1. Brassy cough

    2. Coarse, bronchial breath sounds in periphery of lungs

    3. May have tracheal tenderness on examination

- Diagnostic Tests/Findings

    1. Diagnosis primarily based on history and physical

    2. Chest radiograph may be normal or show peribronchial thickening

    3. Pulmonary function tests (PFT) may be normal or may indicate an obstructive pattern; PFT may or may not improve after bronchodilator

- Management/Treatment

    1. Avoidance of irritants

    2. Expectorants, increase fluid intake; avoid cough suppressants

    3. Bronchodilators

    4. Inhaled steroids may be indicated for chronic bronchitis

    5. Antibiotics are not usually helpful for viral illnesses; however, antibiotics (with efficacy against mycoplasma and chlamydia species) are useful if bacterial etiology is suspected and cough is > 10-14 days; children with chronic pulmonary disease other than asthma may benefit from antibiotics for acute exacerbations; consider pertussis if immunizations incomplete

    6. Prevention

        a. Frequent hand washing with careful disposal of nasal and oral drainage

        b. Avoid overcrowding

        c. Avoid exposure to environmental tobacco smoke

Bronchiolitis

- Definition: An acute viral infection of the smaller airways

- Etiology/Incidence

    1. Primarily caused by RSV

    2. Parainfluenza, adenovirus, rhinovirus, influenza less common

    3. Almost all children will have had one episode of bronchiolitis before age two

    4. Those more likely requiring hospitalization include premature or young infants and those with cardiorespiratory disease (especially bronchopulmonary dysplasia) or immunodeficiency

5. Most commonly occurs in mid-winter to early spring

6. More severe disease in boys and with lower socioeconomic status

- Signs and Symptoms

    1. Initial symptoms—rhinorrhea, congestion, cough, and low-grade fever

    2. Progresses to increased work of breathing, tachypnea, decreased appetite or poor suck; change in level of consciousness or activity level

    3. May present as apnea, lethargy, irritability, or poor feeding in very young or premature infants

- Differential Diagnosis

    1. Bacterial or chlamydia pneumonia

    2. Aspiration pneumonia

    3. Asthma

    4. Foreign body aspiration

- Physical Findings

    1. Symptoms of rhinorrhea, otitis, conjunctivitis, and/or pharyngitis

    2. Often afebrile, or low-grade fever

    3. Tachypnea, retractions, nasal flaring, prolonged expiratory phase

    4. Wheezing, crackles

- Diagnostic Tests/Findings

    1. Diagnosis primarily based on history and physical

    2. Chest radiograph—peribronchial thickening, air trapping, patchy or segmental atelectasis especially in right middle and right upper lobes

    3. Pulse oximetry—hypoxemia with significant disease

    4. White blood cell count with differential—may or may not be increased

    5. Viral culture with rapid diagnostic techniques—may be positive for RSV

- Management/Treatment

    1. Careful monitoring of respiratory status, use oxygen therapy if hypoxemic

    2. Mechanical ventilation rarely necessary in previously healthy infants, but may be required in high-risk groups

    3. Fluid and nutritional support

    4. Bronchodilators—discontinue if not beneficial

    5. Corticosteroids for those with underlying chronic conditions

    6. Ribavirin use is generally not recommended; use based on clinical condition and physician experience (AAP, 2003)

7. Prevention

   a. Palivizumab (preferred) or RSV-Immune Globulin Intravenous (RSV-IGIV) given to children younger than 2 years of age with chronic lung disease receiving medical intervention in the last 6 months; also for infants 28 to 32 weeks gestational age (GA) and less than 6 months, infants less than 28 weeks GA and less than 12 months, or infants 32 to 35 weeks GA and multiple risk factors and less than 6 months of age (AAP, 2003)

   b. Strict contact precautions (gown, gloves) in hospitalized children, decrease exposure to contagious settings for high-risk infants, avoid tobacco smoke exposure, and careful hand washing

Pneumonia

- Definition

  1. Infectious pneumonia—infection which usually involves small airways in children, but may also infect the larger airways and/or the alveoli

  2. Aspiration pneumonia—caused by the ingestion of food, saliva, gastric contents, or other substances into air passages

- Etiology/Incidence

  1. Common viral agents—RSV; parainfluenza; influenza A and B; and adenovirus; usually involves the small airways

  2. Newborns—most common bacterial causes include group B streptococcus, gram-negative enteric bacilli, *Chlamydia trachomatis,* ureaplasma, and rarely syphilis

  3. Infants and young children ≤ 6 years of age—*Streptococcus pneumoniae* is primary cause of bacterial pneumonia; incidence of *Haemophilus influenzae* pneumonia has dramatically decreased since introduction of HIB vaccine

  4. Older children and adolescents—*Streptococcus pneumoniae* most likely bacterial cause, more rarely *Staphylococcus aureus,* anaerobes

  5. Mycoplasma and chlamydia may be most common nonviral organisms in children from preschool to young adulthood

  6. Immunocompromised or malnourished children—consider opportunistic organisms, such as *Pneumocystis carinii,* yeasts

  7. Dimorphic soil fungi should also be considered

  8. Aspiration pneumonia occurs in specific settings—most frequently in children with upper airway abnormalities or neurologic deficits; severe gastroesophageal reflux and other esophageal problems; may also occur subsequent to the inhalation of smoke or hydrocarbons; following near drowning, or ethanol ingestion by adolescents

  9. Incidence—4% in preschool children and 1% to 2% in school age years

- Signs and Symptoms
    1. Cough, occasionally productive or associated with emesis
    2. Wheezing (frequent in viral etiology)
    3. Fever
    4. Chest or abdominal pain; nausea $\pm$ vomiting
    5. May have tachypnea, retractions, expiratory grunting, nasal flaring, cyanosis, and rash
    6. May have change in level of consciousness and/or activity
- Differential Diagnosis
    1. Bronchiolitis
    2. Foreign body aspiration
    3. Asthma
    4. Cystic fibrosis
    5. Tuberculosis
    6. Immunodeficiency
    7. Swallowing dysfunction
- Physical Findings
    1. Fever
    2. May have tachypnea; substernal, supraclavicular, and intercostal retractions; grunting, nasal flaring; pallor or cyanosis
    3. May have wheezing, crackles, diminished or tubular breath sounds on auscultation
    4. If pleural effusion present, may have decreased breath sounds with dullness to percussion
- Diagnostic Tests/Findings
    1. Chest radiograph
        a. Atelectasis (frequently misread as pneumonia)—opacification, intrathoracic structures will shift toward the atelectatic area; hemidiaphragm on affected side may be elevated and intercostal spaces on that side may be narrow
        b. Viral pneumonia usually begins with scattered perihilar and peribronchial infiltrations; in later stages, more localized infiltrations
        c. Bacterial pneumonias—characterized by patchy infiltrates in infants; lobar consolidation is most common with *Streptococcus pneumoniae* or *Haemophilus influenzae;* hilar adenopathy is most common with *Haemophilus influenzae* or *Staphylococcus aureus;* pleural effusion may be present

d. Acute aspiration pneumonia usually develops in portion of lung that is dependent at time of aspiration; otherwise, radiograph typically shows diffuse or localized mottled infiltrates with or without atelectasis

2. White blood cell count may or may not be elevated with increased number of neutrophils or lymphocytes

3. Viral cultures of nasopharyngeal secretions; rapid identification with immunofluorescent assay

4. Blood cultures—if bacterial pneumonia is suspected (frequently negative); positive in 10% to 15% of cases

5. Sputum cultures—warranted if cough is productive; rarely beneficial in younger children

6. Positive cold agglutinin screen or titer > 1:32, positive mycoplasma I$_g$M and/or I$_g$G suggestive of *Mycoplasma pneumonia*

7. Pulse oximetry—decreased O$_2$ saturations with severe disease

- Management/Treatment

1. Most often viral (> 80%) and self limited

2. Antimicrobial treatment based on etiology and age of the child

   a. Intravenous (IV) ampicillin/gentamycin or cephalosporin for hospitalized birth to -3 week old child; IV cephalosporin with or without a macrolide for hospitalized 3-12 week old child; IV cephalosporin or high dose ampicillin for hospitalized 4 months to 4 year old or macrolide or high dose amoxicillin with or without a cephalosporin for outpatient 4 month to 4 year old child; IV cephalosporin with or without azithromycin for hospitalized 5years or older child and macrolides for outpatient 5 years or older child

   b. All ages consider *Staph aureus* if rapidly toxic, >50% with effusions

   c. For infants consider B. *pertussis* if immunizations incomplete or C. trachomatis if mother infected

   d. Consider anerobes if aspiration pneumonia and treat with clindamycin

3. Bronchodilators and chest physiotherapy may improve airway clearance

4. Influenza and/or pneumococcal vaccine for high risk groups

5. Other supportive therapy may include additional fluids and/or oxygen

6. Pneumonia in immunocompromised hosts can progress rapidly; should be managed in a monitored setting, with aggressive diagnostic measures (bronchoalveolar lavage) and appropriate broad-spectrum antimicrobial coverage

7. Refer to pulmonary specialist if recurrent disease without known cause

Pleurisy, Pleural Effusion, and Empyema

- Definition

    1. Pleurisy (pleuritis)—inflammation of the pleural lining

    2. Pleural effusion (pleurisy with effusion)—accumulation of fluid in pleural space

    3. Empyema—pleural inflammation and purulent exudate

- Etiology/Incidence

    1. Parapneumonic effusions (inflammation of pleural space resulting from infection of lung) may complicate pneumonia

    2. Inflammation of pleural lining—caused by a disease process elsewhere in body such as malignancy, trauma, rheumatologic disease, pulmonary vascular obstruction, systemic granulomatous disease; peritoneal inflammation

    3. Conditions causing edema or ascites (eg. renal or hepatic disease) may lead to fluid accumulation in the pleural space

- Signs and Symptoms

    1. Chest pain, particularly with inspiration or cough; chest tightness; dyspnea

    2. High fever, chills, vomiting, anorexia, lethargy (all more likely with infectious etiologies)

    3. Effusions which abut the diaphragm may cause abdominal pain, shoulder pain

- Differential Diagnosis

    1. Tuberculosis

    2. Neoplasm

    3. Connective tissue or collagen disorders

    4. Sarcoidosis

- Physical Findings

    1. Unilateral decrease in chest expansion during inspiration

    2. Pleural rub or decreased breath sounds over affected area

    3. Splinting toward the affected side

    4. Dullness to percussion

- Diagnostic Tests/Findings

    1. Chest radiograph—obliteration of the costophrenic space; supine films may show increased radiodensity of a hemithorax; decubitus films reveal layering of fluid; organized exudates (empyema) unlikely to layer or shift

    2. Thoracentesis for evaluation of the pleural liquid—varies according to type of effusion or exudate

    3. PPD skin test—positive if tuberculosis

4. Blood cultures

5. Pulse oximetry—evaluate hypoxemia

- Management/Treatment: Treat any underlying systemic illness; parapneumonic effusions often resolve with appropriate treatment of pneumonia, but tube drainage may shorten hospital course if organized or loculated; suspected empyema should be referred to subspecialist, may require tube drainage or surgical management, prolonged (4-6 weeks) antibiotics

Cystic Fibrosis (CF)

- Definition: Autosomol recessive disorder of cystic fibrosis transmembrane regulation (CFTR), causing defective epithelial ion transport, which results in dehydrated, viscous secretions which obstruct the exocrine ducts (with subsequent destruction and scarring) in the respiratory, hepatobiliary, gastrointestinal, and reproductive tracts

- Etiology/Incidence

    1. Caused by mutations in a single gene on the long arm of chromosome 7 which directs the production of CFTR

        a. CFTR is the principal chloride channel of epithelial cells and controls other ion transport

        b. Defective CFTR results in increased sodium reabsorption; decreased chloride secretion; and dehydrated, highly viscous secretions in all exocrine ducts which causes disease

        c. There are over 800 mutations of the CFTR gene causing CF, although 22 mutations are the most common in the U.S., with ΔF508 causing 70% of CF

    2. Incidence—most common fatal, autosomal recessive genetic disorder affecting Caucasian population; less frequent among other racial groups

    3. Median life expectancy—32.5 years (in 2002) with respiratory failure leading cause of death; life expectancy slowly increasing as treatments are refined

- Signs and Symptoms

    1. Extremely viscid meconium (newborns), with delayed passage

    2. Poor growth despite normal to increased appetite

    3. Recurrent and chronic respiratory infections (sinuses and lower airways); dyspnea on exertion which progresses to dyspnea at rest as disease progresses

    4. Large, bulky, foul-smelling, greasy stools

    5. Frequent flatulence or abdominal pain

    6. Chronic cough, varies in character, but usually productive, blood-streaked mucus not uncommon, but major hemoptysis can be life threatening

7. Recurrent or persistent wheezing

8. Salty-tasting skin

9. Distal small bowel obstruction

10. Recurrent pancreatitis

11. CF-related diabetes mellitus (50% over 30 years of age)

12. Salt loss syndromes

13. Heat prostration with hypernatnemia dehydration

14. Male infertility (98% of men sterile) and women have reduced fertility

- Differential Diagnosis

    1. Asthma

    2. Immunologic deficiencies

    3. α_1-antitrypsin deficiency (rare)

    4. Airway abnormalities, e.g., airway stenosis, vascular ring, etc.

    5. Gastroesophageal reflux with or without aspiration

    6. Other causes of malabsorption and/or failure to thrive

- Physical Findings

    1. Wheezing and air trapping with increased anteroposterior diameter of the chest (barrel chest) as disease progresses

    2. Crackles

    3. Increased work of breathing with accessory muscle use

    4. Nasal polyps

    5. Failure to thrive from maldigestion and malabsorption (90% of patients)

    6. Abdominal pain and distention

    7. Enlarged liver and spleen

    8. Cholelithiasis

    9. Rectal prolapse

    10. Digital clubbing

    11. Delayed puberty

- Diagnostic Tests/Findings

    1. Pilocarpine iontophoresis sweat test—two tests with a sweat chloride in excess of 60 mEq/L from at least 75 mg of collected sweat; test should be performed by a Cystic Fibrosis Foundation-approved laboratory

2. Genetic testing for mutation analysis; certain countries and states include genetic analysis in newborn screening; prenatal screening available

3. Milder, atypical presentations are being identified by expanded diagnostic criteria

4. Chest radiograph—hyperinflation, increased peribronchial markings, cystic lesions, atelectasis, mucus retention (often right upper lobe)

5. Pulmonary function tests—demonstrates obstructive pattern; decreased flow rates and vital capacity as disease progresses

6. Sputum culture—typical CF pathogens: *Staphlococcus aureus, Pseudomonas aeruginosa, Haemophilus influenzae, Burkholderia cepacia*

7. Oximetry—decreased oxygen saturation with exacerbation and worsening disease

8. Hyponatremia, hypoproteinemia, hypochloremic alkalosis

9. Elevated liver enzymes (AST or ALT)

10. Fat soluble (A, E, and K) vitamin deficiencies

11. Glucose testing

12. Sinus CT—chronic inflammation/disease

- Management/Treatment

    1. Referral to Cystic Fibrosis Care Center for long-term care

        Cystic Fibrosis Foundation
        6931 Arlington Road
        Bethesda, Maryland 20814
        (301) 951-4422
        Fax: (301) 951-6378
        1-800-FIGHT CF (1-800-344-4823) for list of approved centers
        www.cff.org.

    2. Interdisciplinary management involving intensive education, airway clearance techniques, replacement of pancreatic enzymes, nutritional support, prevention and treatment of infection, and psychosocial support

    3. Antibiotic therapy based on sputum culture and sensitivity

        a. Given early in course of disease to delay onset of chronic colonization with *P. aeruginosa*

        b. Once colonized, given to slow decline in pulmonary function

        c. Intravenous courses given for pulmonary exacerbations to restore pulmonary function and reduce symptoms

    4. Isolation—standard precautions for all patients, contact and droplet precautions when indicated, minimize contact with other CF patients to avoid spread of infections

5. Role of primary care provider—annual influenza vaccine, more liberal use of antibiotics for respiratory infections, be alert for CF complications

Asthma

- Definition: Chronic lung disease characterized by:
  1. Airway inflammation
  2. Airway hyper-responsiveness to a variety of stimuli
  3. Variable airway obstruction that is partially or completely reversible either spontaneously or with treatment

- Etiology/Incidence
  1. Airway inflammation plays a central role
     a. Inflammation causes airway narrowing and increased airway secretions
     b. Inflammation contributes to airway hyper-responsiveness
     c. Broad variety of factors trigger inflammation
     d. Causes recurrent acute episodes
  2. Triggers—factors that provoke airway inflammation and acute episodes
     a. Respiratory infections—viral respiratory infections most common trigger for young child
     b. Indoor allergens—dust mites, roaches, mold, animal saliva/ dander
     c. Outdoor allergens—seasonal trees, grasses, weeds, pollens, molds
     d. Weather/humidity changes
     e. Exercise (cold, dry air)
     f. Gastroesophageal reflux
     g. Irritants—tobacco smoke, pollution, strong odors
     h. Food allergies—nuts, shellfish, sulfites (shrimp, dried fruit, beer or wine)
     i. Medications—aspirin, beta-blockers, nonsteroidal anti-inflammatory drugs
     j. Strong emotions
  3. Approximately 5% to 6% of children affected—incidence and mortality increasing worldwide
     a. Increased incidence in childhood; especially among males, lower socio-economic groups, urban African-Americans and Hispanics, and those with family history of asthma or allergies
     b. Leading cause of hospitalization and school absenteeism
     c. Asthma changes over time—some children have recurrent wheezing associated

with viral infections in infancy and early childhood, with subsequently normal airway function

4. Under-diagnosis and inappropriate treatment are *major* contributors to morbidity and mortality

5. Chronic inflammation can lead to chronic airway remodeling with irreversible structural changes and progressive loss of pulmonary function

- Signs and Symptoms

    1. Recurrent episodes of cough, wheezing, mucus production, chest tightness, breathlessness, and decreased endurance

    2. Symptoms often display an initial response (bronchospasm) to a trigger, then a late (inflammatory) phase response in 4 to 8 hours that is more severe and prolonged than the earlier response

    3. Symptoms often worse at night, early morning and during or after exercise

    4. Some patients may have severe, life-threatening exacerbations separated by long periods of normal lung function and no symptoms

    5. A subset of patients present with chronic (usually nighttime) cough without wheezing or exercise intolerance

- Differential Diagnosis

    1. Aspiration

    2. Cystic fibrosis

    3. Cardiac or anatomical defects

    4. Upper or lower respiratory tract infections

    5. Gastroesophageal reflux (can occur coincidentally and exacerbate asthma)

- Physical Findings

    1. Cough

    2. Diffuse wheezes (initially heard at the end of the expiratory phase) with decreased air flow and prolonged expiratory phase

    3. Respiratory distress and hypoxia increases as severity increases

    4. Allergic appearance—allergic "shiners", nasal crease, mouth breathing, and nasal edema; nasal polyps (consider CF especially in younger child)

    5. Skin—atopic dermatitis

    6. Concurrent respiratory infection—viral respiratory illness, sinusitis

    7. Barrel chest—chronic hyperinflation

- Diagnostic Tests/Findings

    1. Thorough history is vital to diagnosis and management, with special emphasis on

triggers, severity of previous episodes, response to medications, and family history of asthma or allergy

2. Spirometry

   a. Lower airway obstruction—forced expiratory volume in 1 second (FEV_1) < 80% predicted

   b. Reversibility—FEV_1 increases at least 12% after using a short-acting inhaled $beta_2$ agonist

   c. May also challenge with exercise, histamine, or methacholine if symptomatic, but initial spirometry normal

3. Chest radiograph

   a. Bilateral hyperinflation with peribronchial thickening

   b. Plate-like atelectasis (often misread as pneumonia)

   c. May be normal

   d. Unnecessary on each acute episode once diagnosis established and responding to therapy

4. Evaluation of other factors contributing to asthma severity

   a. Allergy testing

      (1) Complete blood count—eosinophilia

      (2) Immunoglobulin E—elevated, values age dependent

      (3) Nasal smear for eosinophilia— > 10% considered significant

      (4) Radioallergosorbent test (rast)—serum test which identifies possible allergic responses to various environmental substances

      (5) Refer for allergy evaluation and skin testing as indicated to improve allergy/asthma control

   b. Nasal and sinus evaluation—identify and treat allergic rhinitis, sinusitis

   c. Gastroesophageal reflux assessment

5. Pulse oximetry—evaluate hypoxemia during an acute episode

- Management/Treatment: National Asthma Education and Prevention Program: Expert Panel Report II and Update of Selected Topics (National Heart, Lung and Blood Institute [NHLBI], 1997, 2002) and Pediatric Asthma Promoting Best Practice (American Academy of Allergy, Asthma, and Immunology [AAAAI], 1999)

   1. Diagnose asthma and initiate partnership with family

   2. Classify severity of asthma according to frequency of day and nighttime symptoms

      a. Mild intermittent (symptoms ≤ 2/week daytime or ≤ 2/month nighttime)

      b. Mild persistent (symptoms > 2/week daytime or 3-4/month nighttime)

      c. Moderate persistent (symptoms daily daytime or $\geq$ 5/month nighttime)

      d. Severe persistent (symptoms continual daytime or frequent nighttime)

  3. Medication classification

      a. Long-term control medicines—taken daily

          (1) Inhaled corticosteroids (beclomethasone, budesonide, flunisolide, fluticasone, triamcinolone)—delivered by nebulizer, dry powder inhaler, or meter dose inhaler; preferred treatment for persistent asthma; dose of drug matched to level of disease severity

          (2) Leukotriene modifiers (montelukast, preferred drug with children)

          (3) Long-acting beta$_2$ agonists—salmeterol, inhaled

              (a) Effect lasts 12 hours, helps nocturnal symptoms

              (b) Not to be confused with quick relief medications

              (c) Prevent exercise-induced bronchospasm

              (d) Not to be used as monotherapy—combine with inhaled steroids for moderate or severe persistent asthma

          (4) Cromolyn sodium or nedocromil (inhaled)

          (5) Methylxanthines

          (6) Oral corticosteroids (if severe, chronic asthma, not to exceed 60 mg/day)

      b. Quick relief medications—taken as needed to provide prompt reversal of acute airflow obstruction and relief of bronchoconstriction; not for daily long-term use

          (1) Inhaled short-acting beta$_2$ agonists (albuterol, pirbuterol)

          (2) Anticholinergics (ipratroprium bromide, inhaled)

          (3) Short course systemic corticosteroids (oral or parenteral)

  4. Prescribe medications according to severity (refer to NHLBI, 1997, 2002 and AAAAI, 1999)

      a. Anti-inflammatory medications to all patients with persistent asthma—inhaled steroids preferred treatment

          (1) Symptoms > 2 times a week

          (2) Nocturnal symptoms > 2 times a month

          (3) FEV_1 below 80% predicted (off medication)

      b. Give all patients an inhaled short-acting beta$_2$ agonist for as-needed use to relieve acute symptoms

      c. Increase medication according to severity of asthma and response to therapy

   d. Decrease medication as tolerated once good control demonstrated over 3-6 months

   e. Minimize side effects, use lowest dose of anti-inflammatory that maintains good control

   f. Antibiotics helpful if concurrent bacterial infection

   g. Nasal anti-inflammatory medication (corticosteroids, cromolyn) and antihistamines to treat concurrent rhinitis

   h. Consider referral to allergist for allergy immunotherapy

5. Identify and reduce child-specific triggers

6. Provide clear written instructions; problem solve with family for appropriate solutions for trigger control and medication options

7. Educate child/family to monitor and treat symptoms early

   a. Moderate and severe persistent asthma—should monitor peak expiratory flow (PEF) at home; before morning medication and with acute symptoms

   b. Develop a written ''action'' plan for acute episodes for all patients

      (1) 20% drop in PEF—increase medication

      (2) 50% drop in PEF—severe exacerbation

   c. Treat mild exacerbations with inhaled short-acting $beta_2$ agonist every 4 to 6 hours

   d. Add short course of oral corticosteroids early in course of moderate to severe exacerbations

8. Long-term care (every 1 to 6 months, depending on severity)

   a. Review attainment of treatment goals

      (1) Prevent chronic, nocturnal, and troublesome symptoms

      (2) Maintain normal activity levels (including exercise)

      (3) Prevent recurrent exacerbations and minimize the need for emergency department visits, hospitalizations, or school absenteeism

      (4) Meet family's expectations of asthma care

   b. Assess lung function with objective measures—spirometry or peak flow meter

   c. Adjust medication use, screen for side effects and consistent use—long-term adherence to daily medicines difficult for most families

   d. Review management plan (including trigger control and acute episodes)

   e. Check child's technique with inhaled medications and peak flow meter

   f. Provide asthma treatment plan for school or day care

9. Provide smoking cessation counseling as needed

    a. Identify all tobacco smokers in child's environment

    b. Strongly advise all smokers to quit

    c. Identify all smokers willing to attempt to quit

    d. Assist cessation by:

        (1) Clinician delivered social support

        (2) Nicotine replacement therapy

    e. Arrange follow-up contact

10. High risk for asthma related deaths—refer to specialist

    a. History of life-threatening exacerbations—intensive care admission or intubation

    b. ≥ 2 hospitalizations/year; ≥ 3 emergency department visits/year

    c. Prolonged course of oral steroids or > 2 bursts of oral steroids/year

    d. Overuse of inhaled short-acting $beta_2$ agonist (> one canister/month)

    e. Poor adherence to treatment plan

    f. Young child with moderate or severe persistent asthma

Bronchopulmonary dysplasia (BPD)

- Definition: Any child requiring supplemental oxygen at 36 weeks or greater (post-conceptual age) with radiographic changes of chronic lung disease

- Etiology/Incidence

  1. Birth weight single most predictive factor; highest incidence in infants < 1000 g at birth

  2. 90% following respiratory distress syndrome; other causes include persistent pulmonary hypertension, meconium aspiration, severe lower respiratory infection, maternal infection (amnionitis), or chronic aspiration

  3. Leading cause of chronic lung disease in infants

  4. Multifactorial—lung immaturity, oxygen toxicity, barotrauma from mechanical ventilation, infections, malnutrition, or fluid overload

  5. Mild to severe disease possible (decreased lung compliance and increased airway resistance)

- Signs and Symptoms

  1. Respiratory distress; may have cough and wheeze

  2. Poor growth and poor feeding skills

  3. Fussy with decreased endurance

- Differential Diagnosis

    1. Congenital cardiac or pulmonary defects that result in supplemental oxygen requirement

    2. Upper airway obstruction

    3. Lower airway abnormalities (structural/anatomic, extrinsic compression, tracheomalacia)

    4. Pulmonary hypertension

    5. Metabolic disorders

    6. Respiratory infections/immunodeficiency

    7. Chronic gastroesophageal reflux

    8. Chronic aspiration

- Physical findings—vary with severity of disease

    1. Tachypnea with retractions

    2. Diffuse inspiratory or expiratory crackles and/or wheezes

    3. Pale with cyanotic episodes

    4. Findings consistent with cardiac insufficiency or fluid overload

    5. Fluid sensitivity

    6. Associated findings consistent with sequelae of prematurity and/or chronic lung disease

- Diagnostic Tests/Findings

    1. Oximetry on room air—hypoxemia

    2. Overnight oxygen saturation monitoring—identifies significant, prolonged desaturations (< 90%) with sleep and assists with weaning schedule

    3. Growth curve—often FTT even after corrected for prematurity

    4. Serum electrolytes

        a. Carbon dioxide retention

        b. Chloride and potassium depletion, metabolic alkalosis—with diuretic use

    5. Arterial blood gases (on room air) -- compensated respiratory acidosis

        a. pH—low/normal

        b. $PaO_2 < 70$ mm Hg

        c. $PaCO_2 > 45$ mm Hg

    6. Chest radiograph—diffuse haziness, increased interstitial markings; hyperinflation common, may be normal

    7. Other studies as indicated to monitor and manage associated findings

- Management/Treatment

  1. Maintain adequate oxygenations (92% or greater) to prevent cor pulmonale and promote growth

     a. Provide supplemental oxygen—wean as tolerated, expect gradual improvement with growth

     b. Desaturation commonly occurs during sleeping and feeding

     c. More severe BPD may need long-term mechanical ventilation and tracheotomy

     d. Delayed improvement may indicate undiagnosed complicating factors (structural heart disease, gastroesophageal reflux)

  2. Adequate nutrition and fluids

     a. Achieve 15 to 30 g of growth per day

     b. High calorie formulas with additives often needed; avoid excessive carbohydrate load; nutrition referral

     c. Occupational therapy intervention for feeding skills

     d. Gastrostomy or supplemental tube feedings as needed

     e. Balance nutrition volume with fluid restriction when fluid sensitive

     f. Treat gastroesophageal reflux

  3. Medications

     a. Bronchodilators—if beneficial

     b. Diuretics—as needed for acute fluid overload; avoid chronic use if possible

     c. Inhaled anti-inflammatories—limited usefulness

        (1) Long-term daily use of inhaled corticosteroids; cromolyn or nedocromil

        (2) Ipratropium bromide may be useful during acute illness or in chronic management

        (3) Post-natal steroids only to be used in severe, respiratory failure, not for chronic use

  4. Protective care to avoid lung re-injury

     a. Immunizations

     b. Smoke free environment

     c. RSV precautions—administer Palivizumb (Impact—RSV Study Group, 1998) or RSV intravenous immunoglobulin in high risk population (AAP, 2003)

     d. Avoid high density day care settings

     e. Good hand-washing and other infection control precautions

     f. Avoid elective procedures, especially during winter months

g. Higher incidence of Sudden Infant Death in this population

5. Family education, support, and follow-up

   a. "Rooming in" prior to discharge to demonstrate caregiver competency with home equipment and infant care

   b. Close follow-up (every 1 to 3 months), to determine adequate oxygenation and growth

   c. Higher incidence of rehospitalization in early years due to exacerbations

6. Monitor for associated findings, manage/refer as needed—airway disorders, hypertension, gastroesophageal reflux, heart failure, neurodevelopmental problems, ophthalmology or renal complications

7. High risk for neurologic, developmental, or academic concerns throughout childhood

8. Referrals

   (1) Early intervention for developmental assistance and monitoring

   (2) Financial assistance and counseling

   (3) Home nursing and equipment companies

   (4) Family counseling and support groups

   (5) Community rescue services

   (6) Case management

9. Prevention—reduce incidence of premature births

Apnea

- Definition

1. Respiratory pause lasting > 20 seconds or associated with cyanosis, bradycardia, marked pallor, or hypotonia; may be central, obstructive or mixed

2. Central apnea—cessation of airflow and respiratory effort

3. Obstructive sleep apnea syndrome (OSAS)—cessation of airflow at the nose and mouth with continued respiratory effort; usually caused by upper airway obstruction

4. Mixed—central apnea followed by respiratory movement without airflow

5. Apnea of infancy—pathologic apnea in infants that are > 37 weeks gestation at onset

6. Apnea of prematurity—periodic breathing with pathologic apnea in a premature infant < 37 weeks gestation

7. Apparent Life Threatening Event (ALTE)—an episode that an observer believes is life-threatening, characterized by some combination of apnea, change in skin color, marked change in muscle tone, choking or gagging and requires significant intervention to restore normal breathing

- Etiology/Incidence

  1. Apneas vary significantly depending on underlying etiology

  2. ALTE occurs in 3% of population

     a. When etiology unidentified, sudden infant death risk increases significantly

     b. Subsequent episodes occur commonly

  3. Obstructive sleep apnea syndrome

     a. 3 to 6 years peak age (peak adenotonsillar hypertrophy)

     b. Familial tendency

     c. Increased risk with craniofacial anomalies, obesity, Down syndrome

- Signs and Symptoms

  1. During event, respiratory pause accompanied by marked pallor, cyanosis, hypotonia, and bradycardia

  2. OSAS—loud, habitual snoring; apnea followed by gasping, choking, and arousal; restless sleep, and diaphoresis

  3. Behavioral changes, poor school performance, daytime sleepiness, hyperactivity, growth delay, heart failure, or hypertension may be signs of chronic OSAS

- Differential Diagnosis (ALTE)

  1. Sepsis/meningitis

  2. Respiratory syncytial virus infection

  3. Seizures

  4. Metabolic defects

  5. Cardiac defects

  6. GER

  7. Munchausen syndrome by proxy (MSP)

- Physical Findings

  1. Often normal at time of examination

  2. OSAS—mouth breathing; upper airway narrowed/obstructed from inflammation or structural defects; allergic stigmata; congestive heart failure; obese, normal weight, or failure to thrive, adenotonsillar hypertrophy

  3. Lungs usually clear

  4. May have physical findings of cardiac insufficiency or fluid overload with long-standing, severe obstruction

- Diagnostic Tests/Findings

  1. Complete history—emphasize circumstances surrounding the event, medical and family history

  2. Complete physical examination with detailed neurodevelopmental assessment

  3. Based on history, examination, and age of child

     a. Arterial blood gas—indicate severity of event and current stability

     b. Pulse oximetry—likely normal; may show hypoxemia

     c. Electroencephalogram—seizure disorder

     d. Viral respiratory panel—RSV infection

     e. Complete blood count, blood culture—indicative of sepsis, polycythemia (chronic hypoxemia), anemia

     f. Fluid balance profile—metabolic status, elevated bicarbonate (chronic respiratory insufficiency)

     g. Lumbar puncture—meningitis

     h. Electrocardiogram—cardiac arrythmias

     i. Chest radiograph—evaluate structure and anatomy, heart size

     j. Sleep study (overnight polysomnogram)—definitive test to identify significant apneas and differentiate type of apneas

- Management/Treatment (based on history and physical findings)

  1. Admit to hospital for close observation and monitoring for ALTE

  2. Institute treatment and referrals based on diagnostic findings, history, and physical examination

  3. If cause unclear, decision is more complex, but should include:

     a. Frequent follow up visits with serial measurements of:

        (1) Height, weight, and head circumference

        (2) Developmental assessment

     b. Emotional support and parental counseling

     c. Apnea monitor recommendations with a specific clinical indication

        (1) Use monitor with an event recorder

        (2) Monitor only detects episodes of central apnea

        (3) Monitoring does not prevent all deaths

        (4) Monitoring is stressful (false alarms, child safety, travel cumbersome, and financial burden)

        (5) Requires close supervision and plan for monitor termination

      d. CPR instruction for family and other caregivers

  4. OSAS

      a. Referrals as indicated for adenotonsillectomy, weight loss, or continuous positive airway pressure device with sleep

      b. Repeat sleep study after adenotonsillectomy (may have persistent obstruction despite resolution of snoring)

Tuberculosis (TB)

- Definition: A chronic, granulomatous infection which may cause pulmonary, extrapulmonary, or disseminated disease

- Etiology/Incidence

  1. Caused by *Mycobacterium tuberculosis*

  2. Primary mode of transmission is inhalation of aerosol droplets through person to person contact; virtually all cases of pediatric TB are acquired through contact with an infected adolescent or adult

  3. Tuberculosis is classified as primary infection or tuberculosis disease

      a. Latent tuberculosis infection (LTBI)—positive tuberculin skin test without clinical, radiographic, or laboratory evidence of active disease

      b. Tuberculosis disease

         (1) Pulmonary—hilar adenopathy with or without parenchymal lesion; children younger than 4 years of age increased incidence of miliary disease; pneumonia and pleural effusion may occur in older children; cavitary disease rare in children; airway obstruction with atelectasis may occur

         (2) Extrapulmonary—miliary tuberculosis may involve any organ of the body, most frequently seen in lymph nodes and central nervous system; meningitis more likely in infants

  4. TB rates for all ages in U.S. are highest in urban, low-income areas and in non-white racial and ethnic groups

  5. Increased TB risk associated with

      a. Contacts of persons with confirmed or suspected infectious TB

      b. Minority groups—immigrants from high-risk countries in Asia, Africa, Latin America, and The Middle East; children with travel to these countries; significant contact with persons from these countries

      c. Homeless, migrant, institutionalized, or prison populations

      d. Other—recent skin test conversion, immunodeficiency (HIV) or immunosuppression, IV drug use, certain diseases or some chronic illnesses

- Signs and Symptoms

  1. Usually asymptomatic

  2. Cough, wheezing, dyspnea

  3. Abdominal pain, diarrhea, poor weight gain or weight loss, anorexia or poor suck

  4. Fever, lethargy, night sweats, chills

  5. May present with clinical symptoms of meningitis

  6. Late clinical presentations include symptoms of TB of middle ear and mastoid, bones, joints, skin, and kidneys

  7. Drug resistant TB is clinically indistinguishable from drug-susceptible disease

- Differential Diagnosis

  1. Histoplasmosis

  2. Atypical mycobacteria

  3. Pneumonia

  4. Lung abscess

  5. Foreign body aspiration

  6. Sarcoidosis

  7. Neoplasm

- Physical Findings

  1. Usually asymptomatic

  2. Dry, hacking, or brassy, paroxysmal cough

  3. Localized wheezing or crackles

  4. Lymphadenopathy

  5. Failure to thrive

  6. Low-grade fever

- Diagnostic Tests/Findings

  1. Tuberculin skin test (TST)—Mantoux test recommended, multiple puncture test lacks adequate specificity and sensitivity

     a. All children should have a routine assessment of their risk of exposure to TB. Skin test only those children with increased risk

     b. Skin test immediately any child identified as a contact of a person with confirmed or suspected infectious TB; any child with clinical or radiographic findings suggestive of TB, any child immigrating from an endemic area or traveling in endemic areas or having significant contact with persons from endemic areas

     c. Skin test annually any child with HIV or living with an HIV-infected person; an incarcerated adolescent

     d. Skin test every 2 to 3 years any child exposed to high-risk persons (refer to #5 etiology/incidence section)

     e. Skin test should be considered at 4 to 6 and 11 to 16 years of age for any child living in high-prevalence areas, travel to high-prevalence areas, or with household contacts from high-prevalence areas

     f. A positive TST indicates likely infection—a reaction of 15 mm or greater is considered positive in any population; reactions of 5 to 14 mm may be considered positive in certain high risk groups

2. Chest radiograph with lobar or segmental parenchymal lesion or collapsed consolidation, lymphadenopathy, pleural effusion, or miliary disease (characterized by snowflake appearance)

3. Positive acid fast bacillus culture obtained from sputum or early morning gastric aspirate

- Management/Treatment

1. Diagnosing a child with TB infection or disease represents recent transmission of TB in the community; every effort should be made to identify and treat the source case and others infected by the source case; all cases should be reported to local health department. Epidemiological investigation, isolation, compliance with therapy, and evaluation of the resolution of disease are crucial in controlling spread of disease; prescribing provider and public health authorities are both responsible for treatment completion

2. Referral to appropriate specialist

3. Guidelines for chemotherapy vary widely depending on the sensitivity of the organism, the condition of the patient, and the location of disease; refer to most recent edition of AAP *Red Book* for a complete list of drug dosages and side effects as well as therapeutic regimens; commonly used medications are isoniazid, rifampin, pyrazinamide, streptomycin, rifapentine

4. For LTBI, 9 months treatment with isoniazid is regimen of choice; prolonged therapy for immunocompromised conditions

5. For newborns exposed to household contact infected with TB, recommendations vary based on categorization of infection of household contact; refer to most recent edition of AAP *Red Book*

6. Directly observed therapy and patient-centered case management are recommended for treatment of people with tuberculosis disease

7. Children younger than 12 with primary pulmonary disease are usually not contagious; older children and adults suspected of having TB require TB isolation until proved noncontagious (AAP, 2000)

8. Bacillus Calmette-Guerin (BCG) vaccine—live vaccine from attenuated strains of

Mycobacterium bovis; recommended only in limited and select circumstances in U.S.; recommended internationally by World Health Organization for administration at birth to help prevent disseminated and other life-threatening diseases caused by *Mycobacterium tuberculosis;* indications, adverse reactions, contraindications, and interpretations of Mantoux skin tests in persons who have received BCG described in AAP *Red Book*

9. Management plan should be tailored to promote adherence to the drug regimen

10. Obtain suptum culture at completion of initial phase of treatment to identify patients at increased risk of relapse; extended treatment is recommended for patients with drug susceptible pulmonary TB and cavitation and positive sputum culture after two months of treatment

11. High risk of dissemenated TB in infants and children less that 4 years of age—start treatment as soon as TB is suspected

Questions
Select the best answer

1. Shelby, a 4 week old, presents to your office in mid-January with a one week history of nasal congestion and occasional cough. On the evening prior to this visit Shelby developed a temperature of 102° F; refused to breast-feed; had paroxysmal coughing, and noisy, labored breathing. On exam, you note an ill-appearing infant who is lethargic with tachypnea and intercostal retractions. Shelby does not attend day care but has a 3-year old sibling who is in day care and who recently had a ''cold''. Considering the clinical presentation, what is the most likely cause of Shelby's illness?

   a. Mycoplasma pneumonia
   b. RSV bronchiolitis
   c. Aspiration pneumonia
   d. Streptococcal infection of the pharynx

2. In the above scenario, which of the following would be the treatment of choice?

   a. Antihistamine, decongestant and cough suppressant
   b. Oral antibiotics and follow up chest radiograph in two weeks
   c. Bronchoscopy with lavage, chest physiotherapy, and respiratory isolation
   d. Hospitalization, bronchodilators, supplemental oxygen, and nutritional support

3. Of the following children, which one should not have tuberculin skin testing?

   a. Richard, a 14-year-old, whose uncle was recently granted parole after five years in prison and is currently living with Richard's family
   b. Theresa, a 2-year-old who was infected with RSV three months ago and is currently asymptomatic
   c. Han, a 3-month-old whose family immigrated to the U.S. from Cambodia one month ago
   d. Chris, an 18-month-old whose mother is infected with HIV

4. Which of the following clinical presentations least warrants sweat chloride testing?

   a. 10-year-old female sibling of a patient newly diagnosed with cystic fibrosis; sibling is without pulmonary problems and growth parameters are at 50% for age
   b. 2-year-old male with recurrent pneumonia and growth parameters at 5% for age
   c. 4-year-old female with nocturnal cough which resolves after treatment with bronchodilators and short-term steroids; growth parameters at 10% for age
   d. 7-year-old female with nasal polyps, mildly hyperexpanded lungs, growth parameters at 25% for age

5. Of the following diagnostic findings, which one should be referred to a specialist immediately?

   a. Suspected foreign body aspiration
   b. Sweat chloride results of 30 mEq/L
   c. Pulmonary function tests of 85% predicted
   d. Chest radiograph with hyperexpansion

6. What is the most common agent for nonviral pneumonia from older preschool to young adulthood?

    a. *Mycoplasma/Chlamydia aureus*
    b. *Staphylococcus aureus*
    c. *Ureaplasma*
    d. *Haemophilus influenzae*

7. Which one of the following diagnoses would not be part of the differential for recurrent lobar pneumonia in a 2 year old?

    a. Cystic fibrosis
    b. Foreign body aspiration
    c. Atelectasis
    d. Bronchitis

8. The most common clinical presentation of pneumonia includes:

    a. Cough, fever, tachypnea, and abdominal pain
    b. Hemoptysis, putrid breath, and weight loss
    c. Sudden chest pain, cyanosis
    d. Retractions, stridor

9. In addition to airway hyper-responsiveness and reversible airway obstruction, asthma is a chronic lung disease characterized by:

    a. Bronchiectasis
    b. Inflammation
    c. Pleural effusion
    d. Pulmonary edema

10. The most common trigger for an acute asthma episode in the very young child is:

    a. Respiratory infections
    b. Exercise
    c. Tobacco smoke
    d. Outdoor allergens

11. Luke has mild persistent asthma. Appropriate daily medication should include:

    a. An inhaled low-dose corticosteroid
    b. Short-acting beta$_2$ agonists
    c. An oral systemic corticosteroid
    d. A cough suppressant

12. Which of the following is not a goal of appropriate asthma management?

    a. Limited activity and exercise
    b. Prevent recurrent exacerbations

    c. Prevent chronic troublesome symptoms
    d. Maintain near normal pulmonary functions

13. Deon is a 4-year-old African-American male with a history of atopic dermatitis and recurrent pneumonias according to his mother. He presents with a persistent night time cough. His most likely diagnosis is:

    a. Asthma
    b. Foreign body aspiration
    c. Croup
    d. Cystic fibrosis

14. The most typical chest radiographic finding consistent with the diagnosis of asthma is:

    a. Normal chest film
    b. Diffuse airway edema
    c. Right upper lobe infiltrate
    d. Hyperinflation

15. When providing asthma education regarding the use of a long-acting beta$_2$ agonist, it is important to stress:

    a. It should not be used as a quick-relief medication
    b. May be given every 30 minutes times three for rescue therapy
    c. May be most beneficial for exercise-induced asthma
    d. Should never be taken while also using inhaled corticosteroids

16. Claire is an 8-year-old with moderate persistent asthma who is still having a daily cough. She reports three times a day use of a short-acting inhaled beta$_2$ agonist and cromolyn sodium at her clinic visit. Your management plan should be altered to include:

    a. Broad spectrum antibiotics and recheck in two weeks
    b. Addition of systemic corticosteroids for five days
    c. Replace cromolyn sodium with inhaled cortiocosteroids and when symptoms resolve reduce short-acting beta$_2$ agonist to as-needed use
    d. Addition of an inhaled anticholinergic

17. Ben is a 10-year-old who has recently been diagnosed with mild intermittent asthma. Which of the following is not a routine part of his clinic management?

    a. Spirometry evaluation
    b. Metered dose inhaler technique demonstration
    c. Environmental triggers and control methods review
    d. School excuse to not participate in physical education activities

18. Major contributors to asthma morbidity and mortality are:

    a. Under-diagnosis and inappropriate treatment
    b. An increase in indoor allergens
    c. Overuse of anti-inflammatory medications
    d. An increase in air pollution

19. The primary treatment for bronchopulmonary dysplasia is:

    a. Pancreatic enzymes
    b. Surgical repair
    c. Adequate oxygenation
    d. Chest physiotherapy

20. The single most predictive factor in the development of bronchopulmonary dysplasia is:

    a. Birth weight
    b. Maternal age
    c. Maternal educational level
    d. Respiratory infections

21. The classic radiographic finding in croup is:

    a. Hyperinflation
    b. Perihilar lymphadenopathy
    c. Thumb sign
    d. Steeple sign

22. Unilateral wheezing is a finding suggestive of:

    a. Croup
    b. Asthma
    c. Foreign body aspiration
    d. Cystic fibrosis

23. Which of the following is not characteristic of an apparent life-threatening event (ALTE):

    a. Change in muscle tone
    b. Fever
    c. Change in skin color
    d. Apnea

24. Following an ALTE, management and treatment are based on findings from:

    a. A thorough history and physical exam
    b. An electroencephalogram
    c. A chest radiograph
    d. A sleep study

25. The predominant characteristic of a young infant with bronchopulmonary dysplasia is:

    a. Prolonged fevers
    b. Hypoxemia on room air
    c. Recurrent pneumonias
    d. Chronic hypoinflation

Answers

1. b	10. a	19. c
2. d	11. a	20. a
3. b	12. a	21. d
4. c	13. a	22. c
5. a	14. d	23. b
6. a	15. a	24. a
7. d	16. c	25. b
8. a	17. d	
9. b	18. a	

Bibliography

Agertoft, L., & Pedersen, S. (2000). Effects of long-term treatment with inhaled budesonide on adult height in children with asthma. *New England Journal of Medicine*, 343, 1064-1069.

Allen, J., Zwerdling, R., Ehrenkranz, R., et. al. (2003). Statement on the care of the child with chronic lung disease of infancy and childhood. *American Journal of Respiratory & Critical Care Medicine*, 168(3), 356-385.

American Academy of Allergy Asthma & Immunology (AAAAI). (1999). Pediatric asthma promoting best practice: *Guide for managing asthma in children.* Milwaukee: AAAAI.

American Academy of Pediatrics. (2003). *Red book 2003: Report of the committee on infectious diseases* (26th ed.). Elk Grove Village, IL: Author.

Ampofo, K. K., & Saiman, L. Pediatric tuberculosis. *Pediatric Annals,* 31(2), 98-108.

Anderson, J. E., Jorenby, D. E., Scott, W. J. & Fiore, M. C. (2002). Treating tobacco use and dependence: An evidence-based clinical practice guideline for tobacco cessation. *Chest,* 121(3), 932-41.

Blackmon, L. R., Batton, D. G., Bell, E. F. et. al. (2003). American Academy of Pediatrics Policy Statement: Apnea, sudden infant death syndrome, and home monitoring. *Pediatrics,* 111(4), 914-917.

Blackmon, L. R., Bell, E. F., Engle, W. A., et. al. (2002). Postnatal corticosteroids to treat or prevent chronic lung disease in preterm infants. *Pediatrics,* 109(2). 330-338.

Blumberg, H. M., Hopewell, P. C., O'Brine, R. J., et. al. (2003). American Thoracic Society/ Center for Disease Control and Prevention/Infectious Diseases Society of America: Treatment of tuberculosis. *American Journal of Respiratory & Critical Care Medicine,* 167(4), 603-662.

Bressler, K., Green, C., & Holinger, L. (1999). Foreign body aspiration. In L. Taussig, L. Landau (Eds.), *Pediatric Respiratory Medicine* (pp. 430-435). St. Louis: Mosby.

Cohn, D. L., O'Brien, R. J. (2000). Targeted tuberculin testing and treatment of latent tuberculosis infection. *American Journal of Respiratory and Critical Care Medicine,* 161, 5221-5247.

Ewing, J. M. (2002). Croup. *Pediatric Annals,* 31(2), 125-130.

Gaton, B. (2002). Pneumonia. *Pediatrics in Review,* 23(4)132-140.

Gibson, R. L., Burns, J. L., & Ramsey, B. W. (2003). Pathophysiology and management of pulmonary infections in cystic fibrosis. *American Journal of Respiratory & Critical Care Medicine,* 168(8), 918-951.

Gjona, S., Green-Hernandez, C., & Aronzon, D. Z. (2001). Chronic Pulmonary Diseases. In C. Green-Hernandez, J. K. Singleton & D. Z. Aronzon (Eds.). *Primary Care Pediatrics* (pp. 681-702). Philadelphia: Lippincott, Williams & Wilkins.

Goodman, M. H., & Brady, M. A. (2000). Respiratory disorders. In C. E. Burns, M. A. Brady, A. M. Dunn & N. B. Starr (Eds.). *Pediatric Primary Care: A Handbook for Nurse Practitioners* (2nd ed., pp. 858-890). Philadelphia: W. B. Saunders.

Grad, R. (1998). Acute infections producing upper airway obstruction. In V. Chernick & T. F.

Boot (Eds.). *Kendig's Disorders of the Respiratory Tract in Children* (6th ed., pp. 452-455). Philadelphia: W. B. Saunders Company.

Hogan, M. B., & Wilson, N. W. (2003). Asthma in the school-aged child. *Pediatric Annals, 32*(1), 20-25.

Kuman, R. (2003). The wheezing infant: Diagnosis and treatment. *Pediatric Annals, 32*(1), 30-36.

Lasley, M. V. (2003). New treatments for asthma. *Pediatrics in Review, 24*(7), 222-232.

Lima, J. A., & Fischer, G. B. (2002). Foreign body aspiration in children. *Paediatric Respiratory Reviews, 34*(4), 303-7.

McCarthy, C. A., & Hall, C. B. (2003). Respiratory syncytial virus: Concerns and control. *Pediatrics in Review, 24*(9), 301-08.

Marcus, C. L., Chapman, D., & Ward, S. (2002). Clinical practice guideline: Diagnosis and management of childhood obstructive sleep apnea syndrome. *Pediatrics, 109*(4), 704-12.

Montgomery, M. (1998). Air and liquid in the pleural space. In V. Chernick & T. F. Boat (Eds.), *Disorders of the Respiratory Tract in Children* (6th ed., pp. 389-411). Philadelphia: W. B. Saunders Company.

National Heart, Lung, and Blood Institute. (2002). Expert panel report: *Guidelines for the diagnosis and management of asthma—update of selected topics*. National Asthma Education and Prevention Program. (NIH Publication No. 02-5075). Bethesda, MD: US Department of Health & Human Services.

National Heart, Lung, and Blood Institute. (1997). *Expert panel report II: Guidelines for the diagnosis and management of asthma*. National Asthma Education and Prevention Program. (NIH Publication No. 97-4051). Washington, DC: US Government Printing Office.

Ngai, P., & Bye, M. R. (2002). Bronchiolitis. *Pediatric Annals, 31*(2), 90-97.

Orstein, D. M., Winnie, G. B., & Altman, H. (2002). Cystic fibrosis: A 2002 update. *Journal of Pediatrics, 140*, 156-164.

Phipantanakul, W. (2003). Environmental indoor allergens. *Pediatric Annals, 32*(1), 40-48.

Pongracic, J. A. (2003). Asthma delivery devices: Age-appropriate use. *Pediatric Annals, 32*(1), 50-54.

Ritchie, S. K. (2002). Primary care of the preterm infant discharged from the neonatal intensive care unit. *Maternal Child Nursing, 27*(2), 76-86.

Saiman, L., Marshall, B. C., Mayer-Hamblett, N., et al. (2003). Azithromycin in patients with cystic fibrosis chronically infected with *Pseudomonas aeruginosa* a randomized controlled trial. *Journal of the American Medical Association, 290*(13), 1749-1757.

Schechter, M. S., Marcus, C. L., Chapman, D., et. al. (2002). Technical report: Diagnosis and management of childhood obstructive sleep apnea syndrome. *Pediatrics, 109*(4), e69.

Sheares, B. J. (2002). Recurrent pneumonia in children. *Pediatric Annals, 31*(2), 109-114.

Starke, J. R. (2001) Transmission of *Mycobacterium tuberculosis* to and from children and adolescents. *Seminars in Pediatric Infectious Diseases,* 12(2), 115-123.

The Childhood Asthma Management Program Research Group (2000). Long term effects of budesonide or nedocromil in children with asthma. *New England Journal of Medicine,* 343, 1054-1063.

The Impact—RSV Study Group. (1998). Pavilzumab, a humanized respiratory syncytial virus monoclonal antibody, reduces hospitalization from respiratoy syncytial virus infection in high-risk infants. *Pediatrics,* 102(3), 531-537.

Vaucher, Y. E. (2002). Bronchopulmonary dysplasia: An enduring challenge. *Pediatrics in Review,* 23(10), 349-357.

Vaughn, D., & Katkin, J. (2002). Chronic and recurrent pneumonia in children. *Seminars in Respiratory Infections,* 17(1), 72-84.

Wright, R. B., Pomerantz, W. J., & Luria, J. W. (2002). New approaches to respiratory infections in children: Bronchiolitis and croup. *Emergency Medicine Clinics of North America,* 20(1), 93-114.

Dermatologic Conditions

Beverly Bigler

Newborn Exanthema

Cutis Marmorata

- Definition: Transient mottling of the neonate's skin with a lacy bluish appearance
- Etiology/Incidence
    1. Physiologic response of uneven blood flow which results in constriction of small blood vessels while others dilate
    2. Often precipitated by exposure to cold
    3. More common in premature infants
    4. Persistence after neonatal period found in Down syndrome
- Signs and Symptoms: Generalized lacy, reddish-blue appearance to the skin
- Differential Diagnosis
    1. Cutis marmorata telangiectatica congenita
    2. Cyanosis
    3. Erythema toxicum neonatorum
- Physical Findings: Generalized reddish-blue reticulated pattern to most of body surface
- Diagnostic Tests/Findings: None
- Management/Treatment
    1. Keep neonate at an even warm temperature
    2. Reduce exposure to cold environment
    3. Don't overdress or keep environment overly warm

Erythema Toxicum Neonatorum

- Definition: Transient benign skin rash with lesions of varied morphology; erythematous macules; wheals, vesicles, and pustules
- Etiology/Incidence:
    1. Unknown cause
    2. Occurs in 50% to 60% of neonates
    3. More common in full-term and post-term neonates
    4. More common in neonates with birth weight > 2500 g
    5. Onset usually within first 24 to 48 hours of life, but occasionally present at birth
- Signs and Symptoms
    1. Yellow-white lesions on reddish-pink base; may be blotchy

2. Extent of rash varies from minimal to most of body surface; palms and soles are usually spared

- Differential Diagnosis
    1. Congenital candidiasis
    2. Incontinentia pigmenti
    3. Miliaria rubra
    4. Neonatal pustular melanosis
    5. Urticaria pigmentosa
    6. Bacterial infestation

- Physical Findings
    1. Lesions of varied morphology—erythematous macules 2 to 3 cm in diameter appear first, followed by wheals, vesicles, and rarely pustules
    2. Lesions usually arise from erythematous base with macular erythema fading within 2 to 3 days
    3. Occurs predominately on the trunk, however, may occur anywhere on body except soles and palms
    4. Number of lesions varies from few to many
    5. Spontaneous resolution in 5 to 7 days

- Diagnostic Tests/Findings: Wright's stained smear of pustules identifies presence of eosinophils rather than neutrophils which rules out neonatal pustular melanosis

- Management/Treatment
    1. Obtain detailed history of onset, duration, and progression
    2. Describe and monitor lesions in terms of morphology/structure, size, shape, number, color, location, distribution
    3. No treatment necessary
    4. Educate regarding characteristics of condition and expected resolution
    5. Refer for evaluation if condition does not improve

Milia

- Definition: Benign condition of small yellow-white inclusion cysts filled with cheesy keratinous material on face of newborn

- Etiology/Incidence
    1. Caused by superficial keratinous material accumulated within developing pilosebaceous follicle
    2. Occurs in 50% of newborns

- Signs and Symptoms: Numerous small yellow-white raised lesions on face of newborn
- Differential Diagnosis: Sebaceous hyperplasia
- Physical Findings
  1. Numerous firm pearly yellow-white 1 to 2 mm inclusion papular cysts on the cheeks, forehead, and nose; predominantly on face; may be found on other body surfaces
  2. Oral counterpart are yellow papular lesions on hard palate known as Epstein's pearls
  3. Condition resolves spontaneously without treatment within a few weeks as lesions exfoliate
- Diagnostic Tests/Findings: None
- Management/Treatment
  1. Describe and monitor lesions in terms of morphology/structure, size, shape, number, color, location, distribution
  2. No treatment necessary
  3. Educate regarding characteristics of condition and expected resolution

Sebaceous Hyperplasia

- Definition: Numerous small pale yellow macules or papules at the openings of pilosebaceous follicles on face of newborn
- Etiology/Incidence: Caused by sebaceous gland enlargement and overgrowth due to maternal androgenic hormonal influence
- Signs and Symptoms: Numerous small yellow-white flat and raised lesions on newborn's face
- Differential Diagnosis: Milia
- Physical Findings
  1. Numerous small yellow-white macular and/or papular lesions on cheeks, forehead, nose and upper lip of newborn
  2. Condition resolves spontaneously without treatment as lesions gradually decrease in size and finally disappear within first month of life
- Diagnostic Tests/Findings: None
- Management/Treatment
  1. Describe and monitor lesions in terms of morphology/structure, size, shape, number, color, location, distribution
  2. No treatment necessary
  3. Educate regarding characteristics of condition and expected resolution

Vascular Lesions

Salmon Patch (Nevus Simplex)

- Definition: Benign flat light red to orange vascular birthmark on head and face
- Etiology/Incidence
  1. Caused by overgrowth of blood vessels within dermis skin layer
  2. Seen in approximately 40% to 50% of newborns
  3. More common in girls
- Signs and Symptoms: Flat light red to orange lesions on face and head of newborn
- Differential Diagnosis
  1. Contact irritation or chronic rubbing
  2. Nevus flammeus
  3. Child abuse
- Physical Findings
  1. Single or multiple irregular light red to orange macular lesions on eyelids, nape of neck, glabella, and/or occiput; vary in size
  2. Lesions gradually fade and disappear spontaneously with time
     a. Eyelid lesions fade first resolving completely within 3 to 6 months
     b. Nape of neck lesions fade but may persist into adulthood
     c. Other lesions resolve completely by 7 years of age
- Diagnostic Tests/Findings: None
- Management/Treatment
  1. Describe and monitor lesions in terms of morphology/structure, size, shape, number, color, location, distribution
  2. No treatment necessary
  3. Educate regarding characteristics of condition and expected resolution

Nevus Flammeus

- Definition: Benign permanent flat dark red to purple vascular lesion predominately on head and face
- Etiology/Incidence
  1. Caused by proliferation of dilated capillaries in the dermis
  2. Lesions may be associated with other conditions
     a. Lesions covering entire half of face or bilateral; may be associated with Sturge-Weber syndrome

    b. Lesions on extremities may be associated with hypertrophy of soft tissue and bone

    c. Lesions on the back, especially crossing the mid-line, may be associated with defects in the spinal cord and vertebrae

   3. Seen in approximately 0.4% of newborns

- Signs and Symptoms: Flat dark red or purple lesions on body surface

- Differential Diagnosis: Child abuse

- Physical Findings

   1. Irregular dark red or purple macular lesions occurring on any body surface, predominately on face and head

   2. Size varies from less than 1 cm to more than 20 cm

   3. May initially appear pink in infancy and gradually become darker

   4. Lesion never fades and may become raised in adulthood

- Diagnostic Tests/Findings: None

- Management/Treatment

   1. Describe and monitor lesions in terms of morphology/structure, size, shape, number, color, location, distribution

   2. Refer for MD evaluation to rule out Sturge-Weber syndrome and other associated conditions

   3. No treatment necessary

   4. Later in childhood

    a. May be camouflaged later in childhood with water resistant cosmetics

    b. Refer for MD evaluation and consideration of pulsed dye laser treatment

    c. Counseling as needed for related psychological concerns

   5. Educate regarding characteristics of condition

Capillary Hemangioma (Strawberry Nevus)

- Definition: Bright red or blue-red nodular lesions of varying sizes and shape with a rubbery and rough surface predominately on head and face

- Etiology/Incidence

   1. Caused by proliferation of capillary endothelial cells which may be superficial or deep

   2. Seen in approximately 2.5% of newborns

   3. More common in girls

   4. More common in light-skinned infants

- Signs and Symptoms: Red or blue-red lesions on skin surface
- Differential Diagnosis
    1. Cystic hygroma
    2. Neonatal hemangiomatosis
    3. Blue rubber bleb nevus syndrome
- Physical Findings
    1. Often is not present at birth, however, area of eventual lesion is blanched or slightly colored
    2. Size varies from less than 1 cm to over 4 cm
    3. Pattern of growth and resolution
        a. Grows quickly within 2 to 4 weeks to a red or blue-red, protuberant nodule
        b. Gradual resolution usually begins between 12 to 15 months with gray areas developing, followed by flattening from center to periphery
        c. A flat or involuted area of hyperpigmentation often remains following dissolution of the lesion
    4. Complications may occur resulting from size, location, and depth of lesion
        a. Lesions involving eye area and orbit may cause visual disturbances
        b. Lesions of head and neck may be associated with subglottic hemangiomas causing airway obstruction
        c. Lesions may cause cardiovascular disturbances through compression
    5. Complication of thrombocytopenia may occur resulting from trapped platelets within lesion
    6. Lesions resolve spontaneously and completely disappear with age
        a. 50% are cleared by 5 years of age
        b. 90% are cleared by 10 years of age
        c. Remainder clear during adolescence
- Diagnostic Tests/Findings: None
- Management/Treatment
    1. Describe and monitor lesions in terms of morphology/structure, size, shape, number, color, location, distribution
    2. Refer for MD evaluation to rule out involvement with vital organs
    3. No treatment necessary
    4. Educate regarding characteristics of condition and expected resolution

Melanocyte Cell and Pigmentation Conditions

Café au lait Spots

- Definition: Light to medium brown pigmented macular lesions of varying sizes and shapes found anywhere on the body; the color of coffee with milk from which the name is derived

- Etiology/Incidence

  1. Caused by increased pigmentation activity of melanocyte cells

  2. Overall incidence is higher in dark-skinned populations than light-skinned

  3. Lesions larger than 1.5 cm occur in 10% of light-skinned population and 20% of darker-skinned populations

  4. Lesions are usually present at birth however, may develop at any age

  5. Lesions are present throughout life, however, color intensity may fade

  6. Six or more lesions and/or lesions larger than 1.5 cm in diameter may be associated with neurofibromatosis or Albright's syndrome (Hay, Groothuis, Hayward, & Levin, 1997; Hurwitz, 1993). (see Neurological Disorders chapter.)

- Signs and Symptoms: Flat light brown lesions on skin; may be deeper in color in dark-skinned populations

- Differential Diagnosis: None

- Physical Findings

  1. Macular light to medium brown lesions on any skin surface

  2. Size varies from less than $\frac{1}{2}$ cm to 20 cm in diameter

  3. May be single or multiple

  4. Vary in shape, frequently oval

  5. Six or more lesions and/or lesions larger then 1.5 cm may be associated with neuro-fibromatosis or Albright's syndrome

- Diagnostic Tests/Findings: None

- Management/Treatment

  1. Describe and monitor lesions in terms of morphology/structure, size, shape, number, color, location, distribution

  2. If suspected that lesions may be associated with any other condition, refer to MD for further evaluation

  3. No treatment necessary

  4. Educate regarding characteristics of condition

Mongolian Spots

- Definition: Blue-black and gray macular lesions of irregular shape and varying sizes usually on sacrococcygeal region, buttocks, and lumbar areas but may also involve extremities, upper back and shoulders

- Etiology/Incidence

    1. Lesions consist of migrating spindle-shaped pigmented/melanocyte cells deep within dermis layer

    2. Occurs in 90% of darker skinned infants; 5% of light-skinned infants

- Signs and Symptoms: Blue-black or gray lesions of irregular shape and varying size on lower aspect of back

- Differential Diagnosis: Child abuse

- Physical Findings

    1. Blue-black or gray macular lesions of irregular shapes

    2. Vary in size from < 2 cm to > 10 cm

    3. Located on dorsal body surface, predominately on sacrococcygeal area of buttocks, and lumbar areas, but also on upper back, shoulders, and extremities

    4. Lesions not seen on palms or soles

    5. Lesions resolve spontaneously without treatment

        a. Most fade completely during childhood and adolescence

        b. Some may still be evident in adulthood

- Diagnostic Tests/Findings: None

- Management/Treatment

    1. Describe and monitor lesions in terms of morphology/structure, size, shape, number, color, location, and distribution

    2. No treatment necessary

    3. Educate regarding characteristics of condition and expected resolution

Malignant Melanoma

- Definition: Lethal form of skin cancer involving melanocyte cells; may occur on any skin surface

- Etiology/Incidence

    1. Caused by abnormal growth within melanocyte cells

    2. Severe sunburn or excessive exposure to the sun before the age of 10 years predisposes developing melanoma later in childhood or in adult life

        a. Sun damaged skin cells may be dormant for years

   b.   Melanocyte cells provide mechanism to activate malignant process

3.   Melanoma cells spread through the lymphatic system and invade other skin surfaces and organs

   a.   90% survival rate with localized condition

   b.   20% survival with metastasis

4.   Increasing incidence in general population

5.   More common in males and light-skinned individuals

6.   Increased incidence with family history (Cohen, 1999)

7.   More lethal and faster growing than basal cell or squamous cell cancers

- Signs and Symptoms

1.   Localized change in skin color or increase in size of existing nevus

2.   May have itching with bleeding and tenderness

- Differential Diagnosis: Other skin cancers

- Physical Findings

1.   Asymmetrical lesion with irregular, ragged and blurred borders

2.   Uneven color with shades of blue, black, brown, tan, and red; all colors may exist within same lesion

3.   More common on arms and lower legs of females and on chest of males

4.   Single or multiple (clusters) lesions may be found in distant areas with metastasis

5.   Bleeding and ulceration—usually late signs

- Diagnostic Tests/Findings: Skin biopsy confirms diagnosis

- Management/Treatment

1.   Obtain detailed history of onset, duration, and progression

2.   Refer to MD for evaluation immediately if suspected; surgical excision is indicated

3.   Educate regarding characteristics of condition, treatment and expected prognosis

4.   Educate regarding specific preventive measures

   a.   Protect skin from exposure to sunlight

      (1)   Cover-up clothing and hats

      (2)   Sunglasses

      (3)   Water resistant sunblocks that protect against UVB and UVA ultraviolet light with > 15 sun protection factor (SPF)

   b.   Avoid exposure to sunlight especially during 10 a.m. to 3 p.m.

   c.   Avoid sun lamps

Albinism

- Definition: Inherited congenital defect of total or partial lack of pigmentation in which affected body parts lack normal color
    1. Total form—affects entire skin, hair, and retina
    2. Partial or localized forms—confined to specific area of skin, hair (forelock of hair), or eyes (pupil or retina)
- Etiology/Incidence
    1. Metabolic process within melanocyte cells required for melanin production is impaired—melanin, giving skin its distinctive color, is not secreted
    2. Occurs in all ethnic groups
- Signs and Symptoms
    1. Milky-white skin (localized or generalized)
    2. Light sensitivity
- Differential Diagnosis
    1. Vitiligo
    2. Phenylketonuria
- Physical Findings
    1. Skin is milky-white, hair is white or yellow, iris is usually blue, pupil usually appears red and becomes darker in adulthood
    2. Skin is sensitive to light and sunburns easily
    3. Other symptoms not involving skin include decreased visual acuity, photosensitivity
- Diagnostic Tests/Findings: None
- Management/Treatment
    1. Describe skin and areas of hypopigmentation and monitor routinely for any skin changes that may occur including development of lesions
    2. Educate regarding need to protect from exposure to sunlight
        a. Cover-up clothing and hats
        b. Sunglasses
        c. Water resistant sunblocks that protect against UVB and UVA ultraviolet light with > 15 SPF
    3. Educate regarding characteristics and prognosis of condition
    4. Counsel as indicted regarding
        a. Related psychologic effects
        b. Genetic counselling related to potential inheritance factors

   5. Refer to dermatologist for evaluation if skin changes occur

   6. Refer to ophthalmologist for evaluation of vision and eye involvement

Vitiligo

- Definition: Acquired condition involving patches of hypopigmentation on skin surface and in mouth and genitalia

   1. Segmented form—unilateral involving two dermatones

   2. Generalized form—involves more than two dermatones, often has bilateral distribution

- Etiology/Incidence

   1. Unknown cause

      a. Affected areas of hypopigmentation have loss or destruction of melanocyte cells

      b. May be associated with autoimmune conditions—diabetes mellitus, Addison's disease, or thyroiditis

   2. Occurs in approximately 4% of all ethnic populations

   3. Onset is usually before 20 years of age

- Signs and Symptoms: Milky-white patches on skin

- Differential Diagnosis

   1. Albinism

   2. Pityriasis alba

   3. Pityriasis rosea

   4. Tinea versicolor

- Physical Findings

   1. Milky-white patches of hypopigmentation occur in unilateral or bilateral pattern on skin of normal texture

   2. Shape varies from round, oval, to irregular

   3. Size varies from less than 2 cm to well over 20 cm

   4. Varies in number from one to many

   5. Condition is often permanent without repigmentation

- Diagnostic Tests/Findings: None

- Management/Treatment

   1. Obtain detailed history of onset, duration, severity, progression, and possible precipitating factors

2. Describe skin and areas of hypopigmentation and monitor for any skin changes that may occur including development of lesions

3. Protect skin from exposure to sunlight especially during 10 am to 3 pm

   a. Use cover-up clothing, hats, and sunglasses

   b. Apply water resistant sunblocks that protect against UVB and UVA ultraviolet light with > 15 SPF

4. Refer for MD evaluation and treatment to stimulate repigmentation

   a. Topical steroid applications and controlled ultraviolet light exposure

   b. Repigmentation efforts have varying degrees of success

5. Educate regarding characteristics and expected prognoses

6. Recommend camouflage with water resistant cosmetics for adolescent

7. Counsel regarding

   a. Related psychological impact of condition

   b. Serious need for protection to reduce risk for skin cancer and sunburn

8. Refer for MD evaluation if complications develop

Pityriasis Alba

- Definition: Acquired condition of scaly hypopigmented lesions of varying sizes and shapes with indistinct borders occurring predominately on cheeks

- Etiology/Incidence

  1. Unknown cause

  2. May be associated with overdrying of skin causing inflammation and hypopigmentation

  3. Occurs most often in children ages 3 to 12 years

  4. Occurs more commonly in dark-skinned populations

- Signs and Symptoms

  1. Scaly white patches on cheeks

  2. May be pruritic

- Differential Diagnosis

  1. Pityriasis rosea

  2. Tinea corporis

  3. Vitiligo

- Physical Findings

1. Scaly hypopigmented lesions of varying sizes or shapes with non-distinct borders occurring predominately on cheeks, less commonly on other skin surfaces

2. Some lesions may be slightly erythematous

3. Number of lesions varies from one to many

4. Exposure to sunlight may exacerbate lesions, making them more pronounced

5. Repigmentation occurs as condition resolves spontaneously in 3 to 4 months

- Diagnostic Tests/Findings: KOH preparation to rule out tinea corporis

- Management/Treatment

    1. Obtain detailed history of onset, duration, severity, progression of symptoms, and possible precipitating factors

    2. Describe and monitor lesions in terms of morphology/structure, size, shape, number, color, location, distribution

    3. Educate child and parents regarding need to protect skin from exposure to sunlight especially during 10 a.m. to 3 p.m.

        a. Use cover-up clothing, hats, and sunglasses

        b. Apply water resistant sunblocks that protect against UVB and UVA ultraviolet light with > 15 SPF

    4. Use bland moisturizer to reduce overdrying

    5. Educate regarding characteristics and expected prognoses

    6. Recommend camouflage with water resistant cosmetics for adolescent

    7. Refer for MD evaluation if condition does not improve

Papulosquamous Conditions

Pityriasis Rosea

- Definition: Acquired common mild inflammatory condition characterized by scaly, pale, salmon-pink lesions predominately on the trunk, upper arms and upper thighs

- Etiology/Incidence

    1. Unknown cause

    2. Possible viral association

    3. Occurs more often in fall and spring months

    4. Occurs especially in older children of all ethnic groups

- Signs and Symptoms

    1. Scaly pink marks on skin

    2. Periodic pruritus of varying degrees of severity especially at onset

3. Lack of energy and low grade fever before onset of rash

- Differential Diagnosis

    1. Pityriasis alba

    2. Seborrheic dermatitis

    3. Secondary syphilis

    4. Tinea corporis

- Physical Findings

    1. Scaly, pink to salmon lesions with progressive pattern

        a. "Herald" patch of 1 cm to 5 cm on trunk or buttocks usually occurs 5 to 10 days before generalized rash

        b. Round and oval macular to papular lesions develop over two week period on skin lines and in parallel fashion suggestive of a Christmas tree pattern

        c. Individual lesions clear in central to peripheral pattern

    2. On darker-skinned populations lesions are more predominant on neck, axillary and inguinal regions

    3. Condition is self-limiting and resolves spontaneously in 3 to 4 months

- Diagnostic Tests/Findings

    1. KOH test to rule out tinea corporis

    2. VDRL to rule out secondary syphilis, especially in sexually active individuals

- Management/Treatment

    1. Obtain detailed history of onset, duration, severity, progression of symptoms, and possible precipitating factors

    2. Describe and monitor lesions in terms of morphology/structure, size, shape, number, color, location, distribution

    3. Educate regarding characteristics of condition and prognosis

    4. Use symptomatic treatment for pruritus

        a. Topical calamine lotion on lesions

        b. Oral antipruritic agents for severe pruritus, e.g., diphenhydramine

        c. Cool bath or compresses on lesions

    5. Educate regarding medication dosage, signs of irritation, sensitivity

    6. Use controlled and limited sunlight exposure to shorten resolution time

    7. Refer for MD evaluation if condition worsens or does not resolve

Psoriasis

- Definition: Acquired chronic condition characterized by thick silver-gray-white scales
  1. Psoriasis vulgaris—large lesions occurring predominately on elbows and knees
  2. Psoriasis guttate—small lesions occurring predominately on trunk, upper arms and thighs
- Etiology/Incidence
  1. Specific cause is unknown
  2. Associated with overproduction and too rapid migration of epithelial cells to skin surface; cells migrate in 3 to 4 days in comparison to usual 28 days
     a. Psoriasis vulgaris—often associated with constant rubbing, or with trauma to the affected area known as Koebner's response
     b. Psoriasis guttate—often follows streptococcal infection
  3. Occurs in over 33% of children
  4. More common in light-skinned than dark-skinned populations
  5. More common in males
  6. Positive family history in approximately $\frac{1}{3}$ of cases suggests familial or environmental connection
- Signs and Symptoms
  1. Silvery, gray-white scaling of skin mainly on trunk or extremities, especially elbows and knees; less commonly on scalp and face
  2. Bleeding may occur if scales are picked at or removed
  3. Changes in nails—thickening with pits and ridges
- Differential Diagnosis
  1. Atopic dermatitis
  2. Candida
  3. Pityriasis rosea
  4. Seborrhea
  5. Secondary syphilis
  6. Tinea corporis
- Physical Findings
  1. Psoriasis vulgaris—large 5 to 10 cm lesions with thick silvery-white scales located on elbows and knees
  2. Psoriasis guttate—small 3 to 10 mm multiple teardrop round or oval papular lesions which become covered by a silvery-gray-white scale on trunk and proximal extremities

3. Bleeding occurs when scale is removed

4. Nail plates may be thicker and show signs of pits, ridges, splinter hemorrhages; not all nail plates are involved

- Diagnostic Tests/Findings

    1. VDRL to rule out secondary syphilis

    2. KOH to rule out fungal infections

- Management/Treatment

    1. Obtain detailed history of onset, duration, severity and progression of symptoms, and possible precipitating factors

    2. Describe and monitor lesions in terms of morphology/structure, size, shape, number, color, location, distribution

    3. Reduce hypertrophy of lesion

        a. Use controlled and limited sunlight exposure

        b. Apply topical steroids, e.g., hydocortisone, triamcinolone

        c. Apply mineral oil and moisturizers to decrease drying

    4. Educate regarding medication dosage, signs of irritation, sensitivity

    5. Educate regarding characteristics of condition and prognosis

    6. Refer for MD evaluation if condition does not improve

Dermatitis Conditions

Atopic Dermatitis

- Definition: Common skin disorder with lesions of varied morphology commonly known as eczema

    1. Acute form—occurs predominately in infants

    2. Chronic form—occurs predominately in children and adolescents

- Etiology/Incidence

    1. Specific cause is unknown

    2. May be associated with a disorder of immunity in some cases due to elevated levels of IgE

    3. Positive family history may be predisposing factor in some cases

    4. Occurs in approximately 10% to 15% of children

    5. Up to 50% of affected infants develop asthma and/or other respiratory manifestations, e.g., allergic rhinitis, hay fever and progress to chronic form

6. Up to 25% of children and adolescents continue to have symptoms throughout adulthood

- Signs and Symptoms
    1. Skin changes
        a. Infant—red, swollen skin rash with crusted areas
        b. Older children—areas of darker, thickened, leathery skin
    2. Pruritus for both, worsens with sweating
- Differential Diagnosis
    1. Contact dermatitis
    2. Psoriasis
    3. Seborrheic dermatitis
    4. Scabies
    5. Impetigo or other secondary bacterial infection
- Physical Findings
    1. Acute form in infants usually develops between ages of 2 to 6 months with 50% cases resolving by 3 years and remainder progressing to chronic form
        a. Lesions erupt on reddened and edematous skin of face, head, trunk and extensor surfaces
        b. Lesions of varied morphology, e.g., papules, vesicles, crusts, dry scales are present in various locations
    2. Chronic form develops in children and adolescents between ages 3 to 10 years; may continue into adulthood
        a. Skin is hyperpigmented, leathery, and thickened in the flexor surfaces of the neck, antecubital areas, wrists, popliteal area, ankle, fingers and toes
        b. Scratch marks on affected areas
    3. Other findings include:
        a. Circles under eyes
        b. Facial pallor
        c. Nasal crease on top of nose from frequent rubbing
        d. Dry hair
    4. Pustules may be present as sign of secondary bacterial infection
- Diagnostic Tests/Findings
    1. No specific test confirms diagnosis—serum level of IgE may support diagnosis in some cases

2. Skin scraping to rule out scabies

- Management/Treatment

    1. Obtain detailed history of onset, duration, severity/progression of symptoms, and possible precipitating factors

    2. Describe and monitor lesions in terms of morphology/structure, size, shape, number, color, location, distribution

    3. Treat secondary infections if present

        a. Oral antibiotics, e.g., erythromycin, cefaclor, cefadroxil, cephalexin, nafcillin, penicillin

        b. Topical antibiotics for localized infection—of little value with the exception of mupirocin; others may lead to sensitivity reactions

    4. Reduce and prevent pruritus with oral antipruritics, e.g., hydroxyzine, diphenhydramine

    5. Use topical steroids to reduce inflammation, immune response, and pruritus, e.g., hydrocortisone, triamcinolone

    6. Rehydrate skin if lesions are weeping and oozing

        a. Wet compresses and baths using

            (1) Aluminum acetate preparations

            (2) Oatmeal preparations

        b. Avoid skin drying agents such as harsh soaps, perfumes, lotions

        c. Apply cream emollients and lubricants, e.g., petroleum jelly

    7. Educate regarding medication dosage, signs of irritation, sensitivity

    8. Use mild soaps for general bathing and hygiene habits

    9. Eliminate exposure to all substances and agents that may dry or irritate the skin and exacerbate condition; individually determined

        a. Soaps, perfumes, hand and body lotions, makeup, household cleaning agents, bleach, chlorine, turpentine

        b. Materials and fabrics such as wool, feathers, polyesters, stuffed animals and other fabric toys

        c. Food substances such as cow's milk, eggs, nuts, citrus fruits

        d. Pets and other animals

        e. Dust and dust mites

    10. Monitor environment

        a. Maintain cool temperature to reduce sweating

        b. Increase humidity

11. Educate regarding characteristics of condition and expected prognosis

12. Refer for MD evaluation if condition does not resolve

Contact Dermatitis

- Definition: Allergic response to local contact with an allergen manifested by development of skin eruptions at site of contact

- Etiology/Incidence

  1. Caused by hypersensitivity to an allergen

     a. Initial contact—allergic response usually delayed for several days

     b. Re-exposure—allergic response usually occurs within 24 hours due to prior sensitization

  2. Numerous substances are associated with producing hypersensitivity reactions in sensitive individuals with the most common including:

     a. Perfumes, soaps, cosmetics, fabric dyes,

     b. Topical medications, e.g., neomycin

     c. Animal products—animal dander, feathers, fur, wool, leather

     d. Plastics, synthetics—latex, rubber

     e. Plants—poison sumac/ivy/oak

     f. Metals—jewelry

- Signs and Symptoms

  1. Redness and swelling at site of contact

  2. Pruritus with varying degrees of intensity

- Differential Diagnosis

  1. Bacterial infection

  2. Candida

  3. Diaper dermatitis

  4. Seborrhea dermatitis

- Physical Findings

  1. Erythema and edema with development of lesions of varying morphology—papules, vesicles, and denudation

  2. Lesions confined to area of direct contact with allergen

  3. Pruritus with varying degrees of intensity

  4. Excoriation/scratch marks and bleeding

  5. Chronic exposure may produce areas of hyperpigmentation and lichenification

- Diagnostic Tests/Findings: Skin testing to determine allergen hypersensitivities after acute stage

- Management/Treatment

  1. Obtain detailed history of onset, duration, severity, progression of symptoms, and possible precipitating factors

  2. Describe and monitor lesions in terms of morphology/structure, size, shape, number, color, location, distribution

  3. Avoid contact with allergen if sensitivity is known; if unknown, consider skin testing after acute phase to determine allergen

  4. Cool compresses of Burow's solution to affected areas

  5. Steroids to reduce inflammation, immune response, and pruritus

     a. Apply topical steroids to affected areas, e.g., hydrocortisone, triamcinolone

     b. Oral steroids for severe cases, e.g., hydrocortisone

  6. Oral antihistamines for pruritus, e.g., hydroxyzine, diphenhydramine

  7. Oral antibiotics if secondary infection present, e.g., erythromycin, dicloxicillin

  8. Educate regarding medication dosage, signs of irritation, sensitivity

  9. Educate regarding characteristics of condition and expected resolution

  10. Refer to MD for:

      a. Evaluation if condition does not show improvement in 2 days

      b. Consideration of skin testing for hypersensitivities after acute episode to identify specific allergens

Diaper (Irritant) Dermatitis

- Definition: Common disorder of genital-perineal area due to skin breakdown, characterized by erythema and other skin lesions

- Etiology/Incidence

  1. Breakdown of skin associated with:

     a. Exposure to chemical irritants in soaps, bleach, water softeners, skin lotions, diaper cleansing tissues

     b. Excessive contact with urine, feces; lax hygiene habits (primary irritant)

  2. Occurs in over 95% of all infants

  3. Peak incidence is 9 to 12 months of age

  4. Monilial rash caused by *Candida albicans*

  5. May persist until completion of toilet training

- Signs and Symptoms
  1. Redness, sores in diaper area, blisters
  2. Fiery red rash with monilial
  3. May have general irritability and/or crying especially after elimination
- Differential Diagnosis
  1. Atopic dermatitis
  2. Allergic/contact dermatitis
  3. Psoriasis
  4. Secondary bacterial infection
  5. Child abuse
- Physical Findings
  1. Erythema with varying degrees of severity which may be generalized to entire area or localized to small area
  2. Lesions of varied morphology may develop—papules, vesicles, crusts, erosions and ulcerations
  3. Pustules may be present signaling secondary bacterial infection
  4. Monilial rash—fiery red, papular lesions within folds and on genitals; may also be pustular; may have associated oral thrush
  5. Poor genital hygiene may be present in some children
- Diagnostic Tests/Findings: No specific test confirms diagnosis
- Management/Treatment
  1. Obtain detailed history of onset, duration, severity, progression of symptoms, and possible precipitating factors
  2. Describe and monitor lesions in terms of morphology/structure, size, shape, number, color, location, distribution
  3. Treat secondary bacterial infection if present with topical antibiotics, e.g., bacitracin, mupirocin
  4. Treat present diaper dermatitis
     a. Mild erythema—emollients to affected areas with each diaper change, e.g., petroleum jelly, zinc oxide
     b. Erythema with papules—topical steriods, e.g., hydrocortisone, triamcinolone
     c. Severe erythema and edema with papules, vesicles, and ulcerations—wet dressings may be soothing, e.g., Burow's compresses; topical antibiotics may be indicated

d. Monilial rash—topical nystatin, clotrimazole, ketoconazole; oral nystatin for thrush

e. Avoid occlusive diapers and plastic pants

f. Expose diaper area to air as often as possible

g. Use appropriate preventive measures

5. Educate regarding medication dosage, signs of irritation, sensitivity

6. Preventive measures

a. Expose diaper area to air several times each day

b. Increase oral fluids to make urine less irritating

(1) Water for infant under 12 months

(2) Cranberry juice for older child

c. Change diaper immediately after soiling

d. Wash diaper area with nonirritating agents after each diaper change, e.g., mild soap and water

e. Avoid occlusive diapers and plastic pants

f. Diaper selection and care

(1) Home laundry—mild soap and double rinse using 1 ounce of vinegar per gallon of water in last rinse

(2) Disposable diapers—select alternate brand if sensitivity occurs

g. "Diaper-wipes", may need to be avoided because of irritation or sensitivity

h. Use lubricating ointment when diaper area skin is overly dry, e.g., petroleum jelly

7. Refer for MD evaluation if no improvement within 2 to 3 days or if condition worsens

Seborrhea Dermatitis

- Definition: Chronic inflammatory condition usually on scalp and face

1. Newborn and young infant—cradle cap

2. Adolescents—dandruff

- Etiology/Incidence

1. Associated with over production of sebum in areas abundant with sebaceous glands

2. Increase in sebaceous gland activity may be connected with hormonal stimulation at times when hormonal influence is highest

3. Occurs more often in spring and summer months

- Signs and Symptoms
  1. Newborns and infants—areas of redness under yellow crusts and greasy scales on scalp and face
  2. Adolescents—white flakes and greasy scaling on scalp, forehead, eyebrows, and face
- Differential Diagnosis
  1. Atopic dermatitis
  2. Bacterial infection
  3. Candida
  4. Contact dermatitis
  5. Psoriasis
- Physical Findings
  1. Newborns and infants—areas of underlying erythema with yellow crusts and greasy scaling on scalp and face; in more severe cases lesions may be present on trunk and in diaper area
  2. Adolescents—white flakes and greasy scaling on scalp, forehead, eyebrows, and face; severity varies from simple dandruff to extensive, giving appearance of psoriasis; mild underlying erythema may be present
- Diagnostic Tests/Findings: No tests necessary to confirm diagnosis
- Management/Treatment
  1. Obtain detailed history of onset, duration, severity, progression of symptoms, and possible precipitating factors
  2. Describe and monitor lesions in terms of morphology/structure, size, shape, number, color, location, distribution
  3. Treat existing condition
     a. Shampoo and wash affected areas with antiseborrheic soaps and shampoos
     b. Mineral oil with brushing to loosen crusts prior to washing
     c. Topical steroid creams for extreme cases to reduce inflammation, e.g., hydrocortisone
  4. Educate regarding medication dosage, signs of irritation, sensitivity
  5. Educate regarding characteristics of condition and expected prognosis
  6. Refer for MD evaluation if condition persists without improvement

Burn Conditions

Burns

- Definition: Injury of skin from exposure to hot surfaces and agents

    1. Classified according to depth of injury to skin layers

        a. First degree/superficial burns—involve epidermis layer only

        b. Second degree/partial thickness burns—involve epidermis and part of dermis which may be superficial dermis or deep dermis

        c. Third degree/full thickness burns—involve epidermis, dermis, and dermal appendages

    2. Classified also according to extent of affected area

        a. Minor burns—less than 10% of body surface if burn is superficial, and less than 2% if burn is partial or full thickness

        b. Major burns—10% or more of body surface if burn is superficial and 2% or more if burn is partial or full thickness

        c. Major burns—hand, feet, face, eyes, ears, and perineal burns are always considered major burns, regardless of extent of body surface affected

- Etiology/Incidence

    1. Caused by exposure to hot chemicals, electrical and thermal substances and materials including electrical cords and outlets, irons, sun, flames, fireworks, hot water and foods, cigarettes, light bulbs

    2. Affected cells in epidermis, dermis, or subcutaneous skin layers are injured and no longer capable of providing protective, electrolyte storage, sensory, and other functions of normal skin cells

    3. Third leading cause of death in children and adolescents

        a. More common in toddlers and males

        b. Commonly occurs in kitchen in late afternoon during dinner preparation

        c. Approximately 10% of burns are thought to be intentional in infant, toddler, and young child

- Signs and Symptoms: According to degree, appearance, and healing time

    1. Superficial—red, swollen, and dry areas with tenderness

    2. Partial thickness and superficial burns—red, swollen, moist, and blistered areas with tenderness

    3. Partial thickness and deep burns—white, dry areas with loss of sensation

    4. Full thickness burns—white, brown, black, swollen dry areas with loss of sensation

- Differential Diagnosis

1. Child abuse

2. Staphylococcal scalded skin syndrome

- Physical Findings

    1. Superficial burns—erythema, mild edema, dryness, tenderness, and general discomfort of affected areas

    2. Partial thickness and superficial burns—erythema, edema, moist, few vesicles/blisters may develop, sensitive to touch and air

    3. Partial thickness and deep burns—white, dry, decreased sensitivity to touch, pain, temperature, and may blanch with pressure

    4. Full thickness burns—white, brown, to black; swollen, dry; lack full touch, pain, temperature sensitivity

    5. Physical findings associated with secondary bacterial infection may be present

- Diagnostic Tests/Findings

    1. Electrolyte studies especially if burn is extensive

    2. Culture to determine causal agent if secondary bacterial infection is present

- Management/Treatment

    1. Obtain detailed history of onset, duration, severity and symptom progression

    2. Describe and monitor burn area in terms of morphology/structure, extent of burn area, location, distribution

    3. Inpatient hospital management for all children with major burns, suspected abuse, esophageal and airway burns, and/or injuries such as fractures

    4. Outpatient management for children in stable environment with minor burns

        a. Partial thickness burn if < 10% of body surface area (BSA) or full thickness burn is < 2% BSA

        b. Monitor daily healing process by documenting changes

        c. Cool compresses to affected areas

        d. Medication for pain control, e.g., acetaminophen, ibuprofen

        e. Topical antimicrobial agents to prevent infection on open blistered areas, e.g., silver sulfadiazine (except on face due to potential for hyperpigmentation), bacitracin, mupirocin

        f. Do not excise vesicles/blisters

        g. Fluids to reduce possibility of dehydration, e.g., water, juices

        h. Topical emollients if skin is dry, e.g., petroleum jelly

    5. Educate regarding need to protect skin from exposure to sunlight especially during 10 a.m. to 3 p.m.

     a.   Cover-up clothing, hats, and sunglasses

     b.   Water resistant sunblocks that protect against UVB and UVA ultraviolet light with > 15 SPF

6.   Educate regarding medication dosage, signs of irritation, sensitivity

7.   Educate regarding characteristics of condition and prognosis

8.   Educate regarding measures to prevent further burn episodes and injuries

9.   Refer for MD evaluation if condition does not show improvement

Sunburns

- Definition: Thermal burn due to excessive sunlight exposure

- Etiology/Incidence

  1. Exposed skin results in altered cell function and properties

     a. Increased blood flow

     b. Increased melanin production

  2. Fair-skinned populations are most sensitive

  3. Other factors involving sensitivity include high altitude, nearness to equator, and exposure to sun during hours of 10 a.m. and 3 p.m. when UVB waves are strongest

- Signs and Symptoms

  1. Redness, swelling, blisters, and tenderness of sun exposed areas

  2. Fatigue, chills, and headache after sun exposure

- Differential Diagnosis

  1. Child abuse

  2. Photosensitivity from medications

  3. Systemic viral exanthema

  4. Systemic drug reaction

- Physical Findings

  1. Dependent on degree of exposure and injury; develops within several minutes to several hours after exposure

     a. First degree burns—erythema and tenderness

     b. Second degree burns—increased intensity of erythema and tenderness with edema, some vesicles/blisters

     c. Third degree burns—increased intensity of erythema, tenderness, edema, and vesicles/blisters

  2. Systemic symptoms of malaise, fever, headache may be evident especially in younger child with second and third degree burns

3. Epidermis cells scale and desquamate within 3 to 7 days after injury

4. Exposed areas may become hyperpigmented with development of freckles and moles

- Diagnostic Tests/Findings: None used to confirm diagnosis

- Management/Treatment

1. Obtain detailed history of onset, duration, severity, progression of symptoms and precipitating factors

2. Describe and monitor location, color, and degree of burn, and symptoms

3. Treat existing condition

   a. Remove from sunlight exposure

   b. Cool water or saline compresses to affected areas

   c. Do not use warm or hot showers/baths

   d. Increase oral fluids to prevent dehydration

   e. Oral pain medications, e.g., acetaminophen, ibuprofen

   f. Topical emollients for dry skin, e.g., petroleum jelly

4. Educate regarding medication dosage, signs of irritation, sensitivity

5. Educate regarding measures of prevention

   a. Risk factors of sun exposure

      (1) Teach early signs of skin cancer

      (2) Teach regarding individuals most vulnerable to sun exposure

   b. Use sun screens and blocks with 15 or greater SPF

      (1) Apply at least 20 minutes before exposure

      (2) Apply frequently if sustained exposure—every hour

      (3) Use waterproof agents when in water

      (4) Discontinue if sensitivity is suspected

      (5) Avoid use in infants under 6 months

   c. Use cover-up clothing and hats designed to block UVB waves

6. Refer for MD evaluation if condition does not improve or becomes worse

Bacterial Conditions

Cellulitis

- Definition: Localized infection often precipitated by an insect bite (spider, mosquito, flea) or trauma that penetrates the protective skin barrier

- Etiology/Incidence: Caused when surface streptococci, *Haemophilus influenzae,* or *Staphylococcus aureus* bacteria invade all skin layers—epidermis, dermis, and subcutis, after a break in the skin has occurred

- Signs and Symptoms

    1. Irregular-shaped areas of skin with redness, swelling

    2. Warm and tender to touch

    3. Fever, chills, and malaise may be present

- Differential Diagnosis

    1. Influenza

    2. Furuncle

- Physical Findings

    1. Erythema and edema with ill-defined, irregular borders

    2. Tenderness and warmth

    3. Regional lymphadenopathy may be present

    4. Fever, chills, and malaise indicates systemic involvement

    5. Facial, periorbital, or orbital involvement is vulnerable to development of more severe conditions

- Diagnostic Tests/Findings: Blood culture to confirm causal agent

- Management/Treatment

    1. Detailed history of onset, duration, severity, progression of symptoms and precipitating factors

    2. Describe and monitor

        a. Affected skin areas in terms of morphology/structure, size, shape, color, location, distribution

        b. Systemic signs and symptoms of fever, chills, and malaise

    3. Hospitalization for severe cases and those involving face and eyes

    4. Treat with intramuscular, intravenous, and/or oral antibiotics according to severity of condition, organism, and site of involvement

        a. If streptococcus suspected—penicillins

        b. If *Haemophilus influenzae* suspected—amoxicillin

        c. If *Staphylococcus aureus* suspected—dicloxacillin

    5. Educate regarding medication dosage, signs of irritation, sensitivity

    6. Educate regarding characteristics of condition and expected prognosis

    7. Refer for MD evaluation if condition shows no improvement

Impetigo

- Definition: Localized infection of skin often precipitated by insect bites (spider, mosquito, flea) or other trauma that breaks protective skin barrier; predominately involves face and less commonly other body surfaces including perineum

- Etiology/Incidence

  1. *Staphylococcus aureus* and streptococci bacteria invade epidermis after break in skin

  2. Highly communicable with incubation period of 1 to 10 days

  3. Autoinoculable

- Signs and Symptoms

  1. Itching and tenderness may be present

  2. Areas of red swollen skin, blisters and/or moist honey-colored crusts

- Differential Diagnosis

  1. Eczema

  2. Herpes simplex

- Physical Findings

  1. Two major forms

     a. Nonbullous—underlying erythema with vesicles that erupt resulting in honey/serous colored crusts with erosion of epidermis

     b. Bullous—underlying erythema with pustules and vesicles that erupt resulting in smooth shiny appearance

  2. Regional adenopathy with tenderness

- Diagnostic Tests/Findings: Culture will confirm diagnosis and causative organism

- Management/Treatment

  1. Obtain detailed history of onset, duration, severity, progression of symptoms and precipitating factors

  2. Describe and monitor lesions in terms of morphology/structure, size, location, distribution

  3. Apply compresses of Burow's solution several times daily to aid in cleaning and removing crusts

  4. Apply topical antibiotics to areas of involvement, e.g., bacitracin, mupirocin, neosporin

  5. Prescribe oral antibiotics according to specific bacterial cause (Hay, Groothuis, Hayward & Levin, 1997; Bernstein & Shelov, 1996)

     a. For staphylococci—dicloxacillin

    b. For streptococci—penicillin or erythromycin

6. Educate regarding medication dosage, signs of irritation, sensitivity

7. Educate regarding characteristics of condition, treatment regime, prognosis, and good hygiene for prevention

8. Exclude from school and other public programs until treated for 48 hours due to high communicability

9. Refer for MD evaluation if condition does not improve

Staphylococcal Scalded Skin Syndrome

- Definition: Systemic bacterial infection with skin manifestations; also known as staphylococcal scarlet fever

- Etiology/Incidence

    1. Caused by effects of toxin produced by *Staphylococcus aureus* bacteria

    2. Occurs any season

    3. More common in neonates and infants than older children

    4. Incubation is variable, commonly 3 to 10 days

- Signs and Symptoms

    1. May present with abrupt onset of fever, irritability, and general malaise

    2. Bright, red, painful rash more pronounced around eyes, mouth, neck, underarms, elbow, groin, and knees

    3. Pain on pressure

    4. Blistering and/or scaling of skin

- Differential Diagnosis

    1. Streptococcal scarlet fever

    2. Burns

    3. Child abuse

    4. Drug toxicity

- Physical Findings

    1. Abrupt onset of fever and general malaise

    2. General exanthema with erythema and swelling; more pronounced in perioral, periorbital areas, flexure surfaces of neck, axilla, antecubital, groin, and popiteal areas

    3. Light pressure causes extreme pain and exfoliation of top epidermal layers

    4. After peeling, skin appears glistening and scalded

    5. Vesicles/bullae may occur in more toxic cases

- Diagnostic Tests/Findings
    1. Blood culture to confirm *Staphylococcus aureus*
    2. Culture secretions to confirm *Staphylococcus aureus*
- Management/Treatment
    1. Obtain detailed history of onset, duration, severity, progression of symptoms and precipitating factors
    2. Describe and monitor in terms of morphology/structure, size, shape, number, color, location, distribution
    3. Hospitalization is indicated for all neonates; treat more severe cases with IV antibiotics and monitor fluid and electrolytes
    4. Outpatient management may be considered with less toxic cases if environment is stable
        a. Oral antistaphylococcal antibiotics, e.g., dicloxacillin
        b. Oral antipyretics and analgesics for fever and pain control, e.g., acetaminophen, ibuprofen
        c. Increase fluids to maintain hydration and prevent dehydration, e.g., water, juices
    5. Educate regarding medication dosage, signs of irritation, sensitivity
    6. Educate regarding characteristics of condition, treatment, and prognosis
    7. Refer for MD evaluation if condition does not improve

Bacterial Conditions Involving Pilosebaceous Unit

Acne

- Definition: Inflammatory chronic skin disorder involving the pilosebaceous follicle unit
    1. Occurs predominately on the face, neck, chest and upper back skin surfaces; less commonly in other areas
    2. Often occurs in cyclic periods of exacerbation and remission
- Etiology/Incidence
    1. Specific cause is unknown
        a. Associated with breakdown of follicle wall
        b. Cells combine with sebum and plug follicle
        c. Enzymes from *Corynebacterium acnes* mix with trapped debris causing edema and irritation
    2. Proven factors which may contribute to acne development
        a. Increased androgenic hormonal influence

b. Positive family history

c. Stress

3. Unproven factors with questionable and unsubstantiated contribution

a. Food—nuts, eggs, cheese, chocolate

b. Poor hygiene

4. Affects more than 70% of adolescents with varying degrees of severity

a. Onset parallels puberty

b. More common in females

c. More males develop severe acne

d. More females experience continuation of acne into adult years

- Signs and Symptoms

1. Open and closed pimples/bumps

2. Soreness at site of lesions

3. Scars at site of previous lesions

- Differential Diagnosis

1. Folliculitis

2. Contact dermatitis

3. Urticaria

4. Allergic drug reaction

- Physical Findings

1. Lesions of varying morphology

a. Mild acne—lesions are scattered covering small areas

(1) Open comedones/blackheads—lesions filled with dry oxidized sebum; brown in color

(2) Closed comedones/whiteheads—lesions filled with follicle cells and sebum

b. Moderate acne—lesions are more numerous covering large areas

(1) All lesions of mild acne

(2) Pustules—lesions filled with follicle cells, sebum, and white blood cells

c. Severe acne—lesions are much more numerous covering larger areas

(1) All lesions of mild and moderate acne

(2) Erythema with papules and pustules

(3) Nodules and cysts—deep dermal lesions filled with follicle debris often with communicating tracks to other cysts

2. Increased oiliness of hair and skin

3. Scarring especially when

   a. Lesions at any stage have been manipulated and squeezed

   b. Cysts have erupted deep within the dermis

4. Signs of related psychological distress/depression may be present

- Diagnostic Tests/Findings: None; clinically determined diagnosis

- Management/Treatment

   1. Obtain detailed history of onset, duration, severity and progression of symptoms and possible precipitating factors

   2. Describe in terms of morphology/structure, size, shape, number, color, location, distribution

   3. Wash and dry face and affected areas with mild non-oil base soap

   4. Apply warm compresses

   5. Use topical exfoliates and comedolytic preparations

      a. Mild acne—tretinoin

      b. Moderate acne—benzoyl peroxide

      c. Severe acne: tretinoin and benzoyl peroxide

   6. Use topical antibiotics for moderate to severe acne, e.g., clindamycin, erythomycin

   7. Add oral antibiotics for persistent and unresponsive cases of moderate and severe acne

      a. Tetracycline, erythromycin, doxycycline, minocycline

      b. Oral clindamycin contraindicated due to adverse GI side effects

   8. Consider using isotretinoin for unresponsive, persistent severe acne

      a. Contraindicated in pregnancy

      b. For sexually active females, birth control measures indicated

   9. Educate regarding medication dosage, signs of irritation, sensitivity

   10. Consider counseling for signs of psychological distress and depression

   11. Educate regarding characteristics of condition, treatment regime, and expected prognosis

      a. Condition may become worse with treatment before improvement

      b. Treatment will improve but not cure most cases; may take months

      c. Treatment must be consistent to be effective

12. Monitor progress every 2 to 4 weeks initially; less often as indicated when improvement is evident

13. Refer for MD evaluation if condition does not meet prognostic expectations

Folliculitis/Furuncle

- Definition: Infectious condition involving pilosebaceous follicle occurring on any skin surface where hair follicles are present but predominately on face, neck, scalp and buttocks

    1. Folliculitis—superficial involvement of upper follicle

    2. Furuncle or boil—deeper involvement of follicle and dermal appendages

- Etiology/Incidence

    1. Caused most often by *Staphylococcus aureus*; less commonly by streptococcus bacteria

    2. Also seen with some tinea infections

    3. More common in males

- Signs and Symptoms

    1. Areas of redness and swelling

    2. Nodules may be present with deep-seated furuncles

    3. Tenderness and warmth at site

- Differential Diagnosis

    1. Candida

    2. Impetigo

- Physical Findings

    1. Localized areas of erythema and edema with papular or pustular lesions on face, scalp, neck, buttocks and other areas

    2. Nodules are present with deep-seated furuncles

    3. Tenderness and warmth may be present

    4. Regional adenopathy may be present

- Diagnostic Tests/Findings: Culture confirms specific bacterial agent

- Management/Treatment

    1. Obtain detailed history of onset, duration, severity, progression of symptoms and possible precipitating factors

    2. Describe and monitor lesions in terms of morphology/structure, size, shape, number, color, location, distribution

    3. Wash with antimicrobial soap and apply warm moist compresses to affected areas

4. Topical antibiotics, e.g., bacitracin, mupirocin, neosporin

5. Oral antibiotics

   a. For staphylococci—use dicloxacillin

   b. For streptococci infection—penicillin or cephalosporin, erythromycin for penicillin allergic patients

6. Educate regarding medication dosage, signs of irritation, sensitivity

7. Educate regarding characteristics of condition, treatment regime, prognosis, and good hygiene measures

8. Refer for MD evaluation if condition does not follow prognostic expectation

Viral Conditions

Herpes Simplex/Common Cold Sore

- Definition: Contagious infection predominately of lips and oral mucosa, commonly known as fever blisters

  1. Initial infectious state—more severe, lasts longer, and is more painful

  2. Dormant state—virus lives on ending of selected nerves, asymptomatic

  3. Secondary infectious state—activated at times of increased stress, illness, fatigue, sun exposure, menses

- Etiology/Incidence

  1. Herpes simplex virus type 1—most common cause

  2. Herpes simplex virus type 2—considered in situations of oral sex

  3. Incubation varies, commonly 2 to 12 days

- Signs and Symptoms

  1. Redness with small blisters and crusting on lips

  2. Redness and swelling with painful white ulcerated patches inside mouth

  3. Fever, generalized malaise, and sore throat may occur

  4. Mild itching, tingling, pain, and burning may precede blisters

- Differential Diagnosis

  1. Erythema multiforme

  2. Hand-foot-mouth disease

  3. Candida

  4. Localized bacterial infection

  5. Sexual abuse

- Physical Findings
    1. Lip lesions—grouped or singular vesicles on an erythematous base erupt and form crusts; usually can be found on mucocutaneous border of lips
    2. Oral cavity lesions—erythema and edema of mucous membranes with singular or multiple vesicles and white ulcerations; may include tongue, palate, and gums
    3. Regional adenopathy may be present
    4. Halitosis may be present with oral lesions
    5. Lesions are present 10 to 14 days, gradually resolving
    6. Secondary infection may be present—most caused by staphylococcus bacteria
- Diagnostic Tests/Findings
    1. Tzanck smear confirms presence of multinuclear giant cells indicative of herpes
    2. Culture to confirm causal agent
- Management/Treatment
    1. Obtain detailed history of onset, duration, severity and progression of symptoms, and precipitating factors
    2. Describe and monitor lesions in terms of morphology/structure, size, shape, number, color, location, distribution
    3. Treat lip lesions
        a. Burow's compresses to alleviate discomfort
        b. Topical antiviral applications, e.g., acyclovir, for recurrent disease
    4. Treat oral lesions
        a. Avoid spicy and acid foods
        b. Cool, bland fluids especially when lesions are most painful
        c. Anesthetic mouth rinses, e.g., lidocaine (with caution), or diphenhydramine
    5. Oral antiviral medication with recurrent disease at first sign of prodrome (skin tingling), e.g., acyclovir
    6. Oral antibiotic to treat secondary bacterial infection, e.g., erythromycin, dicloxacillin, cefadroxil, cephalexin
    7. Educate regarding medication dosage, signs of irritation, sensitivity
    8. Educate regarding cause, characteristics of condition, communicability, and prognosis
    9. Educate regarding preventive measures
        a. Avoid direct exposure of others to lesions (kissing)
        b. Wash hands before and after applying topical medications or touching lesions

      c. Avoid sharing personal items—cosmetics, cups, eating utensils

10. Refer for MD evaluation if condition does not improve

Molluscum Contagiosum

- Definition: Common infectious, self-limiting skin condition characterized by waxy firm papules which may occur on any skin surface predominately on face, axillae, abdomen, and arms

- Etiology/Incidence
  1. Caused by a poxvirus
  2. Most common in children and adolescents
  3. Common in children with HIV or AIDS
  4. Incubation is usually 2 to 8 weeks but may be up to 6 months
  5. Period of communicability uncertain
     a. May persist as long as lesions are present
     b. Spread by direct contact and through autoinoculations

- Signs and Symptoms
  1. Mild itching may be present
  2. Few or multiple small, firm, raised pinkish-white or skin colored lesions

- Differential Diagnosis
  1. Warts
  2. Closed comedones
  3. *Condylomata acuminata*

- Physical Findings
  1. Papular pink-white, or skin colored lesions of 1 to 5 mm in size usually on face, neck, axillae, abdomen, and arms
  2. Occasionally lesions grow to 1 to 2 cm
  3. Secondary bacterial infection may be present
  4. Lesions may become umbilicated (central pitting, dimpled, or depressed)
  5. Lesions are self-limiting but may be present for 2 to 3 years if left untreated
  6. May occur in genital area in sexually active and sexually abused

- Diagnostic Tests/Findings
  1. Usually not necessary
  2. Wright or Giemsa stain of papule core will show characteristic intracytoplasmic inclusions

- Management/Treatment

  1. Obtain a detailed history of onset, duration, severity and progression of symptoms, and precipitating factors

  2. Describe and monitor lesions in terms of morphology/structure, size, shape, number, color, location, distribution

  3. Rule out child abuse if lesions in genital area

  4. Treatment options:

     a. Lesions may resolve spontaneously without treatment over time

     b. Curretage removal of lesions provides more expedient resolution; not recommended for facial lesions due to potential scarring

     c. Topical application of keratolytics; not recommended for lesions near eyes

        (1) Tretinoin cream

        (2) Cartharidin

     d. Topical antibiotics for secondary bacterial infection, e.g., erythromycin, bacitracin, mupirocin

  5. Education regarding medication dosages, signs of irritation, sensitivity

  6. Education regarding cause, characteristics of lesions, communicability, and prognosis

  7. Education regarding preventive measures

     a. Avoid direct exposure of others to lesions

     b. Wash hands before and after application of topical medications and/or touching lesions

     c. Avoid sharing personal items—cosmetics, towels, cups, eating utensils

  8. Refer for MD evaluation if condition does not resolve with selected treatment

Verruca (Warts)

- Definition: Common self-limiting skin condition characterized by firm, well-circumscribed smooth to irregular, singular or multiple papules, predominately on fingers, palms, and soles of feet; commonly known as warts

- Etiology/Incidence

  1. Human papillomaviruses with more than 50 identified types

  2. Virus enters skin through minor trauma

  3. Occurs in 10% of children and adolescents with school-age children having the highest incidence

  4. Incidence may be increased with ongoing exposure to moisture

  5. Period of incubation varies widely, and estimated from 2 months to 2 years

     6. Period of communicability unknown

        a. May persist as long as lesions are present

        b. Spread by direct and indirect contact and through autoinoculations

- Signs and Symptoms

     1. Raised gray, brownish to skin colored, smooth to rough, singular or multiple lesions on hands

     2. Painful flat ingrown lesions on soles

     3. Bleeding may occur with trauma or picking

- Differential Diagnosis

     1. Molluscum contagiosum

     2. Calluses

- Physical Findings

     1. Common verruca—gray, brown or skin colored, rough singular or multiple papular lesions, most common on hands and fingers

     2. Flat verruca—skin colored, smooth round multiple lesions slightly elevated; most common on the face and extremities

     3. Plantar verruca—skin colored, irregular, single or multiple lesions that appear flush with sole of foot and grow inward

     4. May occur in genital area of sexually active and sexually abused

     5. Lesions are self-limiting, usually 6 to 9 months but due to reinfection through auto-inoculation; condition may persist for several years

- Diagnostic Tests/Findings: Excision and histological examination may confirm diagnosis

- Management/Treatment

     1. Obtain a detailed history of onset, duration, severity, progression of symptoms, and possible precipitating factors

     2. Describe and monitor lesions in terms of morphology/structure, size, shape, number, color, location, distribution

     3. Rule out child abuse if genital lesions are present

     4. Consider treatment options

        a. No treatment is usually necessary due to self-limiting condition

           (1) Ideal treatment has not been established

           (2) Frequently recur regardless of treatment choice

        b. Topical applications of keratolytics, e.g., cantharidin, tretinoin

        c. Applications of waterproof plastic tapes treated with keratolytics

    d. Excision of lesions except those on face due to potential scarring

5. Topical antibiotics to treat secondary bacterial infection, e.g., erythromycin, bacitracin, mupirocin, neosporin

6. Educate regarding medication dosages, signs of irritation, sensitivity

7. Educate regarding cause, characteristics of condition, communicability, and prognosis

8. Consider congenital or acquired immunodeficiency if no resolution and/or widespread (Cohen, 1999)

9. Refer for MD evaluation if condition does not improve or bleeds with light trauma

Fungal Infections

Tinea Capitis (Ringworm of the Scalp)

- Definition: Superficial dermatophyte (parasitic) fungal skin infection of the scalp
- Etiology/Incidence
    1. Caused predominately by *Trichophyton tonsurans* (90%); also by *Microsporum canis, Microsporum audouinii,* and *Trichophyton mentagrophytes* (less common)
    2. Dermatophytes attach to epidermis skin layer of host's scalp and multiply within stratum corneum; do not involve lower layers of epidermis or dermis
    3. Spreads through direct and indirect contact with infected individuals, animals, caps, combs, brushes, glasses and other personal articles
    4. *Microsporum canis* may be transmitted through contact with infected dogs or cats
    5. Occurs more often in hot humid climates
    6. More common in darker skinned individuals; boys more than girls
    7. Incubation period is unknown, possibly 10 to 14 days
    8. Communicability occurs as long as lesions with dermatophytes are present
- Signs and Symptoms
    1. Itching with varying degrees of severity
    2. Slightly raised round or angular scaly areas with pink borders
    3. Some yellow honey-comb crusts
    4. Broken hairs and balding may be present
- Differential Diagnosis
    1. Impetigo
    2. Eczema
    3. Seborrhea dermatitis

4. Psoriasis

5. Trichotillomania

- Physical Findings

    1. Several presentations may occur singularly or at the same time

        a. Diffuse scaly plaques of varying sizes with or without alopecia

        b. Pustules, papules with areas of honey-comb crusts

        c. Tender erythematous areas with broken hairs at scalp level leaving a "black-dot" appearance

    2. Regional adenopathy may be present, especially occipital nodes

- Diagnostic Tests/Findings

    1. Wood's lamp will fluoresce the *Microsporum canis* only and is of limited use in confirming tinea capitis

    2. KOH scraping from the areas of scalp with alopecia, "black dots," or broken hairs will confirm hyphae and spores of dermatophytes

- Management/Treatment

    1. Obtain detailed history of onset, duration, severity and progression of symptoms, and precipitating factors

    2. Describe and monitor lesions in terms of morphology/structure, size, shape, number, color, location, and distribution

    3. Treat with oral antifungal medication

        a. Griseofulvin

        b. May require treatment up to 6 weeks before resolution

        c. Topical antifungal medications are ineffective

    4. Shampoo 2 to 3 times weekly with selenium sulfide to reduce spore count and infectivity

    5. Although condition is communicable, exclusion from school and other groups is not indicated unless treatment is refused or not followed

    6. Educate regarding medication dosage, signs of irritation, sensitivity

    7. Educate regarding characteristics of condition, treatment regime, and prognosis

    8. Educate regarding communicability and prevention

        a. Avoid sharing personal items of caps, combs, brushes, towels, pillows, glasses, razors; wash these items frequently

        b. Wash hair immediately after barbershop or salon haircut

        c. Maintain personal hygiene, wash hands before/after treatment

d. Avoid touching or scratching affected areas

9. Refer for MD evaluation if condition does not improve

Tinea Corporis (Ringworm of the Body)

- Definition: Superficial dermatophyte (parasitic) fungal skin infection of less-hairy surfaces of body and face; commonly known as "ring worm" due to pattern of healing centrally while spreading peripherally

- Etiology/Incidence

  1. Primary source—*Trichophyton rubrum, Trichophyton mentagrophytes,* as well as *Microsporum canis,* and *Epidermophyton floccosum*

  2. Dermatophytes attach to epidermis skin layer of host and multiply within stratum corneum; do not involve lower layers of the epidermis or dermis

  3. Spreads through direct and indirect contact with infected individuals, animals, shower stalls, benches, and other articles

  4. *Microsporum canis* may be transmitted through contact with infected dogs or cats

  5. Occurs more often in hot humid climates

  6. Incubation period is unknown, possibly 4 to 14 days

  7. Communicability occurs as long as lesions with dermatophytes are present

- Signs and Symptoms

  1. Mild itching at site of affected areas

  2. Slightly raised round or angular scaly areas with pink borders

- Differential Diagnosis

  1. Contact dermatitis

  2. Eczema

  3. Psoriasis

  4. Pityriasis rosea

- Physical Findings

  1. Typical lesions are scaly plaques of varying sizes from less than 5 mm to more that 3 cm with mild erythematous active borders

  2. Lesions spread peripherally as they heal centrally

  3. Lesions may be singular or several; numerous lesions are uncommon

- Diagnostic Tests/Findings

  1. Wood's lamp will fluoresce the *Microsporum canis*

  2. KOH scraping of lesion border—confirms hyphae and spores

  3. Dermatophyte test medium (DTM)—confirm diagnosis

- Management/Treatment

  1. Obtain a detailed history of onset, duration, severity, progression of symptoms, and precipitating factors

  2. Describe and monitor lesions in terms of morphology/structure, size, shape, number, color, location, and distribution

  3. Treat with topical antifungal medications

     a. Clotrimazole, miconazole, econazole, terbinafine, tolnaftate, naftifine, ciclopirox, ketoconazole

     b. May require treatment up to 8 weeks before resolution

  4. Treat with oral antifungal medication for extensive, recurrent, and unresponsive conditions, e.g., griseofulvin

  5. Educate regarding medication dosage, signs of irritation, sensitivity

  6. Educate regarding characteristics of condition, treatment regime, and prognosis

  7. Educate regarding communicability and prevention

     a. Avoid sharing personal items of clothing, towels, pillows, razors and wash these items frequently

     b. Maintain personal hygiene and wash hands before and after applying treatment

     c. Avoid touching or scratching affected areas

     d. Avoid or shower after using public pools

     e. Wash clothing touching affected areas after each use

  8. Refer for MD evaluation if condition does not improve

Tinea Cruris (Jock Itch)

- Definition: Superficial dermatophyte (parasitic) fungal skin infection of the groin, upper thighs, and/or inguinal folds; commonly called "jock-itch"

- Etiology/Incidence

  1. Caused by *Epidermophyton floccosum, Trichophyton rubrum,* and *Trichophyton mentagrophytes*

  2. Dermatophytes attach to epidermis skin layer of host and multiply within stratum corneum; lower layers of epidermis or dermis are not involved

  3. Occurs more often during hot humid weather with increased sweating

  4. More common in adolescents, athletes, obese children, and males

  5. Spreads through direct and indirect contact with infected individuals, including sexual contact

  6. Incubation period is unknown, possibly 4 to 14 days

  7. Communicability occurs as long as lesions with dermatophytes are present

- Signs and Symptoms
    1. Pain and tenderness with varying degrees of severity
    2. Itching with varying degrees of severity reported especially during healing
    3. Red slightly raised scaly areas with defined borders
    4. Blisters may also be present
- Differential Diagnosis
    1. Contact dermatitis
    2. Eczema
    3. Intertrigo
    4. Psoriasis
    5. Seborrheic dermatitis
- Physical Findings
    1. Erythematous scaly red to brown lesions of varying sizes with well defined raised borders
        a. Small vesicles, central clearing, and peripheral spreading may or may not be present
        b. Affected areas may be singular or multiple
        c. In chronic cases, lichenification may be present
    2. All areas of the groin may be affected including scrotum, gluteal folds, buttocks, inner aspect of thighs
    3. Painful to touch and with movement
    4. Often concurrent with tinea pedis
- Diagnostic Tests/Findings
    1. KOH scraping of lesion border—confirms hyphae and spores
    2. DTM—confirms diagnosis
- Management/Treatment
    1. Obtain a detailed history of onset, duration, severity, progression of symptoms, and precipitating factors
    2. Describe and monitor lesions in terms of morphology/structure, size shape, number, color, location, and distribution
    3. Treat with topical antifungal medications
        a. Clotrimazole, haloprogin, miconazole, terbinafine, tolnaftate, ciclopirox, econazole, ketoconazole, naftifine, oxiconazole, sulconazole
        b. May require treatment up to 4 to 6 weeks before resolution

4. Treat with oral antifungal medication for extensive, recurrent, and/ or unresponsive conditions, e.g., griseofulvin

5. Educate regarding medication dosage, signs of irritation, sensitivity

6. Educate regarding characteristics of condition, treatment regime, and prognosis

7. Educate regarding communicability and prevention

    a. Avoid sharing undergarments—pants, jock straps,

    b. Wash personal undergarments frequently

    c. Maintain good daily personal hygiene and dry well after bathing

    d. Wash hands before and after applying topical treatment

    e. Avoid touching or scratching affected areas

    f. Avoid or shower after using public pools

    g. Launder clothing touching affected areas after each use

    h. Don't wear tight clothes next to affected area including jeans and undergarments

    i. Use cotton undergarments and change daily

8. Refer for MD evaluation if condition does not improve

Tinea Pedis (Athlete's Feet, or Ringworm of the Feet)

- Definition: Superficial dermatophyte (parasitic) fungal skin infection of toes and feet
- Etiology/Incidence

1. Caused by *Trichophyton rubrum, Trichophyton mentagrophytes,* and *Epidermophyton floccosum* fungal dermatophytes

2. Dermatophytes attach to epidermis skin layer of host and multiply within stratum corneum; do not involve lower layers of epidermis or dermis

3. Occurs more often during hot humid weather with increased sweating

4. Occurs worldwide; more common in adolescents, athletes, and males

5. Spreads through direct and indirect contact with infected individuals, public baths, swimming pools, and locker rooms

6. Incubation period is unknown

7. Communicability occurs as long as lesions with dermatophytes are present

- Signs and Symptoms

1. Pruritus of affected areas

2. Reddened, scaly and occasionally blistered areas anywhere on foot; cracks and scaling between toes

3. Stinging or pain if cracks between toes

- Differential Diagnosis
    1. Atopic dermatitis
    2. Contact dermatitis
    3. Candida
    4. Eczema
- Physical Findings
    1. Erythematous scaly lesions of varying sizes
        a. Small vesicles, central clearing, and peripheral spreading may or may not be present
        b. Affected areas may be anywhere on foot, most commonly on lateral and planter portions
    2. Lesions on or between toes are scaly with mild erythema
        a. Interdigital fissures are present
        b. One or multiple toes may be involved, most commonly between third and fourth toes
    3. Dystrophy of toenails may be present
- Diagnostic Tests/Findings
    1. KOH scraping of lesion border confirms hyphae and spores
    2. DTM of skin scraping or nail clippings confirms diagnosis
- Management/Treatment
    1. Obtain a detailed history of onset, duration, severity, progression of symptoms, and precipitating factors
    2. Describe and monitor lesions in terms of morphology/structure, size, shape, number, color, location, and distribution
    3. Treat with topical antifungal medications
        a. Clotrimazole, haloprogin, miconazole, econazole, ciclopirox, terbinafine, tolnaftate, ketoconazole, naftifine, oxiconazole, sulconazole
        b. May require treatment up to 4 to 6 weeks before resolution
    4. Treat vesicular and fissured lesions with compresses of Burow's solution
    5. Use absorbent antifungal powder
    6. Treat with oral antifungal medication for extensive, recurrent, and unresponsive conditions, e.g., griseofulvin
    7. Educate regarding medication dosage and signs of irritation and sensitivity
    8. Educate regarding characteristics of condition, treatment regime, and prognosis

9. Educate regarding communicability and prevention

   a. Avoid sharing personal items of shoes, socks, and towels

   b. Wash personal items frequently

   c. Maintain good daily personal hygiene and dry well after bathing

   d. Wash hands before and after applying topical treatment

   e. Avoid touching or scratching affected areas

   f. Avoid using public pools or shower after each use

   g. Launder clothing touching affected areas after each use

   h. Don't wear tight and closed shoes

   i. Use cotton socks instead of nylon or polyester

10. Refer for MD evaluation if condition does not improve

Insect Conditions

Common Insect Bites

- Definition: Wound inflicted by bite of a blood sucking arthropod
- Etiology/Incidence
   1. Caused when mosquitos, fleas, chiggers, and bedbugs feed on human blood

      a. Are attracted to host's moisture, odor, and warmth

      b. Serve as vectors for diseases such as malaria

   2. Pet dogs and cats act as hosts for some fleas that are also attracted to humans

   3. More bites occur:

      a. In warm and humid weather

      b. Around stagnant water

      c. In outside grassy and sandy areas

      d. On uncovered body areas

   4. Itching caused by sensitivity to insect's saliva

- Signs and Symptoms

   1. Itching is major symptom—may persist 5 to 7 days after exposure

   2. Pain—variable

   3. Single or multiple pink/red raised lesions on legs, abdomen, and exposed areas of upper body

- Differential Diagnosis

   1. Folliculitis

2. Insect sting

3. Spider bite

4. Scabies

- Physical Findings

    1. Single or multiple erythematous papules and wheals on lower extremities, abdomen, and exposed upper body parts

    2. Lesions from bed bug and chigger bites are smaller, more erythematous and more numerous

    3. Vesicles may develop signaling greater sensitivity

    4. Excoriation may be present with intense pruritus

    5. Pustules may develop indicating secondary bacterial infection

- Diagnostic Tests/Findings: Culture of pustules confirms causal organism of secondary infection

- Management/Treatment

    1. Obtain detailed history of bite, progression of symptoms, and precipitating factors

    2. Describe and monitor lesions in terms of morphology/structure, size, shape, number, color, location, and distribution

    3. Provide symptomatic treatment of pruritus

        a. Cool compresses

        b. Topical histamines, e.g., hydroxyzine, diphenhydramine

        c. Oral antihistamines if topical treatment is ineffective, e.g., hydroxyzine, diphenhydramine

    4. Topical steroids to reduce inflammation and immune response, e.g., hydrocortisone, triamcinolone

    5. Treat secondary bacterial infection

        a. Use topical antibiotics, e.g., bacitracin, mupirocin, neosporin

        b. Treat with oral antibiotics if extensive, recurrent, or unresponsive, e.g., erythromycin, cefadroxil, cephalexin

    6. Educate regarding characteristics of condition, treatment regime, and prognosis

    7. Educate regarding medication dosage, signs of irritation, sensitivity

    8. Educate regarding prevention

        a. Outside environmental controls—clearing areas, pesticide spraying, removing stagnant water

        b. Inside environmental controls—routine cleaning, vacuuming

        c. Bathe flea-infested pets

    d.   Wear cover-up clothing

    e.   Wear insect repellants

    f.   Avoid wearing fragrances that may attract

    g.   Avoid scratching to prevent infection

9.   Refer for MD evaluation if condition does not resolve

Spider Bites

- Definition: Wound inflicted by spider characterized by both local and systemic manifestations

- Etiology/Incidence

1.   Most spider bites are harmless, causing small localized reaction at site of bite

2.   In U.S. bites from two non-aggressive venomous spiders produce severe toxic reactions in some individuals

    a.   Black widow

       (1)   Mature female is shinny, black, gray or brown with an orange hour glass marking on the ventral surface

       (2)   Overall size is 2.5 to 4.5 cm including legs

       (3)   Male is smaller with fangs that can not penetrate human skin

       (4)   Most common in Ohio, South, Southwest, and West coast

       (5)   Likes dry, warm, dark areas; found in grass, wood piles, gardens, sheds, basements, closets, and trunks

       (6)   Spin irregular asymmetrical web to catch flies and other prey

    b.   Brown recluse

       (1)   Mature spider is gray, or varying shades of red to pale brown with a violin shaped marking on cephalothorax

       (2)   Overall size is 1.5 to 2.5 cm including legs

       (3)   Most common in the Midwest and South

       (4)   Likes trunks, carpets, old shoes, old clothes, closets, crates, shelves

3.   Most bites are in self-defense when spider feels threatened

4.   Most bites occur in warmer months

5.   Infants and small children are most vulnerable to developing serious reactions

- Signs and Symptoms

1.   Black widow

    a.   Initial sensation of pinch or sting is often unnoticed

b. Later within 1 hour of the bite

    (1) Dull burning or pain at site of bite

    (2) Two red puncture marks surrounded by white area with bluish-red border

    (3) Muscle cramps and sweating

    (4) Muscle spasms can spread to rest of body

    (5) In severe cases can progress to shock, coma, and death

2. Brown recluse

    a. Initial sensation of bite is most often unnoticed or moderately painful

    b. Later within 2 to 7 hours

        (1) Mild localized tingling

        (2) Redness or blanching

    c. After 48 to 72 hours

        (1) Blister surrounded by blue-gray area

        (2) Flu-like symptoms may be experienced

3. Reactions from bites of both spiders may become more intense and last for days with more serious life-threatening signs/symptoms developing in a few cases

- Differential Diagnosis—Black widow and Brown recluse

  1. Other insect bites (both)

  2. Tetanus (black widow)

  3. Appendicitis (black widow)

  4. Diabetic ulcers (brown recluse)

  5. Stevens-Johnson syndrome (brown recluse)

- Physical Findings—specifics vary by type of spider

  1. Black widow spider bite

    a. Symptoms begin within one hour

    b. Dull, burning or pain at site

    c. Two red puncture marks surrounded by a blanched area with bluish erythematous border

    d. Muscle spasms, hypertension, tachycardia, diaphoresis

  2. Brown recluse spider bite

    a. Initial symptoms begin within 2 to 7 hours

        (1) Mild, localized tingling

    (2)   Erythema or blanching at site

  b. Delayed symptoms after 48 to 72 hours

    (1)   Hemorrhagic vesicle surrounded by bluish, gray areas of developing necrosis

    (2)   Flu-like symptoms

3. Both (black widow and brown recluse)

  a. Reactions may last for days to weeks

  b. Potential to become serious and life-threatening with major renal, respiratory, cardiovascular, and neurological system involvement

- Diagnostic Tests/Findings

1. No tests confirm specific diagnosis

2. Dead spider specimen may help to confirm specific species

- Management/Treatment

1. Obtain detailed history of onset, duration, severity and progression of symptoms, and precipitating factors

2. Describe and monitor symptoms, and lesions in terms of morphology/structure, size, shape, number, color, location, and distribution

3. If bite from black widow or brown recluse spider is suspected

  a. Apply cold compresses to site of bite

  b. Refer immediately for MD evaluation and hospitalization due to potential risk of severe reaction

4. If bite from another less harmful spider is suspected

  a. Apply cool compresses to site of bite

  b. Use oral antihistamines to reduce severe pruritus, e.g., hydroxyzine, diphenhydramine

  c. Monitor for hypersensitivity reaction

5. Educate regarding characteristics of condition, treatment regime, and prognosis

6. Educate regarding medication dosage, signs of irritation, sensitivity

7. Educate regarding prevention

  a. Outside environmental controls—clearing areas, pesticide spraying

  b. Inside environmental controls—routine cleaning, vacuuming

  c. Avoid and/or be observant around areas of natural habitat

  d. Wear protective clothing and hats

    e. Wear gloves when cleaning closets and trunks

    f. Inspect clothing and shoes prior to wearing

Insect Stings

- Definition: Wound inflicted by sting of an insect, characterized by systemic and/or local manifestations
- Etiology/Incidence
  1. Caused by bees, hornets, wasps, yellow-jackets, and fire ants
  2. Hypersensitivity to venom develops after initial exposure with more severe reactions upon subsequent exposures
     a. Mild reactions occur in 90% of children
     b. Anaphylaxis occurs in approximately 7% of general population
  3. Most stings occur in self-defense when insect feels threatened
  4. Most stings occur in warmer months
  5. Multiple stings may occur when around nests or swarms of insects
- Signs and Symptoms
  1. Usual reaction after initial exposure lasts up to 24 hours
     a. Pain with varying degrees of severity
     b. Redness and swelling at site of sting
  2. More pronounced reaction after re-exposure
     a. Nausea and abdominal pain
     b. Sneezing and coughing
     c. Itching
     d. Larger area of redness and swelling
  3. Anaphylactic reaction may occur after initial or re-exposure
     a. Early signs within minutes of exposure
        (1) Dizziness
        (2) Swelling of lips and throat
        (3) Difficulty breathing
        (4) Difficulty swallowing
     b. Later signs
        (1) Weakness and collapse
        (2) Confusion

(3) Coma

- Differential Diagnosis
    1. Spider bites
    2. Other insect bites

- Physical Findings
    1. Usual reaction after initial exposure may last up to 24 hours
        a. Pain with varying degrees of severity
        b. Erythema and edema surrounding central punctum at site of sting
    2. Thin white to gray stinger may project from center
    3. More pronounced reaction may last several days especially after re-exposure
        a. Nausea, abdominal pain
        b. Sneezing, coughing
        c. Pruritus
        d. Larger area of redness, swelling
    4. Anaphylactic reaction may occur after initial or re-exposure
        a. Could result in ultimate collapse and death
        b. Early signs within minutes of exposure
            (1) Dizziness
            (2) Swelling of lips and throat
            (3) Difficulty breathing
            (4) Difficulty swallowing
        c. Later signs
            (1) Weakness and collapse
            (2) Confusion
            (3) Coma
            (4) Stridor

- Diagnostic Tests/Findings: None

- Management/Treatment
    1. Obtain detailed history of onset, duration, severity, progression of symptoms
    2. Describe and monitor area in terms of size, color, and location
    3. If known sensitivity, life threatening, and/or severe reaction
        a. Administer epinephrine as indicated

        b.   Apply cool compresses

        c.   Refer immediately for MD evaluation and hospitalization

4.   If mild reaction

        a.   Remove stinger by flicking off, do not squeeze

        b.   Apply cool compresses to site of sting

        c.   Use oral antihistamines to reduce severe pruritus, e.g., hydroxyzine, diphenhydramine

        d.   Monitor for hypersensitivity reaction

5.   Provide emotional support as needed to child and family

6.   Educate regarding characteristics of condition, treatment regime, and prognosis

7.   Educate regarding medication dosage, signs of irritation, sensitivity

8.   Educate regarding prevention

        a.   Outside environmental controls—clearing areas, pesticide spraying

        b.   Inside environmental controls—routine cleaning, vacuuming

        c.   Avoid and/or be observant around areas of natural habitat

        d.   Wear protective clothing, hats and gloves

        e.   Avoid wearing bright clothing when hiking around natural habitat

        f.   Avoid wearing perfumes when around natural habitat

        g.   If known sensitivity wear medical alert tag and carry epinephrine kit

Insect Infestations

Scabies Infestation

- Definition: Highly contagious condition caused by parasitic mite infestation

- Etiology/Incidence

  1.   Caused by the *Sarcoptes scabiei* (itch mite); gravid female mite burrows into stratum corneum to lay ova which hatch in 4 to 14 days

  2.   Incubation period of 4 to 6 weeks with initial exposure; 1 to 5 days with re-exposure causing intense itching

  3.   Worldwide distribution in all population groups regardless of hygiene

  4.   Major infestations have occurred in cyclic patterns of every 15 to 30 years

  5.   Spreads through direct contact with infected person or indirect contact with clothing, bed linens, and other personal items

6. Communicability is present until all mites, larva, and ova are destroyed on body surface and in surrounding environment

- Signs and Symptoms

  1. Irritability in infants

  2. Intense itching especially at night in older children and adolescents

  3. Red bumps, blisters, pustules, and small burrow marks which may be obliterated by scratch marks

- Differential Diagnosis

  1. Insect bites

  2. Impetigo

  3. Secondary bacterial infection

- Physical Findings

  1. Intense itching

  2. Fine gray to skin-colored superficial 2 to 8 mm linear curved burrows with small papule at proximal end; burrows may be obliterated by scratch and excoriation marks due to scratching

  3. Infants—typically have red-brown papular, vesicular lesions on head, neck, palms and soles

  4. Older child and adolescent—typically have red papular lesions on webs of fingers and folds of wrists, elbows, axillae, waist, buttocks, groin, umbilicus, abdomen, knees, ankles

  5. Pustules indicate secondary bacterial infection

  6. Regional adenopathy may be present

- Diagnostic Tests/Findings

  1. Skin scrapings of burrow or papule material and microscopic examination for body parts of mite, ova, or feces

  2. Culture of pustule will confirm agent of secondary infection

- Management/Treatment

  1. Obtain a detailed history of onset, duration, severity and progression of symptoms

  2. Describe and monitor lesions in terms of morphology/structure, size shape, number, color, location, and distribution

  3. Bathe and dry skin, then treat with topical medication

     a. Infants and young children—permethrin 5% (drug of choice)

     b. Older children and adolescents—permethrin 5%; lindane, crotamiton 10%, sulfur in petrolatum

4. Use topical steroids to reduce inflammation, immune response, and pruritus, e.g., hydrocortisone, triamcinolone

5. Use oral antihistamines to reduce pruritus, e.g., hydroxyzine, diphenhydramine

6. Treat secondary bacterial infection

   a. Use topical antibiotics, e.g., bacitracin, mupirocin, neosporin

   b. Use oral antibiotics if extensive, recurrence, or unresponsive, e.g., erythromycin, dicloxacillin, cefadroxil, cephalexin

7. Educate regarding medication dosage, signs of irritation, sensitivity

8. Treat household and other close contacts

9. Wash clothes, bed linens, towels, and hats with hot water and dry in hot dryer

10. Store non-washable items in plastic bags for one week; do not use

11. Educate regarding characteristics of condition, treatment regime, and prognosis

12. Educate regarding medication dosage and signs of irritation and sensitivity

13. Educate regarding communicability and prevention

    a. Avoid sharing personal items of clothes, linens, towels, and wash these items frequently

    b. Maintain good daily personal hygiene and dry well after bathing

    c. Wash hands before and after applying topical treatment

    d. Avoid touching or scratching affected areas

14. Refer for MD evaluation if condition does not improve

Pediculosis Infestation (Lice)

- Definition: Highly contagious parasitic louse infestation affecting hairy body surfaces
- Etiology/Incidence

  1. Caused by several species of lice

     a. *Pediculus capitis*—affects scalp

     b. *Pediculus humanus*—affects less hairy body surfaces

     c. *Phthirus pubis*—affects pubic, and axilla areas, eyelashes, eyebrows

  2. Worldwide distribution in all population groups regardless of hygiene practices

  3. More common in school age and adolescents due to sharing of personal items

  4. More common in Caucasians, less common in African-Americans

  5. Spreads through direct contact with infected person or indirect contact with clothing, bed linens, and other personal items

6. Incubation of 6 to 10 days from laying of eggs to hatching; hatched lice mature in 2 to 3 weeks

7. Communicability present until all lice, neophytes, and ova are destroyed on body surface and environment

- Signs and Symptoms
  1. Itching
  2. White flakes on hair
  3. Red blotches and bumps (rare)

- Differential Diagnosis
  1. Bites from other insects
  2. Bacterial infection
  3. Dandruff
  4. Hair casts
  5. Scabies

- Physical Findings
  1. Small white nits (eggs) on hair strands—$\frac{1}{4}$ inch from skin surface; difficult to remove
     a. Head lice most common on back of head, behind ears
     b. Body lice most common in seams of clothing
  2. Macular, papular lesions with mild erythema and excoriation
  3. Pustules secondary to scratching (secondary bacterial infection)
  4. Regional adenopathy may be present

- Diagnostic Tests/Findings
  1. Clinical examination of hair shaft for ova is usually sufficient to confirm diagnosis
  2. Microscopic examination of ova may confirm questionable diagnosis

- Management/Treatment
  1. Obtain detailed history of onset, duration, severity and progression of symptoms
  2. Describe and monitor lesions in terms of morphology/structure, size, shape, number, color, location, and distribution
  3. Treat infestation with topical antiparasitics to destroy louse and ova, e.g., permethrin, pyrethrins; lindane indicated for treatment failures or for those who do not tolerate permethrin or pyrethrins
  4. Educate regarding medication dosage, signs of irritation, sensitivity
  5. Remove ova/nits after topical treatment

    a. Head lice—manually with fine tooth comb

    b. Vinegar and water preparation may help soften cement

    c. Eye lashes—may coat with petroleum jelly for several days

6. Use topical antibiotics to treat secondary bacterial infection antibiotics, e.g., bacitracin, mupirocin, neosporin

7. Treat other infested family members

8. Remove infestation from surrounding environment

    a. Wash clothes, bed linens, towels, and hats with hot water and dry in hot dryer

    b. Wash personal items such as combs and brushes with pediculocide

    c. Vacuum and store nonwashable items 10 days in plastic bag

    d. Vacuum drapes, rugs, floors, and furniture (beds, chairs, sofa)

9. Educate regarding characteristics of condition and prognosis

10. Educate regarding communicability and prevention

    a. Avoid sharing personal items of towels, hats, hair brushes, combs; wash these items frequently

    b. Maintain personal hygiene, wash hands before/after treatments

    c. Avoid touching or scratching affected areas

11. Refer for MD evaluation if condition does not resolve

Miscellaneous Conditions of Hypersensitivity

Drug Reactions

- Definition: Acute condition of the skin involving an allergic hypersensitivity reaction to a drug characterized predominately by a morbilliform generalized rash
- Etiology/Incidence
  1. Caused by release of histamine in reaction to immune system's response to drug allergen
  2. Most common drugs
     a. Sulfates
     b. Penicillins
     c. Barbiturates
     d. Dilantin
  3. Onset usually occurs within first week of exposure; may be delayed for more than 2 weeks and/or after drug has been discontinued

    4. Recurrences are frequent with re-exposures—response varies depending on antigen exposure

- Signs and Symptoms
    1. Intense generalized and localized itching
    2. Generalized red rash beginning on trunk and progressing to extremities
- Differential Diagnosis
    1. Scarlet fever
    2. Contact dermatitis
    3. Erythema multiforme
    4. Rubeola
    5. Urticaria
- Physical Findings
    1. Generalized and localized pruritus
    2. Generalized morbilliform erythematous rash occurring first on trunk and progressing to extremities; initially macular becoming papular and confluent
    3. Wheals are less typical, and less frequent
- Diagnostic Tests/Findings: None
- Management/Treatment
    1. Obtain detailed history of onset, duration, severity, progression of symptoms, and possible precipitating factors
    2. Describe and monitor lesions in terms of morphology/structure, size, shape, number, color, location, distribution
    3. Discontinue contact with drug/medication allergen if known sensitivity
    4. Oral steroids to reduce inflammation and immune response in severe and extensive cases, e.g., hydrocortisone
    5. Oral antihistamines for pruritus, e.g., hydroxyzine, diphenhydramine
    6. Educate regarding medication dosage, signs of irritation, sensitivity
    7. Educate regarding characteristics of condition, cause, treatment prognosis, and recurrence
    8. Refer to MD for evaluation if condition does not improve in 2 days or if becomes more severe at any time

Erythema Multiforme Minor

- Definition: Acute condition of the skin involving hypersensitivity reaction characterized by multi-morphology skin and mucous membrane eruptions; lasts approximately 2 to 3 weeks with spontaneous resolution

- Etiology/Incidence
    1. Hypersensitivity caused by exposure to variety of substances
        a. Infectious organisms—most common are enteroviruses, *Mycoplasma pneumoniae,* and herpes simplex especially in recurrent conditions
        b. Drugs—most common are barbiturates, sulfa, and penicillin drugs
        c. Other substances—food reactions
    2. More common in adults, however, approximately 20% of cases are in children and adolescents
    3. Recurrent episodes occur in approximately $\frac{1}{3}$ of cases
- Signs and Symptoms
    1. Itching may be present
    2. Pain especially in mouth
    3. Redness and swelling may present with blisters and/or ulcers on hands, elbows, knees, ankles, feet, eyes, lips, mouth
    4. Develop in crops over period of 1 to 2 weeks with each crop lasting 1 week
- Differential Diagnosis
    1. Allergic vasculitis
    2. Kawasaki disease
    3. Urticaria
    4. Varicella or other viral infections
- Physical Findings
    1. Pruritus and pain may be present at site of lesions, especially those in oral cavity
    2. Redness and swelling with lesions progressing from macules, to papules, blisters, and petechiae
    3. Lesions occur on bilateral exposed areas predominately—includes hands, elbows, knees, ankles, feet, eyes, lips, oral mucous membranes, tongue, oral cavity; and less commonly on chest and trunk
    4. Lesions develop in crops over period of 1 to 2 weeks with each crop lasting 1 week
    5. Target or "bull's-eye" lesions may be present which have three distinct characteristics—a necrotic or vesicular center, a pale middle macular ring and an outer erythematous peripheral ring
    6. Lasts from 2 to 3 weeks with spontaneous resolution
- Diagnostic Tests/Findings
    1. Chest radiograph to rule out *Mycoplasma pneumoniae*
    2. Tzanck test to rule out herpes simplex

- Management/Treatment
    1. Obtain detailed history of onset, duration, severity and progression of symptoms, and possible precipitating factors
    2. Describe and monitor lesions in terms of morphology/structure, size, shape, number, color, location, distribution
    3. Cool compresses for pain and pruritus
    4. Antihistamines for pruritus, e.g., hydroxyzine, diphenhydramine
    5. Oral analgesics for generalized pain, e.g., ibuprofen, acetaminophen
    6. Topical anesthetics and mouth washes for oral lesions, e.g., lidocaine
    7. Maintain hydration with cool fluids, e.g., water, nonirritating juices
    8. Determine underlying trigger and remove or treat as indicated
    9. Educate regarding medication dosages, signs of irritation, sensitivity
    10. Educate regarding characteristics of condition, cause, prognosis, and recurrence
    11. Refer for MD evaluation if:
        a. Condition does not improve
        b. Systemic symptoms of fever and malaise develop

Erythema Multiforme Major (Stevens-Johnson Syndrome)

- Definition: Skin condition involving hypersensitivity reaction characterized by multi-morphology mucous membrane and skin eruptions with associated systemic involvement; also known as Stevens-Johnson Syndrome
- Etiology/Incidence
    1. Hypersensitivity caused by exposure to a variety of substances
        a. Infectious organisms—most common are enteroviruses, *Mycoplasma pneumoniae,* and herpes simplex especially in recurrent conditions
        b. Drugs—most common are barbiturates, sulfa, and penicillin
        c. Other substances—food reactions
    2. More common in adults, however, approximately 20% of cases are in children and adolescents
    3. Recurrent episodes occur in approximately $\frac{1}{3}$ of the cases
    4. Can be life threatening; approximately 5% mortality of diagnosed cases
- Signs and Symptoms
    1. Fever, fatigue, sore throat, headache, nausea, vomiting, diarrhea, muscle pain, and/or joint pain
    2. Skin rash develops in 2 to 3 days after generalized symptoms

a. Areas of redness and swelling

b. Variety of skin reactions on hands, elbows, knees, ankles, feet, eyes, lips, mouth, chest and/or trunk

3. Itching may be present

4. Pain, especially in mouth

- Differential Diagnosis

    1. Gingivostomatitis

    2. Pemphigus

    3. Toxic epidermal necrolysis

    4. Urticaria

    5. Varicella

    6. Staphlococcal scalded syndrome

- Physical Findings

    1. Sudden onset of prodromal state—high temperature, malaise, weakness

    2. Multimorphology rash develops in progressive pattern

        a. Macular erythematous with edematous areas

        b. Progress to papules, vesicles, erosions, and petechiae

    3. Pruritus and pain, especially lesions in oral cavity

    4. Lesions occur on bilateral exposed areas predominately—includes hands, elbows, knees, ankles, feet, eyes, lips, oral mucous membranes, tongue; less common on chest and trunk

    5. Target or herald lesions may be present which have three distinct characteristics— necrotic or vesicular center, pale middle macular ring, and an outer erythematous peripheral ring

    6. Lesions develop in crops over period of 1 to 2 weeks with each crop lasting 1 week

    7. Condition may progress to more severe stage involving the respiratory, renal, and gastrointestinal systems

- Diagnostic Tests/Findings

    1. Chest radiograph to rule out *Mycoplasma pneumoniae*

    2. Tzanck to rule out herpes simplex

    3. Skin biopsy to confirm diagnosis

- Management/Treatment

    1. Obtain detailed history of onset, duration, severity and progression of symptoms, and possible precipitating factors

2. Describe and monitor lesions in terms of morphology/structure, size, shape, number, color, location, distribution

3. Immediate MD referral for evaluation and hospitalization due to potential life threatening situation

4. Educate regarding characteristics of condition, cause, and prognosis

Urticaria

- Definition: Acute or chronic condition of the skin involving an allergic hypersensitivity reaction characterized by pale or skin colored skin lesions

- Etiology/Incidence

    1. Caused by release of histamine as reaction to immune system's response to an allergen

        a. Foods

        b. Temperature changes of heat and cold

        c. Viral infections

        d. Vibrations and scratching

        e. Emotional elation or stress

        f. Insect bites

        g. Materials and fabrics

    2. Symptoms may last for minutes or up to 24 hours after initial exposure to antigen

    3. Recurrences are frequent with re-exposure to allergen; response is varied

- Signs and Symptoms

    1. Intense generalized and localized itching

    2. Mild redness and swelling of irregular shaped hives—may involve eyelids, lips, hands, feet, mouth, and genitalia

- Differential Diagnosis

    1. Atopic dermatitis

    2. Contact dermatitis

    3. Erythema multiforme

- Physical Findings

    1. Intense generalized and localized pruritus at site of lesions

    2. Mild erythema and swelling with irregular shaped wheals on any skin surface

        a. May have swelling of eyelids, lips, hands, feet, and genitalia

        b. May have swelling and redness of mucous membranes

3. Individual lesions range in size from under 1 cm to over 15 cm

4. Distribution pattern is generalized and scattered

5. Become more pronounced with heat

6. Will blanch with pressure

7. Excoriation due to scratching secondary to severe pruritus

- Diagnostic Tests/Findings: No tests confirm condition

- Management/Treatment

  1. Obtain detailed history of onset, duration, severity and progression of symptoms, and possible precipitating factors

  2. Describe and monitor lesions in terms of morphology/structure, size, shape, number, color, location, distribution

  3. Discontinue contact with allergen if known sensitivity

  4. Cool compresses of Burow's solution for comfort

  5. Topical steroids to reduce immune response and pruritus, e.g., hydrocortisone, triamcinolone

  6. Oral steroids for severe and extensive reactions, e.g., hydrocortisone

  7. Oral antihistamines for pruritus, e.g., hydroxyzine, diphenhydramine

  8. Educate regarding characteristics of condition

  9. Educate regarding medication dosages, signs of irritation, sensitivity

  10. Teach measures for prevention, e.g., avoid known allergens

  11. Refer to MD for evaluation:

      a. If acute episode does not improve

      b. Consideration of skin testing for hypersensitivities after acute episode resolves

Questions:
Select the best answer

1. J.D. is a postterm infant with lesions of varying morphology including wheals, vesicles, and pustules on her trunk. You suspect J.D. has:

   a. Cutis marmorata
   b. Erythema toxicum neonatorum
   c. Milia
   d. Sebaceous hyperplasia

2. In order to confirm your diagnosis of J.D., you order a Wright's stained smear. If your diagnosis is correct, what are the expected results of the smear?

   a. Presence of eosinophils
   b. Presence of neutrophils
   c. Presence of keratinous material
   d. Presence of staphylococcus bacteria

3. In addition to monitoring the skin for any changes, what is the best management for J.D.?

   a. Topical antibiotics on lesions
   b. Topical steroids on lesions
   c. A moisturizer on lesions
   d. No treatment necessary since J.D.'s condition will resolve spontaneously in 5 to 7 days

4. You examine C.C., a newborn, and observe numerous white papular lesions on the cheeks, forehead, and nose. You suspect either milia or sebaceous hyperplasia. Which physical finding helps to confirm a diagnosis of milia?

   a. Papular lesions are intermixed with pale yellow macules.
   b. Papular lesions have an erythematous circular ring at the base
   c. Papular lesions are surrounded by lacy-blue area with erythematous mottling
   d. Papular lesions, yellow in color, are observed on the hard palate

5. Newborn K.T. is three weeks premature and you observe a macular erythematous lacy appearance to her skin when you undress her. K.T. has which condition?

   a. Curtis marmorata
   b. Erythema toxicum neonatorum
   c. Salmon patch
   d. Nevus flammeus

6. In addition to monitoring the skin for any changes, what is the best management for K.T.?

   a. Keep K.T. warm
   b. Decrease the environmental temperature.
   c. Use a moisturizer on affected skin areas
   d. Do nothing as condition will resolve spontaneously in 5 to 7 days without intervention

7. Newborn W.R. has a vascular lesion that will not fade as she gets older. What is your diagnosis?

    a. Salmon patch
    b. Capillary hemangioma
    c. Café au lait
    d. Nevus flammeus

8. W.R.'s parents are concerned about her appearance and the psychological effect on their daughter as she becomes aware of her condition. In educating the parents, you tell them about several options that will be available when W.R. is older. Which of the following is not an appropriate management or treatment consideration for W.R.?

    a. Application of topical steroids to the affected area to prevent pruritus
    b. Camouflage affected areas with cosmetics
    c. Pulsed laser treatment of affected area
    d. Counseling for psychological concerns

9. Which condition is thought to be more common in darker skinned individuals?

    a. Tinea corporis
    b. Psoriasis
    c. Pityriasis alba
    d. Pityriasis rosea

10. J.R., an eight year old boy, has scaly pale salmon lesions predominately on his trunk. One lesion on the buttocks is larger than all the other lesions and measures 4 cm in diameter. What is your likely diagnosis?

    a. Psoriasis
    b. Eczema
    c. Pityriasis alba
    d. Pityriasis rosea

11. What symptom is commonly experienced in J.R.'s condition?

    a. Pruritus
    b. Pain at site of lesions
    c. Nausea
    d. Headache

12. What management would you not recommend for J.R. with his condition?

    a. Cool bath or cool compresses to lesions
    b. Topical steroids to lesions
    c. Oral antihistamine
    d. Monitored and controlled daily sunlight exposure

13. You have diagnosed D.L. with acute atopic dermatitis. Which of the following is not correct regarding the incidence of this condition?

    a. D.L. is most likely an infant
    b. D.L. has a greater chance of developing asthma later in childhood than the average individual
    c. D.L. has a greater chance of developing malignant melanoma in adulthood than the average individual
    d. D.L. has a condition associated with familial predisposition

14. Which of the following management measures or treatments would you not recommend for D.L.?

    a. Topical steroids to affected areas
    b. Wet compresses to affected skin areas
    c. Maintain a dry warm environment
    d. Eliminate all substances that dry the skin

15. In addition to having atopic dermatitis, you have diagnosed D.L. with a secondary bacterial infection at the site of several lesions. What is the best management for the infection?

    a. Topical antibiotics to affected areas
    b. Oral antibiotics
    c. Hot compresses to affected areas
    d. Monitored and controlled daily sun exposure until lesions resolve

16. Many skin conditions have lesions that may be oozing, weepy, crusting and itchy. Which of the following would you routinely recommend?

    a. Dry the affected skin areas with topical preparations
    b. Apply topical antibiotics to lesions to prevent secondary bacterial infection
    c. Increase the room temperature to enhance drying of lesions
    d. Wet dressings/compresses to soothe the skin and relieve itching

17. You see B.D. for the first time at age six weeks. B.D. has a bright red raised rubbery lesion of irregular shape and 2 cm in diameter on the occiput. What condition do you suspect B.D. has?

    a. Malignant melanoma
    b. Nevus flammeus
    c. Capillary hemangioma
    d. Burn

18. Which of the following is not characteristic of the lesion B.D. has?

    a. It was not present at birth, however, B.D.'s mother noticed site was blanched
    b. It will continue to gradually grow for the first 12 to 15 months of B.D.'s life
    c. It will begin to gradually resolve when B.D. is between 12 to 15 months
    d. It is expected to completely resolve by the time B.D. is ten years

19. You notice ten macular tan lesions of varying sizes on D.D. and refer him for a medical evaluation to rule out neurofibromatosis or Albright's syndrome. What kind of lesion does D.D. have?

    a. Malignant melanoma
    b. Café au lait spots
    c. Mongolian spots
    d. Vitiligo

20. What is characteristic of the lesion that D.D. has?

    a. More common in Caucasians than dark-skinned individuals
    b. More common in males than females
    c. Lesions are usually present at birth, however, more lesions may develop at any age
    d. Lesions usually fade spontaneously and completely resolve in adult life

21. Which condition is not more common in dark-skinned populations?

    a. Café au lait spots
    b. Mongolian spots
    c. Pityriasis alba
    d. Atopic dermatitis

22. You suspect that A.F., age nine years, has either pityriasis alba or vitiligo. Which of the following would not confirm the diagnosis of pityriasis alba?

    a. A.F.'s skin would be normal in all aspects except for areas of hypopigmentation
    b. A.F.'s skin would have one or more scaly areas of hypopigmentation
    c. A.F. complains of mild itching in areas of hypopigmentation
    d. A.F.'s lesions became more pronounced when she was exposed to sunlight

23. A.F. was diagnosed with pityriasis alba. Which of the following is proper management of A.F.'s condition?

    a. Bland moisturizers to reduce overdrying
    b. Topical steroids to the affected areas
    c. Expose affected areas to short periods of sunlight each day
    d. Burow's wet compresses to affected areas

24. Patient education is a major part of the PNP's role. What would you teach A.F. and her parent regarding the progress and prognosis of pityriasis alba?

    a. A.F. will continue to develop lesions until she completes puberty
    b. A.F.'s condition should clear completely in three to four months
    c. A.F.'s condition is permanent and affected areas will not repigment
    d. A.F.'s condition will resolve completely, however, the affected areas will become slightly reddened when exposed to sunlight

25. Malignant melanoma is a form of much dreaded skin cancer. Which of the following is not characteristic of this condition?

    a. Occurs in all ethnic groups but more commonly in light-skinned individuals
    b. Severe sunburn or excessive exposure to sunlight before the age of ten years predisposes developing melanoma later in childhood or in adult life
    c. Spreads through the lymphatic system and invades other distant skin surfaces and organs
    d. Spreads primarily by invading skin surfaces that surround the major lesion

26. Which of the following does not characterize the lesion of malignant melanoma?

    a. Irregular asymmetrical nodule with blurred borders
    b. Raised with distinct symmetrical borders
    c. Uneven coloring in which blue, black, brown, tan, and red may all be present in the same lesion
    d. Bleeding, ulceration in later stages

27. Patient education regarding prevention of malignant melanoma is essential. Which of the following is not considered best prevention education?

    a. Avoid sunlight especially during the hours of 9:00 a.m. and 1:00 p.m.
    b. Avoid sun tanning lamps
    c. Use cover-up clothing, hats, and sunglasses
    d. Use sun blocks that protect against ultraviolet exposure with > 15 SPF

28. You suspect M.N. as having chronic psoriasis. Which of the following is characteristic of her lesions if she has psoriasis vulgaris?

    a. Scaly red small areas 3 to 10 mm in diameter
    b. Round or oval in shape
    c. Large scaly silver-white areas 5 to 10 cm in diameter
    d. Located mainly on her trunk

29. M.N.'s condition of psoriasis is common in approximately 33 percent of children. Which of the following is not correct regarding the etiology or incidence of this condition?

    a. Occurs more commonly in dark-skinned ethnic individuals
    b. Associated with constant rubbing or trauma to exposed affected areas such as elbows
    c. Associated with overproduction of epithelial cells
    d. Associated with epithelial cells that migrate to the skin surface much more quickly than normal

30. What would you not advise regarding the management or treatment of M.N.'s condition?

    a. Excise lesions
    b. Apply topical steroids
    c. Apply mineral oil and moisturizers
    d. Expose to monitored short periods of sunlight

31. You have diagnosed Jale as having contact dermatitis. Which symptom is most characteristic of his condition?

    a. Headache
    b. Difficulty breathing
    c. Pruritus at site of affected areas
    d. Pain at site of affected areas

32. Which of the following is not characteristic of Jale's condition?

    a. He has hypersensitivity to a substance within his environment when direct contact is made
    b. He may experience a delayed reaction of several days with re-exposure to an allergen
    c. His dermatitis may be caused by direct contact with topical medications, soaps, cosmetics, fabrics, and plants
    d. Typical response is redness and edema at the site of contact which may progress to papules and vesicles

33. What would you not recommend as management and treatment of Jale's condition?

    a. Skin testing during the acute episode to determine if Jale has an allergy
    b. Cool compresses of Burow's solution to affected areas
    c. Topical steroids to affected areas for five days
    d. Oral antihistamines

34. You diagnose Kelli, age seven months, with diaper dermatitis. Which of the following should not be included in the differential diagnosis?

    a. Atopic dermatitis
    b. Child abuse
    c. Contact dermatitis
    d. Pityriasis alba

35. What management measure would you not prescribe to treat Kelli's condition?

    a. Oral antihistamines
    b. Emollients such as petroleum jelly to mildly affected areas
    c. Topical steroids to severely affected areas with erythema and papules
    d. Topical antibiotics to severely affected areas with ulcerations

36. What would not be an appropriate recommendation to prevent Kelli from having subsequent episodes of diaper dermatitis?

    a. Expose diaper area to air several times each day
    b. Increase oral fluids using orange juice to dilute urine
    c. Make diaper changes immediately after soiling
    d. Use a double rinse of vinegar and water for home-laundered diapers

37. Seborrhea dermatitis is common in both infants and adolescents. Which of the following is not correct of this condition?

    a. Occurs more often in the spring and summer months
    b. Is associated with an over production of sebum in areas abundant with sebaceous glands
    c. The condition in infants is known as "cradle cap" in which lesions have erythematous base with yellow crusted areas and greasy scales
    d. The condition in adolescents is known as acne with comedomes, papular, and pustular lesions

38. What is the best treatment of seborrhea in the infant?

    a. Mineral oil to loosen crusts prior to washing affected areas with an antiseborrheic shampoos
    b. Topical antibiotics
    c. Oral antibiotics in severe cases
    d. Oral steroids for severe cases

39. F.P., age three years, sustained a burn when she pulled a pan of boiling water over on her. Since burns are classified according to the depth of injury to the skin layers and the amount of area involved, how would you rate burn if 5 percent of her body surface is burned involving the epidermis and upper part of the dermis?

    a. She has a minor first and second degree burn
    b. She has a major second degree burn
    c. She has a major full thickness burn
    d. She has major first and second degree burns

40. F.P.'s burn should appear:

    a. Dry, with mild edema and erythema
    b. Dry whitish areas that blanch with pressure
    c. Dry whitish to brownish areas with edema
    d. Moist with edema, erythema and a few vesicles

41. What is the best treatment for F.P.'s burn?

    a. Warm compresses to affected areas and mild analgesic for discomfort
    b. Topical emollients to affected areas
    c. Butter to affected areas
    d. Refer for MD evaluation and hospitalization

42. Jerry has been diagnosed as having folliculitis, an inflammatory condition involving the pilosebaceous follicle. What is the most common cause of this condition?

    a. *Microsporum canis tinea*
    b. Poxvirus
    c. *Staphylococcus aureus*
    d. Streptococcus group A

43. Jerry has a condition that most commonly occurs on which body surface?

    a. Neck and scalp
    b. Upper arms
    c. Chest and abdomen
    d. Legs

44. You order a culture and the results confirm that Jerry's condition is caused by the most common organism for this condition. What treatment do you prescribe?

    a. Oral penicillin
    b. Dicloxacillin
    c. Tinactin
    d. Tretinoin

45. Sandra, age twelve years, has several vesicles and honey colored crusted lesions on her face above the right nares. She has a history of having had a scratch in the same area several days ago. What condition do you suspect?

    a. Acne
    b. Impetigo
    c. Herpes simplex
    d. Eczema

46. Judy, age fifteen years, has been diagnosed as having acne. Which of the following is not true of this condition?

    a. Poor hygiene is a contributing factor
    b. Associated with increased androgenic hormonal activity
    c. Mild acne is more common among females
    d. Severe acne is more common among males

47. Judy has a history of remission and exacerbation that has followed the pattern of menses for two years. However, the condition over the last six months has worsened to a moderate degree of severity and has been chronic and persistent. You prescribe antibiotic therapy. Which of the following antibiotics would you not consider?

    a. Topical clindamycin
    b. Topical erythomycin
    c. Oral clindamycin
    d. Oral tetracycline

48. K.C., age thirteen years, has several firm, small (2 mm) white or skin-colored umbilicated papules on her neck. The lesions have been present for three months and have increased in number. What is your diagnosis?

    a. Acne
    b. Molluscum contagiosum
    c. Warts
    d. Cellulitis

49. What is the cause of K.C.'s condition?

    a. *Microsporum canis* tinea
    b. Poxvirus
    c. *Staphylococcus aureus*
    d. Streptococcus group A

50. Which treatment would you not recommend for K.C.'s condition?

    a. Curettage lesions
    b. Topical antibiotics
    c. Topical steroids
    d. Tretinoin applications

51. Paul has four superficial lesions on his anterior lower abdomen of one week duration. The lesions are 4 cm in diameter scaly irregular shaped plaques with skin colored centers and erythematous borders The affected areas are slightly pruritic. What condition do you suspect Paul has?

    a. Psoriasis
    b. Eczema
    c. Tinea corporis
    d. Pityriasis rosea

52. You performed two tests to confirm your diagnosis of Paul's condition. The KOH scraping was positive for the presence of hyphae. The Wood's lamp did not fluoresce the lesions. You are sure that Paul's condition was not caused by which organism?

    a. *Epidermophyton floccosum*
    b. *Microsporum canis*
    c. *Trichophyton tonsurans*
    d. *Trichophyton rubrum*

53. You see Paul after eight weeks of treatment with a topical antifungal preparation. The original lesions have almost resolved, however, the condition has worsened with the development of several other larger lesions on the abdomen and groin area. Which of the following would you not consider?

    a. Oral antifungal medication, griseofulvin
    b. Topical antibiotic preparation
    c. Continue with the topical antifungal applications
    d. Educate again regarding not sharing personal items

54. Dale, age 7 years, is complaining of pain and burning on his right leg where you observe two small red puncture marks surrounded by a blanched area with an erythematous border. He had been playing with his dog all morning outside in a grassy wooded area near his home and was wearing shorts. You suspect he has been bitten by which insect?

    a. Mosquito
    b. Bee

c. Recluse spider

d. Black widow spider

55. Which of the following is not true of insect stings from bees, wasps, and fire ants?

    a. Greater reaction of hypersensitivity occurs most often with the initial exposure than with subsequent exposures

    b. For mild reactions cool compresses to the site of injury is the usual management

    c. Occurs more often during the spring and summer months

    d. Most stings occur in self-defense when the nonaggressive insect feels threatened or irritated

56. You diagnose W.A. with scabies. Which of the following is not characteristic of this condition?

    a. He has several erythematous papular, pustular, and crusted lesions on his face

    b. He has several excoriated scratched areas around the umbilicus and waist area

    c. He has several linear curved lines approximately 4 mm in length with a papule at the proximal end linear line

    d. He complains of severe pruritus which is worse at night

57. Which of the following is not recommended as a management and treatment strategy for W.A.?

    a. Put nonwashable items in a plastic bag and store for one week

    b. Prescribe topical antifungal applications

    c. Prescribe topical antiparasitics

    d. Prescribe topical steroids and/or oral antihistamines for pruritus

58. Pediculosis is a highly communicable common condition in children. Which of the following is not correct of pediculosis humanus?

    a. Caused by an insect that does not fly or jump

    b. Gravid females lay ova in seams of clothing

    c. Likes hairy areas of the body better than the non-hairy body surfaces

    d. Same medication used for scabies may be used to effectively eradicate this condition

59. Hypersensitivity may occur to a variety of substances causing a variety of reactions. It is important to determine if the body's hypersensitivity reaction will cause erythema multiforme condition. Which of the following is not typical of the erythema multiforme reaction?

    a. Target "bulls-eye" lesion with a necrotic center surrounded by a pale macular middle area and then by a erythematous peripheral ring

    b. Itching at site of affected skin areas

    c. Pain at site of affected areas, especially in the oral cavity

    d. Lesions which all have the same morphology on the trunk

60. You see D.Y. in your clinic and suspect she has a form of erythema multiforme. Erythema multiforme minor must be differentiated from erythema multiforme major. Which of the following

is the most important confirming evidence for making a diagnosis of erythema multiforme major?

    a. Presence of deeper lesions within the dermis
    b. Presence of lesions on the exposed areas of the body
    c. Presence of pustules indicating a secondary infectious process
    d. Occurrence of prodromal systemic symptoms of fever, malaise, sore throat, headache, nausea, and/or vomiting

61. You suspect D.Y. has erythema multiforme major. What treatment or management is most indicated?

    a. Prescribe topical antibiotics due to secondary infection
    b. Prescribe topical steroids to lesions for pruritus
    c. Refer for medical evaluation
    d. No treatment is indicated as condition will resolve spontaneously in one week

62. Urticaria is a hypersensitivity allergic reaction to a variety of substances and agents. You suspect W.P. has urticaria due to the typical morphology of lesions on her trunk and arms which are:

    a. Erythematous papules
    b. Vesicles
    c. Pustules
    d. Wheals

63. During W.P.'s acute episode of urticaria which of the following is not considered an appropriate management or treatment measure?

    a. Oral antibiotics to prevent secondary infection
    b. Oral antihistamines for pruritus
    c. Topical steroids to affected areas to reduce the immune response
    d. Cool compresses to affected areas

Answers

1. b	22. a	43. a
2. a	23. a	44. b
3. d	24. b	45. b
4. d	25. d	46. a
5. a	26. b	47. c
6. a	27. a	48. b
7. d	28. c	49. b
8. a	29. a	50. b
9. c	30. a	51. c
10. d	31. c	52. b
11. a	32. b	53. b
12. b	33. a	54. d
13. c	34. d	55. a
14. c	35. a	56. a
15. b	36. b	57. b
16. d	37. d	58. c
17. c	38. a	59. d
18. b	39. d	60. d
19. b	40. d	61. c
20. c	41. d	62. d
21. d	42. c	63. a

Bibliography

American Academy of Pediatric. (2003). In L. K. Pickering (Ed.). *Red Book 2003: Report of the committee on infectious diseases* (26th ed.) Elk Grove Village, IL: Author.

Barnhill, R. (2004). *Textbook of Dermatopathology.* St. Louis, MO: McGraw-Hill.

Burns, C. E., Barber, N., Brady, M. A., & Dunn, A. M. (2004). *Pediatric primary care: A handbook for nurse practitioners.* Philadelphia, PA: W. B. Saunders.

Cohen, B. A. (1999). *Pediatric dermatology* (2nd ed.). Philadelphia, PA: Mosby Year Book.

Crowson, A. N., Magro, C. M., & Mihm, M. C. (2001). *The melanocytic proliferation: A comprehensive textbook of pigmented lesions.* New York, NY: John Wiley & Sons.

Fitzpatrick, T., Johnson, R. A., Wolff, K., Suurmond, D., & Wolf, K. (2000). *Color atlas and synopsis of clinical dermatology* (4th ed.). St. Louis, MO: McGraw-Hill.

Goldman, M. P., & Hooper, B. J. (1999). *Primary dermatologic care.* St. Louis, MO: Mosby Year Book.

Hay, W. W., Groothuis, J. R., Hayward, A. R., & Levin, M. J. (Eds.). (2002). *Current pediatric diagnosis and treatment* (20th ed.). Norwalk, CT: Appleton & Lange.

Gastrointestinal Disorders

Victoria A. Weill

Gastroesophageal Reflux In Infancy (GER)

- Definition: Reflux of gastric contents into esophagus due to dysfunction of lower esophageal sphincter
- Etiology/Incidence
  1. Etiology unclear
  2. Begins in early infancy
  3. Physiologic GER
     a. 80% to 90% of healthy infants
     b. Often caused by overfeeding or incomplete burping
  4. Pathologic GER
     a. 5% of infants
     b. Males > females
- Signs and Symptoms
  1. Physiologic GER
     a. Occasional, effortless, painless spitting often within 40 minutes of eating
     b. 40% show improvement by 3 months
     c. 85% resolve between 6 to 12 months with more erect posture and introduction of solids
  2. Functional GER
     a. Frequent, large volume, effortless, nonprojectile regurgitation; no choking or color changes
     b. 70% asymptomatic by 18 months of age
     c. Normal growth—growth chart is key
     d. For functional and physiologic GER—feeding history may indicate excessive intake; burp heard during vomiting may indicate incomplete burping
  3. Pathologic GER
     a. Reflux may cause other physical complications, such as:
        (1) Failure to thrive (FTT)—caused by long term, forceful regurgitation
        (2) Esophagitis—causing irritability, anemia and guaiac positive stools or hematemesis; dysphagia
        (3) Aspiration—pneumonia, wheezing, apnea
        (4) Sandifer syndrome—abnormal posturing of head and neck
     b. May be "silent GER"—no overt vomiting, but complications may be presenting symptom

    c. 60% show improvement by 16 months; 30% may remain symptomatic up to 4 years

  4. Secondary GER

    a. Handicapped, especially neurologically impaired child

    b. Pre-existing condition

- Differential Diagnosis

  1. Pyloric stenosis

  2. (Partial) anatomical obstruction

  3. Formula intolerance

  4. Gastroenteritis

  5. Infections—urinary tract infection (UTI); otitis media (OM); pneumonia

  6. Increased intracranial pressure (ICP)/neurological disorder

- Physical Findings

  1. May have wheezing or respiratory symptoms with aspiration

  2. Abdominal examination normal—no masses, olive or peristaltic waves

  3. Neurological examination normal—no signs of increased ICP

- Diagnostic Tests/Findings

  1. Diagnosis often made by observation and history; testing only to determine if reflux is causing problems since vomiting indicates reflux

  2. UGI to ligament of Treitz—only evaluates anatomy; to rule out anomalies sensitive to reflux; nearly all babies will show reflux; should be done if using prokinetic medication

  3. pH probe—indicates amount of reflux occurring; does not confirm diagnosis; not good postprandial because food acts as buffer; can be outpatient procedure

  4. Upper endoscopy—especially good for esophagitis and inflammation due to *Helicobacter pylori*

  5. Manometry—research tool

  6. Scintigraphy—"Milk scan"; evaluates motility and aspiration

  7. Guaiac stool/emesis—positive for occult blood if abnormal

  8. Empiric medical therapy—trial of medication to relieve specific symptoms (Rudolph, Mazur, et al., 2001)

- Management/Treatment

  1. Conservative therapy

    a.   Positioning—(most important) postprandial, prone position for 1 to 2 hours; infant seats/swings worsen by increasing intra-abdominal pressure; caution with diapering/playing postfeeding

    b.   Breast-feeding or predominately whey formula

    c.   A 1-2 week trial of hypo-allergenic formula may be warranted if vomiting or other symptoms severe enough to consider drug treatment

    d.   Thickening agents such as rice cereal have not been proven to decrease reflux but may decrease vomiting

    e.   Avoid over-feeding—age in months plus 3 equals number of ounces every 3 to 4 hours for most infants

    f.   Small feedings with frequent burping

    g.   Reassure parents with growth charts

    h.   Decrease anxiety in mother-infant interaction

    i.   Monitor for problems—aspiration/esophagitits

    j.   Since the risk of SIDS is greater than the risk of aspiration from birth-12 months, non-prone position (preferably supine) during sleep to prevent SIDS is the recommendation of the AAP except in very severe cases of GER

2.   Medications: (if conservative therapy has failed)

    a.   H$_2$ blockers (1st line); protein pump inhibitors (2nd line), and antacids (short term) if irritable from esophagitis

    b.   Cisapride has been removed from market for most patients

    c.   Metoclopramide may be cautiously considered for severe reflux under the supervision of a physician or gastroenterologist—newer studies are indicating a decreased effectiveness in children

3.   Surgery—Nissen fundoplication

Pyloric Stenosis

- Definition: Obstruction due to thickening of circular muscle of the pylorus

- Etiology/Incidence

1.   Unknown cause, possibly hereditary

2.   Occurs in 1:500 infants; male > female; unclear if more likely in first born

3.   Familial predisposition—25% chance if mother had pyloric stenosis, 15% chance if other family member, 22% if identical twin

4.   More common in Caucasians than African-Americans or Asians

5.   Symptoms occur later in breast fed infants; greater muscle thickness required to obstruct smaller-sized breast milk curd

6.   Delayed timing in premature infants

- Signs and Symptoms

    1. Not present at birth; may occur in first week; average age of presentation from 3 to 6 weeks through 3 to 4 months of age

    2. Vigorous, non-bilious vomiting after eating; with time becomes projectile with brownish color

    3. "Hungry" after emesis; progressing to lethargy and irritability

    4. Weight loss or poor weight gain

    5. Constipation

    6. Dehydration develops over time

- Differential Diagnosis

    1. Overfeeding

    2. Gastroesophageal reflux

    3. Milk protein allergy

    4. Gastroenteritis

    5. Malrotation/volvulus if bilious emesis

- Physical Findings

    1. Visible peristaltic waves progressing from left to right across abdomen—darken room, shine bright light on abdomen of naked, supine baby; feed bottle of sugar water; peristaltic waves visible

    2. Palpable pyloric "olive" after vomiting—palpate epigastrium in RUQ deep under liver edge; need very relaxed abdomen; hard, smooth, mobile, non-tender mass may be palpable

    3. Dehydration as obstruction increases

- Diagnostic Tests/Findings

    1. Abdominal ultrasound to determine size of pylorus—preferred test

    2. Upper GI—avoid due to risk of barium aspiration; shows "string sign"; elongated pyloric channel and delayed gastric emptying

    3. Electrolytes to determine dehydration status

- Management/Treatment:

    1. Surgical treatment after correction of fluid and electrolyte deficits

    2. Post-operative monitoring for hypoglycemia

    3. Excellent prognosis

Acute Infectious Gastroenteritis

- Definition: Illness of rapid onset, includes diarrhea with possible nausea, vomiting, fever, or abdominal pain
- Etiology/Incidence
  1. 70% to 80% caused by viral agents; 25% by rotavirus
  2. < age 3 years 1.3 to 2.3 episodes/year; higher if in day care
  3. Predisposing factors (see Table 1)
     a. Day care
     b. Poor sanitation—improper hand washing, food preparation or water quality
     c. Recent travel especially to endemic areas
     d. Ill contacts—animals or humans
     e. Immunocompromised children at risk
     f. Recent antibiotic use
- Signs and Symptoms
  1. Rotavirus—URI symptoms, low fever, frequent vomiting, mild to profuse watery diarrhea
  2. Adenovirus—low fever; vomiting, diarrhea severe enough to cause dehydration, rare respiratory symptoms
  3. Norwalk—nausea, fever, abdominal pain; vomiting more frequent than diarrhea
  4. Shigella—high fever, headache, abdominal pain and tenderness; large, watery stools in which blood and mucus may be seen; can lead to dehydration

Table 1

Most Common Causative Agents in U.S.

Agent	Source/Transmission	Risk Factors	Incubation	Duration
VIRUS				
Rotavirus	Infected persons; contaminated toys, hard surfaces	< 3 years; day care; low SES* winter	1-3 days	5-10 days
Adenovirus	Infected person; contaminated toys; hard surfaces	< 4 years; daycare; winter months	3-10 days	5-12 days
Norwalk	Infected persons; contaminated food or water	older children & adults	12 hrs-4 days	12-48 hrs

Table 1 (*Continued*)

Most Common Causative Agents in U.S.

Agent	Source/Transmission	Risk Factors	Incubation	Duration
BACTERIA				
Shigella	Infected persons; contaminated food, water, objects; houseflies	1-4 years; daycare; crowding; poor sanitation; summer/ fall months, need very few organisms for transmission	1-7 days	48-72 hours even without treatment
Salmonella	Contaminated foods (poultry, red meat, eggs, milk, fruits); contaminated water; infected persons or animals	< 5 years; especially first year	6-72 hrs	2-7 days
Campylobacter jejuni	Contaminated poultry; unpasteurized milk; pets	All ages; summer months	1-7 days	5-7 days
PARASITIC				
Giardia lamblia	Infected persons, animals, contaminated food or water	Daycare, institutions; campers, CF	1-4 weeks	May be long-term
Cryptosporidium	Infected persons, animals, contaminated water supplies	Parasite is chlorine-resistant	2-14 days	10-14 days
Entamoeba histolytica	Amebic cysts; contaminated food and water	Tropical areas; crowding; poor sanitation	1-4 weeks	May be long-term
TOXIN				
S. Aureus	Ingestion of contaminated food products: ham, poultry, salads (egg and potato), cream filled pastries	Inadequate cooking, refrigeration	½-6 hrs	12 hours
E. coli (0157:H7)	Infected persons or carriers; contaminated foods (undercooked ground beef, apple cider, raw vegetables, salami, yogurt, water)	Day care; poor sanitation; inadequate cooking; poor handwashing; travel to developing countries	3-4 days, up to 8 days	Varies

Table 1 (*Continued*)

Most Common Causative Agents in U.S.

Agent	Source/Transmission	Risk Factors	Incubation	Duration
Clostridium difficile	Infected persons or hospital environment	Hospitals, daycare, normal intestinal flora altered— antibiotics; enema, prolonged NG tube; intestinal surgery; c.dif disease rare < 12 months	Unknown	May improve with discontinuation of antibiotic if cause

*SES—socioeconomic status

5. Salmonella—fever, abdominal pain and cramps; watery, mucoid or bloody stools

6. *Campylobacter jejuni*—fever, malaise, appendicitis-like abdominal pain, bloody stools

7. *Giardia lamblia*—flatulence, abdominal pain, failure to thrive, anorexia, range of stools, e.g., asymptomatic carrier to foul, steatorrhea, consider in persistent diarrhea (> 7 days)

8. *Cryptosporidium parvum*—frequent watery stools most common symptom with abdominal pain, anorexia and weight loss, fever, vomiting common; consider in persistent diarrhea (> 7 days)

9. *Entamoeba histolytica*—asymptomatic, mild symptoms, e.g., abdominal distention, constipation, occasionally loose stools; *or* severe abdominal pain with increasingly severe bloody and mucoid diarrhea, weight loss, fever in approximately $\frac{1}{3}$ of patients

10. *Staphylococcus aureus*—abrupt onset of nausea, vomiting, abdominal pain, watery stools

11. *Escherichia coli* (EHEC 0157:H7)—fever < $\frac{1}{3}$ of cases, severe abdominal pain, cramping, watery diarrhea, stools usually progress to grossly bloody, or occult; hemolytic uremic syndrome (HUS) can occur 1 week or more after diarrhea

12. *Clostridium difficile*—abdominal pain and cramps; pseudomembranous colitis, stools bloody with leukocytes, mucus, pus; symptom free carrier state common < 1 year

- Differential Diagnosis

  1. Urinary tract infection (UTI)

  2. Other infections—otitis media, streptococcal pharyngitits

  3. Inflammatory bowel disease

  4. Malabsorption (lactose intolerance, celiac disease, cystic fibrosis)

5. Milk protein allergy

6. Chronic diarrhea

7. If only vomiting:

    a. Trauma

    b. Congestive heart failure

    c. Toxic ingestion

    d. Metabolic disorder

    e. Increased intracranial pressure

- Physical Findings

1. Assess hydration—see Table 2

2. Recent weight (wt) very helpful, but often not available

$$\frac{\text{Pre-illness wt minus wt today}}{\text{Pre-illness wt}} \times 100 = \text{fluid deficit as \% body wt loss}$$

TABLE 2

Assessment of Dehydration

Variable	Mild, 3%-5%	Moderate, 6%-9%	Severe ≥ 10%
Blood pressure	Normal	Normal	Normal to reduced
Quality of pulses	Normal	Normal or slightly decreased	Moderately decreased
Heart rate	Normal	Increased	Increased*
Skin turgor	Normal	Decreased	Decreased
Fontanel	Normal	Sunken	Sunken
Mucous membranes	Slightly dry	Dry	Dry
Eyes	Normal	Sunken orbits	Deeply sunken orbits
Extremities	Warm, normal capillary refill	Delayed capillary refill	Cool, mottled
Mental status	Normal	Normal to listless	Normal to lethargic or comatose
Urine output	Slightly decreased	< 1 mL/kg/hr	<<1 mL/kg/hr
Thirst	Slightly increased	Moderately increased	Very thirsty or too lethargic to indicate

Note. From "Practice Parameters: The management of acute gastroenteritis in young children", by Provisional Committee on Quality Improvement, Subcommittee on Acute Gastroenteritis, 1996, *Pediatrics*, 97(3), p.427. Copyright 1996 by the American Academy of Pediatrics. Reprinted with permission.

    The percentages of body weight reduction that correspond to different degrees of dehydration will vary among authors. The critical factor in assessment is the determination of the patient's hemodynamic and perfusion status. If a clinician is unsure of the category into which the patient falls, it is recommended that therapy for the more severe category be used.

*Bradycardia may appear in severe cases

- Diagnostic Tests/Findings
  1. Testing not necessary unless:
     a. Blood or mucus in stools—test for specific organism
     b. No improvement in symptoms > 5 to 6 days
     c. Signs of severe dehydration—BUN, specific gravity, electrolytes
  2. Test for specific organism
     a. Virus—EIA, rarely necessary
     b. Bacterial—stool culture; specific testing for *E. coli* 0157:H7 if bloody stools
     c. Giardia—giardia antigen (more specific); stools for ova and parasites
     d. Cryptosporidium—stools for ova and parasites, specify cryptosporidium
     e. *Clostridium difficile—Clostridium difficile* toxins
  3. Persistent vomiting as only sign; diarrhea lasting longer than 10 days or with failure to thrive (FTT) need more extensive testing

- Management/Treatment:
  1. Self-limiting in most healthy children
  2. Increased risk associated with dehydration with fever; prematurity, infancy and adolescent mothers
  3. Assess degree of dehydration and correct deficit following the guidelines suggested by the AAP Subcommittee on Acute Gastroenteritis (1996)
     a. Oral rehydration therapy (ORT) can safely and effectively treat mild to moderate dehydration in otherwise healthy child
     b. Maintenance solutions have 45 to 50 mmol/L of sodium, suitable for rehydration; continue for a maximum of 24 hours
     c. Determine replacement volume; give over 4 hour period
        (1) 50 cc/kg for mild dehydration
        (2) 80 to 100 cc/kg for moderate to severe
        (3) Plus replace ongoing losses:
            (a) 5 to 10 cc/kg for each diarrheal stool
            (b) 2 cc/kg for each episode of emesis
     d. Small frequent feedings are key—1 teaspoon every 1 to 2 minutes initially; if tolerated amount may be advanced; do not allow child to drink large amounts quickly; process is labor intensive; parent or staff needs to be available to administer
     e. Home remedies such as juice or sports beverages are non-physiologic and should be avoided in the treatment of young children with dehydration

f. Once rehydrated or in children with diarrhea but no dehydration, feeding with age-appropriate diet should be encouraged; rice, wheat, potatoes, bread, cereals, lean meats, yogurt, fruits and vegetables; early refeeding promotes healing of the GI mucosa and decreases stool output; old practice of "bowel rest" may worsen condition

g. In a change from earlier recommendations, once dehydration is corrected, full strength formula or milk can be given; monitor for the 20% of patients who develop transient (4 to 8 weeks) lactose intolerance.

h. Breast milk may be continued

i. Antidiarrheal medications are not appropriate and may be dangerous

j. UA and CBC with smear, BUN and creatinine to monitor E. coli (0157:H7) infection for changes indicative of HUS (AAP, 2003); may develop microangiopathic hematologic changes and/or nephropathy; close follow-up essential because potential long term sequalae so severe

4. Antimicrobials only in select cases, (AAP, 2003)

a. Shigella—disease generally self-limiting within 48-72 hours; antibiotics will shorten course of diarrhea and decrease shedding of organisms; children in day care, large group settings, immunosuppressed or who have severe disease should be treated; sensitivities must be done due to increased resistance; TMP/SMX (first line) or azithromycin (in TMP/SMX resistant areas) for 5 days; no return to day care until 2 repeat cultures at least 24 hours apart, 48 hours after antibiotics completed are negative; household contacts must be cultured also

b. Salmonella—only for infants < 3 months or patients with suspected sepsis or immunosuppressed since antibiotics can prolong excretion; amoxicillin, TMP/SMX, cefotaxime or ceftriaxone

c. *Campylobacter jejuni*—only helpful if caught in early stages; erythromycin or azithromycin 5 to 7 days; doxycycline > age 8

d. *Giardia lamblia*—metronidazole (drug of choice) 15mg/kg/day in 3 divided doses for 5 days; furazolidone 6 mg/kg/day in 4 divided doses for 7 to 10 days is less effective, but available in liquid form for children; contraindicated with G6PD deficiency and neonates; albendazole (available as liquid) for children > age 2, 400 mg every day for 5 days; all giardia treatments are potential teratogens in pregnant teens; paromomycin (less effective) useful in pregnancy, 25 to 35 mg/kg/day in 3 doses for 7 days; nitazoxanide, 12 months to 47 months 100 mg every 12 hours for 3 days, 4 to 11 years 200 mg every 12 hours for 3 days.

e. *Entamoeba histolytica*—metronidazole 35 to 50 mg/kg/day in 3 divided doses for 7 to 10 days followed by iodoquinol or paromomycin

f. *E. coli* (0157:H7)—antibiotics may not prevent hemolytic uremic syndrome (HUS); may increase risk but studies are inconclusive, AAP recommends no antimicrobial treatment (AAP, 2003)

    g. *Clostridium difficile*—stop causative antibiotics: if no improvement; metronidazole 30 mg/kg/day (maximum 2g/day) in four divided doses for 7 to 10 days.

    h. *Cryptosporidium parvum*—self limiting diarrhea, average 10 days; nitazoxanide 12 months to 47 months 100 mg every 12 hours for 3 days, 4 to 11 years 200 mg every 12 hours for 3 days

5. Severe dehydration/HUS requires physician referral

6. Prevention

    a. Teach children importance of frequent, thorough hand washing

    b. Encourage mothers to breast feed

    c. Day care centers need strict policies for hand washing and food preparation; surfaces and fomites need frequent cleaning with chlorine based disinfectant

    d. Careful food preparation and storage

    e. E. coli (0157:H7), shigella, amebiasis (entamoeba histolytica), campylobacter, cryptosporidiosis, giardiasis and salmonella require public health involvement particularly for day care attendees; may vary from State to State

    f. Teach parents signs/symptoms of dehydration and early at home measures

Pinworms (*Enterobiasis vermicularis*)

- Definitions: Nematode parasite with infestation of intestines and rectum
- Etiology/Incidence

    1. Human pinworm is ubiquitous; adult worm lives in rectum, comes out at night to lay eggs on perianal skin and dies causing pruritus; scratching and finger to mouth contact transfers eggs to intestine; these develop into mature worms and repeat cycle (approximately 2 weeks)

    2. Found in children of all socioeconomic classes

    3. Eggs float easily in air and can be swallowed by others

- Signs and Symptoms

    1. Nocturnal anal itching

    2. Vaginal itching (pinworm crawls into vagina)

    3. Insomnia (itching)

    4. Worm like-"threads"—seen in toilet or on underwear

- Differential Diagnosis

    1. Vulvovaginitis secondary to local irritation

    2. Poor hygiene

- Physical Findings

    1. Excoriation of perianal and perineal area

2. Thread-like worms will be seen on visualization of anus (early morning using flashlight)

- Diagnostic Test/Findings: Adhesive cellophane tape "paddle" with kits available for parental use; or can be made with clear scotch tape and glass slide; prior to arising and bathing, paddle is pressed against anus and then examined for eggs

- Management/Treatment

    1. Medication (over age 2)

        a. Pyrantel pamoate 11 mg/kg one dose (maximum dose 1g); repeat in 2 weeks

        b. Mebendazole 100 mg single dose (same dose for all ages and weights); repeat in 2 weeks

    2. Reassure parents ubiquitous nature of organism; reinfection likely

    3. Test other family members and treat at same time if infected

    4. Prevention

        a. Keep nails clean and short

        b. Bathing will remove eggs from skin and decrease pruritus

        c. Excellent hand washing

Inflammatory Bowel Disease (IBD)

- Definition: Chronic intestinal inflammation with two specific entities of ulcerative colitis (UC) and Crohn's disease; may have extraintestinal symptoms and acute or insidious onset

    1. Location of inflammation in GI tract—Crohn's occurs any part of GI tract, terminal ileum typical; UC more likely in colon

    2. Pattern of inflammation—Crohn's skip pattern; discrete areas of inflammation interspersed with normal; UC mucosal and submucosal inflammation, diffuse and continuous

- Etiology/Incidence (for both types of IBD)

    1. Etiology unclear

    2. Unclear genetic link; 10% to 20% positive family history

    3. Occurs more often in Caucasians than African-Americans and Asians; highest in descendents of Ashkenazic Jews

    4. Age of onset 10 to 20 years; of these 20% to 40% < 12 years of age

- Signs and Symptoms

    1. Symptoms may be acute or unrecognized for years, dependent on location of lesions; more variability with Crohn's disease since any part of GI tract can be involved

    2. Diarrhea

  a. Crohn's—loose with blood if colon involved, or can have pain but no diarrhea

  b. UC—mild to profuse bloody diarrhea

 3. Weight loss/delayed pubertal maturation—often due to inadequate food intake because eating causes cramps, bloating, diarrhea

  a. Growth failure may be presenting problem especially in Crohn's

  b. Weight loss and delayed puberty more common with Crohn's

 4. Abdominal pain

  a. Crohn's —located in right lower quadrant sometimes as fullness or mass; food related

  b. UC—left lower abdomen

 5. Severe cramps, low grade fevers, anorexia

- Differential Diagnosis (based on area of bowel involved)

 1. Ulcerative Colitis

  a. Enteric infection (particularly those involving bloody diarrhea)

  b. Irritable bowel syndrome

 2. Crohn's (particularly if manifested as extraintestinal symptoms)

  a. Rheumatoid arthritis

  b. Acute appendicitis

  c. Lupus erythematosus

  d. Lactose intolerance

  e. Celiac disease

- Physical Findings (common to both UC and Crohn's unless noted)

 1. Weight deceleration

 2. Diffuse abdominal pain or no tenderness

 3. Extraintestinal symptoms

  a. Fever of unknown origin (FUO)

  b. Short stature

  c. Uveitis/iritis

  d. Aphthous stomatitis

  e. Arthritis/arthralgias

  f. Inflammatory lesions of skin

  g. Liver disease

  h. Perianal fissures/tags/abscesses especially with Crohn's disease

- Diagnostic Tests/Findings

    1. Blood studies—CBC with differential shows microcytic anemia, increased WBC; sedimentation rate (ESR) elevated; chemistry panel shows low serum total protein and albumin; findings suggest IBD and indicate the need for further studies for both Crohn's and UC

    2. Stool studies—infectious agents that cause bloody diarrhea for both Crohn's and UC

    3. Colonoscopy with biopsy—to differentiate Crohn's vs. UC

    4. Upper GI with small bowel—shows IBD changes and extent of disease

    5. Endoscopy with biopsy

- Management/Treatment

    1. Refer to pediatric gastroenterologist

    2. Nutritional therapy to ensure adequate growth and pubertal development; total parenteral nutrition (TPN) or elemental formula may be necessary and can improve clinical symptoms; in milder cases high protein, high carbohydrate, normal fat diet providing 75 to 90 kcal/ kg/day; avoid overly restrictive diets

    3. Anti-inflammatory agents—short term corticosteroids, sulfasalazine, mesalamine for mild Chron's disease in colon

    4. Long term patients may need colectomy/ostomy; curative for UC

    5. At higher risk for colorectal cancer

    6. Need emotional support to deal with chronic illness with reassurance that emotional factors are not primary cause

Malabsorption

- Definition: Impaired intestinal absorption of nutrients and electrolytes

- Etiology/Incidence: Classified according to stage of digestion affected

    1. Intraluminal phase—maldigestion; need enzymes (cystic fibrosis, see Lower Respiratory Disorders chapter)

    2. Abnormalities of mucosal surface area—absorption; infections can damage mucosa

        a. Secondary lactose malabsorption

            (1) Most common cause of malabsorption in children

            (2) Can be up to 20% post-gastrointestinal infection

            (3) Primary lactose intolerance rare < age 4; 80% Asian, African-American adults

        b. Infectious—bacterial, viral, parasites, e.g., *Giardia lamblia*

        c. Celiac disease—intestinal intolerance to gluten; rate in population 1:1000; more common in children with Irish, Swedish heritage

3. Decreased conjugated bile acids

    a. Biliary atresia

    b. Hepatitis

    c. Short bowel syndrome

- Signs and Symptoms:

1. Failure to thrive

2. Adequate intake per dietary history

3. Severe, chronic diarrhea

4. Bulky, foul, pale, steatorrhea stools

5. Abdominal distention

- Differential Diagnosis

1. Renal disease

2. Poor dietary intake

3. Failure to thrive

- Physical Findings: Disease specific findings

1. Lactose intolerance—persistent diarrhea after infectious diarrhea

2. Cystic fibrosis—recurrent pulmonary infection, "salty" taste to skin; nasal polyps; rectal prolapse

3. Celiac disease—vomiting, abdominal pain, irritability, anorexia, pallor; protuberant abdomen

- Diagnostic Tests/Findings

1. Stool—(most important) inspection, culture, microscopic examination

    a. Hemoccult test—intestinal mucosa damage

    b. Ova and parasite; giardia antigen to test for giardia and other parasites

    c. pH reducing substances—to rule out carbohydrate malabsorption

    d. Sudan stain for fat (microscopic examination of stool for fat)

2. Urinalysis/culture

3. CBC, electrolytes, ESR

4. Sweat test > 60 mEq/L chloride—cystic fibrosis

5. Hydrogen breath test—increased with lactose intolerance

- Management/Treatment:

1. Refer to gastroenterologist

2. Lactose intolerance—avoid lactose containing foods

3. Celiac disease—gluten free diet; no wheat, oats, rye, barley

4. Cystic fibrosis—pancreatic enzyme replacement

Intussusception

- Definition: Acute episode of prolapse of one portion of intestine into the lumen of the adjoining part

- Etiology/Incidence
    1. Unknown cause—95% idiopathic; may be caused by adenovirus, Henoch Schönlein purpura, celiac disease, CF; Meckel diverticulum of small intestine, no abdominal pain, but causes bleeding; primary cause in older children
    2. Greater incidence in males than females
    3. 60% occur before first birthday; 80% by 2 years

- Signs and Symptoms
    1. Healthy infant/child presents with sudden cycle of inconsolable screaming, flexing of legs; colicky abdominal pain
    2. 90% have nonbilious vomiting after pain
    3. Periods of quietness or sleepiness between episodes; lethargy if intussusception not reduced
    4. Eventually shocklike state develops
    5. Within 12 hours of onset, "currant jelly" (blood with mucus) stool is passed; late presentation

- Differential Diagnosis
    1. Gastroenteritis
    2. Incarcerated hernia
    3. Volvulus/obstruction

- Physical Findings
    1. Abdomen soft between episodes; may palpate sausage shaped mass RUQ
    2. Distention and tenderness increased as obstruction increases
    3. Guaiac positive or grossly bloody stool
    4. If not reduced, develops perforation and peritonitis leading to fever and shock.

- Diagnostic Tests/Findings
    1. Radiography only to clarify diagnosis—no gas RLQ, air fluid levels consistent with obstruction
    2. Barium enema—diagnostic and results in reduction
    3. CBC and electrolytes—dehydration and anemia

4. Ultrasound—tubular mass longitudinal image, doughnut on transverse view

- Management/Treatment

    1. Reduction via barium/air enema; air becoming more common

    2. Emergency surgery

    3. Can recur; fatal if untreated

Appendicitis

- Definition: Acute inflammation of the appendix

- Etiology/Incidence

    1. Cause—obstruction of lumen by fecaliths or parasites

    2. Most common in late childhood and early adolescence with average age of 12 years

    3. Incidence in males greater than females

    4. Seasonal distribution—Autumn and Spring

    5. Increased incidence following gastrointestinal infection

    6. Most common cause of pediatric abdominal surgery

- Signs and Symptoms

    1. Young child may not appear ill or have severe pain particularly in early phase

    2. Abdominal pain—earliest symptom

        a. Vague, possibly midline, constant pain for several hours

        b. Pain eventually localized in RLQ; in some, pain may begin in RLQ

        c. Can wake at night over time with increasing severity of pain

        d. Pain on ambulation

        e. Pain precedes vomiting

    3. Anorexia, nausea and vomiting

    4. Variable changes in bowel patterns—constipation or diarrhea may be noted

    5. Afebrile to very low-grade fever in early phase

- Differential Diagnosis

    1. Gastroenteritis—especially if high fever (early stage) and/or diarrhea

    2. Mittelschmerz

    3. Ovary cyst/ovary torsion/ruptured follicle

    4. Lower lobe pneumonia

    5. Pelvic inflammatory disease (PID)

    6. Constipation

7. UTI/pyelonephritis

8. Ruptured ectopic pregnancy

9. Inflammatory bowel disease

10. Intussusception

11. Perforated peptic ulcer

- Physical Findings: Depends upon the stage of appendicitis

    1. Observe child—may be motionless, with legs flexed

    2. Tenderness localized to RLQ; intense at McBurney's point halfway between umbilicus and anterior superior iliac crest

    3. Rebound tenderness

    4. Rovsing's sign—pain RLQ with left-side pressure; highly indicative of appendicitis in children

    5. Local, right-sided tenderness or mass on rectal examination

    6. Won't jump/difficulty ambulating

    7. Obturator sign—rotating thigh may produce pain in RLQ

    8. Complete examination to rule out other causes of abdominal pain, especially throat, chest, testicles

    9. Perforation and peritonitis within 24 to 48 hours

        a. Rigidity

        b. Higher fever

        c. Pain improves

        d. Generalized tenderness

        e. Increased vomiting

        f. 40% incidence in young children

- Diagnostic Tests/Findings

    1. Diagnosis based on history and physical; tests often not helpful in diagnosing appendicitis, but can rule out other sources of pain

    2. CBC with differential—may have a mild leukocytosis with left shift

    3. CT—most sensitive and specific; useful, especially in early stages of diagnosis; better to identify other diagnoses; US versus CT often depends upon institution; some will do US because it is quicker and if equivocal proceed to CT scan

    4. Ultrasound—if ovarian condition part of differential or findings unclear

    5. Radiography of abdomen to rule out constipation

6. UA to rule out UTI—UA can be abnormal in appendicitis

- Management/Treatment: Immediate surgical referral

Recurrent Abdominal Pain

- Definition: At least 3 episodes of abdominal pain for three or more months, interfering with routine activities; separated by pain free periods

- Etiolgy/Incidence

    1. Unclear mechanism of pain; may be visceral

    2. Multifaceted problem that includes predisposition aggravated by life events or personality

    3. Most common cause of chronic pain in school-aged and young adolescent; 10% to 15% of school-aged population

    4. Onset before age 3 and after 14 years is very unusual, usually > age 6

    5. Greater incidence in girls than boys; average age for females 9 to 10 years, males 10 to 11 years

    6. Family history of GI complaints and somatization disorders; e.g., migraines, peptic ulcers

    7. Cause of pain

        a. Organic—approximately 10%, e.g., inflammatory bowel disease

            (1) With the increased use of endoscopy more dyspepsia disease (peptic ulcer/esophagitis) identified; positive family history; occurs 12 to 18 years; may be caused by *Helicobacter pylori*

            (2) Pancreatitis—more common if positive family history; corticosteroid use

            (3) Cholecystitis—rare < 9 years of age; increased with obesity; positive family history gall stones; birth control pills

        b. Psychogenic—clear psychological component, e.g., school phobia

        c. Nonspecific—80%; interplay between environment and physiology, e.g., irritable bowel; 50% identified as functional abdominal pain

    8. Psychological component unclear; clearly more stress during pain episode; may be a stress reaction

- Signs and Symptoms

    1. Certain personality traits (anxious, high achiever) and family characteristics (protective parents) more frequent; may affect school performance

    2. No mucus or blood in stool or emesis; no diarrhea with functional pain

    3. Nature of pain

        a. Onset of crampy or dull ache; no radiation of pain

   b. Periumbilical, occasionally suprapubic

   c. Lasts less than one hour; nothing relieves pain

   d. Interferes with activities, but no night wakening; unrelated to meals

   e. Resolves between episodes; not constant nor daily

   f. Related symptoms—nausea, sweating, flush, dizziness, pallor, headache

   g. Occasionally constipation or mild vomiting

   h. If constant, localized, or night pain, or occurs in child < age 6, or weight loss, poor growth or joint pain more likely organic

      (1) Peptic ulcer or esophagitis—epigastric pain 1 to 3 hours after eating, or awakens child; sour burps; blood in stools or vomitus

      (2) Irritable bowel—crampy lower abdominal pain, mucous stools alternating with constipation or diarrhea

      (3) Pancreatitis—dull epigastric, postprandial pain with radiation to back; persistent vomiting; fever; flexion of hips and knees provides relief

      (4) Cholecystitis—RUQ and vague epigastric, postprandial pain, radiating to right shoulder; history of high fat diet

- Differential Diagnosis:

   1. Constipation/chronic stool retention

   2. Irritable bowel

   3. Malabsorption/lactose intolerance

   4. Parasites (especially giardia)

   5. Gastroesophageal reflux

   6. Inflammatory bowel disease

   7. Dysmenorrhea

   8. School phobia

   9. Depression

   10. Peptic ulcer/dyspepsia

   11. Trauma

   12. UTI

   13. Abdominal migraine

   14. Pancreatitis/cholecystitis

   15. PID

   16. Sexual abuse

- Physical Findings: Indicate nonorganic cause
  1. Normal weight
  2. Afebrile, may have slight temperature increase during episode
  3. Abdomen may have diffuse or LLQ tenderness, but no guarding
  4. Normal findings on complete examination
- Diagnostic Tests/Findings: Diagnosis of exclusion
  1. Excellent history and physical examination key to diagnosis; special attention to growth parameters
  2. Guaiac stool—negative; rule out inflammatory bowel disease
  3. Blood tests—CBC with differential; ESR to rule out infection/inflammation
  4. Urinalysis/culture—rule out UTI
  5. Ova and parasites; giardia antigen
  6. Additional/selected studies may be warranted depending on symptoms
     a. Pelvic examination of adolescent female
     b. Endoscopy for esophagitis, peptic ulcer—dysphagia, chest pain, weight loss present
     c. Upper gastrointestinal (UGI) with small bowel—if recurrent vomiting, stool blood to rule out obstructive lesions, Crohn's disease
     d. Hydrogen breath test—increased with lactose intolerance
     e. Pregnancy test
     f. Endoscopy or serology—rule out *Helicobacter pylori*
     g. Abdominal ultrasound—rule out cholecystitis
     h. Amylase/lipase—increased with pancreatitis
- Management/Treatment
  1. Emphasize to child and family—pain is real even though no organic cause can be found; work up should reassure them child is healthy
  2. Reinforce normal behavior; go to school, don't allow secondary gain; may go to school nurse briefly if symptoms severe; if too sick to attend school, follow-up with provider required
  3. Decrease hectic life style and hurried meals
  4. Increasing fiber intake may help
  5. Avoid medications if nonorganic
  6. Try to identify source of stress in patient or family; stress reduction techniques may help such as biofeedback and relaxation techniques

7. Keep pain diary to identify situations associated with symptoms

8. Treat identified organic disease

Constipation

- Definition: Alteration in frequency, passage, size or consistency of stool
- Etiology/Incidence
    1. Functional—5% to 10% of children; stool moves slowly through colon, excess water is absorbed, leading to hard, dry stools; can be caused by family tendencies, diet, drugs or change in routine; painful stools can lead to withholding, creating a cycle
    2. Encopresis (fecal soiling)—chronic withholding leads to impaction and soiling; eventually loses urge to stool and results in megacolon; psychological problem not primary cause
    3. Anatomical abnormalities—anal or rectal abnormalities; problems often seen in immediate newborn period
    4. Intrinsic motor disorder—Hirschsprung's disease (most common), congenital absence of ganglion in segments of colon; 1: 5000 births; 4:1 male to female ratio; increased with positive family history or Down syndrome
    5. Metabolic, e.g., hypothyroidism
    6. Neurologic, e.g., tumors, spinal injury, myelomeningocele
- Signs and Symptoms
    1. Onset
        a. Functional—during infancy, particularly after change from breast milk to formula or starting solids; 1 to 3 years of age after life change, e.g., new sibling, home, introduction of toilet training; most improve by age 4
        b. Encopresis—4 to 7 years, male > female
        c. Hirschsprung's—constipation from birth; often no meconium in first 24 hours; history of failure to have bowel movement without aid of laxative or enema; "partial" or incomplete Hirschsprung's may manifest itself beyond the newborn period
    2. Stools
        a. Functional—hard, dry stools, "pellets"; occasionally stool caliber very large/wide; may be dark or have strong odor
        b. Encopresis—soiled underwear, may appear to be diarrhea; may occur daily
        c. Hirschsprung's—small, ribbon like stools; no leakage

3. Complaints

   a. Functional—abdominal pain, blood streaked stools, straining or "dancing around" indicates withholding

   b. Hirschsprung's—no stooling

- Differential Diagnosis

  1. Tumor

  2. Anatomical deficit

  3. Metabolic

  4. Infantile botulism-(recent onset)

- Physical Findings

  1. Functional—rectal examination may show fissure, ampulla full of stool, normal tone; may have no palpable abdominal mass, may have abdominal pain or cramping, but no distension; normal growth and development

  2. Encopresis—may have impacted stool and/or large, dilated rectal vault, normal tone; abdominal distention with sausage-shaped mass in left pelvis or mid-line

  3. Hirschsprung's—unable to admit finger for rectal examination due to long tight internal sphincter; empty rectum; stool may be guaiac positive; abnormal bowel sounds; abdominal distention

  4. Anal wink, neurological examination, muscle strength and tone should be normal

- Diagnostic Tests/Findings:

  1. Radiograph of abdomen to examine for stool

  2. Unprepped barium enema—rule out Hirschsprung's disease

- Management/Treatment:

  1. Emphasize to parents the definition of constipation; straining with soft stool in infancy is normal

  2. Ensure proper preparation of formula

  3. Mild constipation can be treated with dietary changes; avoid constipating foods, e.g., rice cereal, bananas, apple sauce; introduce more juice and fluids; decrease excessive milk consumption; increase fiber; increase exercise in older child

  4. Infants > 6 months of age—prune juice; malt soup extract $\frac{1}{2}$ to 3 teaspoons twice per day for maximum of 3 days

  5. Constipation causing abdominal pain or encopresis needs more aggressive treatment; withheld stool causes intestinal muscle stretching; multifaceted treatment involves emptying intestines, leading to a return of sensation; preventing recurrence of painful stools and bowel training

  6. Plan for otherwise healthy child

a. If impacted—day 1 mineral enema to soften stool

b. No impaction or day 2—sodium phosphate enema one time per day for two to three days

c. May choose oral medications for impaction

d. After intestines emptied, keep stool soft to prevent recurrence of withholding cycle—emulsified mineral oil 1 to 3 mL/kg per day (Baker, 1999); may need to treat for 6 months or more; do not use in children < 1 year, with GER, or vomiting due to risk of aspiration; needs daily multivitamin

e. Prevent pain cycle—emphasize to child that medicine will prevent painful stools

f. Bowel retraining—child should sit on toilet for one minute per year of age twice per day; don't expect bowel movement every sitting

g. Goal—soft bowel movement every day or every other day; leaking orange oil indicates need to cut back on amount of emulsified mineral oil

7. Hirschsprung's—GI/surgery referral

Hepatitis:

- Definition: Inflammation of the liver

- Etiology/Incidence

  1. Hepatitis A virus (HAV)

     a. Most common form of viral hepatitis in children

     b. Highest rates of symptomatic infection 5 to 14 years; less than 10% of infected children under 6 years are symptomatic

     c. Transmission—fecal/oral, raw shellfish, contaminated water; in U.S. HAV shed from asymptomatic, infected children to adults

     d. Incubation—15 to 50 days, average 25 to 30 days; can infect others up to 2 weeks before onset of illness and 1 week after

     e. High risk populations—Native-Americans, Alaskan natives, homosexuals, IV drug users; some Hasidic, Hispanic communities; travelers to developing countries; children in day care

  2. Hepatitis B virus (HBV)

     a. Most common form of hepatitis in world

     b. Transmission—blood or body fluids; virus can survive more than one week on inanimate objects

     c. Incubation—45 to 160 days, average 120 days

    d. 5% to 10% of infected people become chronic carriers; inverse relationship between age of infection and carrier state; majority of perinatally infected infants become carriers

    e. High risk populations—sexually active; institutionalized; IV drug users; patients with clotting disorders; household contacts of HBV carriers; hemodialysis patients; infants of Alaskan natives or Pacific Islanders; travelers to China, Southeast Asia

3. Hepatitis C virus (HCV)

    a. Very low rates in children under 12 years of age

    b. Transmission—blood and blood products, occasionally blood transfusion

    c. Incubation—6 to 7 weeks, range of 2 weeks to 6 months

4. Hepatitis D (HDV)

    a. Co or super infection with HBV

    b. Transmission—blood or blood products, IV drug use, sexual contact

    c. Incubation—2 to 8 weeks, if simultaneous with HBV average is 120 days

5. Hepatitis E (HEV)

    a. Endemic to Asia, Africa, Mexico; U.S. travelers to those areas at risk

    b. Transmission—fecal/oral route especially contaminated water

    c. Incubation—40 days, range 15 to 60 days

    d. More common in adults than children

- Signs and Symptoms

  1. HAV

    a. Infants and young children—asymptomatic or nonspecific symptoms, e.g., nausea, vomiting, diarrhea; no jaundice; misdiagnosed as gastroenteritis

    b. Adults—fever, malaise, anorexia, nausea, abdominal pain, jaundice; later pruritus

    c. Self-limiting disease—several weeks to occasionally 6 months; no chronic or carrier state

  2. HBV and HDV

    a. Children often asymptomatic—mild to severe disease; macular rash and arthritis (early sign); anorexia, nausea, malaise, arthralgia

    b. Up to 90% of perinatally infected infants can develop carrier state

    c. Chronic carrier state can lead to chronic liver disease or cancer

  3. HCV

  a. Children often asymptomatic; those with symptoms have mild disease; < 25% become icteric; gradual onset of headache, fever, nausea, fatigue, anorexia

  b. 50% to 85% become chronic carriers; can lead to chronic liver disease or cancer

 4. HEV

  a. Acute illness with arthralgia, abdominal pain, jaundice, malaise, anorexia and fever

  b. No carrier state

- Differential Diagnosis

 1. Viral gastroenteritis

 2. Hemolytic-uremic syndrome

 3. Reye's syndrome

 4. Cytomegalovirus illness

 5. Toxin/medication exposure

 6. Fitz-Hugh Curtis syndrome with gonorrheal PID

- Physical Findings

 1. Possible hepatosplenomegaly; RUQ tenderness

 2. If jaundiced, may develop dark urine and light stools, scleral icterus

- Diagnostic Tests/Findings

 1. Non-specific findings

  a. Elevated liver enzymes—AST, ALT

  b. Elevated serum bilirubin

  c. Elevated erythrocyte sedimentation rate (HAV)

 2. Specific serologic antigen/antibody testing

  a. Hepatitis A (HAV)

   (1) AntiHAV IgM—current or recent infection; usually disappears within 4 months

   (2) AntiHAV-IgG—resolved infection and immune status; may last for years following infection; 40 to 45% general population carry Anti-HAV-IgG

  b. Hepatitis B (HBV)

   (1) HBsAg (surface antigen)—earliest marker of acute infection; persistence beyond 6 months indicates carrier status

   (2) AntiHBc-IgM—current or recent acute infection; usually disappears within 6 months

> (3) AntiHBc-IgG—chronic infection of at least 6 months duration
>
> (4) AntiHBs—immune status following resolved infection or immunization (Heptavax)
>
> (5) AntiHBe—recovery phase of infection

c. Hepatitis C (HCV)

> (1) AntiHCV (ELIZA)—may need serial testing due to false negatives up to 5 or more weeks following onset of symptoms
>
> (2) AntiHCV (RIBA)—positive after several weeks; confirms infection sooner than AntiHCV

d. Hepatitis D (HDV)—AntiHDV from reference laboratory

e. Hepatitis E (HEV)—serologic and Polymerase Chain Reaction assays are available experimentally at this time; diagnosis by exclusion of acute hepatitis A, B, C, D and other causes of viral hepatitis

- Management/Treatment

  1. Treatment is supportive, good nutrition, decreased activity, monitor hydration and chronic state

  2. HAV—immunoglobulin (IG) available for decreasing course of disease in early stages or prevention in exposed individuals; not recommended for HCV or HEV; defer measles or MMR immunization for 3 months following administration of immune globulin

  3. Interferon alpha-2B treatment for chronic HBV and HCV infections

     a. Limited improvement (30% to 40% HBV; 10% to 20% HCV)

     b. Expensive

     c. Side-effects

  4. Report to State health department

  5. Prevention

     a. HAV—two inactive HAV vaccines available for use in children > age 2 (see Health Maintenance and Health Promotion chapter); not routinely recommended for children in day care, only if endemic area; Hepatitis A (IG) prophylaxis available for international travelers < age 2

     b. HBV—vaccine available and highly recommended for all newborns and adolescents (See Health Maintenance and Health Promotion chapter)

     c. Cautious intake of food and water when traveling to endemic area

     d. Avoid unprotected sex and drug use

Hernia

- Definition: Abnormal protrusion of abdominal tissue/structures through umbilical ring in umbilical hernia or external inguinal ring in inguinal hernias

- Etiology/Incidence:

    1. Umbilical—due to imperfect closure or weakness of umbilical ring; common in infancy, reported in up to 60% of African-American infants; many umbilical hernias resolve by age 2, but in the African- American population closure can occur as late as 11 years of age

    2. Inguinal—failed closure of processus vaginalis

        a. Congenital defect—can be noticeable at birth

        b. Four to nine times more frequent in males

        c. Greater risk with premature births

        d. Hydrocele can increase risk; indicates opening present

- Signs and Symptoms

    1. Intermittent or constant bulge of abdominal wall or inguinal region that may worsen with crying or straining

    2. Uncomplicated hernias—asymptomatic

    3. Umbilical—incarceration or strangulation extremely rare

    4. Inguinal

        a. Incarcerated—cranky, anorexia, nausea, vomiting; groin discomfort, constipation

        b. Strangulated—area becomes tender, swollen and progressively reddened in addition to above symptoms, possible fever

- Differential Diagnosis

    1. Hydrocele

    2. Lymphadenopathy

    3. Undescended testes

- Physical Findings:

    1. Umbilical hernia—size of defect varies from 1 to 5 cm in diameter

    2. Inguinal hernia

        a. Maneuvers that increase intra-abdominal pressure (sitting up, crying, coughing) will increase visibility of hernia

        b. May be bilateral, if unilateral, right side more common

        c. ''Silk'' sign can be diagnostic; elicited by palpation of the spermatic cord over the pubic tubercle, the layers of the peritoneum rubbing together will have a ''silky feel''

    d. Transillumination of scrotal sac will highlight the presence of bowel

- Diagnostic Tests/Findings: None may be needed; ultrasound if unclear
- Management/Treatment:
  1. Monitor umbilical hernias; reassure parents.
  2. Refer inguinal for surgical correction
  3. Emergency referral if incarcerated/strangulated

Questions
Select the best answer

1. A ten-month-old child has been diagnosed with gastroenteritis. He attends day care. What is the most likely cause of his illness?

   a. *Clostridium difficile*
   b. Rotavirus
   c. Salmonella
   d. Cryptosporidium

2. In a healthy, eight-month-old with diarrhea, but no dehydration, what would be the most appropriate advice to give parents?

   a. Encourage $\frac{1}{2}$ strength formula for 12 hours
   b. Give oral rehydration solution (ORT) for 12 hours
   c. Give only fluids until stools return to normal
   d. Give bananas and cereal as tolerated

3. When evaluating the abdominal pain in a child with recurrent abdominal pain (RAP) what symptom would lead to a likely organic etiology?

   a. Night waking
   b. Pallor
   c. Suprapubic pain
   d. Sweating

4. Vomiting in infancy has a long list of differential diagnoses. Which accompanying symptom would most likely point to pyloric stenosis?

   a. Diarrhea
   b. Appropriate growth
   c. Acts hungry after vomiting
   d. Sausage shaped mass in abdomen

5. Which of the following is the appropriate regimen for pinworm medication?

   a. Daily times 7 days, repeat as needed
   b. Three times a day for 10 days, repeat as needed
   c. Twice daily for 3 days, repeat in 2 weeks
   d. 1 dose/1 time, repeat in 2 weeks

6. Mrs. Doyle is upset. Two-month-old John's frequent vomiting has her convinced that "something serious is wrong." Which of the following is most suggestive of physiologic GER (gastroesophageal reflux)?

   a. He's gained 5 ounces this month
   b. He has a slight wheeze today
   c. He eats hungrily after vomiting
   d. He drinks 7 to 8 ounces every 3 to 4 hours

7. John's vomiting worsens despite conservative measures. Prokinetic medication might be considered. What diagnostic test should be done first?

    a. pH probe
    b. Milk scan
    c. Endoscopy
    d. Upper GI

8. Baby Sally was in your office last week for her 6-month check up. Her weight was 7 kg. Today she presents with diarrhea and vomiting for four days. Today her weight is 6.5 kg. What is her percentage of dehydration?

    a. 5%
    b. 7%
    c. 10%
    d. < 1%

9. What clinical signs would you expect to see in Sally on your examination?

    a. Normal capillary refill
    b. Normal fontanel
    c. Cool mottled skin
    d. Dry mucous membranes

10. Sally's vomiting and diarrhea has stopped. If she needs oral replacement therapy (ORT) today, what would be the appropriate amount to recommend?

    a. 325 - 350 cc over 4 hours
    b. 600 - 700 cc over 4 hours
    c. 600 - 700 cc over 12 hours
    d. 325 - 350 cc over 8 hours

11. Pinworms can cause which of the following?

    a. Constipation
    b. Anal itching
    c. Abdominal pain
    d. Diarrhea

12. In evaluating Billy, a child with bloody diarrhea, which of the following would not be an appropriate first action?

    a. Check growth chart
    b. Stool culture
    c. Upper GI
    d. Hemoccult test stools

13. Billy's family eats at fast food restaurants 4 to 5 times each week. If the you suspect the diarrhea is infectious in nature, what is a likely causative organism?

    a. Adenovirus
    b. *E. Coli*
    c. *Giardia lamblia*
    d. *S. aureus*

14. Which of the following conditions would be most likely to occur in a four-year-old boy?

    a. Pyloric stenosis
    b. Recurrent abdominal pain
    c. Intussusception
    d. Giardia infection

15. Which of the following findings could be expected to occur in a baby with intussusception?

    a. Inconsolable screaming
    b. Olive shaped mass
    c. Left to right peristaltic waves
    d. Weight loss

16. Which of the following may occur with suspected appendicitis?

    a. Pain not relieved with ambulation
    b. Young children appear very ill in the early phase
    c. Fever is 102 - 103° F
    d. Leukopenia with left shift

17. In the U.S., parasitic gastroenteritis is most commonly caused by which organism?

    a. *Enterobius vermicularis*
    b. *Entamoeba histolytica*
    c. *Cryptosporidium parvum*
    d. *Giardia lamblia*

18. Which of the following serological findings indicates a carrier state for HBV?

    a. HBs Ag negative for 6 months
    b. IgM anti-HBc negative and HBsAg positive
    c. Anti-HBc positive
    d. Anti-HBs positive

19. Children in day care run the greatest risk of being exposed to which of the following infections?

    a. HAV
    b. HBV
    c. HCV
    d. HDV

20. Infant immunization for hepatitis B often raises many parental questions about the disease. Which of the following is not true about hepatitis B virus?

    a. It can survive for more than 1 week on fomites.
    b. It is the most common form of hepatitis in the world.
    c. Contaminated water and shellfish are the major source
    d. Perinatally infected infants are likely to become carriers

21. Two-day-old baby Jamie is in the hospital nursery and still has not passed meconium. This is a red flag for what condition?

    a. Intussusception
    b. Hemolytic uremic syndrome
    c. Pyloric stenosis
    d. Hirschsprung's disease

22. Consistent with the condition in question 21, Jamie's findings on rectal examination would be which of the following?

    a. Tight anal ring with no stool in vault
    b. Impacted stool with fissure
    c. Large, dilated rectum
    d. Soft stool, normal tone

23. What treatment would be appropriate for Jamie's condition?

    a. Emulsified mineral oil ½ tablespoon per day
    b. Referral to gastroenterologist/surgeon
    c. Malt soup extract 2 teaspoons for 3 days
    d. Rectal dilatation with thermometer

24. When evaluating a child with suspected IBD which of the following diagnostic tests would not be helpful?

    a. Amylase and lipase
    b. ESR
    c. Serum total protein and albumin
    d. CBC with differential

25. Your patient has inflammatory bowel disease. Which finding is most consistent with ulcerative colitis?

    a. Occult blood
    b. Perirectal abscess
    c. Aphthous ulcers
    d. Left sided abdominal pain

26. Antimicrobials will improve the condition of a four-year-old child with diarrhea caused by which of the following organisms?

    a. Salmonella
    b. Rotavirus
    c. Shigella
    d. *E. coli* (0157:H7)

27. Katie has functional abdominal pain. When counseling her family on management of painful episodes, you would recommend which of the following?

    a. Take ibuprofen 200 mg for pain
    b. Stay home from school during episode
    c. Decrease milk products
    d. Go to school during episode

28. Which of the following would not be consistent with a diagnosis of functional constipation in an infant?

    a. Vomiting
    b. Anal fissure
    c. Straining
    d. Starting solids

29. A child has developed her second perirectal abscess in six months. She should be evaluated for which condition?

    a. *Giardia lamblia*
    b. Crohn's disease
    c. Ulcerative colitis
    d. Enterobiasis

30. Which of the following symptoms are most common in the early phase of appendicitis in children?

    a. Abdominal pain after eating
    b. Fever and diarrhea
    c. Severe localized RLQ pain with pallor and sweating
    d. Anorexia, vague, diffuse pain

31. Steatorrhea is not consistent with which of the following?

    a. *C. difficile*
    b. *Giardia lamblia*
    c. Celiac disease
    d. Cystic fibrosis

32. Jamil continues with the third day of diarrhea. His mother calls concerned. Which of the following would not be helpful advice?

    a. Monitor stool for blood or mucus
    b. Encourage solid food
    c. Avoid milk products
    d. Monitor for urination at least every 6 hours

33. Of the following advice, which would be most helpful for the parents of a baby with gastro-esophageal reflux?

    a. Most babies continue to vomit until they are walking; at around one year of age
    b. Laying prone after eating will decrease the amount of vomiting
    c. Increase the interval between feedings to a minimum of four hours
    d. Medications are generally necessary to prevent further problems

34. Which of the following foods would be appropriate for a child with celiac disease?

    a. Oatmeal for breakfast
    b. Boiled rice with butter
    c. Commercially baked bread
    d. Cream of wheat

35. A parent requests that her child receive immunoglobulin (IG) as protection against hepatitis A prior to international travel. Which of the following does this parent need to know?

    a. After IG administration, a 3 month interval is needed prior to the next measles vaccine
    b. There is no impact on future immunizations
    c. No immunizations can be given for 1 year
    d. Since children do not have symptoms with hepatitis A, IG is not necessary

Answers

1. b	13. b	25. d
2. d	14. d	26. c
3. a	15. a	27. d
4. c	16. a	28. a
5. d	17. d	29. b
6. d	18. b	30. d
7. d	19. a	31. a
8. b	20. c	32. c
9. d	21. d	33. b
10. b	22. a	34. b
11. b	23. b	35. a
12. c	24. a	

Bibliography

American Academy of Pediatrics. (2003). *Red Book 2003: Report of the Committee on Infectious Diseases* (26th ed.). Elk Grove Village, IL: Author.

American Academy of Pediatrics. Committee on Quality Improvement, Subcommittee on Acute Gastroenteritis. (1996). Practice parameter: The management of acute gastroenteritis in young children. *Pediatrics, 97,* 424–435.

Baker, S. S., Liptak, G. S., Colletti, R. B., Croffie, J. M., DiLorenzo, C., Ector, W., & Nurko, S. (1999). A medical position statement of the North American Society for Pediatric Gastroenterology and Nutrition. Constipation in infants and children: Evaluation and treatment. *Journal of Pediatric Gastroenterology and Nutrition, 29,* 612–626.

Buzby, M. (1997). Differential diagnosis. Acute diarrheal illness in children. *Lippincott's Primary Care Practice,* 1(3), 252–269.

Carroll, A. E., Garrison, M. M., Christakis, P. H. (2002). A systematic review of nonpharmacological and nonsurgical therapies for gastroesophageal reflux in infants. *Archives of Pediatric and Adolescent Medicine,* 156, 109–113.

Fishman, L. N., Jonas, M. M., & Lavine, J. E. (1996). Update on viral hepatitis in children. *Pediatric Clinics of North America, 43,* 57–74.

Garcia-Peña B. M., Taylor G. A., Fishman S. J., et al (2000). Costs and effectiveness of ultrasonagraphy and limited computed tomography for diagnosing appendicitis in children. *Pediatrics,* 106, 672–676.

Gremse, D. A., & Sacks, A. (1997). Evaluation of dyspepsia. *Pediatric Annals, 26,* 251–259.

Hillemeier, A. C. (1996). Gastroesophageal reflux. Diagnostic and therapeutic approaches. *Pediatric Clinics of North America, 43,* 197–209.

Hofmann, A. D., & Greydanus, D. E. (1997). *Adolescent Medicine* (3rd ed.). Stamford, Ct: Appleton & Lange.

Markowitz, J. F. (1996). Inflammatory bowel disease: The pediatrician's role. *Contemporary Pediatrics, 13*(5), 25–46.

McCollough, M., & Sharieff, G. Q., (2003). Abdominal surgical emergencies in infants in young children. *Emergency Medical Clinics of North America,* 21, 909–935.

Preud'Homme, D. L., & Mezoff, A. G. (1996). Helicobacter pylori: A pathogen for all ages. *Contemporary Pediatrics, 13*(11), 27–49.

Rudolph, C. D., Mazur, L. J., Liptak, G. S. et al. (2001). Pediatric gastroesophageal reflux clinical practice guidelines: Guidelines for evaluation and treatment of gastroesophageal reflux in infants and children. *Journal of Pediatric Gastroenterology & Nutrition,* 32, S1–S31.

Talusan-Soriano, K., & Lake, A. M. (1996). Malabsorption in childhood. *Pediatrics in Review,* 17, 135–142.

Winesett, M. (1997). Inflammatory bowel disease in children and adolescents. *Pediatric Annals,* 26, 227–234.

Infectious Diseases

Nancy E. Kline

Septicemia (Sepsis)

- Definition: A generalized systemic response to infection; usually severe and associated with presence of pathogenic microorganisms or associated toxins (usually bacterial) in blood stream; neonates are most susceptible due to immature immune system

- Etiology/Incidence
  1. Etiologic agents vary by age, immunologic status and mechanism of transmission
     a. Newborn (< 3 days)—placental transfer of pathogens from infected maternal blood stream or from vaginal mucosa during birth
        (1) Group B streptococcus (GBS)—high mortality
        (2) *Escherichia coli*—most common gram negative organism
        (3) *Listeria monocytogenes*
     b. Postnatal (1 to 3 weeks)—cross-contamination in nurseries or other crowded conditions; poor hand washing and housekeeping
        (1) *Staphylococcus aureus*—most common
        (2) Klebsiella
        (3) Enterococci
        (4) Pseudomonas
     c. Older infants in the community can be at increased risk for sepsis due to inadequate immunization status—*Haemophilus influenzae* type B
     d. Hospitalized immunosuppressed children at risk for nosocomial sepsis—cancer, post-operative, and patients with HIV/AIDS
  2. Leading cause of morbidity and mortality among hospitalized patients due to associated hemodynamic changes affecting tissue perfusion and oxygenation; if not treated, may lead to septic shock
  3. Increased risk of septecemia
     a. High risk, premature infants
     b. Males > females
     c. Invasive procedures—IV, intubation
     d. Bottle feeding—breast milk may be protective
     e. Immunocompromised children and adolescents

- Signs and Symptoms
  1. Neonates—symptoms may be vague and non-specific, e.g., poor feeding, color changes (pallor, mottling), changes in muscle tone, apnea, cyanosis
  2. Other immunosuppressed children—fever may be only sign; reports by caregiver that child "isn't him or herself"

3. Older children (rarer) with normal immune function—fever, irritability, anorexia, general toxic appearance

- Differential Diagnosis

    1. Viral sepsis

    2. Fungal infection

    3. Rocky mountain spotted fever

    4. Toxic shock syndrome

    5. Non-infectious causes—hemorrhagic, anaphylactic, or neurogenic shock

- Physical Findings

    1. Neonates—hyper or hypothermia; bradycardia or tachycardia; hepatosplenomegaly, jaundice

    2. Older children—irritability, stiff neck

    3. Later phase—lethargy, delayed capillary refill, hypotension and subsequent septic shock

- Diagnostic Tests/Findings

    1. CBC with differential—WBC > 15,000 with increased neutrophils

    2. Chest radiograph to rule out pneumonia

    3. Positive blood cultures identifying source of infection

    4. Cerebral spinal fluid (CSF)—pleocytosis, decreased glucose, increased protein, positive culture

    5. Coagulation studies—prolonged prothrombin time; decreased fibrinogen levels

- Management/Treatment

    1. Medical referral for hospitalization

    2. Close observation, monitoring, and supportive care

    3. IV fluids to maintain hemodynamics

    4. Broad spectrum parenteral antibiotics for gram positive and negative organisms pending culture and sensitivities

    5. Vasoactive medication if septic shock ensues

Diphtheria

- Definition: Highly contagious acute infection of the upper respiratory tract and/or trachea that is relatively rare in the U.S. but may still occur in under-immunized or unimmunized children

- Etiology/Incidence

    1. Caused by *Corynebacterium diphtheriae*

2. Transmission through direct contact with infected person, carrier, or contaminated food/objects

3. Rare in the U.S. due to DTaP/dT immunization; approximately 5 cases reported annually

4. Increased risk among unimmunized children living in crowded conditions

5. Fall/winter incidence most common

- Signs and Symptoms
  1. Sore throat
  2. Low-grade fever
  3. Nasal discharge
  4. Bloody nose
  5. Hoarseness or cough
  6. Difficulty breathing (severe cases)

- Differential Diagnosis
  1. Acute streptococcal pharyngitis
  2. Nasal foreign body
  3. Mononucleosis
  4. Viral croup
  5. Epiglottitis

- Physical Findings
  1. Greyish-white pseudomembrane found at location of infection—nasopharynx, pharynx or trachea
  2. Other findings vary by location of membrane
  3. Toxin-related severe complications include—myocarditis, Guillain-Barré type neuritis and paralysis

- Diagnostic Tests/Findings
  1. Positive culture of *C. Diphtheriae*
  2. CBC—normal or slight leukocytosis and thrombocytopenia

- Management/Treatment
  1. Hospitalization
  2. Evaluation of sensitivity to horse serum; if negative, single dose of equine antitoxin
  3. Antibiotic treatment—erythromycin or penicillin G; antimicrobial treatment is not a substitute for antitoxin
  4. Respiratory isolation

5. Report to State health department

6. Identification of contacts for follow-up care, immunization and treatment according to current American Academy of Pediatrics *Red Book* recommendations

7. Prevention through universal immunization

Pertussis (Whooping Cough)

- Definition: Highly contagious bacterial infection involving the respiratory tract; characterized by prolonged coughing episodes ending in an inspiratory "whoop"

- Etiology/Incidence

    1. Caused by *Bordetella pertussis*

    2. Infection occurs following person to person contact via aerosolized droplets from respiratory tract

    3. 35% of cases occur in infants less than 6 months of age and these children have the highest mortality

    4. Incubation period is 6 to 20 days, usually 7 to 10 days

    5. Infectivity is highest in catarrhal stage

- Signs and Symptoms

    1. Catarrhal stage—mild URI symptoms with cough for approximately two weeks; low-grade fever

    2. Paroxysmal stage—severe coughing episodes with inspiratory "whoops"that may persist for weeks; vomiting, sucking or crying precipitates coughing episodes; poor feeding

- Differential Diagnosis

    1. Pneumonia (bacterial, viral, chlamydial)

    2. Acute bronchitis

    3. Croup

    4. Upper respiratory infection

    5. Foreign body aspiration

    6. Cystic fibrosis

- Physical Findings

    1. Catarrhal stage—mild URI symptoms

    2. Paroxysmal stage—severe coughing episodes with inspiratory "whoops", cyanosis

- Diagnostic Tests/Findings

    1. Chest radiograph—may reveal thickened bronchi and evidence of atelectasis and bronchopneumonia

2. WBC count reveals marked leukocytosis—usually presents during paroxysmal period and persists for 3 to 4 weeks

3. Nasopharyngeal culture of direct fluorescent antibody stain (DFA)—positive in initial phase of illness

- Management/Treatment

  1. Medical referral is necessary

  2. Antibiotic therapy—erythromycin (40 to 50 mg/kg/day divided four times a day for 14 days; maximum 2 g/day)

  3. Hospitalized children should remain in isolation until they have received five days of erythromycin

  4. Children receiving oral erythromycin at home should not attend day care or school until they have received five days of therapy

  5. Supportive treatment for children who cannot tolerate oral intake due to paroxysmal coughing episodes—intravenous hydration, oxygen supplementation, ventilatory support

  6. Report cases of pertussis to State health department

  7. Prevention

     a. Appropriate pertussis immunization according to schedule

     b. Children less than 7 years of age, with close contact with infected individual, who are unimmunized or have received fewer than four doses of pertussis vaccine, should complete the series with the minimal intervals

     c. If the third dose of vaccine was received six months or more prior to the exposure, should be given a fourth dose at time of exposure

     d. Children who have not received a vaccine within past three years or those ≥ 6 years of age, should receive a booster dose of pertussis vaccine at time of exposure

     e. Erythromycin (40 to 50 mg/kg/day divided four times a day for 14 days; maximum 2 g/day) is recommended for all household contacts and other close contacts, regardless of vaccination status

Influenza

- Definition: Highly contagious, viral illness characterized by sudden onset of fever, chills, malaise, headache, myalgia and dry cough

- Etiology/Incidence

  1. Epidemic influenza caused by types A and B

  2. Transmission occurs by direct person-to-person contact, via airborne droplet or by articles contaminated with nasopharyngeal secretions

3. During outbreak, school-aged children are most frequently infected and infect household contacts

4. Period of highest infectivity 24 hours prior to onset of symptoms and while symptoms are most severe

5. Incubation period 1 to 3 days

6. Influenza season mid-October through mid-February

- Signs and Symptoms
    1. Fever
    2. Chills
    3. Malaise
    4. Headache, myalgia
    5. Dry cough
    6. Anorexia
    7. Rhinorrhea
    8. Sore throat

- Differential diagnosis
    1. Upper respiratory infections
    2. Pneumonia

- Physical Findings
    1. Listlessness
    2. Nonproductive cough
    3. Rhinorrhea
    4. Rigors
    5. Fever
    6. Conjunctivitis
    7. Pharyngitis

- Diagnostic Tests/Findings
    1. Nasopharyngeal cultures obtained within first 72 hours of illness may reveal influenza
    2. Diagnosis is usually made based on clinical signs and available prevalence data

- Management/Treatment
    1. Management of influenza is primarily supportive
        a. Bed rest

    b. Acetaminophen or ibuprofen for fever (avoid aspirin-containing products due to risk of developing Reye's syndrome)

    c. Adequate hydration

2. Rimantadine and oseltamivir diminishes severity of influenza A but is not effective in treatment of influenza B

    a. Not approved for use in infants < 12 months of age

    b. Dosages—Rimantadine 5 mg/kg/day (not to exceed 150 mg/day for children 1 year to 9 years of age; for children ≥ 10 years of age give 5 mg/kg/day if < 40 kg, or 200 mg/day if ≥ 40 kg. Oseltamivir ≤ 15 kg—30 mg orally for 5 days; 16-23 kg—45 mg orally for 5 days; 24-40 kg—60 mg orally for 5 days; Children > 40 kg and adults 75 mg orally for 5 days

3. Secondary bacterial infection may occur with influenza

4. Persons in high risk groups (e.g., HIV, cancer, cystic fibrosis, sickle cell disease) should be vaccinated yearly, as should household contacts. The intranasal influenza vaccine is only intended for healthy children, adolescents and adults ages 5 through 49

Rubella (German Measles)

- Definition: An acute, contagious, viral disease characterized by a minor or absent pro-drome, swelling of suboccipital, postauricular and cervical nodes

- Etiology/Incidence

1. Caused by an RNA virus

2. Postnatal transmission occurs via contact from nasopharyngeal secretions

3. Incubation period ranges from 14 to 21 days

4. Preventable by active immunization

- Signs and Symptoms

1. History of inadequate immunization

2. Rash starts on face and spreads over trunk and extremities; disappears by 3rd day

3. Associated signs and symptoms

    a. Malaise, low-grade fever

    b. Transient joint pain

    c. Bruising (rare)

- Differential Diagnosis

1. Rubeola

2. Scarlet fever

3. Erythema infectiosum

4. Adenovirus

5. Rocky mountain spotted fever

6. Roseola

- Physical Findings

    1. Generalized erythematous, maculopapular discrete rash—usually first indication of illness

    2. Listlessness

    3. Postauricular and suboccipital lymphadenopathy—usually precedes rash

    4. Purpura/petechiae (rare)

    5. Meningeal signs (rare)

- Diagnostic Tests/Findings

    1. Presence of rubella specific IgM antibody indicates recent postnatal infection or congenital infection in newborn

    2. Refer to current American Academy of Pediatrics *Red Book* for further information on available assays for detecting rubella infection

- Management/Treatment

    1. Management of uncomplicated infection is primarily supportive—includes fever and pain (in lymph nodes) control with acetaminophen or ibuprofen

    2. Determine contacts that may require immunization

    3. Infected children should limit contact with susceptible persons, including women of childbearing age

    4. Educate adolescent females regarding teratogenic nature of rubella in pregnancy

    5. Educate caretakers regarding complications of arthritis, and rarely thrombocytopenia and encephalitis

Rubeola (Red measles)

- Definition: An acute, highly contagious viral disease characterized by prodrome of upper respiratory manifestations followed by generalized maculopapular eruptions

- Etiology/Incidence

    1. Caused by a morbillivirus, in *Paramyxovirus* family

    2. Transmitted by direct contact with infected secretions or via airborne droplets

    3. Infected individuals are contagious 3 to 5 days before appearance of rash, to four days after appearance of rash

    4. Increased incidence during winter and spring

    5. Preventable by active immunization

- Signs and Symptoms
    1. History of inadequate immunization
    2. Acute onset of fever, coryza, cough, conjunctivitis, malaise, anorexia
    3. Confluent, erythematous, maculopapular rash 3 to 4 days after initial symptoms; progresses in caudal direction
- Differential Diagnosis
    1. Roseola or rubella
    2. Viral infections (e.g., echovirus, coxsackievirus, adenovirus)
    3. Infectious mononucleosis
    4. Scarlet fever
    5. Rickettsial diseases
    6. Serum sickness
- Physical Findings
    1. Confluent, erythematous maculopapular rash; after 3 to 4 days, rash assumes a brownish appearance
    2. Profuse coryza
    3. Conjunctivitis
    4. Pulmonary findings (crackles, rhonchi)
    5. Koplik spots (red eruptions with white centers on buccal mucosa) prior to appearance of rash
- Diagnostic Tests/Findings: Presence of measles specific IgM antibody suggests recent infection
- Management/Treatment
    1. Medical referral necessary
    2. No specific antiviral therapy available
    3. Management of uncomplicated measles is primarily supportive—bedrest, adequate hydration; acetaminophen or ibuprofen for fever; antitussive therapy
    4. Otitis media is most common complication of measles infection— treated with same antibiotics as in standard otitis media
    5. Educate caretakers regarding complications including otitis media, encephalitis and pneumonia

Roseola (Exanthem Subitum)

- Definition: An acute contagious disease characterized by high fever, and appearance of a rash with simultaneous decrease in fever

- Etiology/Incidence
    1. Caused by human herpesvirus 6 (HHV-6)
    2. Mode of transmission not known
    3. Incubation period is 5 to 15 days
    4. Period of infectivity is thought to be during the febrile episode, prior to appearance of the rash
    5. Most commonly occurs in children 6 to 24 months of age
    6. Most cases occur in spring and summer
- Signs and Symptoms
    1. Abrupt onset of high fever (102 to 105° F) lasting 3 to 5 days
    2. Appearance of a rash follows resolution of fever
    3. Associated symptoms include irritability and swelling of eyelids
- Differential Diagnosis
    1. Rubeola
    2. Scarlet fever
    3. Rubella
- Physical Findings
    1. Generalized erythematous, maculopapular rash; starts on trunk and spreads to arms, and neck with less involvement of face and legs
    2. Irritability
    3. May have mildly inflamed edematous conjunctiva
- Diagnostic Tests/Findings: Progressive leukopenia during febrile period
- Management/Treatment
    1. Acetaminophen or ibuprofen for fever
    2. Medical referral if meningeal signs appear, or if fever persists
    3. Education
        a. Potential for febrile seizures
        b. Reassurance that appearance of rash is sign of recovery

Fifth Disease (Erythema Infectiosum - EI)

- Definition: A contagious, usually afebrile, exanthematous disease
- Etiology/Incidence
    1. Human parvovirus B19

    2.   Typically seen in 5 to 14-year-old children

    3.   Outbreaks occur most often during spring months

    4.   Incubation period between 4 and 14 days

    5.   Mode of transmission includes respiratory secretions and blood

- Signs and Symptoms

    1.   No prodromal symptoms

    2.   Rash

        a.   Begins as bilateral erythema on cheeks ("slapped cheek" appearance)

        b.   Spreads to upper arms, legs, trunk, hands and feet

        c.   Palms and soles are spared

        d.   Lacy-reticular exanthem appears as facial erythema begins to diminish

        e.   May reappear when skin is exposed to sunlight, temperature extremes

        f.   Rash lasts from 2 to 39 days, average 11 days

    3.   Low grade fever may occur

    4.   Can cause aplastic crises in young children, and in patients with hemolytic diseases

- Differential Diagnosis

    1.   Drug reactions

    2.   Rubella, atypical measles

    3.   Enteroviral diseases

    4.   Systemic lupus erythematosus

- Physical Findings

    1.   Early—bilateral erythema on cheeks ("slapped cheek" appearance)

    2.   Late—erythematous rash on upper arms and legs, trunk, hands and feet; palms and soles are spared

    3.   Late—lacy-reticular exanthem appears as facial erythema begins to diminish

- Diagnostic Tests/Findings

    1.   Parvovirus B19 IgM antibody confirms current infection, or infection within past several months

    2.   Parvovirus B19 IgG antibody indicates previous infection and immunity

- Management/Treatment

    1.   None indicated

    2.   Reassure parent of benign nature of disease

    3.   Avoid sunlight as exposure may exacerbate the condition

4. Period of high infectivity in persons with EI is prior to onset of symptoms; unlikely to be infectious after rash develops; conversely patients with aplastic crises are highly contagious prior to the onset of symptoms and through week of onset, or longer

Varicella-Zoster Virus (VZV) (Chickenpox)

- Definition: An acute contagious disease caused by a herpesvirus; characterized by a short or absent prodrome and usually a sequential rash consisting of papules, vesicles, pustules and crusts

- Etiology/Incidence
    1. VZV is a herpesvirus
    2. Transmission occurs by direct contact with varicella lesions or by airborne droplet infection
    3. Susceptible individuals can contract chickenpox from patients with varicella zoster (shingles)
    4. Incubation period between 10 and 21 days
    5. Infected individual contagious for 24 to 48 hours prior to outbreak of lesions, until lesions have crusted over
    6. Most cases occur between ages of 5 and 10 years
    7. VZV occurs commonly in late winter and early spring

- Signs and Symptoms
    1. Early lesions appear as faint erythematous macules that progress to papules, followed by appearance of vesicles primarily on trunk, scalp, face; lesions eventually crust over
    2. Lesions continue to erupt for 3 to 4 days and may be present in various stages
    3. Associated symptoms may include fever, pruritus, malaise, anorexia, joint pain

- Differential Diagnosis
    1. Herpes zoster
    2. Bullous impetigo
    3. Insect bites
    4. Urticaria

- Physical Findings
    1. Crops of skin lesions that may appear as maculopapular (early), vesicular, pustular with eventual crusts; many maculopapular lesions may progress to vesicular stage and resolve without crusting
    2. Rash usually present on scalp, face, trunk and extremities; most lesions on face and trunk
    3. Hepatomegaly (rare)

4. Meningeal signs (rare)

5. Pulmonary findings—crackles, wheezes (rare)

- Diagnostic Tests/Findings: None routinely performed

- Management/Treatment

1. VZV is a self-limited disease lasting 7 to 10 days

2. Supportive treatment

   a. Control of pruritus with oatmeal baths, diphenhydramine, calamine lotion

   b. Acetaminophen for fever (*avoid aspirin-containing products due to risk of developing Reye's syndrome*)

3. Oral acyclovir is beneficial in reducing duration of new lesion formation, and total number of lesions (20 mg/kg/dose, four times a day; maximum 800 mg four times a day); should be started within 24 hours of onset for maximum benefit

4. Oral acyclovir not usually recommended in healthy children with uncomplicated varicella

5. Varicella-zoster immune globulin (VZIG) should be given to immune suppressed contacts to provide passive protection

6. Medical referral necessary for immune suppressed children

7. Education

   a. Avoid contact with elderly, pregnant women, neonates and immunocompromised children

   b. Live-attenuated varicella vaccine is available in U.S. and is recommended for all healthy children age 12 months to 13 years who lack a reliable history of varicella (AAP, 2000)

   c. Signs and symptoms of complicated varicella infection—meningeal signs, respiratory distress, dehydration, ocular involvement, secondary bacterial infection, thrombocytopenia, pneumonia

   d. Signs and symptoms of Reye's syndrome—persistent vomiting, lethargy, agitation, disorientation, combativeness, coma

Mumps

- Definition: A contagious, systemic, viral disease characterized by swelling of the salivary glands

- Etiology/Incidence

1. Caused by paramyxovirus

2. Spread by direct contact via respiratory airborne droplet and fomites contaminated with infected saliva

3. Incubation period between 12 to 25 days after exposure

4. Infected individual is contagious for as many as 7 days prior to, and as long as 9 days after onset of symptoms

5. Infection occurs throughout childhood; rarely during adulthood

6. More common in late winter and spring

- Signs and Symptoms
    1. History of inadequate immunization
    2. Swelling of salivary glands (specifically parotid gland), pain with swallowing
    3. Malaise, fever
    4. Scrotal swelling and pain

- Differential Diagnosis
    1. Submandibular or preauricular lymphadenitis
    2. Salivary duct obstruction
    3. Infectious mononucleosis
    4. Epididymitis

- Physical Findings
    1. Swelling of salivary glands (specifically parotid gland)
    2. Listlessness
    3. Scrotal swelling and pain

- Diagnostic Tests/Findings: Serum for complement fixation (CF)—positive test for complement-fixing antibody against mumps virus suggests recent infection

- Management/Treatment
    1. Acetaminophen for pain and fever
    2. Warm compresses for salivary gland swelling
    3. Soft or liquid diet
    4. Education
        a. Complications include pancreatitis, oophoritis, meningitis, orchitis
        b. May return to day care or school when all symptoms have resolved or 9 days after onset of symptoms
    5. Report cases to State health department

Cat Scratch Disease (CSD)

- Definition: An infection characterized by regional lymphadenopathy in an otherwise healthy person, following contact with an infected cat, as a result of a cat bite or scratch, or contact with cat saliva on broken skin or the conjunctivae of the eye

- Etiology/Incidence

  1. Most cases are caused by *Bartonella* spp., which include the former genus *Rochalimaea*

  2. More than 24,000 cases per year occur in the U.S. (Stechenberg, 2000)

- Signs and Symptoms: Mild systemic symptoms

  1. History of cat exposure

  2. Usually do not appear ill

  3. Swollen lymph nodes

  4. May have low-grade fever; general malaise; headache

  5. Anorexia

  6. May have rash

- Differential Diagnosis

  1. Bacterial lymphadenitis

  2. Lymphoma

  3. Tularemia

  4. Lymphogranuloma venereum

- Physical Findings

  1. Papule or pustule at site of cat scratch or bite, followed in 1 to 3 weeks by enlargement of an associated lymph node

  2. Lesion may be present for several days to several months

- Diagnostic Tests/Findings

  1. May have elevated ESR

  2. Immunofluorescence assay (IFA) detects antibody to CSD

  3. Warthin-Starry silver stain used to identify CSD in lymph node, skin or conjunctival tissue

- Management/treatment

  1. CSD is a self-limited disease lasting 2 to 4 months

  2. Supportive Treatment

     a. Analgesics for discomfort and fever

     b. Limited activity

     c. Needle aspiration of painful, suppurative nodes questionable; may result in chronic draining sinus tract

     d. No treatment required for animal that transmitted CSD

Rocky Mountain Spotted Fever (RMSF)

- Definition: A systemic, febrile illness with characteristic petechial or purpuric rash
- Etiology/Incidence
    1. Caused by *Rickettsia rickettsii*
    2. Transmitted to humans via tick bites
    3. Usually occurs in persons younger than 15 years of age
    4. Widespread in U.S.; most prevalent in southern States
    5. Incubation period ranges from 1 to 14 days
- Signs and Symptoms
    1. Fever, myalgia, nausea and vomiting precede appearance of rash
    2. Erythematous, macular rash (usually appearing before the sixth day of illness), on wrists, ankles, spreading within hours to the trunk
    3. In some cases rash fails to develop, or develops late in the illness
    4. Disease can last 3 weeks with multisystem involvement (e.g., CNS, cardiac, pulmonary, GI, renal)
- Differential Diagnosis
    1. Rubeola
    2. Rubella
    3. Lyme disease
    4. Septicemia
    5. Meningococcemia
- Physical Findings
    1. Characteristic petechial, erythematous, macular rash
    2. Neurologic deficits
    3. Heart murmur
    4. Pulmonary findings (crackles)
    5. Decreased urine output
    6. Jaundice
- Diagnostic Tests/Findings
    1. Culture is not attempted due to transmission risk for laboratory personnel
    2. Renal failure
    3. Elevated liver enzymes

    4.   Increase in antibody titer as established by serologic testing; indirect hemagglutination (IHA) and microimmunofluorescence (micro-IF) are most sensitive

- Management/Treatment

    1.   Medical referral

    2.   Doxycycline or tetracycline is given until patient is afebrile for 2 to 3 days

    3.   Tetracycline not routinely given to children less than 8 years of age; doxycycline is drug of choice

    4.   Education includes preventive measures such as use of tick repellent and protective clothing in tick-infested areas

    5.   Patients with multisystem organ involvement may require rehabilitative services

    6.   Report cases to State health department

Lyme Disease

- Definition:

    1.   An immune-mediated, inflamatory response

    2.   Affects multiple organ systems

    3.   Transmitted primarily via the deer tick

- Etiology/Incidence

    1.   Caused by a spirochete *Borrelia burgdorferi*; is most often transmitted via the deer tick

    2.   Most often seen in Northeast from Massachusetts to Maryland; the Midwest, primarily Wisconsin and Minnesota; and in California; primarily in heavily wooded areas

    3.   Persons of all ages and both sexes are affected

    4.   Most cases occur during June and July

    5.   Incubation period is between 3 to 32 days

- Signs and Symptoms

    1.   Appearance of well-circumscribed, erythematous, annular rash with central clearing (erythema chronicum migrans) at site of recent tick bite

    2.   Fever, malaise, headache, arthralgia, conjunctivitis, or mild neck stiffness

    3.   May initially present as flulike illness if erythema migrans does not occur, or not recognized

    4.   Late signs and symptoms (weeks to months later)

        a.   Migratory pain in joints, muscles and bones

        b.   Transient, but severe, headaches and stiff neck

        c.   Poor memory, mood changes, somnolence

      d.   Muscle weakness and poor coordination

      e.   Chest pain, cardiac abnormalities

      f.   Dizziness/fainting

      g.   Facial palsies

      h.   Joint stiffness

- Differential Diagnosis

  1. Tinea corporis (ringworm)

  2. Insect bite

  3. Cellulitis

  4. Acute rheumatic fever

  5. Influenza

  6. Aseptic meningitis

  7. Juvenile rheumatoid arthritis

  8. Henoch-Schöenlein purpura

- Physical Findings

  1. Well-circumscribed, erythematous, annular rash with central clearing

  2. Malar rash, diffuse erythema or urticaria

  3. Heart murmur

  4. Neurologic findings—seventh cranial nerve palsy

- Diagnostic Tests/Findings

  1. Enzyme-linked immunosorbent assay (ELISA)—detects antibodies against *B. burgdorferi*

  2. Western blot—used to validate a positive or equivocal ELISA

  3. Serum immunoglobulins—IgM, IgG elevated

  4. Culture of erythema migrans lesion—expensive, time to isolation may take four weeks

  5. White blood cell count—normal or elevated

  6. Erythrocyte sedimentation rate (ESR)—elevated

- Management/Treatment

  1. Medical referral is necessary

  2. Early disease

     a. Children > 8 years of age—amoxicillin or doxycycline

     b. Children ≤ 8 years of age—amoxicillin or penicillin V

    c.   For penicillin-allergic patients—cefuroxime or erythromycin may be used, although erythromycin may be less effective

3.   Late disease for persistent arthritis, carditis, neurologic disease—parenteral ceftriaxone or penicillin G

4.   Education/prevention

    a.   Ticks that carry Lyme disease are 4 to 5 mm in diameter

    b.   Prompt removal of ticks from the skin and use of tick repellent decreases the incidence of Lyme disease

    c.   Use blunt-end tweezers to grasp tick as close to skin surface as possible; wear rubber gloves

    d.   Disinfect skin where tick bite occurred

    e.   Early intervention leads to improved prognosis

    f.   Wear protective clothing in heavily wooded areas, check skin closely after outdoor activities

    g.   Report cases of Lyme disease to State health department

Infectious Mononucleosis (IM)

- Definition: An acute disease characterized by fever, exudative pharyngitis, lymphadenopathy, hepatosplenomegaly and atypical lymphocytosis

- Etiology/Incidence

  1. Caused by Epstein-Barr virus (EBV), a herpesvirus

  2. Contact with infected secretions is required for transmission

  3. Incubation period is 30 to 50 days

  4. Commonly diagnosed in adolescents and young adults

- Signs and Symptoms

  1. Fever, malaise, fatigue

  2. Severe sore throat

  3. Rash especially with administration of ampicillin derivatives

  4. Tender lymph nodes

- Differential Diagnosis

  1. Streptococcal pharyngitis

  2. Hepatitis

  3. Influenza or viral illness

  4. Measles

5. Blood dyscrasias, especially leukemia

- Physical Findings
    1. Exudative pharyngitis
    2. May have hepatosplenomegaly
    3. Lymphadenopathy
    4. May have jaundice
    5. May have erythematous, macular, papular rash
    6. Tender posterior cervical nodes
- Diagnostic Tests/Findings
    1. Positive monospot, or positive Epstein-Barr virus titer
    2. WBC count reveals leukocytosis, 10,000 to 20,000 cells/mm^3, with $\geq$ 60% lymphocytes and 20 to 40% atypical lymphocytes
    3. Rapid strep test and throat culture—identifies presence of ß-hemolytic streptococcal infection, if present
- Management/Treatment
    1. IM is a self-limited disease lasting 2 to 3 weeks
    2. Supportive treatment
        a. Bedrest during acute phase
        b. Pain control for pharyngitis and lymphadenitis
        c. Saline gargles for sore throat
        d. Avoid contact sports until spleen is no longer palpable
        e. Antibiotic therapy as needed for pharyngitis—avoid use of ampicillin derivatives such as amoxicillin, and other penicillins; may result in rash

Infant Botulism

- Definition: A neuroparalytic disorder affecting young infants (< 6 months) resulting from ingestion of *Clostridium botulinum* spores with release of toxins as organism colonizes gastrointestinal tract
- Etiology/Incidence
    1. Etiologic agent is *Clostridium botulinum*; disease is caused by toxins produced by this anaerobic bacillus
    2. Toxin inhibits acetylcholine release at myoneural junction resulting in impaired motor activity
    3. *C. botulinum* spores have been associated with honey, reported association with corn syrup not substantiated (AAP, 2000)

    4.   Rural, farm environments associated with increased incidence

- Signs and Symptoms: Evolving symptomatology

    1.   May be asymptomatic

    2.   Constipation (most common presenting symptom)

    3.   Poor feeding

    4.   Weak cry

    5.   Weakness

    6.   Loss of head and neck control

    7.   Generalized floppiness

- Differential Diagnosis

    1.   Sepsis

    2.   Benign congenital hypotonia

    3.   Benign constipation

    4.   Hypothyroidism

    5.   Hirschprung's disease

    6.   Other neuromuscular disorders

- Physical Findings

    1.   Generalized weakness

    2.   Diminished deep tendon reflexes

    3.   Cranial nerve deficits

    4.   Swallowing difficulties

    5.   Loss of muscle tone

- Diagnostic Tests/Findings

    1.   Stool culture positive for *C. botulinum*

    2.   Polymerase chain reaction (PCR) assays—detection of organism in stool

    3.   Blood culture—may or may not be positive for *C. botulinum*

- Management/Treatment

    1.   Equine antitoxin not usually recommended for infant botulism

    2.   Hospitalization; possibility of respiratory arrest

    3.   Stool softener

    4.   Prevention/education regarding honey as potential source of botulism; avoid feeding to infants < 12 months of age

    5.   Report to State health department

Poliomyelitis

- Definition: An acute, contagious, potentially paralytic viral disease
- Etiology/Incidence
    1. Caused by enterovirus (EV)
    2. When susceptible person comes in contact with poliovirus, one of three responses occur
        a. Nonspecific febrile illness (most frequent)
        b. Aseptic meningitis (nonparalytic poliomyelitis)
        c. Paralytic poliomyelitis (least frequent)
    3. Incubation period to onset of paralysis is 4 to 21 days
    4. Preventable by active immunization
    5. Occurs more often in infants and young children
    6. Occurs more commonly in conditions of poor hygiene
- Signs and Symptoms
    1. History of inadequate immunization or recent immunization
    2. Fever, weakness
    3. Anxiety
    4. Urinary incontinence
    5. Meningeal signs
    6. Respiratory compromise
    7. Speech disturbances
    8. Headache
    9. Nausea, anorexia
- Differential Diagnosis
    1. Guillain-Barré syndrome
    2. Meningitis
    3. Encephalitis
    4. Peripheral neuritis or neuropathy
- Physical Findings
    1. Meningeal signs
    2. Respiratory compromise
    3. Inability to speak without frequent pauses
    4. Muscle weakness

- Diagnostic Tests/Findings: EV isolated from feces, throat, urine or CSF in cell culture
- Management/Treatment
    1. Medical referral necessary
    2. Supportive management—bedrest, adequate hydration, pain control, acetaminophen or ibuprofen for fever, respiratory support if paralysis ensues, physical therapy for deficits associated with muscle weakness and paralysis
    3. Education
        a. Educate family regarding potential complications of possible paralysis including respiratory compromise and arrest, hypertension, renal calculi due to immobility
        b. Oral polio vaccine should not be given to persons who reside with immunocompromised individuals; virus is shed in stool and there is risk of contracting poliomyelitis; inactivated poliovirus vaccine (IPV) may be substituted.

Tetanus (Lockjaw)

- Definition: A neurologic disease characterized by severe muscle spasms that can be fatal
- Etiology/Incidence
    1. Caused by neurotoxin produced by anaerobic bacterium *Clostridium tetani* in contaminated wounds
    2. Occurs throughout the world; neonatal tetanus is common in countries where women are not immunized
    3. Incubation period 2 days to 2 months with an average of 10 days; 5 to 14 days in neonates
    4. More common in warmer climates and months
    5. Has dramatically decreased with advent of tetanus vaccine
- Signs and Symptoms
    1. Incomplete tetatus immunization series
    2. History of deep puncture wound, laceration
    3. Insidious onset
    4. Muscle spasms aggravated by stimuli
    5. Muscle rigidity
    6. Increased oral secretions
    7. Respiratory compromise
- Differential Diagnosis
    1. Muscle spasms
    2. Amyotrophic lateral sclerosis (Lou Gehrig's disease)

3. Hypocalcemic tetany

4. Phenothiazine reaction

5. Strychnine poisoning

- Physical Findings

    1. Muscle spasms aggravated by stimuli

    2. Muscle rigidity

    3. Increased oral secretions

    4. Respiratory compromise

- Diagnostic Tests/Findings: Diagnosis made clinically

- Management/Treatment

    1. Medical referral

    2. Supportive management—treatment of muscle spasms, intravenous fluids, respiratory support

    3. Minimize external stimuli (e.g., loud noise, bright light) to prevent aggravating muscle spasms

    4. Tetanus immune globulin (TIG) given to prevent circulating toxin from binding to central nervous system sites

    5. Infection with tetanus does not confer immunity; patient should be reimmunized in convalescent period to prevent future infection

    6. Education—educate family regarding potential complications from tetanus including respiratory compromise, inability to speak

Malaria

- Definition: An infectious disease primarily acquired via mosquito bite characterized by high fever, rigors, sweats and headache

- Etiology/Incidence

    1. Caused by *Plasmodium* spp. and transmitted primarily via mosquito bite; although transmission can be congenital; via transfusions or contaminated needles

    2. Infection by *Plasmodium falciparum* is most serious and potentially fatal

    3. Endemic in tropical areas worldwide; most cases in U.S. reported annually, (approximately 1,000) are acquired during foreign travel

- Signs and Symptoms

    1. History of recent travel to endemic area

    2. Classic paroxysmal symptoms—high fever, rigors, diaphoresis and headache

    3. Fever and other symptoms eventually become synchronized, and depending on the infecting species of *Plasmodium*, fever will occur every other, or every third day

4. Associated symptoms—nausea, vomiting, diarrhea, arthralgia, cough, abdominal and back pain, pallor, jaundice

5. Multisystem involvement can develop with *Plasmodium falciparum* infection; may be fatal

    a. Neurologic—seizures, signs of increased intracranial pressure, confusion, stupor, coma and death

    b. Pulmonary—coarse breath sounds, pulmonary edema

    c. Renal—decreased urine output, oliguria, hematuria

    d. Cardiovascular—absent peripheral pulses, hypotension

    e. Gastrointestinal—diarrhea

    f. Vascular collapse and shock

*   Differential Diagnosis

    1. Influenza

    2. Rocky mountain spotted fever

    3. Septicemia

*   Physical Findings

    1. Early findings—listlessness, rigors, muscle weakness, pallor, jaundice, hepatospleno-megaly

    2. Findings seen in *Plasmodium falciparum* infection—neurologic deficits, pneumonia, elevated liver enzymes, renal failure

*   Diagnostic Tests/Findings: Diagnosis depends on identification of parasite on stained blood films

*   Management/Treatment

    1. Medical referral

    2. Drug therapy based on the infecting *Plasmodium* species; refer to most current American Academy of Pediatrics *Red Book* for varying treatment regimens

    3. Prevention best achieved through prophylactic therapy prior to travel to endemic areas

    4. Education should include natural history of the illness, and specific follow-up or rehabilitation needed after infection with *Plasmodium falciparum*

    5. Report cases to State health department

Questions
Select the best answer

1. Septicemia in the newborn period is most likely caused by which organism?

    a. *Listeria monocytogenes*
    b. *Haemophilus influenzae*
    c. *Neisseria meningitidis*
    d. *Streptococcus pneumoniae*

2. Signs and symptoms of bacterial sepsis in children beyond the neonatal period include:

    a. Cough, fever, abdominal pain
    b. Vesicular rash, pruritus, fever
    c. Irritability, stiff neck, lethargy
    d. Abdominal pain, diarrhea, vomiting

3. Which of the following vaccines provides protection against a common type of sepsis/meningitis?

    a. Smallpox vaccination
    b. Hepatitis B vaccine
    c. *Haemophilus influenzae* vaccine
    d. Inactivated polio vaccine

4. Although relatively rare in the U.S., diphtheria can occur among under-immunized children. Which of the following clusters of signs, symptoms and physical findings would suggest diphtheria in a child presenting with upper respiratory complaints?

    a. Low grade fever, sore throat, nasal discharge, and greyish-white pseudo-membrane in his/her throat
    b. Abrupt onset of high fever, severe sore throat, nasal discharge, and greyish-white pseudo-membrane his/her throat
    c. Low grade fever, abrupt onset of severe sore throat with difficulty swallowing and drooling
    d. Abrupt onset of high fever, severe sore throat, with difficulty swallowing and drooling

5. Infants younger than six-months-of-age with pertussis frequently require hospitalization to manage:

    a. Fever, cough, dehydration
    b. Coughing paroxysms, apnea, cyanosis, feeding difficulties
    c. Coughing paroxysms, dehydration, renal failure
    d. Seizures, fever, pneumonia

6. One of the most appropriate agents used to treat Influenza A is

    a. Acyclovir
    b. Rimantadine
    c. Erythromycin
    d. Tetracycline

7. Which of the following symptoms are characteristic of rubella?

   a. Vesicular, crusted lesions and high fever
   b. Postauricular lymphadenopathy and low grade fever
   c. Intense pruritus, usually in finger webs, buttocks, thighs and ankles
   d. Rough textured maculopapular rash that blanches with pressure

8. Although uncommon, a potential sequela of rubella may include:

   a. Pneumonia and chronic otitis media
   b. Arthritis, thrombocytopenia and encephalitis
   c. Oophoritis and infertility
   d. Arthritis, carditis, and neurological involvement

9. Rubeola is:

   a. Preventable by active immunization
   b. Caused by an RNA virus
   c. Treated with intravenous acyclovir
   d. Not associated with severe complications (e.g., encephalitis, pneumonia)

10. You are examining a child who has fever, coryza, cough, conjunctivitis, malaise, and anorexia. During the oral examination, you observe red eruptions with white centers on the buccal mucosa. What are these eruptions called?

    a. Pastia's spots
    b. Rubeola spots
    c. Koplik's spots
    d. Strawberry spots

11. Which of the following best describes the treatment for roseola?

    a. Acetaminophen or ibuprofen for fever, parental reassurance
    b. Warm compresses for salivary gland swelling
    c. Oral acylovir, 20mg/kg/dose, four times a day
    d. Bedrest, saline gargles for sore throat

12. Fifth disease is usually:

    a. Seen in age 5 to 14-year-old children
    b. Transmitted via the deer tick
    c. Treated with oral erythromycin
    d. Characterized by prolonged coughing episodes

13. Which of the following statements is not true regarding the transmission of chickenpox?

    a. Susceptible individuals can contract chickenpox from patients with varicella zoster (shingles)
    b. Children with chickenpox are infectious only during the period of time when skin lesions are present

c. Children with chickenpox are no longer infectious once crusting of skin lesions has occurred

d. Varicella-zoster immune globulin (VZIG) should be administered to susceptible immuno-compromised individuals who are exposed to a patient with varicella zoster infection

14. A child with chickenpox and temperature of 102° F should receive which medication for fever?

a. Aspirin
b. Amoxicillin
c. Acetaminophen
d. Acyclovir

15. The most appropriate agent for use in treating varicella zoster infection in an immunocompromised host is:

a. Ganciclovir
b. Acyclovir
c. Ceftriaxone
d. Chloramphenicol

16. Varicella zoster infection is most commonly associated with which of the following skin lesions?

a. Vesicle
b. Comedone
c. Nodule
d. Macule

17. Which of the following is not a complication of mumps?

a. Meningitis
b. Pneumonia
c. Oophoritis
d. Pancreatitis

18. What recommendation would you make to a parent whose son has been diagnosed with mumps and wants to know when he can return to day care?

a. He can return once he becomes afebrile and can tolerate eating
b. He can return 9 days after onset of symptoms
c. He can return when he is well enough to participate in activities since infectivity is highest prior to symptoms
d. He can return after a mimimum of 5 days of antibiotic therapy

19. Which of the following are symptoms of cat scratch disease?

a. Joint pain, conjunctivitis, mild neck stiffness
b. Irritability, fever, hypotension
c. Fever, malaise, lymphadenopathy
d. Severe coughing, vomiting, anorexia

20. The following describes a characteristic rash associated with which disease? Initially erythematous and macular, becoming maculopapular and petechial. The rash first appears on the wrists and ankles, spreading proximally to the trunk. The palms and soles are often involved.

    a. Lyme disease
    b. Roseola
    c. Rubeola (measles)
    d. Rocky mountain spotted fever

21. A 10-year-old child manifests symptoms of fever, sore throat, and swollen lymph nodes. Spleen tip is palpable. Throat culture and Monospot test results are negative. The next logical diagnostic test would involve:

    a. Repeat throat culture
    b. Chest radiograph
    c. Bone marrow examination
    d. Epstein-Barr virus titer

22. Which of the following factors is not associated with increased risk for infantile botulism?

    a. Rural environments
    b. Use of honey
    c. Use of corn syrup
    d. Farm families

23. Which of the following interventions would not be appropriate for a 6-month-old infant with a suspected diagnosis of infantile botulism?

    a. Stool and blood cultures
    b. Immediate administration of equine antitoxin
    c. Stool softeners
    d. Supportive care

24. Which of the following are associated with paralytic poliomyelitis?

    a. Lacy, erythematous, pruritic rash
    b. Respiratory compromise, speech disturbances, urinary incontinence
    c. Abdominal swelling, lymphadenopathy and jaundice
    d. Unlocalized abdominal pain, nausea and vomiting

25. Muscle spasms associated with tetanus are aggravated by which of the following?

    a. Fever
    b. Tetanus immuneglobulin
    c. External stimuli
    d. NSAID

26. Classic symptoms associated with malaria include:

    a. Low grade fever, upper respiratory congestion, cough
    b. Annular rash, conjunctivitis, headache, arthralgia
    c. High fever, chills, rigors, sweats, headache
    d. High fever, jaundice, lethargy, vomiting

27. Lyme disease is most closely associated with which of the following skin lesions?

    a. Erythema migrans
    b. Nodule
    c. Scale
    d. Pustule

28. Many infectious diseases present with rashes along with general complaints of fever, malaise, and headaches. Which of the following clusters of symptoms would make you consider Lyme disease as a likely diagnosis?

    a. Fever, malaise, headache, arthralgia and well-circumscribed, erythematous, annular rash with central clearing
    b. Fever, malaise, headache, transient bone pain, and generalized erythematous, maculopapular rash that began on the face and spread to trunk and extremities
    c. Fever, malaise, anorexia, and confluent, erythematous, brownish maculopapular rash
    d. Fever, malaise, anorexia, and erythematous rash beginning on wrists and ankles then spreading to the trunk

29. Which of the following would be included in patient education regarding Lyme disease?

    a. Educate caretakers regarding complications including hypertension and renal calculi due to immobility
    b. Avoid use of aspirin-containing products for fever control due to association with increased risk for Lyme disease
    c. Protective clothing and tick repellent should be worn in heavily wooded areas
    d. Educate caretakers regarding natural history of the illness, and specific follow-up needed after infection with *Rickettsia rickettsii*

Answer key:

1. a	11. a	21. d
2. c	12. a	22. c
3. c	13. b	23. b
4. a	14. c	24. b
5. b	15. b	25. c
6. b	16. a	26. c
7. b	17. b	27. a
8. b	18. b	28. a
9. a	19. c	29. c
10. c	20. d	

Bibliography

Atkinson, W. (2002). *Epidemiology and prevention of vaccine-preventable diseases* (7th ed.). Atlanta: Centers for Disease Control and Prevention.

American Academy of Pediatrics. (2003). *Red Book 2003: Report of the committee on infectious diseases* (25th ed.). Elk Grove Village, IL: American Academy of Pediatrics.

Behrman, R. E., Kliegman, R. M., & Jenson, H. B. (2004). Nelson textbook of pediatrics (17th ed.). Philadelphia: W. B. Saunders.

Feigin, R. D., & Cherry, J. D. (2004). *Textbook of pediatric infectious diseases* (5th ed.). Philadelphia: W. B. Saunders.

Hoekelman, R. A., Adam, H. M., Nelson, N. M., Weitzman, M. L. & Wilson, M. H. (Eds.). (2001). *Primary Pediatric care* (4th ed.). St. Louis: Mosby.

Pizzo, P. A., & Poplack, D. G. (2002). *Principles and practice of pediatric oncology* (4th ed.). Philadephia: J. B. Lippincott.

Musculoskeletal Disorders

Susan Heighway

Torticollis (Wry neck)

- Definition: Abnormal position of head and neck, due to contracture of one of sternoclei-domastoid muscles that may be congenital (most common) or acquired
- Etiology/Incidence
    1. Cause not well-defined, but may be due to:
        a. Compartment syndrome
        b. Soft tissue compression at delivery
        c. Occlusion of venous outflow of sternocleidomastoid muscle
        d. Uterine crowding
        e. Neurogenic myopathy from trauma or ischemia
    2. Neurogenic causes rare
    3. Higher incidence in children with breech presentation and forceps delivery, but occurs with normal births or C-sections
    4. Familial tendency (rare)
    5. 0.4% live births; males more frequently effected
- Signs and Symptoms
    1. Child's head tilted toward side of contracture
    2. Chin rotated away from contracted side (origin of muscle on mastoid process)
- Differential Diagnosis
    1. CNS tumors
    2. Syringomyelia
    3. Arnold-Chiari malformation
    4. Ocular dysfunctions
    5. Paroxysmal torticollis of infancy
- Physical Findings
    1. Contracture of one of sternocleidomastoid muscles
    2. Fusiform, firm mass or "tumor"
        a. In body of contracted muscle
        b. Palpable after 4 weeks of age, then recedes
    3. Plagiocephaly, or asymmetry of face/skull development present with progressive deformity
- Diagnostic Tests/Findings
    1. Cervical radiograph

    a. To rule out congenital spine abnormalities, e.g., hemivertabrae

    b. Normal with muscular torticollis

  2. Other imaging (MRI or CT scan) not indicated—abnormalities not detected unless neurogenic pathology (rare) exists

- Management/Treatment

  1. Conservative measures—initial treatment

    a. Stretching exercises—guided by physical therapist

    b. Encourage infant stretching by placing toys, mobiles, items of interest in infant's line of vision, on the affected side

  2. Surgery recommended when:

    a. Defect persists beyond 1 year of age

    b. Stretching exercises have been unsuccessful

    c. Infant between 1 and 4 years of age; best outcome for surgical release

Developmental Dysplasia of the Hip (DDH)

- Definition: Abnormal development or dislocation of the hip(s), which is congenital, but may not be recognized until ambulation occurs

- Etiology/Incidence

  1. Multifactorial etiology in an otherwise normal child

    a. Intrauterine mechanical factors

      (1) Breech presentation (30% of cases)

      (2) Infants with oligohydramnios

    b. Genetic effects in primary acetabular dysplasia

      (1) Various degrees of joint laxity

      (2) 20% have positive family history

    c. Increased incidence in first born Caucasian infants; tight uterine muscles limit movement

  2. Left hip involved more commonly than right

  3. Sixfold greater incidence in girls (girls more often in breech position)

  4. Incidence 1 to 1.5:1000 live births

- Signs and Symptoms

  1. Newborn

    a. Instability without significant fixed deformity

    b. Detected during newborn examination

2. Sometimes not detected at birth

   a. Untreated dislocation becomes fixed, with less instability, more limitation of movement

   b. Limp noticeable at onset of walking

   c. Afebrile, painless, may have ligamentous laxity

- Differential Diagnosis

  1. Leg length discrepancy

  2. Innocent hip "click"—not associated with movement of femoral head

  3. Arthrogryposis

  4. Cerebral palsy

- Physical Findings

  1. Galeazzi's sign—knee height comparison with infant in supine position with flexed hips/knees

     a. Asymmetry evident in DDH

     b. Shortening of the femoral segment limits abduction and full extension

     c. Not helpful finding for detecting bilateral dislocation

  2. Limited abduction of affected hip in older child

  3. Indicators of hip instability in newborn—test each hip individually

     a. Barlow's sign

        (1) Positive when movement of femoral head can be felt as it slips out onto the posterior lip of acetabulum

        (2) Not diagnostic, but indicates need for surveillance

     b. Ortolani's sign (positive findings)

        (1) Newborn period—sometimes a "click" or "clunk" is heard as femoral head enters or exits acetabulum

        (2) After newborn period—"click" is less apparent and decreased abduction of flexed legs (at hip) is more significant

  4. Three degrees of hip dysplasia

     a. Subluxation

        (1) First degree, least severe

        (2) Femoral head rests in acetabulum

        (3) Can be dislocated partially by examination

     b. Dislocatable

        (1) Second degree

(2) Hip can be dislocated fully with manipulation, but is reducible

c. Dislocated hips

(1) Third degree, most severe

(2) Fixed dislocation

- Diagnostic Tests/Findings

1. Physical examination is most reliable

2. Radiographs

a. Not commonly used before 6 months of age

b. After 6 months of age assess femoral head/acetabulum relationship

3. Ultrasonography

a. Occasional use by experienced clinician

b. Assesses hip stability and acetabular development

- Management/Treatment

1. Identification during newborn period essential for good prognosis

2. Goal is to restore contact between femoral head and acetabulum

3. Subluxation in newborn

a. High incidence of spontaneous improvement in perinatal period

b. Observe and re-examine 3 to 4 weeks after birth

4. Dislocated hips

a. Treat at time of diagnosis

b. Before 6 months of age

(1) If unstable, stabilize with an abduction-flexion device, (e.g., Pavlik harness); triple diapers not effective

(2) If device is ineffective, surgery is indicated

c. If diagnosis made after 6 months of age

(1) Child usually too large and strong to tolerate brace

(2) Surgical reduction indicated

Talipes Equinovarus Congenita (Clubfoot)

- Definition: Common foot deformity that involves the foot and entire lower leg; classified into three groups, (1)congenital, (2) teratologic and (3) positional

- Etiology/Incidence

1. Cause unknown, possible inheritance factors or neuromuscular cause

2. Congenital form—about 75% of all cases

     a. 50% cases are bilateral

     b. 1:700 to 1:1000 live births; more common in males

  3. Teratologic form—associated with neuromuscular disorders, e.g., spina bifida, arthrogryposis, multiple congenital or a syndrome complex

  4. Positional form—normal foot that has been held in deformed position in utero

- Signs and Symptoms

  1. Congenital form

     a. Absence of other congenital abnormalities

     b. Variable rigidity of the foot

     c. Mild calf atrophy

     d. Mild hypoplasia of the tibia, fibula and bones of the foot

  2. Older child—calf and foot atrophy are more obvious than in infant regardless of how well corrected

- Differential Diagnosis

  1. Internal femoral torsion

  2. Internal tibial torsion

  3. Metatarsus adductus

  4. Neuromuscular disorders

- Physical Findings

  1. Small foot with limited dorsiflexion; usually obvious at birth

  2. Combination of deformities

     a. Results in 90 degree rotation of forefoot in all planes

     b. Leg and foot resemble shape of club

  3. Deep crease on medial border of foot

  4. Calf muscles thin and atrophic (more obvious in older child)

- Diagnostic Tests/Findings: Radiographs

  1. Rule out other conditions

  2. Done serially to evaluate progression of treatment

- Management/Treatment

  1. Refer to orthopedist

  2. Serial casting with manipulation begins at birth; usually 3 to 6 months

  3. If further corrections required, surgery indicated

Metatarsus Adductus/Metatarsus Varus

- Definition: Congenital deformity of forefoot
- Etiology/Incidence
    1. Uncertain etiology; often associated with abnormal intrauterine positioning
    2. Most common congenital foot deformity
    3. 10% of children with metatarsus also have developmental dysplasia of the hip
- Signs and symptoms
    1. Toeing-in; "pigeon-toed" gait in older child
    2. No pain
- Differential Diagnosis
    1. Internal femoral torsion
    2. Internal tibial torsion
    3. Equinovarus
- Physical Findings
    1. Adductus—forefoot adducted only; full ROM
    2. Varus—forefoot adducted and inverted; limited ROM
    3. Ankle joint has normal dorsiflexion and plantar flexion
- Diagnostic Tests/Findings
    1. Physical examination—usually sufficient to establish treatment plan
    2. Radiographs
        a. Usually unnecessary
        b. Used when:
            (1) Underlying congenital anomalies are suspected
            (2) Foot is unusually rigid
            (3) Failure of spontaneous improvement with growth
        c. Done serially to evaluate effects of stretching treatment
- Management/Treatment
    1. Supple deformity (adductus)
        a. Parents stretch forefoot in all planes of motion with each diaper change for 4 to 6 months
        b. Observe and follow-up
    2. Rigid deformity (varus)
        a. Serial casting or bracing done until age 2 years

      b. Then straight-laced/outflare shoes fitted for daytime until no chance of recurrence

      c. Surgical intervention required for child older than 4 years if significant residual metatarsus adductus persists

Tibial Torsion (Internal)

- Definition: Abnormal bowing (internal or external rotation) of the tibia
- Etiology/Incidence
  1. Combination of genetic factors and intrauterine position
  2. Usually not pathological
  3. Internal tibial torsion—12% at birth; usually resolves by 2 years
  4. External tibial torsion—develops after birth or by 2 years
- Signs and Symptoms
  1. Toeing-in appearance of child's legs when walking/running
  2. Rarely painful
  3. Tripping and falling may be noticed
- Differential Diagnosis
  1. Metatarsus adductus
  2. Femur anteversion
  3. Neuromuscular disorders
  4. Equinovarus
- Physical Findings
  1. No obvious deformity
  2. Full ROM
  3. Internal rotation of affected leg, flat feet, increased lumbar lordosis
- Diagnostic Tests/Findings
  1. Observation
  2. Angle measurement
     a. Between foot and thigh
     b. With ankle and knee position at 90 degree angle
     c. With child lying in prone position
- Management/Treatment

1. Reassure parents that most children have spontaneous correction with growth and need no treatment

2. Recommend supine sleeping position

Genu Varum (Bowleg)

- Definition: Lateral bowing of the tibia
- Etiology/Incidence
    1. Joint laxity may contribute to deformity
    2. Considered normal until 2 years
    3. May be related to intrauterine position
- Signs and Symptoms
    1. Parental concern common regarding appearance of legs
    2. Physiologic bowing of up to 20 degrees is normal in children until 18 to 24 months of age
    3. Bowing does not generally increase after walking
- Differential Diagnosis
    1. Rickets
    2. Blount disease (tibia vara)
    3. Injury to medial proximal epiphysis of tibia
    4. Osteogenesis imperfecta
    5. Achondroplasia, and other skeletal dysplasias
    6. Extreme physiologic bowing
- Physical Findings
    1. With child standing
        a. Clinically present—space between knees is greater than 5 cm or 2 inches with apposition of medial malleoli
        b. Resolution usually occurs without treatment
    2. Full range of motion
- Diagnostic Tests/Findings: Radiographs used for extreme and/or unilateral bowing
- Management/Treatment
    1. Observation to verify resolution
    2. Avoid unnecessary treatment of mild to moderate bowing
    3. Further evaluation with radiographs necessary if:
        a. Genu varum is present after 2 years of age

b. Progressive after 1 year of age

c. Unilateral involvement

d. Appears to be severe

e. Occurs in a high risk group, e.g., obese; African-American children with early ambulation

Genu Valgum (Knock-knee)

- Definition: Deformity in which the knees are abnormally close and space between the ankles is increased

- Etiology/Incidence

    1. A natural shifting occurs from varum to valgus between 30 to 60 months

    2. Normal alignment about 7 years of age

    3. Underlying bone disease can cause marked bilateral valgum

- Signs and Symptoms

    1. Parental concern common regarding appearance of legs

    2. Associated with pronation; more common in overweight children

- Differential Diagnosis

    1. Injury to lateral proximal tibial epiphysis causes unilateral valgum

    2. Rickets

    3. Hurler Syndrome

- Physical Findings

    1. Knees are together and distance between medial malleoli (ankles) is greater than 3 in. (7.5 cm) when standing

    2. Full range of motion

    3. No pain

    4. Child may walk and run awkwardly

    5. Normal knee alignment usually occurs before 8 years of age

- Diagnostic Tests/Findings: Radiographs used for extreme valgum; standing AP and lateral views

- Management

    1. Observation to verify resolution

    2. Further evaluation with radiographs necessary if:

        a. Genu valgum is present after 7 years of age

        b. Unilateral involvement

Transient (Toxic) Synovitis of the Hip

- Definition: Self-limiting inflammation of hip joint
- Etiology/Incidence
    1. Etiology uncertain; possible immune or viral process
    2. Most common cause of irritable hip
    3. Males affected more often
    4. Occurs most often in 2 to 6 year-olds, but also in 1 to 15 year-olds
- Signs and Symptoms
    1. Painful limp, or hip pain with acute or insidious onset, usually unilateral
    2. Afebrile or low-grade temperature
- Differential Diagnosis
    1. Septic arthritis
    2. Osteomyelitis
    3. Legg-Calve'-Perthes disease
    4. Juvenile monoarthritis
    5. Rheumatoid arthritis
    6. Slipped capital femoral epiphysis
- Physical Findings
    1. Range of motion of hip causes spasm and pain, particularly with internal rotation
    2. No obvious signs on inspection or with palpation
- Diagnostic Tests/Findings
    1. Radiography elicits no abnormal findings
    2. Normal or slightly elevated WBC
    3. Joint fluid aspiration—normal
- Management/Treatment
    1. Hospitalize child
        a. If high fever or severe symptoms are present
        b. To differentiate between transient synovitis and septic arthritis
    2. Analgesics (ibuprofen every 4 to 6 hours)
    3. Bedrest
    4. Benign, self-limiting illness

Legg-Calve'-Perthes Disease (LCPD)

- Definition: Aseptic or avascular necrosis of the femoral head
- Etiology/Incidence
    1. Unknown etiology; possibly due to vascular embarrassment
    2. Generally, slightly shorter stature/delayed bone age compared to peers
    3. Most common in Caucasian boys, ages 4 to 9 years
    4. 15% of cases are bilateral
- Signs and Symptoms
    1. Insidious onset of limp with knee pain
    2. Pain also in groin or lateral hip
    3. Pain less acute and severe than transient synovitis or septic arthritis
    4. Afebrile
- Differential Diagnosis
    1. Transient synovitis
    2. Septic arthritis
    3. Hematogenous osteomyelitis
    4. Various types of hemoglobinopathy
    5. Gaucher's disease
    6. Hypothyroidism
    7. Epiphyseal dysplasias
- Physical Findings
    1. Limited passive internal rotation and abduction of hip joint
    2. May be resisted by mild spasm or guarding
    3. Hip flexion contracture and leg muscle atrophy in long-standing cases
- Diagnostic Tests/Findings
    1. Radiograph studies
        a. Show disease progression and sphericity of femoral head
        b. Used initially for definitive diagnosis
        c. Subsequently used to assess reparative process
    2. Other laboratory studies not indicated
- Management/Treatment
    1. Goal—to restore range of motion while maintaining femoral head within acetabulum

2. Observation only if full ROM preserved

    a. Children < than 6 years of age

    b. Involvement of < than one-half the femoral head

3. Aggressive treatment

    a. Indicated when > one-half femoral head involved and in children older than 6 years

    b. Use of orthosis

        (1) Produce abduction with or without internal rotation

        (2) Document containment with radiographs

        (3) Worn until early reossification seen

        (4) Child allowed activity that is possible while in the brace

    c. Surgical treatment

        (1) Femoral osteotomy, shelf procedure

        (2) Used more commonly as alternative to orthosis

4. Patient/family education—inform family that LCPD lasts 1 to 3 years and is potentially serious if not treated properly

Growing Pains

- Definition: A controversial diagnosis of exclusion for (usually intermittent) lower extremity pain
- Etiology/Incidence
  1. Onset at 3 to 5 years of age, or more commonly, 8 to 12 years of age
  2. Related factors
     a. Rapid growth
     b. Puberty
     c. Fibrositis
     d. Weather
     e. Psychological factors
- Signs and Symptoms: Pain/ache localized to lower extremities; usually intermittent
- Differential Diagnosis
  1. Trauma
  2. Infection
  3. Hematologic causes—sickle cell, hemophilia
  4. Slipped capital femoral epiphysis

  5. Osgood-Schlatter

  6. Osteochondritis dissecans

- Physical Findings (usually none)

  1. No history of traumatic insult

  2. No loss of ambulation or mobility

  3. No systemic changes

  4. No edema or erythema

  5. Full range of motion

- Diagnostic Tests/Findings

  1. All laboratory studies normal—CBC with differential, ESR

  2. Radiograph of affected area normal

- Management/Treatment

  1. Prescribe anti-inflammatory medication

  2. Massage and heating pad to area

  3. Rest during painful episodes, activity as tolerated

Osgood-Schlatter Disease

- Definition: Inflammation of tibial tubercle from repetitive stresses in athletes with immature skeletal development

- Etiology/Incidence

  1. Tiny stress fractures in apophysis likely etiology

  2. Associated with a rapid growth spurt

  3. Occurs 11 to 14 years of age when immature cartilage susceptible to repeated trauma

- Signs and Symptoms: Pain and tenderness localized to tibial tubercle

- Differential Diagnosis

  1. Osteomyelitis

  2. Osteosarcoma

  3. Patellar tendonitis

- Physical Findings

  1. Point tenderness over tibial tubercle

  2. Prominence/enlargement of tibial tubercle compared with unaffected side

  3. 50% have bilateral involvement

- Diagnostic Tests/Findings
    1. Diagnosis accurate by clinical examination
    2. CT and MRI scans rarely indicated
    3. Radiographs
        a. Used to rule out presence of more serious bone pathology
        b. Lateral view
            (1) May demonstrate ossicle between patellar tendon and tibial tubercle
            (2) For pain which persists after skeletal maturity
        c. Rarely useful at follow-up
- Management/Treatment
    1. Self-limiting condition
    2. Conservative and largely symptomatic treatment
    3. Pain resolves with full ossification of tibial tubercle and closure of apophysis
    4. Activity limitations
        a. Complete avoidance of sports activities not recommended
        b. Limit activity to control pain at tibial tubercle
        c. Stretching exercises before activity, icing helpful afterwards
        d. Use knee immobilizer
            (1) Pain relief—briefly to avoid muscle atrophy
            (2) In combination with thigh muscle strengthening
    5. Corticosteroid injections—not recommended; may aggravate apophysitis
    6. Surgery
        a. Indicated if tubercle pain persists after skeletal maturity
        b. Excision of ossicle may ameliorate symptoms

Scoliosis (Idiopathic)

- Definition: Lateral curvature of spine
- Etiology/Incidence
    1. Multifactorial etiology
    2. 70% cases idiopathic
    3. Most common occurrence during adolescent growth spurt
    4. Female to male ratio of 8:1
    5. Mild curves occur equally between the sexes

    6. Positive family history in about 70% of cases

- Signs and Symptoms (usually asymptomatic)
  1. Infancy to school age—parents may notice alteration in back contour
  2. Adolescence—more likely detected on routine screening
  3. Rarely painful
- Differential Diagnosis
  1. Hip disease
  2. Transient synovitis
  3. Legg-Calve' Perthes disease
  4. Slipped capital femoral epiphysis
- Physical Findings: Inspection in standing position
  1. Asymmetry of shoulder height
  2. Uneven hip level
  3. Waistline uneven
  4. Thoracic spinal curve
  5. Rib asymmetry
  6. Unequal arm length
  7. Asymmetry of scapulae
- Diagnostic Tests/Findings
  1. Adams' forward-bending test
     - a. Child bends forward 90° or more, keeping knees straight, dropping head with arms hanging downward, elbows extended, palms together
     - b. Observed from caudal aspect to detect abnormal prominence of thoracic ribs
  2. Radiographs evaluate degree of deformity
- Management/Treatment
  1. If pain occurs, further evaluation required
  2. Treatment mode depends on severity of curve and child's age
     - a. Curves of 25 degrees
       - (1) No further evaluation/treatment if child skeletally mature
       - (2) Follow-up for possible progression if child is still growing
       - (3) Bracing treatment 80% successful
     - b. Curves of 40 to 50 degrees
       - (1) Likely to increase even after growth complete

      (2)   Surgery required for thoracic curve > 50 degrees or lumbar curve > 40 degrees

   3. Clinical pulmonary restriction may occur with thoracic curves > 75 degrees

Sports Injuries

- Definition: Musculoskeletal injuries occurring as a result of participation in athletic activities; most common include sprains/strains, fractures or overuse injuries

  1. Head and neck injuries

     a. Common in football and ice hockey

     b. Generally not severe

     c. Include brachial plexus injuries

     d. Concussions

  2. Back Injuries—low back pain caused by:

     a. Muscle strain

     b. Spondylolysis—overuse from repetitive hyperextension of back as in gymnastics, most likely in lower lumbar area

  3. Upper extremity injuries

     a. Anterior shoulder dislocation, shoulder separation

     b. Overuse injuries

        (1) Impingement syndrome—"pitcher's shoulder", "swimmer's shoulder" or "tennis shoulder"

        (2) Lateral epicondylitis—"tennis elbow"

  4. Lower extremity injuries

     a. Sprains

        (1) Medial collateral ligament sprain

        (2) Anterior cruciate sprain and tear

     b. Overuse injuries

        (1) Iliac apophysitis

        (2) Femoral stress fracture

        (3) Chondromalacia (chronic patellar pain "runner's knee")

- Etiology/Incidence

  1. Leading causes—trauma, improper training

  2. Contributing factors include fatigue and improper nutrition

  3. 20 million children participate in organized athletics

    4. One out of fourteen adolescents treated for athletic injury

    5. Highest frequency in adolescent boys; football and wrestling cause most injuries

- Signs and Symptoms
  1. Fracture
     a. Edema
     b. Erythema
     c. Ecchymosis
     d. Pain
     e. Obvious angulation
     f. Point tenderness
  2. Sprain
     a. Various degrees of pain
     b. Swelling
     c. Difficulty weight bearing
     d. Detectable joint laxity
     e. Decreased ROM
  3. Overuse—various degree of pain with or without activity limitations
- Differential Diagnosis: Possible underlying disease process of metabolic, neoplastic or infectious origins
- Physical Findings
  1. Fracture
     a. Decreased ROM
     b. Pain
     c. Obvious deformity
     d. Swelling
     e. Evidence of injury seen on radiographs at site of injury
     f. Localized tenderness
  2. Sprains—use subjective grading
     a. Grade I
        (1) Few fibers torn within ligament; does not compromise ligament's strength
        (2) Minimal pain and swelling
        (3) Full ROM

(4) No increase in joint laxity

b. Grade II

(1) Tears portion of the ligament

(2) Clinically significant pain and swelling

(3) Impairment of ROM

(4) Detectable increase in joint laxity

c. Grade III

(1) Complete tear of ligament

(2) Marked laxity evident when ligament is stressed

- Diagnostic Tests/Findings

   1. Physical examination and accurate history to evaluate injury

   2. Radiographs

   a. Injured area and contralateral area

   b. View open growth plate

   c. Rule out fracture or tumor

   d. Compare affected with nonaffected area

   3. MRI—utilized to evaluate torn ligaments or damage to cartilage

   4. Ultrasonography

- Management/Treatment

   1. Encourage sports physical examinations prior to participation in athletic events to identify conditions that may interfere/worsen with athletic participation

   2. Fractures—immobilization, ice, pain management, ROM exercise

   3. Sprain/strain

   a. Minimize hematoma and swelling with rest, ice, compression, elevation (RICE)

   b. ROM exercise

   c. Grade III sprains may require surgery

   4. Overuse Injuries

   a. Usually respond to conservative treatment, rest, ice and gradual return to athletic activities

   b. Nonsteroidal anti-inflammatory drugs prescribed to decrease inflammation and pain

   5. Refer to orthopedist

      a. If complex, open fracture

      b. If sprain/strain or overuse injuries not resolving with conservative treatment measures

6. Child can return to athletic activity based on functional evaluation of actions required during the activity

Slipped Capital Femoral Epiphysis

- Definition: Spontaneous dislocation of femoral head (capital epiphysis) both downward and backward relative to femoral neck and secondary to disruption of epiphyseal plate
- Etiology/Incidence
  1. Etiology unknown—thought to be precipitated by hormone changes related to puberty
  2. Generally occurs without severe, sudden force or trauma; sometimes related to trauma
  3. Usually occurs during growth spurt (ages 10 to 17), and before menarche in girls
  4. Rare condition, 1:100,000 to 8:100,000
  5. More common in males and African-Americans
  6. One-quarter to one-third have bilateral involvement, with one side following the other
  7. Incidence greater among obese adolescents with sedentary lifestyles
- Signs and Symptoms
  1. Varies with acuity of the process
  2. Most children have limp
  3. Varying degrees of aching or pain (in groin, often referred to thigh/ knee)
  4. Some have acute, severe pain and inability to walk or move hip
- Differential Diagnosis
  1. Knee complaint with no obvious cause
  2. Trauma
  3. Septic arthritis
  4. Transient (toxic) synovitis
  5. Juvenile arthritis
  6. Legg-Calve'-Perthes disease
- Physical Findings
  1. Unable to properly flex hip as femur abducts/rotates externally
  2. May observe limb shortening, resulting from proximal displacement of metaphysis

- Diagnostic Tests/Findings
    1. Accurate history combined with knowledge of etiological factors
    2. Radiographs
        a. Confirms diagnosis
        b. Shows degree of slipping between femoral head and neck
    3. Laboratory studies
        a. Depend on findings from physical examination and history
        b. Done to rule out associated causes of infection or inflammation
- Management/Treatment
    1. Immediate referral to orthopedist
    2. Treatment goal is to prevent further slippage
    3. No ambulation is allowed
    4. Surgery
        a. Pin fixation, open epiphysiodesis using bone graft
        b. Done to stabilize upper femur and cause growth plate to close
    5. Monitor other hip for same problem

Juvenile Rheumatoid Arthritis

- Definition: Chronic, idiopathic arthritis characterized by presence of chronic synovial inflammation with associated swelling, pain, heat and/or limited ROM
- Etiology/Incidence
    1. Cause unknown, possible etiological factors include infections, autoimmunity, genetic predisposition or stress and trauma
    2. Most common rheumatic disease of childhood
    3. Mean incidence 16:100,000; estimated 65,000 to 70,000 children in U.S. affected
    4. Mean age of onset 1 to 3 years; rarely before 6 months
    5. Females affected twice as often as males
- Signs and Symptoms
    1. Range of severity of disease
        a. May be mild in one joint with no symptoms
        b. May have severe disease in many joints with fever, rash lymphadenopathy, and organomegaly
    2. Signs of joint inflammation
        a. Swelling with heat

      b.   Redness

      c.   Pain

      d.   Limited ROM

   3. May also exhibit

      a.   Morning stiffness, limp, refusal to walk

      b.   Irritability, fatigue

   4. Hallmark of systemic disease is high spiking fever with rash

- Differential Diagnosis

   1. Hip disease

   2. Transient synovitis

   3. Legg-Calve'-Perthes disease

   4. Slipped capital femoral epiphysis

   5. Leukemia

   6. Other rheumatic diseases, e.g., kawasaki, systemic lupus erythematosus (SLE)

- Physical Findings

   1. Diagnostic criteria

      a.   Age of onset < 16 years

      b.   Joint involvement

         (1) Arthritis (swelling/effusion) in one or more joints, or

         (2) Presence of 2 or more of these signs:

            (a) Range of motion limitation

            (b) Tenderness

            (c) Pain with movement

            (d) Increased heat

      c.   Duration of disease 6 weeks or longer

      d.   Further classified by onset type during first 6 months

      e.   Exclusion of other forms of juvenile arthritis

   2. Polyarthritis (polyarticular disease)

      a.   40% to 50% of all cases

      b.   5 or more inflamed joints

      c.   May be acute or gradual onset

      d.   Symmetric pattern

    e. Commonly affects large joints, e.g., knees, wrists, elbows, ankles

    f. May not complain of pain

3. Oligoarthritis (pauciarticular disease)

    a. 40% to 50% of cases

    b. 4 or less joints affected

    c. Gradual onset

    d. Can be painless

    e. Often confined to lower extremity joints, knee or ankles

    f. Usually no systemic signs, except for chronic uveitis

        (1) Early onset (< than 5 years of age)

            (a) Asymmetric involvement

            (b) Large joints commonly affected

            (c) Hips and sacroiliac (SI) joint spared

            (d) Systemic symptoms usually not present

        (2) Late onset

            (a) Asymmetric involvement

            (b) Hips and SI joint involvement present

4. Systemic

    a. 10% to 20% of cases

    b. Occurs in late childhood > 8 years of age

    c. Systemic onset may precede arthritis appearance by weeks, months, or years

    d. High, daily intermittent spiking fevers is hallmark symptom

        (1) Temperature elevations occur once or twice/day

        (2) To 39° C (102° F) or higher with quick return to baseline temperature or lower

    e. Discrete rash present

        (1) Salmon-colored nonpruritic macular lesions

        (2) Commonly on trunk and proximal extremities

        (3) Most characteristic feature is transient nature

    f. Painful multiple joint involvement

    g. Associated findings

        (1) Hepatosplenomegaly

        (2) Lymphadenopathy

(3)   Visceral disease, e.g., pericarditis, hepatitis

(4)   Pulmonary involvement

(5)   CNS

h.   50% of cases have chronic, destructive arthritis

5.   Associated problems

   a.   Periarticular soft tissue edema

   b.   Intra-articular effusion

   c.   Hypertrophy of synovial membrane

6.   Synovitis—painful inflammation of synovial membrane, with fluctuating swelling

   a.   May develop insidiously, existing months to years without joint destruction

   b.   May cause joint damage in relatively short time

- Diagnostic Tests/Findings

1.   No specific laboratory studies, however abnormalities may be found

2.   CBC—characteristics of chronic anemia of inflammation

   a.   Moderately severe anemia; hemoglobin between 7 and 10 g/dL

   b.   Leukocytosis

3.   Synovial fluid WBC count—moderately elevated 10,000/mm^3 to 20,000/mm^3

4.   Rheumatoid factor present in:

   a.   Approximately 15% to 20% of cases

   b.   Child with later onset, or older child

   c.   Child with prominent symmetric polyarthritis with:

      (1)   Involvement of small joints

      (2)   Subcutaneous rheumatoid nodules

      (3)   Articular erosions

      (4)   Poor functional outcome

5.   Antinuclear antibodies (ANA)—seropositivity for antibodies

   a.   Present in about 40% of cases

   b.   Presence correlated significantly with development of chronic uveitis

   c.   Less commonly found in older boys or in systemic disease

   d.   Valuable diagnostic measure for JRA

      (1)   Usually not positive in other childhood illnesses

      (2)   Positive in SLE, scleroderma, transient acute viral disease

6. Radiographs

    a. Early changes

        (1) Soft tissue swelling

        (2) Juxta-articular osteoporosis

        (3) Periosteal new bone apposition

    b. Development of ossification centers may be age accelerated

    c. Stunting of bone growth secondary to premature epiphyseal closure

    d. Cervical spine disease characteristic feature

7. Joint disease may be better evaluated with MRI, CT, bone scans

- Management/Treatment

  1. Goal is to control clinical manifestations and prevent/minimize deformity

  2. Suppress inflammation and fever

    a. Use NSAID (ibuprofen, naproxen) for most children

    b. In severe, progressive disease resistant to therapy

        (1) Methotrexate

           (a) Most successful and safe drug

           (b) 10 to 15 mg/m^2/once a week

           (c) No oncogenic potential or risk of sterility

        (2) Hydroxychloroquine—useful adjunctive agent

           (a) Retinopathy possible adverse reaction

           (b) Low dose, e.g., 5 mg/kg/day

           (c) Frequent ophthalmologic examinations required

        (3) Gold salts—given IM or as oral compound

           (a) Toxicities are hematologic, renal, hepatic

           (b) Must be constantly monitored during treatment

        (4) Glucocorticoid drugs

           (a) Indicated for resistant or life-threatening disease

           (b) Ophthalmic administration for chronic uveitis

           (c) Toxicities, e.g., Cushings syndrome and growth retardation

  3. Maintenance of function and prevention of deformity

    a. Prescriptions for physical and occupational therapies

    b. Balanced program of rest and activity

    c. Selective splinting

    d. Encourage normal play

    e. Avoid high levels of stress on inflamed weight-bearing joints

4. Counsel parents about course of chronic disease with exacerbations

5. Refer to pediatric rheumatologist

Systemic Lupus Erythematosus

- Definition: Multisystem disease characterized by widespread inflammatory involvement of connective tissues with immune-complex vasculitis

- Etiology/Incidence

1. Unknown, but many factors implicated

    a. Excessive sun exposure

    b. Drug reaction

    c. Infection

    d. Hereditary

    e. Immunogenetic

2. Can develop at any age

    a. Usually after 5 years of age

    b. More common during adolescent years

3. Females affected 8 times more often after 5 years of age

4. Relatively more boys affected at younger ages

- Signs and Symptoms:

1. Fever

2. Malaise

3. Weight loss

4. Facial rash

- Differential Diagnosis

1. Juvenile rheumatoid arthritis (JRA)

2. Other forms of acute glomerulonephritis

3. Hemolytic anemia

4. Leukemia

5. Allergic or contact dermatitis

6. Idiopathic seizure disorder

7. Mononucleosis

8. Acute rheumatic fever with carditis

9. Septicemia

- Physical Findings

    1. Onset is usually acute—three quarters of children usually diagnosed within 6 months of symptoms

    2. Diagnosis delayed for others by 4 to 5 years

    3. Early diagnostic suspicion based on:

        a. Episodic, multisystem constellation of clinical disease

        b. Associated with persistent antinuclear antibody (ANA) seropositivity

    4. Severity of manifestations variable

        a. Rapidly fatal illness

        b. Insidious chronic disability with multisystem exacerbation

    5. Each exacerbation of disease tends to mimic previous episodes

    6. Rash

        a. Characteristic of acute onset or exacerbation

        b. Malar erythematous

        c. Butterfly distribution across bridge of nose and over each cheek

    7. Arthritis

        a. Affects majority of children

        b. Involves small joints

        c. Transient and migratory

        d. Never erosive

        e. No permanent deformity in 95% of cases

    8. Pericarditis is most common manifestation of cardiac involvement

    9. Central and peripheral nervous system manifestations

        a. Recurrent headaches

        b. Seizures

        c. Chorea

        d. Frank psychosis

    10. Kidney involvement in all children

- Diagnostic Tests/Findings

    1. Leukopenia—otherwise unexplained, common at onset

2. ANA—positive in most children

3. Coombs test—often positive

4. Rheumatoid factor (RF) and other antitissue antibodies—often positive

- Management/Treatment

  1. Long-term supportive care

     a. Maintain adequate nutrition

     b. Maintain fluid and electrolyte balance

     c. Early recognition and treatment of infections

     d. Control of hypertension

  2. Anti-inflammatory drugs useful for minor manifestations, e.g., myalgia and arthralgia

  3. Counsel parents and child about chronic nature of disease with repeated exacerbations, remissions often prolonged over many years

Osteomyelitis

- Definition: Inflammation of bone caused by a pyogenic organism

- Etiology/Incidence

  1. Causative agents

     a. In all age groups, *Staphylococcus aureus*

     b. Consider also *Streptococcus pneumoniae* and *Haemophilus influenzae*

  2. Peak ages—infancy (less than 1 year) and preadolescence (9 to 11 years)

  3. More frequent in males

- Signs and Symptoms

  1. May appear well

  2. Systemic involvement ranging from malaise to shock

  3. Neonates usually afebrile, swollen or motionless limb early sign

  4. Earliest symptom in child may be refusal to bear weight

- Differential Diagnosis

  1. Neoplasm

  2. Contusion

  3. Non-displaced fracture

  4. Sickle cell crisis

- Physical Findings

1. Early signs

    a. Fever

    b. Local bone tenderness

2. If subperiostal or soft tissue abscess develops, fluctuant mass present

- Diagnostic Tests/Findings

    1. WBC & ESR—elevated, but not diagnostic

    2. Radiographs—at earliest stage may show soft-tissue swelling

    3. Bone scan

        a. May be initially normal

        b. Repeated after 48 hours, may show cold/photopenic areas (indicating avascular sites)

    4. Aspiration—always indicated to identify pathogen

- Management/Treatment

    1. Refer to physician

    2. Delivery of antibiotic to all infected tissue

        a. Broad spectrum antibiotic initially

        b. Follow with antibiotic

            (1) Most effective against isolated organism

            (2) Least toxic antibiotic

            (3) Used for 4 to 6 weeks

    3. Surgery reserved for:

        a. Child with systemic illness

        b. Worsening symptoms under medical treatment

        c. Abscess present

Duchenne Muscular Dystrophy (DMD)

- Definition: Progressive genetic disorder that affects muscles in lower extremities and eventually muscles of upper extremities, chest wall and heart

- Etiology/Incidence

    1. X-linked recessive genetic disorder which results in absence or severe deficiency of cytoskeletal protein known as dystrophin

    2. Most commonly inherited neuromuscular disease in children

    3. Affects 1:3,500 males; 1:1,750 females are carriers

    4. Average age of diagnosis is 3 to 5 years of age

- Signs and Symptoms
  1. At birth—rarely affected clinically
  2. Becomes clinically evident by 3 to 5 years of age
     a. Abnormalities of gait and posture
     b. History of developmental "clumsiness"
     c. Large "muscular" looking calves
     d. Inability to keep up with peers when running
  3. Progresses over next 2 decades—weakness more evident in proximal muscles
  4. Wheelchair dependent by 10 to 12 years of age
     a. Muscles decrease in size
     b. Contractures progress with loss of joint mobility
     c. Kyphoscoliosis develops with respiratory function problems
  5. Complications from:
     a. Cardiac involvement
     b. Nervous system involvement
     c. Musculoskeletal deformities
     d. Compromised respiratory function
  6. Eventual death from cardiac or respiratory failure
- Differential Diagnosis
  1. Hypothyroidism
  2. Carnitine deficiency
  3. Spinal muscular atrophy
  4. Fascioscapulohumeral dystrophy
  5. Other types of muscular dystrophies of childhood
- Physical Findings
  1. Preschooler—3 to 5 years of age
     a. Increasing lumbar lordosis
     b. Pelvic waddling
     c. Gowers' maneuver
        (1) Child may "walk" hands up legs to attain a standing position when arising from floor
        (2) Indication of pelvic girdle weakness
        (3) Distinctive in DMD, but seen in other conditions as well

     d. Proximal muscle strength and ankle reflexes may be depressed

     e. Calf hypertrophy present

  2. Cardiac involvement in all patients

  3. Contractures develop before ambulation is compromised

     a. Iliotibial bands

     b. Hip flexors

     c. Heel cords

- Diagnostic Tests/Findings

  1. Obtain 3-generation family history

     a. May be positive history of muscle disorders, weakness, DMD

     b. Carrier females have symptoms of weakness or cramping of muscles

  2. Laboratory studies

     a. Creatine kinase (CK)—will be markedly elevated in affected males (15,000 to 35,000 IU/L)

     b. EMG—distinctively myopathic

     c. ECG—changes are distinctive

       (1) Tall right precordial R waves

       (2) Deep Q waves in left precordial and limb leads

     d. Muscle biopsy—histopathologic findings

       (1) Groups of necrotic degenerating fibers most prominent

       (2) Variation in fiber size evident

       (3) Dystrophic immunoreactivity confirms DMD

     e. Genetic testing

       (1) Utilizes WBC from blood specimen

       (2) DNA analysis of DMD gene confirms diagnosis

- Management/Treatment

  1. No cure available at present

  2. Goal of treatment is essentially symptomatic aimed at delay of progression and supportive care

  3. Maintenance of strength and mobility

     a. Exercise

     b. Use of ankle/foot orthoses, bracing, spinal support measures and wheelchair as needed

4. Consultation with neuromuscular disease specialty team for diagnosis and for periodic evaluations

5. Refer family for genetic testing/counseling

6. Counsel family regarding course of disease

7. Refer parents

   a. To other families who have children with DMD

   b. To other community resources for support

Questions
Select the best answer:

1. Which of the following disorders is usually associated with adduction of the forefoot?

    a. Internal femoral torsion
    b. Talipes equinovarus congenita
    c. Genu valgum
    d. Internal tibial torsion

2. The most common rheumatoid disease of childhood is:

    a. Systemic lupus erythematosus
    b. Kawasaki disease
    c. JRA
    d. Legg-Calve'-Perthes disease

3. Radiographic findings of disease progression and sphericity of femoral head is helpful in the diagnosis and follow-up of:

    a. Transient synovitis of the hip
    b. Osgood-Schlatter disease
    c. Legg-Calve'-Perthes disease
    d. Slipped capital femoral epiphysis

4. A 4-year-old boy is brought in by his mother concerned about a sudden onset of a painful limp in his right leg 2 days ago. Today he has a low-grade fever. Which of the following diagnoses is most likely?

    a. Osgood-Schlatter
    b. JRA
    c. Osteomyelitis
    d. Transient synovitis of the hip

5. Which of the following would be the most appropriate initial management of a newborn diagnosed with developmental dysplasia of the hip?

    a. Observe and re-examine at 2 week well-child visit
    b. Triple diapering in nursery
    c. Pavlik harness
    d. Surgical reduction

6. A physical finding not usually associated with talipes equinovarus congenita is:

    a. Contracture of the illiotibial bands
    b. Deep crease on medial border of foot
    c. Atrophy of calf muscles
    d. Small foot with limited dorsiflexion

7. A characteristic feature of polyarticular JRA disease is:

    a. The involvement of 5 or more inflammed joints
    b. Confinement to lower extremity joints, knees and ankles
    c. Asymmetric involvement
    d. High, daily intermittent spiking fevers

8. ANA seropositivity for antibodies is:

    a. A valuable diagnostic marker for JRA
    b. Is not positive in any other childhood diseases
    c. More commonly found in older boys or in systemic disease
    d. Present in over 75% of cases

9. Dislocation in the hip of a child six months or older may typically present with:

    a. Asymmetry of skin folds
    b. Atrophied hip muscles
    c. Positive Galeazzi sign
    d. Negative Trendelenburg sign

10. For a newborn, the correct management of hip dislocation should include:

    a. Use of flexion-abduction device, such as Pavlic harness to stabilize hip
    b. Follow and observe closely for 3 to 4 weeks, then refer to orthopedist
    c. Surgical reduction
    d. Traction for 6 weeks

11. Duchenne muscular dystrophy is characterized by which of the following signs and symptoms?

    a. At birth affected infants are notably hypotonic, "floppy" babies
    b. Earliest symptom is often refusal to bear weight
    c. Abnormalities of gait and posture become evident during preschool years
    d. Unable to keep up with peers when running by school-age

12. Most children with Duchenne muscular dystrophy become wheel-chair dependent by what age?

    a. 7 to 9 years of age
    b. 10 to 12 years of age
    c. 14 to 16 years of age
    d. Highly variable depending on response to treatment

13. School-aged children and young adolescents actively involved in athletic activities may not be at increased risk for:

    a. Osgood-Schlatter disease
    b. Chondromalacia
    c. Spondylolysis
    d. Slipped capital femoral epiphyis

14. Management of scoliosis depends on the severity of curve as well as the age of the child. Which of the following would require surgical intervention?

    a. Curves of 25 degrees in a child who is still growing
    b. Thoracic and/or lumbar curve greater than 25 degrees even if growth is complete
    c. Thoracic curve greater than 40 degrees or lumbar curve greater than 50 degrees
    d. Thoracic curve greater than 50 degrees or lumbar curve greater than 40 degrees

15. In performing a diagnostic work-up and management plan for a child with osteomyelitis, which of the following is not accurate or recommended?

    a. Elevated ESR confirms diagnosis
    b. Aspiration is always indicated
    c. Antibiotic treatment for 4 to 6 weeks is recommended
    d. Surgery is recommended if abscess is present

16. A 6-year-old child presents with a limp and knee pain. The PNP finds limited passive internal rotation and abduction of the hip joint on physical examination. The most likely diagnosis is

    a. Slipped capital femoral epiphysis
    b. Osgood-Schlatter disease
    c. Transient synovitis of the hip
    d. Legg-Calve'-Perthes disease

17. Which of the following statements is true about acute osteomyelitis?

    a. Occurs more frequently in females than males
    b. Peak ages are infancy (less than 1 year) and preadolescence (9 to 11 years)
    c. Most common sites are radius and ulna
    d. A self-limiting disorder

18. Which of the following statements is not true of slippped capital femoral epiphysis?

    a. Thought to be precipitated by hormone changes during puberty
    b. Unilateral involvement is more common than bilateral
    c. More common among males and African-Americans
    d. Thought to be caused by repetitive stresses in young athletes prior to growth spurt

19. Genu varum is considered an abnormal condition when:

    a. Extreme knock-knees continues after 7 years of age
    b. Extreme bowing continues after 2 years of age
    c. Parents are concerned about their child's appearance
    d. Evident before 2 years of age

20. Tibial torsion is commonly associated with:

    a. Pain
    b. Restricted ROM
    c. Internal rotation of affected leg
    d. Occurrence in adolescents 13 to 16 years of age

21. Which of the following diagnoses is associated with contracture of one of the sternocleidomastoid muscles?

    a. Lordosis
    b. Torticollis
    c. Scoliosis
    d. Kyphosis

22. Sports injuries are commonly associated with:

    a. Improper training
    b. Higher frequency in females
    c. Scoliosis
    d. Low socioeconomic status

23. Initial treatment of a sprain includes which of the following

    a. Rest, ice, compression, elevation
    b. Heat, ROM exercise, compression, elevation
    c. Rest, heat, compression, elevation
    d. Rest, ice, ibuprofen, compression

24. The most definitive feature(s) for a diagnosis of "growing pains" includes:

    a. Exclusion of other causes of lower extremity pain
    b. Pain, swelling, erythema
    c. Loss of ambulation
    d. Decreased ROM

25. Systemic-onset JRA is most commonly associated with:

    a. High, daily intermittent spiking fevers and rash
    b. Single joint involvement
    c. Positive RF factor
    d. Painless joint involvement

26. Signs and symptoms associated with Duchenne muscular dystrophy are

    a. History of "clumsiness", delayed motor development
    b. Visual-motor disturbance, calf hypertrophy
    c. Delayed motor development, positive Ortolani maneuver
    d. History of "clumsiness", visual-motor disturbance

27. Which of the following are suspected etiologic factors of systemic lupus erythematosis (SLE)?

    a. Excessive sun exposure, drug reaction, infection
    b. Drug reaction, immunogenetic factors, lack of sun
    c. Excessive sun exposure, arthritis, sickle cell crisis
    d. Infection, immunogenetic factors, arthritis

28. Complications of SLE commonly include which of the following?

    a. Pericarditis, arthritis, nephritis
    b. Encephalitis, nephritis, pericarditis
    c. Nephritis, arthritis, rheumatic fever
    d. Nephritis, hemolytic anemia, contact dermatitis

29. Which of the following children need an immediate orthopedic referral?

    a. A 6-year-old with mild bowing of the lower legs
    b. A 6-month-old with internal tibial torsion
    c. A three-week-old with fixed metatarsus adductus
    d. A newborn with a positive Pavlic sign

30. Antonio is a newborn and the NP notes on physical assessment that both his feet turn in. When attempting range of motion, she finds that both feet move relatively freely in all directions. Antonio has:

    a. Clubfoot
    b. Congenital hip dysplasia
    c. Metatarsus adductus
    d. Tibial torsion

31. Which of the following is an appropriate goal for a child being treated for osteomyelitis?

    a. Prohibiting activities
    b. Complete course of antibiotic therapy
    c. Encouraging a high-iron diet
    d. Restricting visitors

32. In a newborn, a diagnosis of hip dislocations is confirmed by:

    a. A longer left leg when both legs are extended
    b. Resistance of the left leg when both legs are flexed and abducted
    c. Flaccidity of the left leg following extension of both legs with return to flexion
    d. Tonic neck reflex in which the left leg is flexed

33. Which of the following statements is true for slipped capital femoral epiphysis?

    a. More common in females
    b. Generally occurs following severe sudden trauma
    c. Incidence more common in athletes
    d. The goal of treatment is to stabilize or improve the position of the femoral head

34. In Legg-Calve'-Perthes disease, which of the following signs and symptoms are seen?

    a. Insidious onset of limp with knee and groin pain
    b. Sudden onset of limp and pain in lateral hip
    c. Fever and insidious onset of limp
    d. Afebrile and sudden onset of limp

35. Which of the following is true for idiopathic scoliosis which occurs primarily in adolescents?

   a. Mild curves occur equally between the sexes
   b. Generally there is no family history
   c. Back pain is usually associated with curves of 35 degrees or greater
   d. Bracing is indicated for thoracic curves of 10 to 25 degrees

Answers

1. b	13. d	25. a
2. c	14. d	26. a
3. c	15. a	27. a
4. d	16. d	28. a
5. c	17. b	29. c
6. a	18. d	30. c
7. a	19. b	31. b
8. a	20. c	32. b
9. c	21. b	33. d
10. a	22. a	34. a
11. c	23. a	35. a
12. b	24. a	

Bibliography

Behrman, R. E., Kliegman, R. M., & Jenson, H. B. (Eds.). (2004). *Nelson's textbook of pediatrics* (17th ed.). Philadelphia: W. B. Saunders.

Berman, S. (1996). *Pediatric decision-making.* (3rd ed.). St. Louis: Mosby.

Cassidy, J. T., & Petty, R. E. (Eds.) (2001). *Textbook of pediatric rheumatology* (4th ed.). Philadelphia: W. B. Saunders.

Hoekelman, R. A., Adam, H. M., Nelson, N. M., Weitzman, M. L. & Wilson, M. H. (Eds.). (2001). *Primary pediatric care* (3rd ed.). St. Louis: Mosby-Year Book.

Kulling, F. A. (2003). Special considerations in the pediatric and adolescent athlete. In J. DeLee & D. D. Oreg's, *DeLee and Oreg's orthopedic sports medicine* (2nd. ed. pp. 615-736). Philadelphia: W. B. Saunders

McIlvain-Simpson, G. (2000). Juvenile rheumatoid arthritis. In P. L. Jackson & J. A. Vessey (Eds.), *Primary care of a child with a chronic condition.* (3rd ed.). St. Louis: Mosby.

McMillan, J., DeAngelis, C., Feigin, R., & Warshaw, J. (Eds.). (1999). *Oskis' pediatrics: Principles and practice* (3rd ed.). Philadelphia: Lippincott Williams & Wilkens.

Morrissy, R., & Weinstein, S. (Eds.). (2001). *Lovell & Winter's pediatric orthopaedics* (5th Ed.). Philadelphia: Lippincott Williams & Wilkins.

Verst, A. (1997). Musculoskeletal system. In J. A. Fox (Ed.). *Primary health care of children* (pp. 628–666). St. Louis: Mosby.

Neurological Disorders

Susan Heighway

Seizure Disorders/Epilepsy

- Definition

  1. Seizures—disturbances of normal nerve cell function characterized by uncontrolled, spontaneous electrical activity in the brain, that may result in loss of consciousness, altered body movements or disturbances of sensation and behavior

  2. Seizure disorder (epilepsy)—condition of recurrent seizures

  3. Status epilepticus—a series of rapidly, repetitive seizures without any periods of consciousness between them

- Etiology/Incidence

  1. Caused by any event with potential to produce insult to the brain

  2. Multiple causes; specific etiologies remain uncertain for 50% of cases

     a. Genetic component or familial predisposition

     b. Genetic disorders—tuberous sclerosis; neurofibromatosis

     c. Hemorrhage (intracranial)

     d. CNS infection (encephalitis, meningitis)

     e. Head trauma

     f. Developmental defects of brain

     g. Biochemical factors (inborn metabolic errors, electrolyte imbalance)

     h. Intracranial tumors

     i. Toxic ingestions—e.g., alcohol

     j. Poor drug compliance or altered drug metabolism because of illness

  3. Incidence varies greatly with age

     a. 1:1000 during first year of life

     b. 50% of all cases of epilepsy occur before age 25

  4. Variation in clinical manifestations due to location of brain involved

- Signs and Symptoms: International Seizure Classification System (1985) used to group seizures with similar clinical presentations

  1. Partial seizures

     a. Simple partial seizures

        (1) Characterized by seizure activity restricted to one side of body

        (2) No loss of consciousness and no postictal state

        (3) Motor—part of body or entire side (e.g., arm, leg, Jacksonian march, postural, vocalizations)

        (4) Sensory—visual, auditory, olfactory, parasthesias

        (5)   Autonomic—e.g., tachycardia, pallor, sweating, flushing

        (5)   Psychic—e.g., fearful or feelings of déjà vu

  b. Complex partial seizures—variety of clinical expressions

        (1)   Limited to impairment of consciousness, for 30 seconds or longer

        (2)   Cognitive symptomatology

            (a)   Abrupt alteration in mental state

            (b)   Involves disruption of time relationships and memory

        (3)   Affective symptomatology—inexplicable feelings, e.g., fear or dread without obvious cause

        (4)   Somatosensory disturbances

            (a)   Distortions of perception or hallucinations

            (b)   May involve taste, smell, vision

        (5)   Automatisms

            (a)   Occur in 50% to 75% of cases

            (b)   Semi-purposeful perseverative movements

            (c)   May involve walking, sucking, lip-pursing or picking at clothing

2. Generalized seizures—involve electrical discharges of both hemispheres of the brain usually with some loss of consciousness

  a. Absence seizures (petit mal)

        (1)   Onset between 4 and 8 years of age, higher incidence in girls

        (2)   Brief generalized, nonconvulsive episode with no aura and no postictal state

        (3)   Characterized by interruption of activity, staring and unresponsiveness

        (4)   Usually lasts between 5 and 15 seconds

        (5)   Episode begins and ends abruptly

        (6)   Child may be unaware of episode

  b. Tonic-clonic (grand mal)

        (1)   Consists of motor manifestations with loss of consciousness

        (2)   May begin with aura

        (3)   Tonic phase

            (a)   Sustained contraction of muscles

            (b)   Person falls to ground

            (c)   Extensor posturing and tonic contraction

            (d)   Lasts less than 1 minute

(4) Clonic phase

(a) Bilateral and rhythmic jerking

(b) May bite tongue

(c) Bowel or bladder incontinence may occur

(d) Stops after several minutes

(5) Postictal phase

(a) Period of cortical inhibition

(b) Vomiting

(c) Confusion and lethargy

(d) Gradual recovery of consciousness

c. Myoclonic seizures

(1) Brief, sudden muscle contractions

(2) May involve only one part of body or be generalized

(3) May occur in clusters

(4) May be no alteration in consciousness

d. Infantile spasms

(1) Onset during first year of life; usually between 4 and 8 months

(2) Brief, symmetric contraction of muscles in neck, trunk and extremities

(3) Spasms may be flexor, extensor or mixed

(4) Often in clusters up to 100 individual spasms

(5) Classified in two groups—infants with cryptogenic spasms have good prognosis whereas those with symptomatic type have a specific etiological factor identified and an 80% to 90% risk of mental retardation

e. Atonic

(1) Also termed "drop" attacks

(2) Characterized by sudden loss of muscle tone, which may result in head nodding or mild flexing of legs

(3) Usually no alteration in consciousness

f. Lennox-Gastaut syndrome

(1) Severe epileptic encephalopathy

(2) Characterized by variety of primary, generalized seizures

(3) Onset between 3 and 5 years of age

(4) Mental retardation and cerebral palsy common prior to onset

(5) Frequently preceded by infantile spasms

- Differential Diagnosis

    1. Breathholding spells—usually under 6 years of age

    2. Sleep disorders, e.g., narcolepsy

    3. Tics

    4. Complicated migraine headaches

    5. Syncope—more common in adolescence

    6. Gastroesophogeal reflux

    7. Benign paroxysmal vertigo

    8. Pseudoseizures

- Diagnostic Tests/Findings

    1. Clinical versus laboratory diagnosis

    2. Complete history

        a. Detailed description of seizure—onset, type, duration

        b. Previous seizures and frequency

        c. Evidence of infection

        d. Abnormal behavior

        e. Previous static or progressive neurologic/developmental dysfunction

        f. Pica; possible ingestion

        g. Trauma

        h. Birth history

        i. Current medication including anticonvulsants

        j. Family history of febrile and nonfebrile seizure

    3. Laboratory studies—to identify possible underlying etiology

        a. Serum fasting glucose, calcium, magnesium and serum electrolyte levels

        b. Seizures and mental retardation suggestive of metabolic problem

            (1) Plasma amino acids

            (2) Blood ammonia

            (3) Blood lactate and pyruvate

            (4) Urinary organic acids

            (5) Cytogenetic analysis

        c. Other studies as determined by history/physical findings

    4. Lumbar puncture—not routine

5. Neuroimaging studies

    a. Skull radiographs—rarely indicated, but helpful to rule out skull fracture

    b. Cranial CT and MRI

        (1) For detection of structural abnormalities

        (2) Indicated for:

            (a) A changing seizure pattern

            (b) Focal or lateralized abnormalities

            (c) History of trauma

            (d) Focally abnormal EEG

            (e) Evidence of increased intracranial pressure

            (f) Known or suspected specific white or gray matter disease

            (g) First seizure in all adolescents

    c. MRI more sensitive for detection of low grade tumors

    d. CT more sensitive to small foci or calcifications

6. EEG—measures physiologic function of brain

    a. Performed on all children, at least initially, to evaluate seizures

    b. Interpret in context of child's age, history, and physical findings

    c. Recorded for 1-hour, during periods of wakefulness and sleeping

    d. Helps to define seizure type

    e. Epileptiform EEG supports diagnosis; normal EEG does not exclude diagnosis

- Physical Findings

1. Physical examination can be abnormal with underlying cerebral pathology

2. Transient abnormal neurologic signs common during and after seizures

    a. Intention tremor

    b. Incoordination

    c. Weakness of one or more extremities

    d. Pathologic exaggeration of reflexes

    e. Confusion

3. Warning signs of serious neurologic problems

    a. Asymmetric pupils

    b. Signs of increased intracranial pressure

    c. Focal deficits

Table 1

Antiepileptic Drugs and Type of Seizures

Type of Seizure	Drug(s) of Choice	Drugs also Used
Generalized tonic/clonic	Carbamazepine Valproic acid	Phenobarbital Phenytoin
Simple/complex partial	Carbamazepine Valproic acid	Phenobarbital
Absence	Valproic acid Ethosuximide	Clonazepam
Myoclonic	Valproic acid	Clonazepam
Lennox-Gastaut	Valproic acid	Ethosuximide
Infantile spasm	ACTH or corticosteroids	Valproic Acid

      d. Unusual physical features, e.g., lesions seen in tuberous sclerosis, that may indicate underlying genetic disorder

      e. Change in seizure pattern

- Management/Treatment: Referral to neurologist for initial management

  1. Antiepileptic drugs

      a. Principles

          (1) Utilize least number of medications

          (2) Maintain maximum level of alertness, with fewest number of seizures

          (3) Select drug effective for specific seizure type (see Table 1)

          (4) Use least toxic, least expensive, requiring least amount of laboratory monitoring

          (5) Begin with single drug, easier to assess side effects

          (6) Obtain baseline of child's physical status

              (a) Complete blood count

              (b) Liver function tests

              (c) Blood urea nitrogen and urinalysis

      b. Factors to consider in choice of drug (See Table 2)

          (1) Type of seizure

          (2) Dosage

          (3) Potential side effects

          (4) Half-life

          (5) Age, sex, weight and physical condition of child

  2. Anticipatory guidance

      a. First aid measures

Table 2
Characteristics of Antiepileptic Drugs

Drug	Oral Dosage (mg/kg/d)	Half-life hours	Side Effects
Carbamazepine	20–30	8–12	Allergic rashes, nausea, lethargy, blurry vision, nystagmus, dizziness, bone marrow suppression, decreased liver function
Valproic acid	30–60	6–12	Nausea, weight gain, tremor, transient alopecia, hepatotoxicity, leukopenia, thrombocytopenia, rash
Ethosuximide	20–40	30	Abdominal discomfort, nausea, rash, hiccups, behavioral problems, drowsiness, dystonias, blood dyscrasias
Phenytoin	3–9	7–42	Rash, hirsutism, nausea, psychomotor slowing, neuropathy, ataxia, gingival hyperplasia, folate deficiency
Phenobarbital	3–5	36–120	Sedation; paradoxical hyperexcitability, rare
Clonazepam	0.05–0.2	18	Ataxia, sedation, drooling, inattention, withdrawal seizures
ACTH	20–40 IU		Cushing syndrome, hypertension, susceptibility to infections, GI bleeding, hypergylcemia

      (1)   Protect child from injury, but do not restrain

      (2)   Assess for adequate airway, breathing and circulatory status

      (3)   Do not insert items in mouth

      (4)   Note time, duration and activity

      (5)   If seizure persists beyond 10 to 15 minutes, seek medical assistance

   b.   Observe for side effects of drugs

   c.   Possible drug interactions

   d.   Guidelines for activities/activity restrictions

      (1)   Avoid activities where seizures may cause dangerous fall (e.g., high diving, rope climbing)

      (2)   Supervised swimming only

      (3)   Discuss other sports participation with parents and child

   e.   Importance of compliance with drug therapy

  3.   Intractable seizures—15% children with epilepsy

   a.   Refer to epilepsy center with interdisciplinary team

   b.   Alternative treatments

      (1)   Ketogenic diet—very restricted, high fat/low carbohydrate diet

      (2)   Epilepsy surgery—approximately half of children with intractable seizures are appropriate candidates for surgical procedures

Febrile Seizures

- Definition: Generalized tonic or tonic-clonic seizures which occur as a consequence of an abrupt and steep rise in body temperature in young children
- Etiology/Incidence
    1. 3% to 4% of otherwise healthy children between 9 months and 5 years of age have one or more febrile seizures; peak onset between 18 and 24 months of age
    2. Exact cause unknown; hereditary influence suspected
    3. Most common non-epileptic seizure disorder
- Signs and Symptoms
    1. Two groups based on clinical features
        a. Simple (benign) febrile seizures
            (1) Duration < 15 minutes
            (2) No focal features
            (3) If occur in series, total duration of less than 30 minutes
        b. Complex febrile seizures
            (1) Duration > 15 minutes
            (2) Focal features or postictal paresis present
            (3) Occur in series with total duration greater than 30 minutes
- Differential Diagnosis
    1. Underlying meningitis or encephalitis
    2. Chills
    3. Underlying metabolic disorder
    4. Epilepsy
- Physical Findings
    1. Often associated with viral or bacterial illness
        a. While fever is rising
        b. Usually above 102° F (39° C)
    2. Associated more frequently with severe constitutional symptoms during illness
- Diagnostic Tests/Findings
    1. Detailed description of seizure
    2. Complete physical assessment with careful neurological examination
    3. Lumbar punctures not routine; but indicated for:
        a. Infants < 1 year of age

    b. If seizure occurs after second day of illness

    c. Rule out meningitis

4. Skull radiographs not routine

5. Blood laboratory studies, EEG, CT or MRI not routine but performed if indicated by history or physical findings

- Management/Treatment

  1. Urgent treatment for unabated seizures of ≥ 10 minutes

  2. Fever control for temperature > 101° F

    a. Sponge baths with tepid water for at least 1 hour; avoid chilling

    b. Antipyretic use, e.g., acetaminophen

  3. A comprehensive search for cause of fever and treatment of underlying illness

  4. Reassurance to parents regarding excellent prognosis

  5. Antiseizure drugs

    a. Short-term or prolonged anticonvulsant prophylaxis not recommended

    b. Oral diazepam safe and effective method of reducing risk of recurrence; at onset of each febrile illness, diazepam 0.3 mg/kg every 8 hours orally is administered for duration of illness (usually 2 to 3 days)

Headaches

- Definition: Head pain
- Etiology/Incidence

  1. Exact etiology unknown; pain may be extracranial and/or intracranial

  2. Difficult to distinguish tension headaches from migraine headaches in many children

  3. Chronic and recurrent headaches are most common neurologic complaints; occur in 3% to 20% of children and adolescents

    a. Migraines—account for 50% of chronic or recurrent headaches; 60% of affected children are male

    b. Cluster headaches

      (1) Briefer in duration and more frequent than migraines

      (2) Begin in teenage years

      (3) More frequent in males

  4. Headache pain is produced by several factors which activate pain fibers

    a. Inflammation

    b. Stretching

    c. Torsion

    d. Contraction of innervated structures

        (1) Large intracranial arteries and veins

        (2) Dural sinuses

        (3) Periosteum of bone

        (4) Muscle/skin of scalp

        (5) Teeth and gums

- Signs and Symptoms

  1. Migraine headaches—recurrent headaches with varied frequency, intensity and duration

    a. Diagnostic criteria: Repeated episodes of headache accompanied by at least 3 of the following symptoms

        (1) Recurrent abdominal pain (with or without headache) or nausea and vomiting

        (2) An aura, usually visual, but may be sensory, motor, or vertiginous

        (3) Throbbing or pounding pain

        (4) Pain restricted to one side of head (although may shift sides from one headache to next); bilateral before puberty

        (5) Relief of pain by brief periods of sleep

        (6) Family history of migraine in one or more immediate relatives

  2. Tension headaches—headaches occurring with most frequency and intensity during periods of increased stress

    a. Tend to involve occipital or temporal regions bilaterally and often extend to the neck, or may be diffuse

    b. Nausea and vomiting may occur, but not as often as with migraine

  3. Intracranial headaches—may have certain distinguishing factors

    a. Severe occipital headache

    b. Exacerbated by straining, sneezing or coughing

    c. Awakens child from sleep

    d. Exacerbated or improved markedly by position changes

    e. Associated with projectile vomiting or vomiting without nausea

    f. Associated with history of focal seizures

    g. Increase in intensity and severity if not treated

4. Sinus headache—chronic or recurrent headaches which occur in about 15% of children with chronic sinusitis

   a. Often occur same time each day, build slowly, with throbbing quality

   b. Accompanied by rhinorrhea, postnasal drip, persistent cough, recurrent ear infections; afebrile

   c. Pain or pressure over frontal or maxillary sinuses

- Differential Diagnosis

  1. Acute, severe headache—distinguish between intracranial and extracranial cause by thorough history and physical examination

     a. Intracranial causes

        (1) Intracranial mass

        (2) Infection—meningitis, encephalitis

        (3) Intracranial hemorrhage

        (4) Post-head injury

        (5) Post-seizure

     b. Extracranial causes

        (1) Sinusitis—rare

        (2) Temporomandibular joint problem

  2. Chronic headaches—stress, anxiety, or tension with resulting muscle contractions

- Physical Findings

  1. Chronic migraine or tension headaches—physical examination generally normal

  2. Acute headache—critical indicators of possible intracranial cause

     a. Meningismus

     b. Focal neurologic signs

     c. Papilledema

     d. Split sutures

     e. Evidence of cranial trauma (including blood in or behind ear)

     f. Depressed level of consciousness

- Diagnostic Tests/Findings: Unnecessary unless history/physical examination suggest intracranial etiology, e.g., infection, bleeding or tumors

- Management/Treatment

  1. Specific treatment determined by etiology

  2. Headaches with suspected intracranial etiology need evaluation by physician/neurologist

  3. Cautious use of medications for pain relief

a. Initial treatment with simple analgesics

b. Acetaminophen

   (1) Under 1 year—60 mg orally every 4 to 6 hours

   (2) 1 to 3 years—60 to 120 mg orally every 4 to 6 hours

   (3) 3 to 6 years—120 to 180 mg orally every 4 to 6 hours

   (4) 6 to 12 years—240 mg orally every 4 to 6 hours

   (5) Older than 12 years—325 to 650 mg orally every 4 to 6 hours

c. If mild analgesics ineffective in children older than 11 years, may progress with caution to:

   (1) Midrin

      (a) Combination of isometheptene mucate 65 mg; acetaminophen 325 mg and dichloralphenazone 100 mg

      (b) 1 to 2 capsules immediately; repeat 1 capsule every hour until relieved to a maximum of 3/day or 5/week

   (2) Ergotamine tartrate—2 mg sublingual

d. Prophylactic treatment:

   (1) With headaches more than once/week and those that interfere with routine activities, e.g., school attendance

   (2) Unresponsive to symptomatic treatment

   (3) Medications used

      (a) Propranolol—.5 to 3.0 mg/kg/day ≥ 11 years of age

      (b) Cyproheptadine hydrochloride—0.25 mg/kg/day ≥ 3 years of age

      (c) Phenobarbital—3 to 5 mg/kg/day every night (3 to 10 years)

      (d) Phenytoin—5 mg/kg/day in 2 doses

      (e) Amitriptyline hydrochloride—1 to 2 mg/kg/day ≥ 11 years of age

4. Stress management and relaxation techniques

5. Eliminate foods which may be triggers, e.g., chocolate, cheese, MSG

6. Refer to specialists for further evaluation if headaches are recurrent, unresponsive, including allergist, psychiatrist, neurologist or pain clinic

Neurofibromatosis (NF)-1 (von Recklinghausen Disease)

- Definition

1. A neurocutaneous syndrome characterized by multiple café-au-lait spots (CLS) on the body; nerve tumors (neurofibromas present within the body and on skin)

2. Most common type of NF

3. Always a progressive disorder

4. Intelligence is usually normal

- Etiology/Incidence
    1. Inherited autosomal dominant disorder; associated with chromosome # 17
    2. Occurs 1:3000 to 1:4000 persons
    3. High variability and severity among individuals and within families
    4. Penetrance (likelihood that mutant gene will express itself at all if it is present) is virtually 100%

- Signs and Symptoms
    1. Skin lesions and/or freckling
    2. Developmental delays
    3. Seizures

- Differential Diagnosis
    1. Benign condition with < 5 or 6 CLSs
    2. McCune-Albright syndrome
    3. Neurolemmoma
    4. Proteus syndrome

- Physical Findings: A diagnosis of NF is made when two or more of the following diagnostic criteria are met (developed by the 1987 National Institutes of Health Consensus Development Conference on NF) are met:
    1. 6 or more CLSs > 5 mm diameter in prepubertal child and > 15 mm in postpubertal adolescent; 5 or more in young child < 5 years is highly suggestive
    2. 2 or more cutaneous and/or subcutaneous neurofibromas, or one plexiform neurofibroma
    3. Axillary or inguinal freckling
    4. Optic pathway glioma
    5. 2 or more iris Lisch nodules
    6. Distinctive osseous lesion (e.g., sphenoid wing dysplasia or thinning of long-bone cortex, with or without pseudarthrosis)
    7. First degree relative (parent, sibling or offspring) with NF-1 diagnosed by above criteria

- Diagnostic Tests/Findings: Additional tests to confirm diagnosis and identify complications
    1. Slit-lamp ocular examination to identify ocular abnormalities (e.g., iris Lisch nodules and signs of optic pathway glioma)
    2. Cranial MRI—to identify gliomas
    3. Radiographs of spine, chest, skull—to identify neurofibromas and other tumors

4. EEG—to detect epileptogenic foci

5. Psychological evaluation of school-age child for school—to determine abilities and deficiencies

6. Audiogram/brain stem evoked response testing—baseline for hearing and detection of acoustic neuromas

- Management/Treatment

    1. Problems associated with NF-1 most likely to require medical treatment

        a. Constipation

        b. Seizures

        c. Headaches

        d. Hyperactivity

        e. Learning disabilities

        f. Anxiety

        g. Renovascular hypertension

    2. Surgery

        a. Removing or debulking tumors

        b. Treating skeletal dysplasia

        c. Correcting scoliosis

        d. Treatment of vascular compromise

    3. Frequent consultation with medical and surgical specialists, social workers, and other health care specialists

    4. Genetic counseling

    5. Referral to support group for NF

Tuberous Sclerosis (TS)

- Definition

    1. Neurocutaneous syndrome with a combination of skin abnormalities, seizures, and cognitive deficits

    2. Progressive disorder with deterioration over time including new lesions and complications with increasing patient age

    3. Majority have ongoing debilitation from TS throughout their lives

    4. Mental retardation and seizures are most common problems

- Etiology/Incidence

    1. Autosomal dominant mutant gene

2. Previously negative family history does not exclude diagnosis

3. Incidence—1:10,000 to 1:50,000

4. Recurrence risk for affected person's children is 50%

- Signs and Symptoms

    1. Hypopigmented skin lesions often noted at birth

    2. Developmental delay

    3. Abnormal movements, particularly myoclonic jerking movements

- Physical Findings

    1. Establishing diagnosis of TS depends on detecting presence of two or more specific abnormalities:

        a. Skin

            (1) Hypopigmented macules, of elliptical shape (ash-leaf spots)

            (2) Fibroadenomas—adenoma sebaceum

            (3) Distinctive brown patch on forehead

            (4) Shagreen patch (characteristic)—raised lesion in lumbosacral region

        b. Teeth—characteristic pitting of enamel

        c. Eye

            (1) Choroidal hamartomas

            (2) Hypopigmented defects of iris

        d. CNS

            (1) Periventricular tubers

            (2) Cerebral astrocytomas

            (3) Nonspecific EEG abnormalities, including hypsarrhythmia

        e. Cardiovascular

            (1) Cardiac rhabdomyomas

            (2) Aortic and major artery constrictions

        f. Kidney—renal angiomyolipomas

        g. Lungs—diffuse interstitial fibrosis

    2. Seizures of all types, particularly myoclonic jerks, and mental retardation most common symptoms

- Differential Diagnosis: Seizures, or mental retardation

- Diagnostic Tests/Findings

    1. MRI scan of brain—virtually diagnostic and must be used in suspected TS

2. Once diagnosis is made, close follow-up surveillance is essential using appropriate clinical laboratory and radiographic techniques to monitor progression and identify new lesions

- Management/Treatment
    1. No specific medical treatment available
    2. Treat seizures and other complications (e.g., heart failure, renal failure) the same as if TS were not present, unless surgery on primary lesions is indicated
    3. Genetic counseling
    4. Psychometric testing and psychoeducational techniques for cognitive needs
    5. Family and individual support and counseling
    6. Refer to tertiary care center for specialized treatment, information, and support

Tic Disorders

- Definition
    1. Tic—repetitive, brief, involuntary, stereotypic muscle movement or vocalizations
    2. Severity ranges from mild and transient to more severe and permanent
    3. Types
        a. Transient tic disorder—duration less than 1 year
        b. Chronic tic disorder—duration more than 1 year, simple or complex
        c. Gilles de la Tourette syndrome—most severe chronic tic disorder; symptoms include multiple motor and vocal tics varying in nature and severity over time
- Etiology/Incidence
    1. Uncertain etiology; possible genetic central nervous system disturbance
    2. Occasionally precipitated by stimulant medications
    3. Transient tics
        a. Occur in 25% of normal children
        b. Often begin in school-age children and can be intensified by anxiety, fatigue, or excitement
    4. Gilles de la Tourette syndrome
        a. Onset between 2 and 15 years of age with mean age 6 to 7 years
        b. Incidence—1:10,000 persons
        c. Males 3 times more frequently affected
- Signs and Symptoms
    1. Characteristics of tics

      a. Variable expression—frequency, intensity, and severity

      b. Exacerbated by stress

      c. Some degree of voluntary control often present

      d. Typically subside during sleep

  2. Simple tics

      a. Movements present that resemble nervous habits

      b. Facial "twitches", head shaking, eye blinking, shoulder shrugging or throat clearing

  3. Gilles de la Tourette syndrome

      a. Simple tics

      b. Complex sequences of coordinated movements (e.g., bizarre gait, kicking, jumping, body gyrations, scratching, and seductive or obscene gestures)

      c. Involuntary vocalizations occur, ranging from simple to complex noises

      d. Expression is gender influenced

        (1) Motor and vocal manifestations more prevalent in boys

        (2) Behavioral problems, such as obsessive-compulsive disorder more common in girls.

- Differential Diagnosis

  1. Chronic tic disorder

  2. Stuttering

  3. Seizures

  4. Medication-induced tics

  5. Pervasive developmental disorder

  6. Psychiatric disorders, e.g., schizophrenia

  7. Medical conditions with associated abnormal movements, e.g., post-viral encephalitis, multiple sclerosis

- Physical Findings

  1. Usually normal

  2. Some degree of voluntary ability to suppress tics is usually present

- Diagnostic Tests/Findings: None

- Management/Treatment

  1. Transient tics—support and education for child and family

  2. Chronic tics/Gilles de la Tourette syndrome

a. Referral to mental health specialist

b. May involve psychotherapy, behavior management, stress management

c. Pharmacologic management

    (1) Consultation and/or referral—pediatric neurologist

    (2) Medications useful to suppress behavioral symptoms interfering with daily functioning

    (3) Pimoxide—beginning dose of 1 mg at bedtime

        (a) Gradual increases (every 5 to 7 days) until symptoms subside

        (b) Maximum dose of 10mg/day in children; 20mg/ day in adolescents

        (c) Side effects—sedation, lethargy, acute dystonic reactions, tardive dyskinesia

        (d) Less frequent side effects than haloperidol

    (4) Haloperidol—beginning dose of 0.25 to 0.50 mg at bedtime

        (a) Gradual increases (every 4 to 5 days) until symptoms subside

        (b) Side effects similar to pimoxide; tardive dyskinesia more common than with pimoxide

    (5) Clonidine—less effective but with fewer side effects is sometime used

Head Injuries

- Definition: Any injury to the meninges, scalp, skull, or any part of the brain; severity of injury ranges from very mild to severe brain-damaging injury

- Etiology/Incidence

    1. Injury resulting from external physical force to the cranium and internal brain structures

    2. Approximately 1 in 25 children receives medical attention each year for head injuries

    3. Twice as frequent in boys

    4. Greatest incidence in children < 1 year and > 15 years

    5. Age specific etiology

        a. Infant—child abuse, falls

        b. One to 4 years of age—falls

        c. School age—falls, motor vehicle accidents, sports/recreation

        d. Adolescents—motor vehicle accidents; athletic injuries

- Signs and Symptoms: Important to determine specific circumstances associated with head trauma

    1. Scalp injuries—contusions and lacerations are most frequent complications

    2. Concussion

        a. Head injury sufficient to cause brief loss of consciousness or amnesia for event

        b. Presence and duration of amnesia is indicative of severity

        c. Usually brief loss of consciousness is followed in minutes by complete return to normal mental status and behavior

        d. Recovery usually complete without complications

        e. Few children experience postconcussional syndrome, several hours after concussion, characterized by:

            (1) Headache

            (2) Drowsiness

            (3) Confusion or irritability

            (4) Symptoms may last for several days

    3. Diffuse Axonal Injury (DAI)

        a. Diffuse injury, usually resulting from violent motion, e.g., motor vehicle accidents

        b. Diagnosis of exclusion associated with:

            (1) Unconsciousness ≥ 6 or more hours

            (2) No other cause for symptoms, such as seizures or hematoma

        c. More serious diagnosis with less favorable prognosis than concussion

        d. Other symptoms depend on severity of injury

            (1) Abnormal movements with abnormal pupillary reaction

            (2) Difficulty regulating respirations and blood pressure

    4. Contusion

        a. Bruising or tearing of cerebral structures

        b. Common locations include frontal, temporal lobes and orbital area

        c. Focal motor signs related to increased intracranial pressure (ICP) may be diagnostic

    5. Hematomas

        a. Epidural hematoma—blood clot formation between skull and dura of the brain

            (1) Most treatable, but potentially most lethal type of head injury

     (2)   Classic clinical sign is delayed onset of symptoms

     (3)   Initial neurological symptoms may be minimal or absent

     (4)   Secondary injury from increased ICP as hematoma enlarges may result in neurological symptoms

          (a)   Headache

          (b)   Confusion

          (c)   Vomiting

          (d)   One-sided weakness

          (e)   Agitation

     (5)   Symptoms may progress to lethargy, coma, and even death if left untreated

     (6)   Prognosis is favorable if surgery is performed before secondary injury becomes irreversible

  b.   Subdural hematoma—blood clot formation on brain surface beneath the duramater

     (1)   Acute presentation

          (a)   Symptoms appear within 48 hours of head injury

          (b)   Signs of intracranial hypertension including irritability or lethargy, vomiting, headache

     (2)   Subacute

          (a)   Symptoms between 2 and 21 days

          (b)   Chronic hematoma with symptoms appearing after 21 days

          (c)   Signs include seizures, motor abnormalities (hypertonicity and agitation), systemic (irritability, vomiting, fever, anemia, poor weight gain)

6. Skull fracture

  a.   Brain damage may not be present, and conversely, brain can be injured without skull fracture present

  b.   Type, severity, symptomatology depend on area involved, age of child, and force of impact

  c.   Linear

     (1)   Fracture in temporoparietal region

     (2)   Most common

     (3)   Frequent in children less than 2 years old who fall from low heights

     (4)   Outcome is usually excellent

    d. Depressed

        (1) Skull is disrupted/depressed at point of impact

        (2) Underlying structures may be bruised or lacerated

    e. Basal

        (1) Diagnosis dependent on recognition of signs including hemorrhage in nose, nasopharynx, middle ear

        (2) Bruising over mastoid bone (Battle sign) or around eyes (raccoon's eye sign)

        (3) Cranial nerve palsy

        (4) Cerebral spinal fluid from ears or nose

- Differential Diagnosis

  1. Seizure disorder

  2. Child maltreatment

- Physical Findings

  1. Alterations in vital signs may indicate shock

  2. Headache, irritability and/or crying may indicate acute pain

  3. Tense anterior fontanel in young child

  4. Alterations in level of consciousness (LOC) vary from irritability, agitation, restlessness to confusion and/or coma

  5. Skull fractures may or may not show bony displacement

  6. Unilateral swelling may present from a possible hematoma

  7. Other signs:

     a. Asymmetry

     b. Focal neurologic deficits

     c. Cranial nerve injuries

     d. CSF rhinorrhea or otorrhea

     e. Ecchymosis

     f. Hearing impairments

  8. With cerebral edema and increasing ICP, may observe:

     a. Changes in level of consciousness

     b. Abnormal respiratory patterns

     c. Loss of protective reflexes (e.g., cough, gag or corneal)

     d. Changes in motor function or posturing

e. Nausea and projectile vomiting.

- Diagnostic Tests/Findings

    1. Skull radiography

        a. Indicated when severity of head trauma includes:

            (1) Loss of consciousness

            (2) Presence of focal neurologic signs

        b. Only 20% of basal skull fractures can be recognized on standard skull radiographs

        c. If depressed skull fracture is suspected, obtain tangential along with standard views

    2. CT scan—useful in detection of intracranial hemorrhage; investigation of localizing neurologic signs

    3. MRI—most useful in evaluation of subacute or chronic rather than acute injuries

- Management/Treatment

    1. For acute injury, rapid, accurate assessment of primary injury and level of severity

    2. Most head trauma is minor, with momentary unconsciousness, then child resumes activity and does not require treatment

    3. Hospital observation may be required for:

        a. More than momentary loss of consciousness

        b. Lethargy, confusion or irritability

        c. Severe headache

        d. Changes in speech or movements in arms and legs

        e. Significant bleeding from wound

        f. Vomiting 1 to 2 hours following injury

    4. Anticipatory guidance

        a. Instructions for home observation

        b. Need to return to health care provider if child exhibits:

            (1) Excessive prolonged sleepiness

            (2) Disorientation

            (3) Confusion

            (4) Persistent vomiting

            (5) Seizure

            (6) Change in swelling of scalp

Meningitis

- Definition—Inflammation of the meninges
- Etiology/Incidence—related to age
  1. Most frequently a result of hematogenous dissemination
  2. Bacterial pathogens—related to age
     a. Newborn
        (1) *Escherichia coli*
        (2) Group B streptococci
        (3) *Listeria monocytogenes* (less frequent)
     b. Etiologic agents responsible for 95% of cases that occur in children over 2 months of age have been:
        (1) *Haemophilus influenzae* type b (decline in incidence with H. influenzae immunization)
        (2) *Streptococcus pneumoniae*
        (3) *Neisseria meningitidis*
  3. Other etiologic agents
     a. Mycobacteria
     b. Fungal infections
     c. Aseptic (viral)
     d. Protozoa
  4. Highest risk—infants between 6 and 12 months of age; 90% of all cases occurr in children between 1 month and 5 years
- Signs and Symptoms
  1. Newborn
     a. Often nonspecific and indistinguishable from those of septicemia
     b. Most frequent signs:
        (1) Temperature instability
        (2) Respiratory distress
        (3) Irritability, lethargy
        (4) Poor feeding
        (5) Vomiting
     b. Seizures present in 40%
  2. Older infants and children

    a. Nausea and vomiting

    b. Irritability, confusion

    c. Anorexia

    d. Headache, back pain, nuchal rigidity

    e. Hyperesthesia, cranial nerve palsy, ataxia

    f. Photophobia

- Differential Diagnosis

    1. Brain abscess

    2. Spinal, epidural, or intracranial abscess

    3. Bacterial endocarditis with embolism

    4. Subdural empyema with or without thrombophlebitis

    5. Brain tumor

- Physical Findings

    1. Newborn

        a. Bulging fontanel (with or without suture diastasis)

        b. Increased ICP

        c. Cardinal signs of meningitis in older children are usually absent in infants

           (1) No stiff neck

           (2) No evidence of Kernig's and Brudzinski's signs

    2. Older infants and children

        a. Common clinical signs associated with meningeal irritation are:

           (1) Kernig's sign:

               (a) Flexion of the leg 90° at hip

               (b) Pain on extension of leg

           (2) Brudzinski's sign—involuntary flexion of legs when neck is flexed

        b. Headache is frequent sign of increased intracranial pressure

- Diagnostic Tests/Findings

    1. Diagnosis based on examination and culture of cerebrospinal fluid (CSF)

    2. Lumbar puncture for CSF analysis

        a. Contraindicated in following conditions

           (1) Cardiopulmonary compromise

           (2) Signs of increased ICP—papilledema

(3) Infection in area overlying lumbar puncture location

b. Adverse reactions—pain, headache, bleeding

3. CSF analysis

    a. Cloudy

    b. Increased cell count (300 to 10,000)

    c. Increased protein

    d. Decreased glucose

- Management/Treatment

1. Hospitalization for bacterial meningitis—first 3 to 4 days are critical

2. Initiate antibiotic therapy once diagnosis is confirmed by clinical findings while awaiting specific CSF and blood culture results

3. Neonates:

    a. Fatality rate is 15% to 30% in neonates

    b. Prognosis depends upon:

        (1) Causative pathogen

        (2) Predisposing risk factors

        (3) Availability of intensive care facilities

    c. Follow-up

        (1) Group B streptococcus

            (a) 15% to 20% have sequelae—spastic quadriplegia; profound mental retardation; hemiparesis; hearing/ visual deficits

            (b) 11% have hydrocephalus

            (c) 13% have seizure disorder

        (2) Gram negative meningitis

            (a) 10% have severe sequelae of developmental delays

            (b) About 25% to 35% have mild to moderate sequelae, which may not interfere with normal development

            (c) Hydrocephalus develops in $\frac{1}{3}$ of infants

    d. Neonatal survivors without major sequelae seem to develop normally

4. Older infants and children

    a. Prognosis depends on several factors:

        (1) Patient's age at onset

      (2)   Duration of disease before appropriate antibiotic therapy initiated

      (3)   Specific microorganism involved and number of organisms

      (4)   Whether disorder is compromising host response to infection

   b.   Mortality rate 1% to 5% beyond the neonatal period

   c.   Up to 50% of survivors have some sequelae

      (1)   10% have hearing deficits

      (2)   15% have language disorder/delay

      (3)   2% to 4% have vision impairment

      (4)   10% to 11% have mental retardation

      (5)   3% to 7% have motor problems

      (6)   2% to 8% have seizures

Brain Tumors

- Definition: Expanding intracranial lesion
- Etiology/Incidence

   1.   Etiology is unknown, may be genetic predisposition, congenital factors, environmental exposures

   2.   Two most common primary tumors in childhood

      a.   Cerebellar astrocytomas (20% of all brain tumors in children)

      b.   Medulloblastoma

   3.   In children between 4 and 11 years, infratentorial (posterior fossa) tumors predominate, including cerebellar and brain stem tumors

- Signs and Symptoms

   1.   In infants with open sutures

      a.   Increased head circumference

      b.   Irritability

      c.   Head tilt

      d.   Loss of developmental milestones

   2.   Older children

      a.   Headache; symptoms usually increase in frequency, becoming more severe in the morning followed by vomiting

      b.   85% of children with malignant tumors have abnormal neurologic or ocular examinations within 2 to 4 months of onset of headaches

    c.   Certain specific neurologic symptoms may occur later and suggest localization of the CNS tumor

        (a)   Ataxia, hemiparesis, cranial nerve palsies

        (b)   Somnolence

        (c)   Seizures

        (d)   Head tilt

        (e)   Diencephalic syndrome—failure to thrive (FTT), emaciation

        (f)   Diabetes insipidus

- Differential Diagnosis
  1. Brain abscess
  2. Intracranial hemorrhage
  3. Nonneoplastic hydrocephalus
  4. Arteriovenous malformations or aneurysm
  5. Indolent viral infections
  6. Subdural hematoma

- Physical Findings: Directly related to anatomic location, size and to some extent the age of the child; may include:
  1. Tense bulging fontanel at rest (in infant)
  2. Cranial enlargement (present in infants and young children)
  3. Papilledema (edema of optic nerve)
  4. Nuchal rigidity
  5. Incoordination or clumsiness
  6. Poor fine motor control
  7. Hypoflexia or hyperflexia
  8. Positive Babinski sign
  9. Spasticity/paralysis
  10. Behavioral changes—may be earliest symptom in child/adolescent

- Diagnostic Tests/Findings
  1. MRI—superior, sensitive neuroimaging technology
  2. CT scan
     a. Without contrast, can detect:
        (1) Whether lesion is cystic or solid
        (2) Presence of calcifications, hemorrhage, edema, and hydrocephalus

      b.   With contrast can detect:

          (1)   Small tumors

          (2)   Differentiation of areas of edema

  3.   Angiography—determines blood supply to affected structures

  4.   Lumbar puncture contraindicated in presence of increased ICP

- Management/Treatment: Therapy selected depends on type and site of tumor

  1.   Surgery (usually treatment of choice)

  2.   Radiation therapy

  3.   Chemotherapy

  4.   Follow-up

      a.   EEG for seizures

      b.   VER for visual problems

      c.   BAER for hearing problems

      d.   Multidisciplinary approach for comprehensive health and developmental needs of child/family

Questions
Select the best answer

1. Which of the following children is most likely to experience a typical febrile seizure?

   a. A 1-year-old with otitis media and a fever of 104° F
   b. A 3-month-old with unequal pupils and bulging fontanels
   c. An 11-year-old with fever of 101° F who is on valproic acid for seizure disorder
   d. A 5-year-old with bacterial meningitis

2. Which of the following responses during a tonic-clonic seizure is most appropriate to teach family members of a child who has these seizures?

   a. Restrain the child
   b. Insert an airway into the mouth to prevent tongue biting
   c. Note the time, duration, and activity of the seizure
   d. Protect child from injury

3. Which of the following is an appropriate strategy to instruct the parents of an 18-month-old child who has just been diagnosed with a febrile seizure and who has a fever of 104° F?

   a. Aspirin every 4 hours for temperature over 101° F
   b. Bathe with cold water mixed with alcohol
   c. Dress warmly to avoid chills
   d. Continue sponge baths with tepid water for at least 1 hour

4. What is the primary method of preventing and controlling the incidence of bacterial meningitis in infants and children?

   a. Keeping infants and young children away from crowded places
   b. Administering antimeningitis vaccines during outbreaks
   c. Immediately isolating all children suspected of having meningitis
   d. Routinely giving infants *H. Influenzae* vaccine

5. Which type of seizure is first seen between 4 and 8 months of age, may be confused with myoclonic seizures and may be associated with serious developmental problems?

   a. Febrile seizures
   b. Infantile spasms
   c. Absence seizures
   d. Tonic-clonic

6. Which of the following would not be associated with a concussion?

   a. Focal motor signs
   b. Brief loss of consciousness
   c. Headache
   d. Confusion or irrritability

7. Which of the following factors is not usually associated with migraine headaches?

   a. Complaints of diffuse occipital pain
   b. Positive family history in immediate relatives
   c.. Pain relieved by brief sleep
   d. Recurrent abdominal pain

8. Sarah is a 13-month-old whose parents are very concerned after she experienced a second febrile seizure. At today's visit, they ask you about the use of medications to prevent any further seizures. Which of the following statements is not true regarding febrile seizure prophylaxis?

   a. Short-term anticonvulsant prophylaxis is not indicated
   b. Prolonged anticonvulsant prophylaxis for preventing recurrent febrile convulsions is controversial and no longer recommended
   c. It may be indicated for children < 12 months with recurrent febrile seizures
   d. Oral diazepam may be used at the onset, and for the duration of the febrile illness to reduce the risk of recurrence of febrile seizures

9. Problems associated with NF-1 most likely to require treatment include which of following?

   a. Learning disabilities
   b. Transient tics
   c. Obsessive-compulsive behavior
   d. Progressive mental retardation

10. An 11-year-old girl is brought in by her mother complaining of severe headaches associated with nausea and vomiting. Which of the following signs and symptoms would lead you to consider a brain tumor as part of your differential diagnoses?

    a. Throbbing pain restricted to one side
    b. Bilateral throbbing pain
    c. Visual aura
    d. More severe in the morning followed by vomiting

11. The National Institutes of Health Consensus conference on NF describes guidelines for diagnosis of NF. Which of the following is not among the diagnostic criteria?

    a. Family history of first degree relative with NF-1
    b. 6 or more CLSs > 5 mm diameter in prepubertal child
    c. 6 or more neurofibromas > 15 mm in postpubertal adolescent
    d. Optic glioma

12. Although meningitis related mortality decreases dramatically after the neonatal period, as many as 50% of survivors experience some sequelae. Which of the following is the most frequent post-meningitis sequelae in older infants and children?

    a. Motor deficits
    b. Seizures

    c. Language delays/disorders

    d. Visual impairments

13. A neonate is being worked up for meningitis after experiencing a seizure preceded by fever, irritability, and poor feeding for one day. On physical examination which of the following findings would be most consistent with a diagnosis of meningitis?

    a. Bulging fontanel

    b. Positive Brudzinski's sign

    c. Nuchal rigidity

    d. Positive Kernig's sign

14. Diagnostic criteria for Gilles de la Tourette syndrome includes which of the following?

    a. Must have both motor and vocal tics

    b. Steady pattern of motor tics

    c. Presence of tics for 6 months

    d. Multiple voluntary motor tics

15. Which of the following statements about Tourette's syndrome is not true?

    a. It is the most severe type of tic disorder

    b. It is more common among males than females

    c. Mean age at onset is between 6 and 7 years

    d. Expression is not gender influenced

16. A prominent feature in simple partial seizures is:

    a. Night terrors

    b. Microcephaly

    c. Bilateral tremor

    d. No loss of consciousness

17. Absence seizures:

    a. Often begin in infancy

    b. Appear as altered awareness and blank stare for brief period

    c. More commonly occur in first-born children

    d. Always progress to a more severe seizure disorder beyond childhood

18. The differential diagnosis for seizures includes which of the following:

    a. Poliomyelitis with paralysis

    b. Schizophrenia

    c. Sleep disorders

    d. Multiple sclerosis

19. The most useful diagnostic tool for diagnosing epilepsy is:

    a. MRI
    b. EMG
    c. EEG
    d. ECG

20. Which of the following drugs are used for treatment of generalized tonic/clonic seizures?

    a. Ethosuximide, carbamazepine, valproic acid
    b. Carbamazepine, valproic acid, phenytoin
    c. Clonazepam, carbamazepine, valproic acid
    d. Clonazepam, valproic acid, phenobarbital

21. Which of the following is included in the diagnostic criteria for migraine headache in children?

    a. Recurrent abdominal pain, throbbing head pain not relieved by sleep
    b. Nausea and vomiting, positive family history, aura
    c. Positive family history, nausea and vomiting, pain not relieved by sleep
    d. Aura, positive family history, diffuse head pain relieved by sleep

22. Headache caused by intracranial factors include which of the following distinguishing features?

    a. Severe occipital headache, awakens child from sleep, and vomiting
    b. Not affected by change in position, severe occipital headache
    c. Severe occipital headache, sleep unaffected, nausea and vomiting
    d. Severe occipital headache, aura, exacerbated or improved with change in position

23. Tuberous sclerosis is progressive, neurocutaneous syndrome in which there is a combination of:

    a. Skin abnormalities, blindness and cognitive deficits
    b. Skin abnormalities, seizures, cognitive deficits
    c. Cerebral palsy, cognitive deficits and skin problems
    d. Skin abnormalities, blindness and cognitive deficit

24. Tuberous sclerosis is caused by:

    a. Autosomal dominant mutant gene
    b. Autosomal recessive mutant gene
    c. Autosomal recessive mutant chromosome
    d. Autosomal dominant mutant chromosome

25. Seizures of all types are associated with tuberous sclerosis, but most commonly:

    a. Tonic-clonic seizures
    b. Simple partial seizures
    c. Myoclonic jerks
    d. Absence

26. For children 1 to 4 years of age, the most common cause of head injury is:

    a. Motor vehicle accidents
    b. Falls
    c. Child abuse
    d. Bicycle accidents

27. A concussion can be identified by which of the following:

    a. Brief loss of consciousness or amnesia with complete return to normal
    b. Usually associated with brief loss of consciousness and poor recovery
    c. Usually associated with sequelae of paralysis and seizures
    d. Usually associated with Battle sign

28. A head injury in which bruising or tearing of the brain occurs is:

    a. Contusion
    b. Concussion
    c. Hematoma
    d. Diffuse axonal injury

29. The most common type of skull fracture in children with an excellent prognosis is:

    a. Depressed
    b. Basilar
    c. Linear
    d. Simple

30. Which of the following is most likely to be the etiologic cause of meningitis in the newborn?

    a. *Neisseria meningitidis*
    b. *Escherichia coli*
    c. *Listeria monocytogenes*
    d. *Haemophilus influenzae*

31. Drug therapy commonly used to treat absence seizures, in addition to valproic acid, includes:

    a. Phenytoin, phenobarbital
    b. Ethosuximide, clonazepam
    c. Phenobarbital, ethosuximide
    d. ACTH, carbamazepine

Answers

1. a	11. c	22. a
2. d	12. c	23. b
3. d	13. a	24. a
4. d	14. a	25. c
5. b	15. d	26. b
6. a	16. d	27. a
7. a	17. b	28. a
8. c	18. c	29. c
9. a	19. c	30. b
10. d	20. b	31. b
	21. b	

Bibliography

American Psychiatric Association. (1994). *Diagnostic and statistical manual of mental disorders* (4th ed.). Washington, DC: Author

Barkin, R. (Ed.). (1997). *Pediatric emergency medicine: Concepts and clinical practice* (2nd ed.). St. Louis: Mosby

Benitz W., & Tatro, D. (1995). *The pediatric drug handbook* (3rd ed.). St. Louis: Mosby.

Behrman, R. E., Kliegman, R. M., & Jenson, H. B. (Eds.). (2004). *Nelson textbook of pediatrics* (17th ed.). Philadelphia: W. B. Saunders.

Berman, S. (1996). *Pediatric decision-making* (3rd ed.). St. Louis: Mosby

Farley, J. A. (2000). Epilepsy. In P. L. Jackson & J. A. Vessey (Eds.). *Primary care of a child with a chronic condition* (3rd ed.). St. Louis: Mosby.

Hoekelman, R. A., Adam, H. M., Nelson, N. M., Weitzman, M. L., & Wilson, M. H. (Eds.). (2001). *Primary pediatric care* (4th ed.). St. Louis: Mosby.

Levine, M. D., Carey, W. B., & Croder, A. C. (Eds.). (1999). *Developmental-behavioral pediatrics* (3rd ed.). Philadelphia: W. B. Saunders.

Marx, J. A. (Ed.) (2002). *Rosen's emergency medicine: Current concepts and clinical practice* (5th ed.). St. Louis: Mosby.

Pellock, J. M., Dodson, W. E., & Bourgeois, B. F. D. (Eds.). (2001). *Pediatric epilepsy diagnosis and therapy* (2nd ed.). New York: DEMOS.

Genitourinary/Gynecological Disorders Adolescent Pregnancy

Sandra L. Elvik
Mary A. Baroni

Urinary Tract Infection (UTI)

- Definition: A generic term referring to the presence of bacterial infection of the urinary tract including the bladder (cystitis), urethra (urethritis), or kidney (pyelonephritis)

- Etiology/Incidence

    1. Multifactorial etiology including agent virulence and host predisposing factors

        a. Agent virulence

            (1) *Escherichia coli*—pathogenic agent in 75% to 90% of all childhood UTIs

            (2) Other enteric bacteria agents—*Klebsiella, Enterobacter sp.*

            (3) *Staphylococcus saprophyticus*—common in males

            (4) Viral agents rare with exception of adenovirus

        b. Host predisposing factors

            (1) Immature kidneys associated with premature and low birth weight infants

            (2) Congenital urologic abnormalities, reflux, neurogenic bladder

            (3) Gender differences in anatomy of urinary tract predisposes females, e.g., short urethra and proximity to anus

            (4) Infrequent voiding—urinary stasis

            (5) Obstruction—constipation, pregnancy

            (6) Trauma/irritants—catheterization, bubble baths, sexual intercourse, sexual abuse, pinworms

    2. Incidence—most common pediatric urinary tract problem

        a. Newborns—1.4 to 5 per 1,000 live births

        b. Accounts for 4% to 8% of infant febrile episodes without apparent source of infection

        c. Infancy—increased incidence in males (5:1) than females in first year of life; 10 fold increased risk in uncircumcised male infants

        d. Increased incidence among females (8:1 to 10:1) after infancy and through adolescence

- Signs and Symptoms

    1. May be asymptomatic or with nonspecific symptoms especially in infancy

    2. Symptom clusters by age group (Todd, 1995)

        a. Newborns—jaundice, hypothermia, fever, vomiting, sepsis, failure to thrive

        b. Infants/preschoolers—diarrhea, vomiting, fever, failure to thrive, strong/foul-smelling urine

    c.   School age/adolescents—fever, vomiting, strong/foul-smelling urine, abdominal pain, frequency, painful urination

- Differential Diagnosis
  1. Acute abdomen—appendicitis, sexually transmitted diseases, ectopic pregnancy
  2. Chemical irritation—soaps, bubble baths
  3. Vulvovaginitis
  4. Dysfunctional voiding—enuresis
  5. Sexual abuse
  6. Foreign body
  7. Pelvic inflammatory disease (PID)

- Physical Findings
  1. May be normal
  2. Infancy—weight loss, jaundice, failure to thrive
  3. Fever and irritability
  4. Blood pressure may be elevated—reflux nephropathology
  5. Abdominal examination—pain, tenderness, guarding
  6. Urethral or vaginal irritation/discharge—with vulvovaginitis due to irritation or STD

- Diagnostic Tests/Findings
  1. Urine analysis—presence of urinary leukocyte esterase, nitrate, and blood suggestive of UTI but NOT diagnostic
  2. Urine culture mandatory for accurate diagnosis—technique for specimen collection depends on age and developmental status of child, severity of condition and urgency of need for unequivocal results

     a. Random voids/bagged urine—minimal usefulness due to high potential for contamination from external genitalia

     b. Clean-catch midstream—often contaminated from external genitalia, especially in girls; more reliable from circumcised males

        (1) Appropriate for mild symptoms or follow-up

        (2) Positive with colonies > 10^5/mL of single organism

     c. Straight catheterization—used with infants/children who cannot void voluntarily; lower risk for nocosomial infection than indwelling catheters

        (1) Appropriate for moderate or severe symptoms

        (2) Positive with colonies > 10^3/mL of single or multiple organisms

     d. Suprapubic aspiration—used with infants/children unable to void voluntarily,

when culture is urgently needed due to severity or equivocal results from alternative techniques

   (1) Appropriate for moderate or severe symptoms

   (2) Positive with colonies > 10^3/mL of single or multiple organisms

3. Blood culture—collected in infants < 12 months with suspected sepsis

4. Radiologic studies—for localizing infection and to rule out urinary abnormalities as part of UTI work up

   a. Indications for imaging studies—recommendations vary but generally include:

      (1) Symptoms of pyelonephritis regardless of age and gender

      (2) UTI in any child < 8 years of age

      (3) Males with first infection and females with second if above criteria are not met

   b. Types

      (1) Bladder and renal ultrasound—usually first step in evaluation of structural and developmental anomalies/disorders

      (2) Voiding cystourethrogram (VCUG)—detects regurgitation (reflux) of urine into ureter; delay 4 to 6 weeks after diagnosis to exclude UTI related reflux; continue antibiotic prophylaxis until after VCUG

      (3) Intravenous pyelogram (IVP) or nuclear renal cortical scans—detects scarring and examines renal function; usually done if VCUG is positive

- Management/Treatment

   1. Antibiotic treatment

      a. Parenteral antibiotics—newborns, infants, or older children with vomiting or severe symptoms

      b. Oral antibiotic

         (1) Generally treated for 10 day regimen

         (2) Short-term treatment regimen (3 to 5 days) gaining greater acceptance for uncomplicated cystitis in girls

         (3) Single dose regimen remains controversial

      c. First-line drugs of choice

         (1) Trimethoprim-sulfamethoxazole (TMP/SMX)—infants > 2 months of age

            (a) TMP 6 to 10 mg/kg/day + SMX 30 to 60 mg/kg/day b.i.d.

            (b) Recommended until sensitivities are available since most UTIs are caused by *E. coli*

         (2) Amoxicillin—30 to 50 mg/kg/day t.i.d.

      (3)   Amoxicillin/clavulanate—40 mg/kg/day t.i.d.

      (4)   Sulfisoxazole—150 mg/kg/day q.i.d.

      (5)   Cephalexin—50 mg/kg/day t.i.d.

2. Follow-up urine cultures

    a. Second culture at 48 to 72 hours after initiating treatment

    b. Third culture one week after completion of treatment

    c. Close monitoring of periodic urine cultures with recurrent infections and/or unexplained fevers

3. Prophylactic antibiotics—vesicoureteral reflux (VUR) trimethoprim-sulfamethoxazole, one-half daily dose usually at bedtime for 6 months to 2 years

    a. Most grades I to III resolve as child grows

    b. Annual VCUG to assess status of reflux

4. Education/prevention

    a. Increased fluid intake

    b. Frequent voiding with complete emptying of bladder

    c. Good perineal hygiene with front-to-back wiping

    d. Avoid bubble baths and other urethral irritants

Enuresis

- Definition: Involuntary urination after child has reached age when bladder control is usually attained; may occur during daytime (diurnal) or at night, especially while sleeping (nocturnal); usually resolves by 5 to 6 years of age

  1. Primary enuresis—child has never attained control

  2. Secondary enuresis—recurrence of incontinence following 3 to 6 months of dryness

- Etiology/Incidence

  1. Many causes suggested

      a. Primary—small bladder capacity; toilet-training problems; delayed maturation of voiding inhibitory reflex; sleep problems ("deep sleeper"); lack of inhibition of antidiuretic hormone (ADH); ingestion of increased amounts of fluid; inattention (too busy to void)

      b. Secondary

        (1)   Diseases—UTI, diabetes, GU abnormalities

        (2)   e.g., Medications—e.g., theophylline, diuretics

        (3)   Family disruptions, stress

  2. Primary enuresis most common form in children—75% to 80%

    3. Over 12 years of age—50% have secondary enuresis

    4. Familial predisposition

       a. One parent—44% increased risk

       b. Both parents—77% increased risk

- Signs and Symptoms

    1. Bed wetting or daytime "accidents"

    2. Odor of urine in clothing

    3. May have withdrawal/isolation from peers

- Differential Diagnosis

    1. UTI

    2. GU anomalies—ectopic ureter

    3. Mechanical obstruction

- Physical Findings: Genitalia

    1. Hypospadias, epispadias

    2. Labial fusion

    3. Dribbling of urine during examination

- Diagnostic Tests/Findings

    1. Urinalysis/urine culture—to rule out UTI

    2. Renal ultrasound/vesicoureterogram—with abnormal urine studies; GU anomaly on examination

- Management/Treatment

    1. Primary nocturnal

       a. Limit fluid intake after dinner

       b. Voiding before bedtime

       c. Avoid punishment/criticism

       d. Usually self-limited; spontaneous resolution of 10% per year after 5 years of age (Rosenstein & Fosarelli, 1997)

    2. Motivational therapy

       a. May be unsuccessful as exclusive treatment

       b. Verbal praise for dryness

       c. Reward system

       d. Dryness calendar

    3. Conditioning therapy—enuresis alarm

a. Triggered by urine

b. Children awakened by alarm

c. Alarm sensitizes child to sensation of full bladder

d. Restrictions

    (1) Expensive—not covered by all insurance plans

    (2) Treatment 2 to 3 months, often up to 6 months for greater success rate

    (3) May awaken other family members

    (4) Child's age, motivation, cooperation, family support important success factors

e. Bladder stretching exercises

    (1) Exercise to increase bladder capacity

    (2) Child given fluid load—child encouraged to hold urine as long as possible

f. Pharmacologic treatment

    (1) Desmopressin acetate

        (a) Synthetic analog of antidiuretic hormone vasopressin

        (b) Dose—oral tablet (0.2 mg to 0.6 mg at bedtime or nasal spray (10 μg/1 spray) in each nostril at bedtime (maximum dose of 40 μg

        (c) Rapid response—1 to 2 weeks once initiated

        (d) Increase or decrease according to response

        (e) Relapse 90% once discontinued

        (f) Side effects—headache, congestion, nasal irritation, epistaxis

    (2) Imipramine (use is becoming controversial)

        (a) Tricyclic antidepressant; unclear mechanism of action; may depress bladder contractions

        (b) Used in children over 6 years of age

        (c) Dose—0.9 to 1.5 mg/kg/day, 1 to 2 hours before bedtime;

        (d) Results seen within a few weeks

        (e) Treat 3 to 6 months, then taper

        (f) Relapse after treatment—75% to 90%

        (g) Side effects—arrhythmias, sedation, dry mouth

4. Secondary enuresis

a. Evaluation of underlying etiology—disease process, medication; modification of current treatment

b. Therapeutic intervention for individual/family stress

Cryptorchidism (Undescended Testes)

- Definition: Absence of one or both testes in scrotal sac due to failure of normal descent from abdomen during fetal development

- Etiology/Incidence

  1. Normal fetal descent of testes

     a. Hormonal mediation of normal testicular descent

        (1) Abdominal descent to inguinal ring—12 to 14 weeks gestation

        (2) Inguinal descent into scrotum—28 to 36 weeks

     b. Increased incidence among premature infants secondary to gestational development

  2. Failure of normal descent associated with hormonal imbalance, chromosomal abnormalities, structural disorders

  3. May be unilateral (usually right-sided) or bilateral

  4. Incidence

     a. Common (20% to 30%) among premature male births with birth weight < 1500 g

     b. Lower incidence (3% to 5%) among full-term male infants

     c. Incidence decreases to approximately 1% by one year due to spontaneous descent in approximately 75% of full-term and up to 95% of preterm cases

- Signs and Symptoms

  1. May be asymptomatic

  2. Family history of undescended testes

  3. Testes may be palpable or nonpalpable

- Differential Diagnosis

  1. Rectractile testes

  2. Ectopic testes

  3. Anorchia

  4. Chromosomal disorders

- Physical Findings

  1. Palpable testes—may be retractile or ectopic

  2. Nonpalpable testes—may be abdominal or absent

3. Presence or absence of testes should always be documented

- Diagnostic Tests/Findings
    1. Unilateral—usually none
    2. Bilateral nonpalpable testes
        a. Karyotyping for chromosomal abnormalities
        b. Follicle-stimulating and luteinizing hormones may suggest anorchia
        c. Imaging studies occasionally utilized

- Management/Treatment
    1. Routine assessment at each well-child visit during first year of life; most spontaneous descents occur by 6 months
    2. Refer to urologist if undescended by one year
        a. Hormonal therapy—human chorionic gonadotropin (hCG); gonadotropin-releasing hormone (GnRH) currently used in Europe but not yet approved for use in U.S.
        b. Surgical intervention—orchiopexy usually recommended when child is between 12 and 18 months
    3. Family education and support regarding potential complications
        a. Infertility—greater risk in bilateral cryptorchism
        b. Testicular malignancy—20 to 25 times increased risk
        c. Hernia

Hydrocele

- Definition: Painless scrotal swelling due to collection of peritoneal fluid within the tunica vaginalis surrounding the scrotum
    1. Noncommunicating type—tunica vaginalis is closed limiting fluid collection to scrotum; size of hydrocele is constant
    2. Communicating type—tunica vaginalis remains open allowing fluid to flow between peritoneum and hydrocele sac; often associated with hernia

- Etiology/Incidence
    1. Incomplete closure of processus vaginalis which usually isolates tunica vaginalis from peritoneum
    2. Most common cause of painless scrotal swelling; uncertain incidence

- Signs and Symptoms
    1. Swelling in scrotum—alternating or fixed
        a. Usually asymptomatic

   b. May become painful, if full or tense, secondary to coughing or straining

   c. Variable size with child's state; larger when active, decreases with rest

   d. Smaller on awakening—enlarges as day progresses

- Differential Diagnosis
    1. Cryptorchidism
    2. Retractile testes
    3. Hernia
    4. Inguinal lymphadenopathy

- Physical Findings
    1. Scrotal swelling or asymmetry—tense appearance; scrotal skin normal, nontender
    2. Fluctuance
    3. Translucent with transillumination

- Diagnostic Tests/Findings: Abdominal ultrasound to differentiate hydrocele from hernia

- Management/Treatment
    1. Noncommunicating
        a. Most resolve spontaneously without intervention
        b. Refer for evaluation:
            (1) Persists beyond one year
            (2) Significant increase in size
            (3) Causes discomfort
    2. Communicating
        a. Occasional spontaneous resolution
        b. Frequently develops into hernia requiring surgical intervention
        c. Refer for surgical evaluation if persists beyond one year

Hypospadias

- Definition: Congenital defect with urethral meatus on ventral surface of penis
- Etiology/Incidence
    1. Urethral folds along midline fail to fuse
    2. Common disorder—1 in 300 newborns
    3. Occurs more frequently in Caucasians
    4. Both genetic and environmental factors have been implicated
- Signs and Symptoms: Deflected urinary stream

- Differential Diagnosis: Ambiguous genitalia; female masculinization
- Physical Findings
    1. Location of urethral meatus
        a. Anterior—glans, corona, anterior shaft
        b. Midshaft
        c. Posterior—scrotal, penoscrotal junction, posterior shaft
    2. Inguinal hernia, undescended tests, incomplete foreskin
    3. Chordee—ventral curvature of penis due to fibrous band of tissue
- Diagnostic Tests/Findings
    1. Radiography if meatus in perineum (severe)
    2. Karyotype for chromosomal analysis
- Management/Treatment
    1. Avoid circumcision—foreskin used for repair
    2. Mild cases—primarily cosmetic surgery
    3. Increasing severity—functional, psychological and cosmetic surgery
        a. Repair early—6 to 18 months
        b. Family preparation for procedure and expected results

Phimosis and Paraphimosis

- Definition
    1. Phimosis—foreskin not fully retractable to expose glans
        a. Newborns normally have adhesions, glans to foreskin
        b. May not be fully retractable until 10 years of age or older
    2. Paraphimosis—inability to replace foreskin over glans after retraction
- Etiology/Incidence
    1. Most childhood phimosis physiologically normal
    2. Phimosis may be due to congenital narrowing/tightness
    3. Phimosis may be due to inflammation/infection under foreskin
    4. Paraphimosis may be due to forcible retraction of foreskin for "cleaning" purposes
- Signs and Symptoms
    1. May be asymptomatic
    2. Painful urination
    3. Weak urine stream

4. Pain/tenderness with paraphimosis

5. Ballooning of foreskin when urinating; may be normal if voiding uncompromised

- Differential Diagnosis

    1. Balanitis (inflammation of glans penis)

    2. Balanoposthitis (inflammation of glans penis and prepuce)

- Physical Findings

    1. Phimosis—unretractable foreskin

    2. Paraphimosis—edema/discoloration of foreskin and glans

- Diagnostic Tests/Findings—none indicated

- Management/Treatment

    1. Maintain good hygiene

    2. Gentle stretch of foreskin during bath—advise family against forceful retraction; scarring and balanitis may occur

    3. Paraphimosis may respond to ice—reduction of swelling to reduce foreskin; may be surgical emergency

    4. Surgery—circumcision in phimosis with urinary obstruction

Meatal Stenosis

- Definition: Narrowing of distal end of urethra

- Etiology/Incidence

    1. Post-circumcision

        a. Mechanical irritation by diaper

        b. Ischemia from frenular artery damage during procedure

        c. Inflammation secondary to dermatitis

    2. Almost never seen in uncircumcised males

- Signs and Symptoms

    1. Penile pain/discomfort with urination

    2. Narrow, dorsally-diverted urine stream

- Differential Diagnosis

    1. Hypospadias

    2. Chordee

- Physical Findings

    1. Inflammation of glans

   2. Slit-like or narrowed meatus—best to observe urination; appearance alone may be misleading

- Diagnostic Tests/Findings: None
- Management/Treatment
  1. Air exposure
  2. Warm soaks/baths
  3. Frequent diaper changes
  4. Meatotomy may be necessary in some cases
  5. Prevention
     a. Care exercised at circumcision to avoid damage to frenular artery
     b. Cover glans following procedure—petrolatum gauze commonly used
     c. Observe for early sign of irritation/inflammation

Testicular Torsion

- Definition: Torsion of the spermatic cord; can result in gangrene of testes (emergency)
- Etiology/Incidence
  1. Abnormal fixation of testis to scrotum—permits testis to twist/rotate; impedes lymphatic and blood flow
  2. Occurs after trauma, physical exertion
  3. Most common between 7 to 12 years of age
- Signs and Symptoms
  1. Acute, progressive unilateral pain of scrotum
  2. Nausea, anorexia, vomiting
  3. Minimal fever, if any
  4. Lack of urinary symptoms is the norm
- Differential Diagnosis
  1. Trauma
  2. Orchitis
  3. Acute epididymitis
- Physical Findings
  1. Enlarged, highly tender testis
  2. Scrotum on involved side edematous, warm, erythematous
  3. Anxious patient, resistant to movement

4. Lifting testis does not relieve pain (Prehn's sign)

5. Solid mass may be visualized with transillumination

- Diagnostic Tests/Findings

    1. Complete Blood Count (CBC)—may see slight increase in white blood count

    2. Doppler ultrasound

    3. U/A—normal

- Management/Treatment: Immediate referral for surgery

    1. Emergently performed within first 6 hours—preservation of fertility great concern; prevention of atrophy and abscess

    2. Untreated torsion can lead to testicular loss

Labial Adhesions (Labial Fusion, Synechia Vulvae, Labial Agglutination)

- Defintion: Generally benign fusion of labial minora

- Etiology/Incidence

    1. Results from tissue irritation/inflammation and hypoestrogenization of labia minora

    2. Potential sources of irritation—trauma, infection, poor hygiene, sexual abuse

    3. Incidence—rarely present at birth; usually occurs after 2 months of age

        a. Estimated incidence is 10% to 20% of all girls in first year

        b. Highest incidence between 2 and 6 years of age, but may occur anytime up to menarche

- Signs and Symptoms

    1. Generally asymptomatic

    2. Parental concern regarding potential anatomic abnormality

    3. Difficulty voiding, general discomfort

    4. Enuresis—primarily diurnal

        a. Pooling of urine behind adhesion after voiding may occur depending upon degree of meatal obstruction

        b. Results in dribbling of urine throughout the day

- Differential Diagnosis

    1. Intersex anomalies

    2. Imperforate hymen

    3. Genital scarring

- Physical Findings: Thin, flat, membrane of variable length found midline extending from clitoris to posterior fourchette when labia majora are gently separated

1. Complete fusion—entire vestibule covered; may see pinpoint opening

2. Partial fusion—much of genital structures visible

- Diagnostic Tests: None indicated

- Management/Treatment

    1. In most cases, parental reassurance and observation for resolution without intervention

    2. Previous practice of mechanical lysis no longer recommended due to high frequency of refusion

    3. Observation for UTI symptoms

    4. Topical application of conjugated estrogen cream twice a day for 2 to 3 weeks results in separation within 8 weeks in 90% of cases

        a. Overuse may stimulate signs of precocious puberty which resolve when cream is discontinued

        b. Following separation

            (1) Maintain good hygiene

            (2) Topical applications of bland creams or petroleum jelly

    5. Inspection of vulvae on routine well-child visits to monitor baseline anatomy, hygiene, sexual development and detect problems

Vulvovaginitis

- Definition: Perineal inflammation and/or infection of the vulva (vulvitis) or vagina (vaginitis) often associated with vaginal discharge

- Etiology/Incidence

    1. Sources of vulvovaginitis may be noninfectious or infectious

    2. Noninfectious vulvovaginitis

        a. Chemical irritation—bubble bath, powder, detergents, soaps, over the counter (OTC) douches

        b. Mechanical irritation—tight clothing, nylon underwear

        c. Foreign body irritation—toilet tissue, retained tampon

        d. Trauma/sexual abuse

        e. Masturbation

    3. Infectious vulvovaginitis

        a. Nonspecific—bacterial overgrowth due to poor hygiene

        b. Specific

       (1) Bacterial—Group A beta hemolytic streptococcus, *Pneumococcus, Enterococcus, Shigella flexneri/sonnie, N. gonorrhea, Chlamydia trachomatis*

       (2) Viral—Herpes simplex virus (HSV)

       (3) Parasitic—*Enterobius vermicularis* (pinworms); *Trichomonas vaginalis*

       (4) Mycotic/fungal—candidiasis (common following antibiotic use)

  4. Uncertain incidence; 30% to 85% are noninfectious/nonspecific inflammation with normal flora

- Signs and Symptoms
  1. Vaginal discharge
  2. Genital discomfort/itching
  3. Dysuria/burning
  4. Erythema/edema of vulva or vagina

- Differential Diagnosis
  1. Physiologic leukorrhea—thin, clear or white discharge
  2. UTI
  3. Dermatologic disorders—psoriasis, seborrheic dermatitis, atopic dermatitis

- Physical Findings
  1. May have no physical findings
  2. Discharge
     a. White to yellow—chemical, mechanical, *Chlamydia trachomatis*
     b. Pale yellow to gray green—trichomoniasis
     c. White, thick, cheesy—candidiasis ("yeast")
     d. Thin white, frothy—bacterial vaginosis
     e. Brown, bloody, foul odor—foreign body
  3. Genital erythema
  4. Lesions
  5. Perianal soiling
  6. Examination techniques—sensitive, gentle
     a. Prepubertal female
        (1) Pelvic examination usually deferred; visual inspection only
        (2) Exploratory procedure under anesthesia may be needed for vaginal bleeding and should be referred

b. Pubescent female

    (1) Pelvic examination—especially if sexually active

    (2) Cervix best site for culture

- Diagnostic Tests/Findings

    1. Urinalysis for presence of WBC, trichomonads

    2. Tape test for pinworms

    3. Saline preparation for wet mount

       a. Clue cells—bacterial vaginosis

       b. Presence of WBC—may indicate bacterial vaginosis in the absence of clue cells/trichomonads

       c. Trichomonads

    4. Potassium hydroxide (KOH) 10% preparation

       a. Hyphae—candidiasis

       b. "Whiff test"—positive (fishy odor of bacterial vaginosis)

- Management\Treatment (see section on sexually transmitted diseases for specific management)

    1. Foundation of treating childhood vulvovaginitis is improvement of local perineal hygiene

    2. Nonspecific vaginitis often resolves without intervention

    3. Discontinue genital irritants—bubble bath, harsh bath soap and laundry detergents

    4. Cotton or cotton-lined underwear—avoid tight fitting clothing (tights, pants, undergarments)

    5. Bacterial vaginosis

       a. Metronidazole—1 g/day orally in two divided doses for 7 days (adolescents/adults) and 15 mg/kg per day (children < 45 kg) with maximum dose of 1 g/day OR metronidazole gel, 0.75%, 5 g (1 applicator) intravaginally daily for 5 days (adolescents) or 15 mg/k per day

       b. Clindamycin cream 2%, 5 g (1 applicator) intravaginally at night for 7 days

       c. Alternative treatments are less effective

       d. Pregnant women should be treated for bacterial vaginitis

    6. Parasitic

       a. Pinworms—mebendazole, pyrantel pamoate, or albendazole in single dose repeated in 2 weeks

       b. Trichomonas vaginalis—metronidazole 15 mg/kg per day orally in 3 divided doses for 7 days (< 45 kg) with maximum of 1 g/day OR 2 g orally in single dose or 1 g/day in 2 divided doses for 7 days (> 45 kg)

7. Fungal—candidiasis may be treated with various topical agents including clotrimazole, miconazole, butoconazole nitrate, terconazole which are more effective than nystatin

8. Foreign body

   a. Prepubertal—attempt irrigation; warm saline via small feeding tube

   b. Postpubertal

      (1) Pelvic examination to locate object

      (2) Moistened cotton-tip applicator or forceps for removal

   c. Unsuccessful irrigation/pelvic or anxious child—refer for examination under general anesthesia

9. Positive cultures suspicious for sexual abuse or sexual activity—see section on sexually transmitted diseases

10. Physiologic leukorrhea

    a. Some benefit from "mini-pads" in underwear to absorb moisture/prevent wetness from staining clothing

    b. Avoid use of douches and creams

Dysmenorrhea

- Definition: Pain during menstrual cycle; usually first 1 to 2 days; cramping discomfort felt mid-to-lower abdomen

  1. Primary dysmenorrhea—no pelvic abnormality; common in adolescents; usually develops 6 to 12 months after menarche; ovulation necessary component

  2. Secondary dysmenorrhea—underlying pelvic pathology

     a. Congenital anomalies (septate uterus)

     b. Cervical stenosis or strictures

     c. Cysts, tumors of ovary or uterus

     d. Endometriosis

     e. Pelvic inflammatory disease

- Etiology/Incidence (Primary Dysmenorrhea)

  1. Increased production of uterine prostaglandins; uterine contractions, ischemia

  2. Ovulation is required for development of primary dysmenorrhea

  3. Most common gynecological complaint

  4. Some degree of pain with menses in over 60% of ovulating women

  a. Significant limitation for 10% to 15% of females

  b. Leading cause of adolescent female school absenteeism—14%

- Signs and Symptoms

  1. Pain usually starts with flow or several hours later or may precede flow by several hours to 2 days

  2. Crampy/spasmodic pain, primarily lower abdominal area; may radiate to inner thighs, lower back

  3. Systemic symptoms

    a. Nausea/vomiting/diarrhea

    b. Lightheadedness/dizziness

    c. Fatigue or general malaise

- Differential Diagnosis

  1. Reproductive system malformations

  2. Endometriosis

  3. PID

  4. Psychogenic problems

- Physical Findings: May be none; defer pelvic examination only if adolescent is not sexually active

  1. Bimanual and rectovaginal exams indicated

  2. Cervical motion tenderness with PID

- Diagnostic Tests/Findings

  1. Suspicion of PID—see section on sexually transmitted diseases

  2. Pelvic ultrasound for palpable masses or concern of GU abnormalities

- Management/Treatment

  1. Primary dysmenorrhea—mild

    a. Heat to abdomen

    b. Exercise

    c. Acetaminophen

    d. Ibuprofen—400 mg orally immediately at onset of pain, then every 4 to 6 hours for 1 to 3 days; take with food, milk, antacid to avoid GI distress

    e. Well balanced diet

    f. Acknowledgment of symptoms, pain is real

  2. Primary dysmenorrhea—moderate to severe; unresponsive to treatment for mild disorder

      a.   Nonsteroidal anti-inflammatory drugs (NSAIDS)

          (1)   Inhibit prostaglandin synthesis

          (2)   Naproxen sodium—500 mg orally at onset, then 250 mg every 6 to 8 hours

          (3)   Mefenamic acid—500 mg orally at onset, then 250 mg every 6 to 8 hours

          (4)   Assess efficacy of NSAIDS after 3 to 4 cycles before using another medication

          (5)   NSAIDS contraindicated in clotting disorders, renal or peptic ulcer disease

3.   Severe dysmenorrhea—unresponsive to NSAIDS alone

      a.   Low-dose combination oral contraceptives (OC); effective in 90% of cases with severe pain

      b.   Minimum 3 to 4 cycles for symptom improvement

      c.   Continuous symptoms after 4 months

          (1)   OC used in conjunction with NSAIDS

          (2)   Consider gynecological referral

4.   Secondary dysmenorrhea—gynecological referral

Premenstrual Syndrome

- Definition: Cluster of symptoms, both physical and behavioral, that occur in second half of menstrual cycle (last week of luteal phase); usually resolve with onset of menses

- Etiology/Incidence

   1.   Numerous mechanisms postulated

      a.   Vitamin B_6 deficiency

      b.   Fluid retention

      c.   Steroid hormone fluctuation

      d.   Alteration in serotoninergic neuronal mechanisms

      e.   Inappropriate prostaglandin activity

      f.   Food/environmental allergies

   2.   Significant complaints from 30% to 70% older adolescents

- Signs and Symptoms

   1.   Onset of symptoms usually within one week of menses

      a.   Breast tenderness

      b.   Headache

      c. Weight gain

      d. Mood swings, lethargy, anxiety

      e. Fatigue

      f. Appetite changes

      g. Lower back pain

      h. Loss of concentration

- Differential Diagnosis

    1. Pregnancy

    2. Primary/secondary dysmenorrhea

- Physical Findings: Pelvic examination normal

- Diagnostic Tests/Findings: None indicated

- Management/Treatment

    1. Diet/nutrition

      a. Frequent small meals

      b. Increase intake—complex carbohydrates, protein, fresh fruits, vegetables, foods rich in pyridoxine (B_6)

      c. Vitamin/mineral supplement—Vitamin B_6, magnesium

      d. Limit intake—refined sugar, salt, red meat, alcohol, coffee, tea, chocolate

    2. Life style

      a. Regular exercise (especially aerobic)

      b. Stress management

      c. Avoid active and passive cigarette smoke

    3. Pharmacological management

      a. Diuretics

      b. NSAID

      c. Selective serotonin reuptake inhibitors (SSRIs), e.g., fluoxetine, sertraline, paroxetine—more useful for emotional rather than somatic symptoms; currently recommended as first line of treatment in adult females (Hofmann & Greydanus, 1997)

      d. Preliminary European study exploring efficacy of herbel remedy "Femal" reported positive results with minimal side effects (Winther & Hedman, 2002)

Genitourinary Trauma

- Definition: Injury to the genitourinary tract; refers to accidental injury (for nonaccidental trauma refer to section on sexual abuse)

- Etiology/Incidence
    1. Blunt insult generally from athletic activities, motor vehicle accidents, falls
    2. No specific incidence—commonly seen; over 50% associated with trauma to intra-peritoneal organs
- Signs and Symptoms
    1. Frank urethral bleeding
    2. Hematuria
    3. Bluish-red mass in perineal area
- Differential Diagnosis
    1. Hemorrhagic cystitis
    2. Vaginitis
    3. Sexual abuse
- Physical Findings
    1. Hematomas—urethral/scrotal/perineal
    2. Periurethral lacerations
- Diagnostic Tests/Findings: Referral necessary if extensive injury suspected
- Management/Treatment
    1. Urethral/vulvar trauma
        a. Mild bruising, superficial lacerations (symptomatic relief)—ice pack, sitz baths, analgesics
        b. Blunt or penetrating trauma—surgical intervention
    2. Testicular trauma—surgical referral
    3. Suspected renal injury—referral
    4. Penetrating injury—immediate surgical exploration

Glomerulonephritis (GN)

- Definition: Disease characterized by diffuse inflammatory changes in the glomeruli; immune-mediated response
    1. Primary acute form—poststreptococcal glomerulonephritis; most common form in children; true incidence unknown
    2. Primary chronic form
        a. Primarily seen with IgA nephropathy
        b. Other types—membranoproliferative glomerulonephritis (MPGN), mesangial proliferative glomerulonephritis

3. Secondary forms—associated with other disorders, e.g., systemic lupus erythematosus, anaphylactoid purpura, vascular problems

- Etiology/Incidence
    1. Multifactorial etiology—not completely understood
    2. Combination of factors induce injury
        a. Immune complex deposits in glomerular basement membrane
        b. Coagulation factors—fibrin deposits
        c. Exogenous nephrotoxins
            (1) Penicillamine, trimethadione, captopril, probenecid
            (2) Heavy metals—gold, mercury
    3. Uncertain incidence
- Signs and Symptoms
    1. Acute disease
        a. Hematuria
        b. Decreased urine output
        c. Edema
        d. Dark urine—acute poststreptococcal glomerulonephritis (APSGN)
    2. Chronic disease
        a. Fatigue
        b. Failure-to-thrive
- Differential Diagnosis
    1. Benign hematuria
    2. Hereditary nephropathy
    3. Lupus erythematosus
    4. Anaphylactoid purpura
- Physical Findings
    1. May be asymptomatic or severely ill depending upon extent of renal involvement
    2. Gross hematuria
    3. Edema—facial (especially periorbital) in the morning
    4. Hypertension
    5. CVA tenderness
- Diagnostic Tests/Findings
    1. Urinalysis

    a. Casts—RBC, leukocytes and/or casts indicate glomerular inflammation

    b. Hematuria

    c. Protein—correlates with degree of hematuria

    d. pH—low

    e. Specific gravity—increased

2. Titers—serum ASO, AHT, anti-Dnase B

3. Cultures—throat, skin; may be negative when signs of nephritis appear

4. Chest radiograph—assess pulmonary edema

5. Serum complement

    a. Returns to normal in APSGN

    b. Chronic elevation in MPGN

- Management/Treatment

1. All treatment is supportive

    a. Hypertension/relieve edema

        (1) Fluid restriction

        (2) Diuretics

        (3) Vasodilators

    b. Antibiotic (penicillin) if throat or skin infection persists

Hydronephrosis

- Definition: Unilateral or bilateral dilation of kidney(s)
- Etiology/Incidence

1. Caused by anatomic block of urine flow from kidney

2. Obstruction in 1 per 1000 births—slight male prevalence

3. Ureteropelvic junction (UPJ)—most common site of blockage

- Signs and Symptoms

1. Nausea

2. Abdominal or flank pain

3. Decreased urine output

- Differential Diagnosis

1. Prune belly syndrome

2. UPJ obstruction

3. Ectopic ureterocele

4. Urethral/ureterovesical obstructions

- Physical Findings

    1. Pain—abdominal/flank

    2. Failure-to-thrive

- Diagnostic Tests/Findings

    1. May have been detected during prenatal ultrasound

    2. IVP—late emptying of renal pelvis

    3. Renal scan—impact of obstruction on total renal function

- Management/Treatment

    1. Surgery to relieve obstruction

    2. Obstruction will lead to destruction of renal parenchyma; early exploration and repair advocated

    3. Must follow-up long term to assess final renal function

Renal Tubular Acidosis (RTA)

- Definition: Defect in normal urine acidification with resulting persistent metabolic acidosis; primary RTA includes 2 types

    1. Type 1 (distal tube)—defect in distal tube secretion of hydrogen ions

    2. Type 2 (proximal tube)—defect in reabsorption of bicarbonate

- Etiology/Incidence

    1. Cellular basis of defect is unknown; distal RTA may have genetic transmission as autosomal dominant disorder

    2. Incidence of primary RTA is unknown

- Signs and Symptoms

    1. Growth failure

    2. Gastrointestinal complaints

    3. Muscle weakness

- Differential Diagnosis

    1. Diarrhea

    2. Diabetes mellitus

    3. Renal failure

    4. Lactic acidosis

- Physical Findings: Growth failure

- Diagnostic Tests/Findings

    1. Urine pH—first morning specimen; pH less than 5.5 supports diagnosis of proximal RTA; 5.8 or greater indicates distal RTA

    2. Serum electrolytes—serum bicarbonate less than 16 mEq; hyperkalemia

- Management/Treatment

    1. Correction of acidosis; balance serum bicarbonate to normal level

        a. Intravenous therapy for infants with severe hyperkalemia/acidosis

        b. Oral therapy for most children

    2. Alkali administration as sodium bicarbonate or sodium citrate

        a. Potassium supplement if needed

        b. Sodium bicarbonate tablets—325 mg and 650 mg

    3. Mineralocorticoid deficiency corrected; diuretics reduce serum potassium

    4. Carnitine supplements if needed

    5. Risk of nephrocalcinosis, renal failure—continuous alkali therapy and long term clinical monitoring

    6. Normal growth resumes with corrected acidosis

Sexually Transmitted Diseases

Gonorrhea

- Definition: Acute infectious process primarily involving genital tract, anorectum, throat and ophthalmic epithelium; street terms—clap, drip, strain

- Etiology/Incidence

    1. *Neisseria gonorrhoeae*—gram-negative diplococcus

    2. Reportable disease in all States; estimated 650,000 new cases per year in U.S.

    3. Highest incidence among females 15 to 19 years of age

    4. Incidence among inner-city, poor adolescents as high as 14% (Hofmann & Greydanus, 1997)

    5. Associated with sexual abuse in children beyond newborn period and nonsexually active adolescents

- Signs and Symptoms

    1. Varies by site and gender; asymptomatic in 10% to 40% males and 50% to 80% females

    2. Vaginal or penile creamy discharge

    3. Perineal discomfort

   4. Menstrual irregularities

   5. Frequent, urgent, painful urination

   6. Rectal pain/itching

   7. Sore throat

   8. Fever, malaise, chills

- Differential Diagnosis

   1. *Chlamydia trachomatis* infection (may be concurrent)

   2. Genital mycoplasmas (may be concurrent)

   3. Bacterial vaginosis (may be concurrent)

   4. Trichomoniasis (may be concurrent)

   5. PID

- Physical Findings

   1. External Genitalia

     a. Erythema, edema

     b. Thick, purulent, greenish-yellow discharge (penile or vaginal)

   2. Female—pelvic examination

     a. Cervical erythema, friability, exudate

     b. Vaginal wall discharge/erythema

     c. Cervical/adnexal tenderness

   3. Male

     a. Thick, creamy penile discharge

     b. Enlarged, tender prostate

     c. Scrotal or groin pain (unilateral)

     d. Tender swelling above testis

- Diagnostic Tests/Findings

   1. Gram stain for presence of gram-negative, intracellular diplococcus

     a. Specimen sites—vagina, urethra, anus, oropharynx

     b. Oldest and least expensive method

     c. Basis of initiating treatment pending culture results

   2. Culture on selective media (Thayer-Martin) to confirm diagnosis

     a. Specimen sites—as above

     b. Most sensitive and specific test

3. Non-culture tests (DNA probes, enzyme immunoassay); not recommended for use in pediatric patients—false positive

4. No useful serologic test available to distinguish current from past infection

5. Evaluate for possible concurrent syphilis, hepatitis B, HIV and *Chlamydia trachomatis*

- Management/Treatment (see AAP *Red Book* for most current treatment guidelines)

1. Uncomplicated infections

   a. Children < 8 years weighing < 100 lb

      (1) Ceftriaxone sodium, 125 mg, IM in single dose (drug of choice) OR spectinomycin, 40 mg/kg (maximum of 2 g) IM in single dose

      (2) Concomitant treatment for possible *Chlamydia trachomatis*

          1. Azithromycin, 20 mg/kg (maximum 1g) orally in single dose OR erythromycin, 50 mg/kg per day (maximum 2 g/day) orally in 4 doses for 14 days

   b. Children/adolescents weighing > 100 lb and older than 8 years

      (1) Ceftriaxone, 125 mg, IM in single dose (drug of choice)

      (2) Flouroquinolones may be alternative treatment for patients over 18 years, non-pregnant or nursing and infections NOT acquired in Asia, Pacific Islands including Hawaii and California

      (3) Concomitant treatment for possible *Chlamydia trachomatis*—azithromycin, 1 g orally in single dose OR doxycycline, 100 mg orally b.i.d. for 7 days

2. Complicated (disseminated) infections

   a. Children < 8 years weighing < 100 lb

      (1) Ceftriaxone, 50 mg/kg/day (maximum 1 g/day) in single dose (IV or IM) for 7 days

      (2) Concomitant treatment for possible *Chlamydia trachomatis* with azithromycin or erythromycin

   b. Children/adolescents weighing > 100 lb and older than 8 years

      (1) Ceftriaxone, 1 g (IV or IM) in single dose for 7 days OR Cefotaxime, 1 g (IV) every 8 hours for 7 days

      (2) IV administration may change to oral antimicrobial agent such as ciprofloxacin (500 mg b.i.d. for 7 days) after 1–2 days of initial improvement

      (3) Concomitant treatment for *Chlamydia trachomatis* with azithromycin, 1 g orally in single dose OR doxycycline, 100 mg, orally b.i.d. for 7 days

3. Prophylaxis after sexual victimization

   a. Antimicrobial prophylaxis no longer recommended for abused prepubertal victims

   b. Prophylaxis for postpubertal females seen within 72 hours of sexual victimization:

   (1) Ceftriaxone, 125 mg IM in single dose

   (2) Concomitant treatment for possible *Chlamydia trachomatis* with

   (a) Azithromycin, 20 mg/kg (maximum of 1 g) orally in single dose for patients weighing < 100 lb

   (b) Azithromycin, 1 g orally in single dose for patients > 100 lb

Chlamydia

- Definition: Most common sexually transmitted disease in U.S. with primary sites of infection being genital tract, cornea and respiratory system

- Etiology/Incidence

   1. *Chlamydia trachomatis;* obligate intracellular bacteria; at least eighteen variants

   2. Reportable disease most states

   3. Incidence among sexually active females 15% to 37%; sexually active males 3%. (Hofmann & Greydanus, 1997, p. 497)

   4. Congenital chlamydia—See Multisystem Disorders chapter

   a. Perinatal transmission from infected mothers to infants estimated from 40% to 70%

   b. Manifestation primarily as conjunctivitis or pneumonia

- Signs and Symptoms: Genital Tract Infection

   1. Often asymptomatic for months to years

   2. Abdominal/pelvic pain

   3. Dysuria/burning

- Differential Diagnosis

   1. Gonorrhea

   2. Genital mycoplasmas

   3. Trichomoniasis

   4. Bacterial vaginosis

   5. PID

- Physical Findings: Genital Tract Infection

   1. May be normal

   2. Erythema of external genitalia

3. Vaginal/penile discharge—yellowish, watery

4. Tenderness on bimanual examination

- Diagnostic Tests/Findings: Judson & Ehret, 1994; Hoffmann & Greydanus, 1997

    1. Tissue culture—"gold standard" method for definitive diagnosis

        a. Culture specimen must contain epithelial cells to be accurate

        b. Only acceptable method for suspected child sexual abuse

        c. Culture processing requires 2 to 3 days; results available in 3 to 7 days depending on laboratory

    2. Alternative nonculture techniques

        a. Direct fluorescence assay (DFA)—stained direct smear of endocervical or urethra cells

            (1) Less expensive with results available within hours

            (2) Requires sufficient specimen collection

            (3) Good specificity but lower sensitivity resulting in false-positives

        b. Enzyme immunoassay (EIA)—genital secretions

            (1) Less expensive with rapid processing

            (2) Good sensitivity and specificity

        c. DNA hybridization—detects both chlamydia and gonorrhea

            (1) Results available within several days

            (2) Good sensitivity and specificity

        d. Polymerase chain reaction (PCR)—nucleic acid amplification

            (1) Good sensitivity and specificity

            (2) Not recommended for infants and young children

        e. Lipase chain reaction (LCR)—for confirmation

- Management/Treatment (See AAP, *Red Book* for additional treatment guidelines)

    1. Antibiotic treatment for uncomplicated genital tract infection

        a. Adolescents—doxycycline, 100 mg b.i.d. for 7 days OR azithromycin 1 g in single dose

            (1) Doxycyline is contraindicated in pregnancy

            (2) Alternative treatment regimen in pregnancy

                (a) Erythromycin base, 50 mg/kg/day q.i.d. for 7 days—may be given in half doses for 14 days if not tolerated well

                (b) Amoxicillin 1.5 g/day in 3 divided doses for 7 days

    b.   Children (6 months to 12 years)—erythromycin, 50 mg/kg/day, q.i.d. for 7 days OR azithromycin 20 mg/kg in single dose

    c.   Infants < 6 months of age

        (1)   Erythromycin, 50 mg/kg/day q.i.d. for 14 days

        (2)   Second course may be required

        (3)   Association between oral erythromycin and infantile hypertrophic pyloric stenosis (IHPS) has been reported in infants < weeks of age which require informing parents of potential risks and careful follow-up

    d.   Identify, examine, test, and treat any sexual contacts

2.   Evaluate for other STDs, e.g., gonorrhea, syphilis and treat as necessary

3.   No need for retest following treatment with doxycycline, azithromycin unless symptoms persist or if possibility of reinfection

4.   Retest may be recommended at 3 or more weeks following treatment with erythromycin, sulfisoxazole or amoxicillin (AAP, 1997)

Acquired Syphilis

- Definition: A contagious systemic infectious disease characterized by three progressive clinical stages

   1.   Primary stage—painless chancres on skin or mucous membranes at site of exposure

   2.   Secondary stage—begins between 1 to 2 months after inoculation characterized by skin rash

   3.   Tertiary stage—multisystem involvement that may occur from years to decades after primary infection including aortitis or gummatous changes of skin, bone or viscera; neurosyphilis may occur at any stage of infection particularly in HIV patients

   4.   Street terms—siff, lues, bad blood

- Etiology/Incidence

   1.   Infectious agent—*Treponema pallidum,* a thin, motile spirochete

   2.   Transmission—sexual contact, transplacental, direct contact with infected tissue (see Multisystem and Genetic Disorders chapter for congenital syphilis)

   3.   Reportable communicable disease in all States

   4.   Increased incidence during later 1980s and early 1990s

      a.   Incidence has begun to decline except in large urban areas and rural south

      b.   10% to 12% of all reported cases are among adolescents between 15 and 19 years of age

- Signs and Symptoms

   1.   Primary stage—one or more painless lesions usually on genitalia but may be on lips, tongue or extremities

    2. Secondary stage—fever, malaise, sore throat, skin rash, hair loss

    3. Tertiary stage—symptoms recur 15 or more years after initial infections; rarely seen among adolescents

- Differential Diagnosis

    1. Primary syphilis

        a. Genital herpes

        b. Condylomata acuminata

        c. Molluscum contagiosum

    2. Secondary syphilis

        a. Pityriasis rosea

        b. Psoriasis

        c. Drug sensitivity reactions

        d. Infectious mononucleosis

- Physical Findings

    1. Primary stage

        a. Chancre—one or more painless ulcers

        b. Most common on genitalia but seen at other sites of inoculation

    2. Secondary stage

        a. Generalized maculopapular/papulosquamous rash—classic if palms and soles included

        b. Round to oval, reddish-brown, "copper-colored" lesions

        c. Lymphadenopathy, arthralgia, fever, malaise

        d. Hypertrophic lesions of vulva/anus—condylomata lata

    3. Latency period follows with recurrences of secondary rash

    4. Tertiary phase

        a. 15 or more years after chancre

        b. Neurosyphilis, aortitis, gummous changes of bone, skin or viscera

- Diagnostic Tests/Findings

    1. Dark-field microscopic tests or direct fluorescent antibody tests (DFA)—presence of spirochetes from scrapings or washings of primary lesions; inexpensive, definitive diagnosis

    2. Serologic tests—presumptive diagnosis

        a. Nontreponemal tests—rapid plasma reagin (RPR), venereal disease research laboratory (VDRL), automated reagin test (ART)

(1) Measure nonspecific antigens

(2) False-positive rate of 1% to 2%

(3) False-negatives with recently acquired infections prior to seroconversion

(4) Serial testing used to monitor response to treatment

b. Treponemal tests—fluorescent treponemal antibody absorption (FTA-ABS, and microhemagglutination assay for antibody to *Treponema pallidum* (MHA-TP)

(1) Detect specific treponemal antigens

(2) Greater specificity than nontreponemal methods

(3) More expensive and time-consuming

(4) Useful to distinguish/confirm positive vs. false-positive nontreponemal results

(5) May show false-positive results in presence of lyme disease, genital herpes, autoimmune disorders, and IV drug use

c. High probability of infection in sexually active person with reactive nontreponemal and trepomenal tests

d. VDRL/RPR screening in early pregnancy and at delivery for all women to prevent transplacental transmission

- Management/Treatment: See AAP *Red Book* for additional treatment guidelines

1. Primary, secondary and early latent syphilis (less than 1 year duration)

a. Children—penicillin G benzathine, 50,000 U/kg IM up to adult dose of 2.4 million units in single dose

b. Adults—penicillin G benzathine, 2.4 million units, IM in single dose

(1) If allergic to penicillin and NOT pregnant—doxycycline, 100 mg orally b.i.d. for 14 days OR

(2) Tetracycline, 500 mg orally q.i.d. for 14 days

2. Late latent (more than 1 year duration) and tertiary syphilis

a. Children—penicillin G benzathine, 50,000 U/kg, IM up to adult dose of 2.4 million units, as 3 single doses administered at 1 week intervals

b. Adults—penicillin G benzathine 7.2 million units total administered as 3 doses of 2.4 million units IM per dose at 1 week intervals

(1) If allergic to Penicillin or pregnant—doxycycline, 100 mg orally b.i.d. for 4 wks OR

(2) Tetracycline, 500 mg orally q.i.d. for 4 wks

3. Neurosyphilis

a. Children—aqueous crystalline penicillin G, 200,000—300,000 U/kg per day given every 4–6 hours for 10–14 days not to exceed adult dose

b. Adults—aqueous crystalline penicillin G, 18–24 million units per day in doses of 3–4 million units, IV every 4 hours for 10–14 days OR penicilling G procaine, 2.4 million units, IM once daily PLUS probencid, 500 mg, orally both for 10–14 days

4. Evaluation of patient and all recent sexual contacts for syphilis and other STDs

5. Prevention and Control

   a. Patient education/discussion of sexuality, contraception and STDs as part of adolescent well-child visits

   b. Counseling regarding safe sexual practices including abstinence and proper use of condoms

Genital Herpes Simplex Virus (HSV)

- Definition: Most common HSV infection among adolescents characterized by clusters of painful lesions of the genital tract, perineum, mouth, lips or pharynx

- Etiology/Incidence

   1. Agent (herpes simplex viruses)—large, DNA viruses of two major types

      a. Type 2 (HSV-2)—primary source of genital herpes, usually affecting skin below the waist

      b. Type 1 (HSV-1)—less common source of genital herpes, usually sites include face, and skin above the waist

   2. Primary transmission through sexual contact and/or direct contact with open lesions; may be transmitted by autoinoculation of HSV-1 to genital area

   3. Transplacental transmission results in congenital herpes—see Multisystem and Genetic Disorders chapter

   4. Genital herpes is rare in prepubertal children except in cases of child abuse

   5. Estimated prevalence of 20% among sexually active adolescents

- Signs and Symptoms

   1. Painful genital lesions

   2. Burning with urination

   3. Tender, swollen lymph nodes

   4. Fever, malaise

- Differential Diagnosis

   1. Chancre of early syphilis

   2. Chancroid

   3. Molluscum contagiosum

   4. Allergic reaction

- Physical Findings

    1. Vesicular/ulcerated lesions—genital tract, perineum, mouth, lips, pharynx

    2. Genital, perianal erythema and/or edema

    3. Cervical friability, discharge

    4. Lymphadenopathy

- Diagnostic Tests/Findings

    1. Tissue culture—standard, most reliable diagnostic test

        a. Sensitivity varies by stage of disease—highest with vesicular lesions; lowest with recurrent infections and crusted lesions

        b. Results available within 1 to 3 days

    2. Newer diagnostic techniques

        a. DNA probe testing—relatively new technique with good sensitivity and specificity; results available within 1 to 3 days

        b. Direct fluorescent antibody/enzyme immunoassay—more rapid results than cultures but less sensitive results

        c. Polymerase chain reaction (PCR)—very sensitive; lower specificity resulting in false-positive results

    3. Serologic testing—may show rise in HSV antibodies; of limited value

        a. May be used to confirm initial diagnosis

        b. Often shows no rise in titers with recurrences

- Management/Treatment: See AAP *Red Book* for additional treatment guidelines

    1. Primary episode of genital infection

        a. Acyclovir, 200 mg, orally, 5 times/day for 7 to 10 days

        b. Initiation of treatment within 6 days of onset of lesions may reduce duration and severity of symptoms

        c. Valacyclovir and famciclovir provide alternatives for adult (pediatric formulations not yet available) treatment with advantage of less frequent dosing

    2. Recurrent episodes—alternative doses/frequency

        a. Acyclovir, 200 mg, orally, 5 times/day for 5 days

        b. Acyclovir, 400 mg, orally, 3 times/day for 5 days

        c. Acyclovir, 800 mg, orally, 2 times/day for 5 days

        d. Acyclovir less effective in treatment of recurrent vs. primary episodes

        e. Valacyclovir and famciclovir are alternatives for recurrent episodes

    3. Topical acyclovir no longer recommended; limited benefit

4. Suppressive therapy—with frequent recurrences of > 6 per year

    a. Acyclovir 400 mg, orally, b.i.d. OR 200 mg, orally, 3 to 5 times/day

    b. Discontinue after one year to reassess recurrences

5. Sitz baths may provide relief

6. Education—recurrences; viral shedding; abstinence when lesions are present; use of condoms during sexual activities

Genital Warts (Condylomata Acuminata)

- Most common symptomatic viral reproductive tract infection in U.S. (Hatcher, 1998); characterized by epithelial warts/tumors of mucous membranes and skin

- Etiology/Incidence

    1. Causative agent—Human papillomavirus (HPV), a small DNA virus with more than 100 subtypes; types 6 and 11 usually cause genital warts and types 16, 18, 31, 33, 35 vaginal, anal and cervical dysplasia (Hatcher, 1998)

    2. Primary mode of transmission is sexual contact; sexual abuse must be considered when present in prepubertal child

    3. Genital HPV infection may be as high as 38% among sexually active female adolescents

- Signs and Symptoms

    1. Firm bumps in anogenital area

    2. Occasional local symptoms—burning, pain, itching, bleeding

    3. Often asymptomatic

- Differential Diagnosis

    1. Chancre of secondary syphilis

    2. Molluscum contagiosum

- Physical Findings

    1. Firm, flesh-colored anogenital lesions resembling cauliflower in configuration

    2. Range in size from few millimeters to centimeters

    3. Males—warts on shaft of penis, meatus, scrotum and perianal areas

    4. Females—warts usually seen on labia and perianal areas

- Diagnostic Tests/Findings

    1. Diagnosis usually based on clinical inspection; no culture is available

    2. Colposcopy to detect cervical lesions—application of 3% to 5% acetic acid (vinegar) causes lesion to blanch; not definitive

    3. Pelvic examination—pap smear for cytological analysis may be diagnostic

4. Biopsy of lesion for histologic examination—may be diagnostic

5. DNA probe—may detect asymptomatic HPV infection

- Management/Treatment

  1. No definitive treatment yet available to eradicate HPV virus; palliative treatment focusing on removal of lesions, symptom relief, and close follow-up for recurrences and sequelae

  2. Spontaneous resolution within 3 months in 25% cases; recurrences are common

  3. External visible lesions

     a. Self-treatment with podophyllum resin solution or gel (contraindicated in pregnancy and not yet tested for safety/efficacy in children)

        (1) Topical application b.i.d. for 3 days; need not be washed off

        (2) First application should be done in office to assure proper technique

        (3) Treatment may be repeated up to 4 cycles with 4 day rest period between cycles

     b. Podophyllin, 10% to 25% in compound tincture of benzoin (contraindicated in pregnancy)

        (1) Weekly treatment up to total of 6 applications

        (2) Must be washed off in 1 to 4 hours

     c. Trichloracetic acid (TCA 80% to 90%)

        (1) Topical application followed by careful drying and application of talc or baking soda

        (2) Weekly treatments up to total of 6 applications

        (3) Causes more local discomfort than podophyllin

     d. Liquid nitrogen or cryotherapy

     e. Laser surgery, cryosurgery, excision, electrodessication—reserved for extensive, severe, and/or resistent cases

  4. Gynecologic referral necessary for cervical warts

  5. Monitoring of Pap smears for increased risk of cervical cancer

     a. Every 3 months during active disease; then every 3 to 6 months for 2 years

     b. Annual Pap smears for all HPV positive asymptomatic females thereafter

  6. Screening serology for syphilis; evaluate for any other concommitent STDs and treat accordingly

  7. Education regarding safe sexual practices

Trichomoniasis

- Definition: Common sexually transmitted infection of the genital tract
- Etiology/Incidence
    1. Causative agent—*Trichomonas vaginalis,* a flagellated protozoan
    2. Transmitted primarily through sexual contact; presence in prepubertal child should alert practitioner to possible sexual abuse
    3. Often associated with other STDs, e.g., gonorrhea, chlamydia
    4. Unknown incidence
- Signs and Symptoms
    1. Females—asymptomatic in 25% to 50% of all cases
        a. Vaginal discharge
        b. Vulvovaginal irritation and itching
        c. Vaginal odor
        d. Difficult urination
    2. Males—usually asymptomatic
        a. Mild dysuria
        b. Itching
- Differential Diagnosis
    1. Candidiasis
    2. Chemical vaginitis
    3. Bacterial vaginosis
    4. UTI
    5. Poor hygiene
    6. Gonorrhea
- Physical Findings
    1. Vaginal discharge—frothy, light yellow to grey-green, musty odor
    2. Pelvic examination—evidence of vaginitis, cervicitis; erythema, edema and pruritus of external genitalia may be present
    3. Males generally asymptomatic
- Diagnostic Tests/Findings
    1. Wet mount of vaginal secretions or spun urine sediment—presence of motile trichomonads
    2. Motile trichomonads may also be seen on Pap smears and urine analysis

3. Other tests—culture (trypticase yeast extract iron serum (TYI) medium); antibody tests using enzyme immunoassay; direct/indirect immunofluorescence techniques are available

    a. More sensitive techniques than wet mount

    b. Rarely needed to make diagnosis

- Management/Treatment: See AAP, *Red Book*, for additional treatment guidelines

    1. Metronidazole—treatment of choice

        a. Prepubertal—15 mg/kg/day orally t.i.d. for 7 days (maximum 2 g for 7 days) or 40 mg/kg (maximum 2 g) orally in single dose

        b. Adolescent—2 g orally in single dose

        c. Avoid alcohol during treatment

        d. During pregnancy—2 g single dose of metronidazole or 7 day regimen

    2. No sexual activity during treatment

    3. Partners should receive concurrent therapy

    4. Evaluate for presence of other STD—treat accordingly

Bacterial Vaginosis (BV)

- Definition: Clinical syndrome characterized by vaginal symptoms, primarily in sexually active adolescents/adults

- Etiology/Incidence

    1. Not an actual infection but classified as a sexually transmitted disease

    2. Results from replacement of normal vaginal flora (*Lactobacillus*) with high concentrations of anaerobes—*Gardnerella vaginalis, Mycoplasma hominis*

    3. Transmission may be sexual or nonsexual

    4. Incidence unknown

- Signs and Symptoms

    1. Profuse vaginal discharge with "fishy" odor

    2. May be asymptomatic

- Differential Diagnosis

    1. Foreign body

    2. Gonorrhea/chlamydia/trichomoniasis

    3. Vulvovaginitis—group A streptococci, shigella organisms

    4. Candidiasis

    5. Physiologic leukorrhea

- Physical Findings
  1. Vaginal/cervical discharge—thin, white, malodorous; adherent to vaginal wall
  2. Itching, swelling, redness of external genitalia
- Diagnostic Tests/Findings
  1. Vaginal secretions
     a. pH greater than 4.5
     b. KOH 10% mixed with vaginal discharge—releases amine, ''fishy odor'' (whiff test)
     c. Saline wet mount—clue cells
  2. Culture available—rarely helpful, expensive
- Management/Treatment (See AAP, *Red Book* for additional treatment guidelines)
  1. Metronidazole
     a. 500 mg, orally, b.i.d. for 7 days OR
     b. 2 g orally, single dose with 2nd dose in 48 hours
  2. Alternative Treatment
     a. Clindamycin cream 2%, one full applicator (5 g) intravaginally at bedtime for 7 days
     b. Metronidazole gel 0.75%, one full applicator (5 g), intravaginally b.i.d. for 5 days
     c. Clindamycin, 300 mg, orally, b.i.d. for 7 days
  3. Clindamycin recommended for pregnant women due to possible teratogenicity of metronidazole
  4. Education regarding possible complications
     a. Increased risk for PID
     b. Pregnancy risk for chorioamnionitis and premature delivery

Contraception

- Abstinence—most effective method
  1. Half of all adolescents select this option
  2. Should be discussed as viable option regardless of prior history
- Male Condoms—most effective barrier method
  1. Mechanism—mechanical barrier preventing semen from entering vagina; some brands provide additional protection with spermicide coating
  2. Types of male condoms—over 100 brands currently on the market

    a. Latex—recommended

    b. Polyurethane (latex-free) if latex sensitive

    c. Natural skin (lambskin)—not recommended (inadequate STD and HIV protection)

  3. Failure rates

    a. Theoretical—3%

    b. Actual—12% primarily due to nonuse/misuse

    c. Combined with spermicide—0.1%; comparable to oral contraceptive

  4. Risks/precautions

    a. Breakage rate— ~1% to 2%

    b. Only water-based lubricants should be used—latex breaks down in contact with petroleum-based products

    c. Latex breakdown over time and/or when exposed to heat

- Vaginal Spermicides—topical creams, jellies, foams, suppositories, and films to prevent pregnancy; used alone or in combination with condoms

  1. Active spermicidal agent—nonoxynol-9 or octoxynol-9

  2. Failure rates— ~6%

  3. Risks/precautions

    a. Few side effects—occasional reports of local burning/irritation

    b. Timing of insertion varies by form used

    c. Must be reapplied with repeated intercourse

- Diaphragm—female barrier contraceptive method

  1. Thin latex dome with flexible ring for vaginal insertion prior to intercourse; positioned with posterior rim on posterior fornix and anterior rim behind pubic bone

  2. Requires pelvic examination for proper fitting for appropriate size

  3. Failure rate among adolescents—10% to 25%

  4. Risks/precautions

    a. Requires technical skill/comfort with body for correct placement

    b. Must be kept in place for 6 hours post-intercourse

    c. Spermicidal agent must be used for subsequent intercourse

    d. Side-effects—UTI, vaginitis

- Oral Contraceptives (OC)

  1. Mechanisms

     a. Prevents ovulation

     b. Increases viscosity of cervical mucus inhibiting sperm penetration

     c. Alters endometrium to resist implantation

2. Estrogen-progestin combinations

     a. Estrogens—ethinyl estradiol and mestranol

        (1) Ethinyl estradiol—1.2 to 1.4 times stronger than mestranol

        (2) Ethinyl estradiol effective at doses as low as 20 μg

        (3) Usually select lowest effective estrogen dose (20 to 35 μg)

     b. Basic progestins—norethindrone, norethindrone acetate, norethynodrel, ethynodiol diacetate, norgestrel

     c. Newer progestins—norgestimate, desogestrel, gestodene

     d. Monophasic, biphasic, or triphasic combinations—deliver constant or progressively increasing progestin during cycle

3. Failure rates—0.5% (theoretical) to 2% to 3% (actual)

4. Risks/precautions

     a. OC-drug—interactions

        (1) Drugs that may reduce OC effectiveness—antibiotics, antifungals, anticonvulsants, antacids

        (2) Drugs that enhance OC effectiveness—ascorbic acid, co-trimoxazole

     b. Major side-effects—thrombosis

     c. Minor side-effect—vaginal spotting, nausea, bloating, irritability

     d. OCs do not protect against AIDS and other STDs

     e. Absolute contraindications for OC use

        (1) History of clotting disorder

        (2) Impaired liver function

        (3) Abnormal vaginal bleeding (undiagnosed)

        (4) Pregnancy

        (5) Estrogen-dependent carcinoma

     f. Relative contraindications for OC use

        (1) Severe hypertension

        (2) Migraines

        (3) Chronic diseases, e.g., diabetes, heart disease, sickle cell etc.

        (4) Rheumatologic disorders

- Long-Acting Progestins (Injectable and Implantable to Inhibit Ovulation)
    1. Depo-medroxyprogesterone acetate (injectable)
        a. Dosage and administration—150 mg/mL intramuscular injection every 3 months during first 5 days of normal period to assure non-pregnant status
        b. Failure rate—0.25%
        c. Precautions/risks
            (1) If > 3 months between injections, pregnancy test as precaution
            (2) Should not be given to postpartum, lactating adolescent mothers
            (3) Spotting, weight gain, bloating, headaches, mood changes
            (4) Risk of decreased bone density
    2. Norplant (subdermal implants)
        a. Six match-stick size tubes filled with levonorgestrel implanted in subcutaneous tissue of upper inner arm
        b. Effective for up to 5 years
        c. Failure rates—0.04% (1st year) to 1.1% (5th year)
        d. Precautions/risks
            (1) Appropriate screening, education and follow-up associated with continued effective use
            (2) Side effects similar to injectable—spotting, weight gain, headaches, and moodiness
- Postcoital or "Morning After" Contraception: Use of oral contraceptive within 72 hours of unprotected intercourse (50 μg ethinyl estradiol and 0.5 mg norgestrel)
    1. 2 tablets initially followed by additional 2 tablets 12 hours later
    2. Simplest, most common method used in U.S.
    3. Side-effects of nausea and vomiting common
    4. Failure rate—1.6%
- Contraceptive Methods Less Suitable for Adolescents
    1. Coitus interruptus—failure rate > 19%
    2. Natural family planning—high failure rate even among motivated adults
    3. Cervical cap—difficulties with proper placement; risk of cervical dysplasia
    4. Intrauterine device (IUD)—risk of PID
    5. Progestin-only mini-pill—failure rates up to 13% among mature adults
    6. Female condom—failure rates of 12% to 20% among adult users

Issues of Pregnancy and Birth for the Adolescent

- Pregnancy: Diagnosis and counseling

    1. Risk factors

        a. Early onset of sexual activity; inadequate concept of fertility and contraception

        b. Low socioeconomic level

        c. Poor academic achievement

        d. Low self-image; few options for future

        e. Early pregnancy in mother or sister

        f. Substance abuse

        g. Physical/sexual abuse

    2. Incidence

        a. U.S. has the highest rates of adolescent pregnancy and births among industrialized nations; estimates of one million each year

        b. More than 4 out of 10 U.S. teens have at least one pregnancy before 20 years of age

        c. Rates have shown a slow decline from 1991 to 1996; overall decline of 12% among 15 to 19 year olds with largest decline among African-American teens

        d. Birth rate among 15 to 19-year-old females—54.7:1000 (1996)

        e. Recidivism common—17% to 40% pregnant again within 1 year, 28% to 50% within 2 years

        f. Only $\frac{1}{3}$ of adolescent mothers complete high school

    3. Signs and Symptoms

        a. First trimester

            (1) Irregular menses/amenorrhea

            (2) GI—nausea, vomiting

            (3) Urinary frequency

            (4) Breast tenderness/tingling

            (5) Other—headache, vertigo, abdominal cramps

        b. Second trimester

            (1) Increased/darkening skin pigmentation

            (2) Fetal movement—"quickening" 16 to 20 weeks

            (3) Contractions—Braxton-Hicks 16 to 27 weeks

        c. Third trimester—increased contractions

4. Physical Findings

   a. First trimester

      (1) Breast—fullness/tenderness, nipple tingling/discharge/darkening areola

      (2) Abdomen—fullness/pelvic mass; uterine fundus at symphysis pubis at 12 weeks

      (3) Pelvic examination

         (a) Softening of uterine isthmus (Hegar sign) 6 to 8 weeks

         (b) Bluish hue to cervix/vaginal epithelium (Chadwick sign) 6 to 8 weeks

         (c) Cervical softening (Goodell sign) 6 to 8 weeks

         (d) Increased leukorrhea

      (4) Weight gain—2 pounds (1 kg)

      (5) Fetal heart tones (FHT)—doppler 10 to 12 weeks

   b. Second trimester

      (1) Stretch marks "striae" on abdomen and breasts

      (2) Fundus midway between symphysis pubis and umbilicus by 14 to 15 weeks, at umbilicus 20 to 22 weeks

      (3) Fetal outline 20 weeks

      (4) Fetal heart tones (FHT) by fetoscope at 20 weeks

      (5) Weight gain—11 pounds (5 kg)

   c. Third trimester

      (1) Colostrum from breasts 28 to 40 weeks

      (2) Fundus between umbilicus and xiphoid 28 weeks; at xiphoid 38 weeks

      (3) Weight gain—11 pounds (5 kg)

      (4) Bloody show—impending labor

      (5) Ruptured membranes

   d. Labor

      (1) Stage 1—effacement and dilatation of cervix

      (2) Stage 2—delivery of fetus

      (3) Stage 3—separation and delivery of placenta

5. Differential Diagnosis

   a. Ectopic pregnancy

   b. Incomplete spontaneous abortion

c. Molar pregnancy

d. PID

e. Corpus luteum cyst (Emans, 1998)

f. UTI

6. Diagnostic Tests/Findings

    a. Urine for human chorionic gonadotropin (hCG)—positive 7 to 10 days after conception

    b. Radioimmunoassay (RIA)—serology; more specific than urine, expensive; positive 7 to 10 days after conception

    c. Cervical cultures—gonorrhea/chlamydia screen

    d. Wet mount—saline, KOH

    e. Papanicolaou smears

    f. Serology—syphilis, hepatitis B surface antigen, blood type/Rh factor, CBC with indices, rubella, human immunodeficiency virus

    g. Urinalysis/culture (if indicated)

    h. Pelvic ultrasound

7. Counseling/Education

    a. Impact on future plans, finances, family structure

    b. Identity and age of father—anticipated involvement

    c. Options

        (1) Continue pregnancy and maintain custody

        (2) Place child for adoption

        (3) Termination of pregnancy

    d. Prenatal care—examinations, adequate diet, vitamins (include folic acid) and iron

    e. Avoidance of medications/drugs/alcohol

- Prenatal Diagnosis: Identify potential inherited/acquired defects

1. Variety of causes—genetic factors (25%); environmental (15%); combination of both genetic and environmental (30%); unaccountable (30%)

2. Incidence—3% to 5% infants in U.S.

3. Risk factors—maternal

    a. Disease—diabetes, thyroid, immune deficiency or compromise

    b. Age—young, especially less than 16 years; over 35 years

    c. Previous child with Down syndrome, anencephaly, meningomyelocele

4. Screening tools

    a. Family pedigree—graphic record, family medical history

    b. Alpha-fetoprotein

        (1) Screens for neural tube defects; Meckel syndrome

        (2) Serum levels less accurate than amniotic fluid analysis but can be done earlier in pregnancy for initial screen

    c. Amniocentesis—collection of amniotic fluid, 15 to 16 weeks gestation; karyotype/chromosomal analysis; inborn errors of metabolism; confirmatory test with abnormal serum alpha-fetoprotein

    d. Chorionic villus sampling—tissue (villus) sample from fetal placenta at 9 to 11 weeks gestation; chromosomal abnormality; usually reserved for women over 35 years

    e. Metabolic disease, hemaglobinopathies from DNA analysis

- Genetic counseling: Communication process regarding risk/problems surrounding certain disorders

    1. Often initiated following birth of affected child

    2. Both parents included—family history, medical/psychological consequences for child/family; possibility of future children affected; options

    3. Utilizes results from prenatal diagnostic tools/tests

- Pregnancy termination

    1. Spontaneous termination—miscarriage

        a. Miscarriage/spontaneous abortion of pregnancy prior to fetal viability

        b. May be complete or incomplete

        c. Occurs in 14% of all pregnancies including adolescents

        d. Often associated with genetic abnormality in fetus

    2. Elective termination—induced abortion

        a. Induced or elective abortion—35% of adolescent pregnancies

        b. Procedural options—dependent on trimester of termination

        c. First trimester abortion options—rule out STD prior to procedure

            (1) Manual syringe evacuation/early suction curettage—4 to 6 weeks of pregnancy

                (a) Cannula positioned into uterus with aspiration or suction of conceptus (menstrual extraction)

                (b) Low risk of genital injury or complications

      (2) Suction curettage/vacuum aspiration—up to 12 to 14 weeks of pregnancy

         (a) Cervical dilation 6+ hours prior to procedure using *Laminaria* (hydrophilic seaweed sticks)

         (b) Cannula position into uterus with suction followed by curettage

         (c) Considered safest first trimester method

      (3) Mifepristone—abortifacient which induces abortion when administered in early pregnancy (49 days or less)

         (a) Acts as antiprogesterone

         (b) Initial dose of 600 mg followed with 400 µg of misoprostol (a prostaglandin) two days later

   d. Second trimester

      (1) Dilatation and evacuation curettage (D&E)—20 to 24 weeks of pregnancy

         (a) Cervical dilation prior to procedure with osmotic dilators

         (b) Conceptus removed via curettage, aspiration, or ring forceps under general anethesia; risk of cervical trauma

         (c) Antibiotics recommended post-procedure

      (2) Prostaglandin suppository technique—16 to 24 weeks of pregnancy

         (a) Cervical dilation with osmotic dilators followed by vaginal suppositories of prostaglandin E; has largely replaced more controversial intraamniotic instillation techniques

         (b) 20 mg prostaglandin suppositories used every 3 to 4 hours induces labor and subsequent abortion within 4 to 60 hours

         (c) Complications include significant flu-like symptoms and possible delivery of live fetus

   e. Referral and follow-up

      (1) Referral to obstetrician-gynecologist or family-planning clinic once decision to terminate pregnancy is made

      (2) Continue supportive care and counseling options on follow-up

- Birthing methods: Greater risk of cesarean delivery due to immature pelvic skeletal development; cephalopelvic disproportion

- Prematurity/Low Birth Weight

   1. Maternal risk factors—maternal age less than 16; poor prenatal care/poor nutrition

   2. Prevention aimed at prenatal management

      a. Good nutrition; avoid dieting—daily calories 2500 to 2700 Kcal/day

    b. Supplements—vitamins (include folic acid), iron (anemia possible), calcium

3. Early/consistent prenatal care

    a. Avoid all medications unless specifically approved by health care provider

    b. Potential for multisystem complications—infant

       (1) Respiratory—respiratory distress syndrome, bronchopulmonary dysplasia, apnea

       (2) Cardiovascular—patent ductus arteriosus, bradycardia, malformations

       (3) Hematologic—hyperbilirubinemia, subcutaneous hemorrhage

       (4) Gastrointestinal—poor motility

       (5) Metabolic/endocrine—hypocalcemia, hypoglycemia or hyperglycemia, hypothermia

       (6) Central nervous system—intraventricular hemorrhage, hypotonia

       (7) Renal abnormalities

       (8) Infections

- Home monitoring/follow-up care

    1. Frequent contact with mother/infant—early discharge follow-up recommended within 48 hours

      a. Infant feeding patterns

      b. Adaptation of mother to sleep changes

      c. Social support—father of baby, mother's family

    2. Follow-up (well-child visits)

      a. Adolescent problems—repeated pregnancy; STD

      b. Optimal health of mother/infant

      c. Future plans—completion of high school, college/technical training, career

- Maternal substance abuse

    1. Use of substances among adolescents high—more likely to stop during and after pregnancy

    2. Drug/alcohol use

      a. Counsel at initial prenatal visit

      b. Reinforce impact of all substances on developing fetus—tobacco, alcohol, marijuana, inhalants

- Screening for potentially abusive parents

    1. Increased risk of battering by partner when pregnant

      a. Assess relationship between girl and partner

      b.   Some states require mandatory reporting of victims of domestic violence

  2. Many risk factors for child abuse

      a.   Parental factors

          (1)   Young and/or immature parents

          (2)   Minimal education

          (3)   Financial stress

          (4)   Lack of social support

          (5)   Unplanned or unwanted pregnancy

          (6)   Unrealistic expectations of parenting

      b.   Infant factors

          (1)   Prematurity

          (2)   Perception as "different/bad"; difficult temperament

          (3)   Congenital defect/malformation

- Perinatal complications of neonate

  1. Low birth weight and prematurity—see earlier section

  2. Infant mortality—almost 6% die in first year

  3. Cognitive/social development—possible low self-esteem, less responsive/expressive, decreased ability to trust others

  4. Sudden Infant Death Syndrome (SIDS)

Questions
Select the best answer

1. Urinary tract infections (UTI) are the most common pediatric urinary tract problems seen in primary care. Which of the following statements is not true regarding UTIs?

   a. Symptoms are often nonspecific especially in infancy
   b. Urine culture is required for definitive diagnosis
   c. Trimethoprim-sulfamethoxazole is drug of choice for most children
   d. Radiologic studies are rarely indicated with first infection

2. A 3-year-old girl presents with symptoms of painful urination, frequency, and occasional incontinence over the past week. When seen in your office, she has a temperature of 101.6° F. Which of the following would be your approach in establishing a definitive diagnosis?

   a. Clean-catch midstream collection of specimen for urine analysis
   b. Clean-catch midstream collection of specimen for urine culture
   c. Straight catheterization collection of specimen for urine culture
   d. Voiding cystourethrogram (VCUG)

3. The most likely organism to cause a UTI in the pediatric population is:

   a. *Staphylococcus saprophyticus*
   b. Klebsiella
   c. Chlamydia
   d. *E. coli*

4. One of the most commonly suggested reasons for primary enuresis is:

   a. Certain medications, such as theophylline
   b. Genitourinary abnormalities
   c. Family disruptions and stress
   d. Delayed maturation of voiding inhibitory reflex

5. Suzanne, a 7-year-old, comes to you for a physical examination prior to participation in soccer. Suzanne's mother is concerned that the child "still has accidents at night." You determine that Suzanne has primary nocturnal enuresis and your first recommendation to her mother is to:

   a. Avoid use of criticism or punishment
   b. Use a sticker/star chart
   c. Treat with medication
   d. Purchase an enuresis alarm

6. The incidence of cryptorchidism at one year of age is about 1%. The best explanation for this is:

   a. Examination of the scrotum begins at this age
   b. A child can usually stand, making palpation of the testes easier
   c. Spontaneous resolution often occurs in first year
   d. Surgical repair can now be done in neonatal period

7. Communicating hydrocele is best differentiated from the noncommunicating type by the fact that:

    a. There is no association with hernia
    b. It usually resolves on its own
    c. The fluid is static in the scrotum
    d. Frequently develops into hernia

8. In counseling parents when their child is diagnosed with mild hypospadias, suggest that the following may be part of the management:

    a. Circumcision
    b. Radiography
    c. Chromosomal analysis
    d. Surgical correction at 2 years of age

9. On physical examination of a 2-year-old uncircumcised male, you note that the foreskin is retracted and discolored. There is swelling of the glans. The most likely diagnosis is:

    a. Phimosis
    b. Balanitis
    c. UTI
    d. Paraphimosis

10. Meatal stenosis, narrowing of the distal urethra, is seen following:

    a. Orchiopexy
    b. Circumcision
    c. Epididymitis
    d. Hypospadias repair

11. During a track meet, a 14-year-old male pole vaulter falls to the ground screaming in pain. He complains of intense, searing pain in his right scrotum. He vomits twice while waiting for the ambulance. He most likely has:

    a. Orchitis
    b. Hydrocele
    c. Acute epididymitis
    d. Testicular torsion

12. Treatment for this disorder is primarily:

    a. Scrotal elevation
    b. Ice
    c. Immediate surgical referral
    d. Bedrest

13. Labial adhesions are a relatively common finding among infants and young girls. Which of the following statements about this condition is true?

    a. Adhesions are usually present at birth but may be missed on examination
    b. Highest incidence is from birth to 3 years
    c. Simple lysis of adhesions is often recommended
    d. Most cases resolve without intervention

14. Which of the following statements is true regarding the use of topical application of conjugated estrogen cream with labial adhesions?

    a. It is highly successful in resolving most adhesions within 2 months
    b. It is no longer recommended because it may stimulate precocious puberty
    c. Topical applications of bland creams or petroleum jelly are equally effective
    d. Mechanical lysis is preferred treatment today

15. Sheryl, a 12-year-old, complains of a vaginal discharge for the past 8 to 9 months. She tells you her underpants are frequently wet. When she wipes after urinating, there is "white stuff" on the tissue. Sheryl denies urinary problems, genital itching or odor. She also denies sexual activity. Her menses have not yet started, but she reports she "started to develop" in her breasts at about age 10. Her vaginal discharge is most likely a result of:

    a. A fungal infection
    b. Poor hygiene
    c. Retained foreign body
    d. Physiologic leukorrhea

16. Your recommendations to Sheryl regarding management of the discharge includes which one of these?

    a. Vinegar and water douche
    b. Placing a sanitary "mini pad" in her underpants
    c. A 10 day course of penicillin or erythromycin
    d. Use of a monilial cream for 1 week

17. Which of the following is not true of dysmenorrhea?

    a. Onset is usually within the first two to three months following menarche
    b. A leading cause of school absenteeism in adolescent females
    c. Systemic symptoms include vomiting and dizziness
    d. Pain is from start of menses to about 24 to 48 hours later

18. Amy, a 16-year-old, has symptoms of premenstrual syndrome. She refuses to take NSAIDS, preferring instead more "natural" treatments. Her options include:

    a. Eating foods rich in sodium and fat
    b. Including more foods or supplements with Vitamin C
    c. Limited fluid intake, to avoid "bloating"
    d. Adequate rest, a healthy diet, and exercise

19. In cases of accidental genitourinary trauma, which of the following is not commonly seen:

    a. Extensive tears of the vaginal wall
    b. Hematuria
    c. Hematoma of the urethra, scrotum, lower abdomen
    d. Periurethral lacerations

20. The most common form of glomerulonephritis in children is:

    a. Mesangial proliferative
    b. Poststreptococcal
    c. Membranoproliferative
    d. Mesangiostreptococcal

21. Which of the following signs/symptoms is not associated with acute forms of glomerulone-phritis:

    a. Edema
    b. Hematuria
    c. Increased urine output
    d. Dark urine

22. One of your male patients presents with weight loss, abdominal pain, and decreased urine output. On examination, you palpate a right-sided mass, noting tenderness in the abdomen and flank. Urinalysis reveals significant leukocytosis. An intravenous pyelogram is ordered, which shows marked delay of emptying from the renal pelvis. The most likely diagnosis is:

    a. Glomerulonephritis
    b. Pyelonephritis
    c. Hydronephrosis
    d. UTI

23. Which of the following is true of renal tubular acidosis—type 1?

    a. Genetically transmitted as autosomal recessive disorder
    b. Distal tube defect affecting secretion of hydrogen ions
    c. Distal tube defect affecting bicarbonate reabsorption
    d. Most children remain short in stature in spite of early treatment

24. Vulvovaginitis may be caused by all of the following except:

    a. Poor hygiene
    b. Herpes simplex virus
    c. Pinworms
    d. Condylomata acuminata

25. Meatal stenosis can be identified by all of these with the exception of:

    a. Crying with urination
    b. Inflammation of glans penis

c. Slit-like meatus

d. Wide urinary stream

26. Trina, age 14, comes in with complaints of headache and nausea. She admits to having a boyfriend, whom she has sex with "once in a while," and sometimes he uses a condom. She had a period last month, but it lasted 2 days instead of the usual seven. Which of the following are not usually perceived as risk factors for adolescent pregnancy?

   a. Early onset of sexual activity

   b. Familiarity with fertility knowledge

   c. Sporadic, if any, contraceptive use

   d. Low self-image

27. Trina's urine pregnancy test is positive and confirmed by serology. Which of the following physical findings is not consistent with a gestation of less than 12 weeks?

   a. Hegar sign

   b. Goodell sign

   c. Doppler auscultation of fetal heart sounds

   d. 4 to 6 pound weight gain

28. Congenital defects are present in approximately 3 to 5% of infants born in this country. Which of the following factors is the lowest contributor to defects?

   a. Genetic

   b. Unknown

   c. Environmental

   d. Combination of environmental and genetic

29. Which of the following is the earliest screening test that you would use in managing Trina's care during her first trimester of pregnancy?

   a. Amniocentesis

   b. Chorionic villus sampling

   c. Serum alpha-fetoprotein

   d. Fetal ultrasound

30. Trina expresses to you that she may want to terminate the pregnancy. She has heard that abortion is a simple procedure, without complications. Your discussion with her is based on the fact that:

   a. Adolescents only choose to terminate pregnancy 10% of the time

   b. Menstrual extraction could be done at this point

   c. The risk is high for hemorrhage and fever

   d. Cervical injury overall from induced abortion is rare

31. You know that if Trina delivers her baby, close follow-up of both is important. What is not a focus of care in the first few weeks after delivery?

   a. Social support for the family

    b. Mother's goals for education

    c. Infant's continued weight gain

    d. Adaptation of mother to sleep changes

32. While child abuse occurs across age barriers, the adolescent parent may be at greater risk for abusing their child because:

    a. The pregnancy may be unplanned or unwanted

    b. Adolescents continue substance abuse after the baby is born

    c. The infant mortality rate is low

    d. Education becomes more important than parenting

33. A thick, purulent vaginal discharge that is greenish-yellow is most likely an infection caused by:

    a. *Chlamydia trachomatis*

    b. Herpes simplex virus

    c. *Neisseria gonorrhea*

    d. Human papillomavirus

34. The primary treatment for this infection would be:

    a. Amoxicillin

    b. Ceftriaxone

    c. Ofloxacin

    d. Penicillin

35. The most common sexually transmitted disease in the United States is:

    a. Gonorrhea

    b. Human immunodeficiency virus (HIV)

    c. Chlamydia

    d. Herpes

36. Which of the following tests provide the most definitive diagnosis for suspected syphilis?

    a. VDRL

    b. ART

    c. Dark-field microscopy

    d. FTA-AB$_s$

37. Which of the following is not true regarding the use of acyclovir in the treatment of herpes simplex virus?

    a. Topical treatment not recommended

    b. Treatment is equally effective for active primary and recurrent lesions

    c. The focus of treatment is decrease in intensity symptom duration, and viral shedding

    d. Therapy is best initiated within 6 days of onset of lesions

38. Your 15-year-old female patient presents with genital lesions. Your work-up is based on the knowledge that:

    a. Human papillomavirus (HPV) is often associated with malignancy
    b. HPV manifests itself as molluscum contagiosum
    c. Most HPV infections cause genital itching and pain
    d. Syphilis serology should be included to distinguish HPV from condylomata lata

39. After your examination, you determine that your patient has condylomata acuminata. Which of the following is not commonly used to treat these lesions?

    a. Topical podophyllum resin
    b. Laser treatment for unresponsive lesions
    c. Topical acyclovir
    d. Treatment is often not needed; many lesions regress spontaneously

40. During your evaluation of Lisa, a 16-year-old female patient, she relates recent, first-time sexual intercourse with her boyfriend. Now she complains of a "frothy" substance in her underwear that "smells weird." She also has slight itching in her vaginal area. You suspect:

    a. Trichomoniasis
    b. Gonorrhea
    c. Chlamydia
    d. Herpes

41. What education needs to be included in prescribing metronidazole to treat trichomoniasis?

    a. It is safe for use during pregnancy
    b. Sexual contact may resume after 48 hours of treatment
    c. Sexual contacts do not require therapy
    d. Alcohol should not be used during treatment

42. A patient with a thin, white, malodorous vaginal discharge most likely has:

    a. Trichomoniasis
    b. Monilia
    c. Bacterial vaginosis
    d. Chlamydia

43. At which point of life is UTI more common in males?

    a. Toddler
    b. Adolescent
    c. School-age
    d. Newborn/infant

44. The organism primarily responsible for UTI is:

    a. Proteus
    b. *E. coli*

    c. Enterobacter

    d. Pseudomonas

45. Most patients with uncomplicated UTI can be treated on an outpatient basis. The first antibiotic you would consider using is:

    a. Amoxicillin

    b. Trimethoprim-sulfamethoxazole

    c. Cephalexin

    d. Amoxicillin/clavulanate

46. Cryptorchidism is more prevalent in:

    a. Term infants

    b. Premature infants

    c. Babies at 1 year of age

    d. Toddlers

47. A 3 year old boy is in the process of toilet-training. The parents come to see you because when the child urinates, all of the urine goes on the floor. You suspect hypospadias because:

    a. It is a rare disorder and would indicate a more serious problem

    b. Normally, the urine stream is directed downward

    c. The child is circumcised

    d. Fusion of the urethral folds has occurred

48. Which of the following is not used in the management of the child with phimosis?

    a. Ice packs

    b. Gentle stretching when bathing

    c. Circumcision in cases of urinary obstruction

    d. Good hygiene

49. Jeanine, an 8-year-old Hispanic girl, presents with a 2 week history of a brownish-red, very foul smelling, vaginal discharge. It is most likely caused by:

    a. Sexual abuse

    b. Accidental genital trauma

    c. Foreign body

    d. Poor hygiene

50. Which of the following is not a proposed etiologic factor in premenstrual syndrome?

    a. Imbalance of water and sodium

    b. Fluctuation in steroids

    c. Vitamin B_{12} deficiency

    d. Synthesis of prostaglandins

51. Treatment of a child with glomerulonephritis would include:

    a. Vasoconstrictors for hypotension
    b. Antibiotics for persistent infection
    c. Increased fluids to maintain hydration
    d. Avoidance of diuretics

52. Which of the following is not a frequent sign of gonorrhea infection:

    a. Diarrhea
    b. Urinary symptoms
    c. Menstrual problems
    d. Fever

53. The most significant finding in the case of chlamydia infection is:

    a. The vaginal discharge is grey and frothy
    b. Most examinations are normal
    c. The external genitalia is markedly inflamed
    d. Infection by *Chlamydia trachomatis* alone is the rule

54. One difference between the lesions of primary syphilis (chancre) and HSV genital lesions that may help in differentiating the two is:

    a. Syphilis chancre is painless while HSV lesions are painful
    b. Syphilis lesions have a flat edge while HSV lesion edges are more raised
    c. Syphilis chancres are more likely to ulcerate than HSV lesions
    d. Erythema and edema is greater with syphilis chancre than HSV lesions

55. Education of sexually active adolescents concerning use of condoms to prevent STDs would include:

    a. Only latex or natural skin condoms should be used
    b. Polyurethane condoms have inadequate STD protection
    c. Condom use is only method to prevent STDs and AIDS
    d. Only petroleum-based lubricants should be used

56. Which of the following contraceptive methods would be least suitable for adolescents?

    a. Condoms with spermicides
    b. Progestin only, mini-pill
    c. Long-acting progestins
    d. Estrogen-progestin combination

57. Which of the following is not an absolute contraindication for oral contraceptives?

    a. Clotting disorder
    b. Impaired liver function
    c. Severe hypertension
    d. Undiagnosed vaginal bleeding

Answers

1. d	20. b	39. c
2. c	21. c	40. a
3. d	22. c	41. d
4. d	23. b	42. c
5. a	24. d	43. d
6. c	25. d	44. b
7. d	26. b	45. b
8. c	27. d	46. b
9. d	28. c	47. b
10. b	29. c	48. a
11. d	30. b	49. c
12. c	31. b	50. c
13. d	32. a	51. b
14. a	33. c	52. a
15. d	34. b	53. b
16. b	35. c	54. a
17. a	36. c	55. c
18. d	37. b	56. b
19. a	38. d	57. c

Bibliography

AAP Committee on Adolescence (1996). The adolescent's right to confidential care when considering abortion. *Pediatrics, 97*(5), 746–751.

AAP Committee on Child Abuse and Neglect. (1998). Gonorrhea in pre-pubertal children. *Pediatrics, 101*(1), 134–135.

AAP Committee on Adolescence (1999). Adolescent pregnancy—Current trends and issues 1998. *Pediatrics, 103*(2), 1516–1520.

AAP Committee on Adolescence (1999). Contraception and adolescents. *Pediatrics, 104*(5), 1161–1166.

American Academy of Pediatrics. (2003). *Red Book 2003: Report of the committee on infectious diseases* (26th ed.). Elk Grove Village, IL: American Academy of Pediatrics.

Barratt, T. M., Avner, E. D., & Harmon, W. E. (1999). *Pediatric nephrology.* Baltimore: Lippincott, Williams, & Wilkins.

Behrman, R. E., Kliegman, R. M., & Jenson, H. B. (Eds.). (2004). *Nelson textbook of pediatrics* (17th ed.). Philadelphia: W. B. Saunders.

Berkowitz, C. D. (Ed.). (2000). *Pediatrics: A primary care approach (2nd ed.).* Philadelphia: W. B. Saunders.

Bukowski, T. P., & Zeman, P. A. (2001). Hypospadias: Of concern but correctable. *Contemporary Pediatrics,* 89–90, 92–94, 97–98, 100, 103–104, 109.

Burns, C. E., Barber, N., Brady, M., & Dunn, A. (Eds.). (2000). *Pediatric primary care: A handbook for nurse practitioners (2nd ed.).* Philadelphia: W. B. Saunders.

Carpenter, S. E., & Rock, J. A. (2000). *Pediatric and adolescent gynecology.* Philadelphia: Lippincott Williams & Wilkins.

Coupey, S. M. (2000). *Primary care of adolescent girls.* Philadelphia: Hanley & Belfus, Inc.

Emans, S. J., Laufer, M. R., & Goldstein, D. P. (Eds.). (1998). *Pediatric and adolescent gynecology* (4th ed.). Philadelphia: Lippincott-Raven.

Friedman, S. B., Fisher, M., Schonberg, S. K., & Alderman, E. M. (1998). *Comprehensive adolescent health care* (2nd Ed.). St. Louis: Mosby.

Gonzales, E. T. (1999). *Pediatric urology practice.* Philadelphia: Lippincott, Williams, & Wilkins.

Hatcher, R. A., Trussell, J., Stewart, F., Cates Jr. W., Stewart, G. K., Guest, F., & Kowal, D. (1998). *Contraceptive technology* (17th rev. ed.). NY: Ardent Media.

Hoekelman, R. A., Adam, H. M., Nelson, N. M., Weitzman, M. L. & Wilson, M. H. (Eds.). (2001). *Primary pediatric care* (4th ed.). St. Louis: Mosby.

Hofmann, A. D., & Greydanus, D. E. (Eds.). (1997). *Adolescent medicine.* Stamford, CT: Appleton & Lange.

Judson, F., & Ehret, J. (1994). Laboratory diagnosis of sexually transmitted infections. *Pediatric Annals, 23*(7), 361–369.

Koo, H. P. (2001). Is it really cyrptorchism? *Contemporary Pediatrics*, (January) 12–18.

Koo, H. P. (2001). Management of undescended testis. *Contemporary Pediatrics* (March), 20–31.

National Campaign to Prevent Teen Pregnancy. (1997). *Whatever happened to childhood? The problem of teen pregnancy in the United States.* Washington, DC: Author.

Perdad, R., Sharma, S., McTavish, J., Imber, C., & Mouriquand, P. D. (1995). Clinical presentation and pathophysiology of meatal stenosis following circumcision. *British Journal of Urology, 75,* 91–93.

Rosenstein, B. J., & Fosarelli, P. D. (1997). Genitourinary disorders. *Pediatric pearls: The handbook of practical pediatrics* (3rd ed., pp. 137–167). St. Louis: Mosby.

Sanfilippo, J. S., Muram, D., Dewhurts, J., & Lee, P. A. (2001). *Pediatric and adolescent gynecology.* Philadelphia: W.B. Saunders Company

Starr Barber, N. (1996). Labial adhesions in childhood. *Journal of Pediatric Health Care, 10,* 26–27.

Todd, J. K. (1995). Management of urinary tract infections: Children are different. *Pediatrics in Review, 16*(5), 190–196.

Winther, K., & Hedman, C. (2002. Assessment of the effects of the herbal remedy Femal on the symptoms of premenstrual syndrome: A randomized, double-blind, placebo-controlled study. *Current Therapeutic Research*, 63 (5): 344–353.

Hematologic/Oncologic/Immunologic Disorders

Juanita Conkin Dale

ABO/Rh Incompatibility

- Definition: Incompatibility between the ABO or Rh blood group of the fetus and mother that may result in isoimmunization and red cell hemolysis

- Etiology/Incidence

    1. Rh incompatibility—mother rhesus antigen (Rh) negative, baby Rh positive

        a. Occurrence in first born—5%

        b. More severe in subsequent sensitized pregnancies

    2. ABO incompatibility—major blood group antigen of mother (type O) is different from the baby (type A, B or AB); 20% of pregnancies are at risk for ABO incompatibility; about 33% of neonates at risk are Coombs' test positive (usually weakly positive), only 20% of the Coombs' test positive neonates develop clinically significant jaundice requiring phototherapy

- Signs and Symptoms

    1. Mild cases—asymptomatic

    2. Severe cases—yellow discoloration of skin, whites of eyes, and gums or inside of mouth

- Differential Diagnosis

    1. Physiologic jaundice—most common

    2. Infection

    3. Hyperbilirubinemia of prematurity

    4. Metabolic disorder

- Physical Findings

    1. Jaundice usually occurring within first 24 hours of life; may be present or appear up to a week later

    2. May have hepatosplenomegaly

- Diagnostic Tests/Findings

    1. Rh incompatibility

        a. Blood type—mother Rh negative, baby Rh positive

        b. Direct Coombs' test (direct antiglobulin test [DAT])—positive

        c. Hemoglobin—below normal, may be very low; hemolysis often continues up to 3 months

        d. Serum indirect bilirubin—markedly elevated

    2. ABO incompatibility

        a. Blood type—mother usually O, baby A, B, or AB

        b. Coombs' test (DAT)—usually positive (often weakly positive)

    c. Hemoglobin—moderately low; hemolysis occasionally occurs up to 2 to 3 months

    d. Serum bilirubin—variably elevated

- Management/Treatment

    1. Rh isoimmunization

       a. Obstetrical

          (1) Rh isoimmunization screen at first prenatal visit to identify "setups"; prevention if pregnancy at risk

          (2) If mother Rh negative, test father; if pregnancy at risk, follow titers and anti-D; consider Rh immunoglobulin at 28 weeks or within 72 hours of delivery

       b. Neonatal

          (1) Cord blood bilirubin, hemoglobin, and DAT

          (2) Hydration—aggressive oral feeding, IV if indicated

          (3) Phototherapy, if indicated

          (4) Exchange transfusion if indicated based on rate of rise in bilirubin and age of baby

    2. ABO isoimmunization

       a. Monitor unconjugated bilirubin levels

       b. Phototherapy if indicated based on bilirubin, gestational and post-delivery age of neonate

Hyperbilirubinemia

- Definition: An increased amount of unconjugated (indirect) or conjugated (direct) bilirubin in the blood associated with a range of conditions and liver dysfunction

- Etiology/Incidence

    1. Unconjugated (indirect) types—may be caused by overproduction of bilirubin, impaired conjugation, transport or uptake of bilirubin

       a. Physiological hyperbilirubinemia—indirect bilirubin 5 to 7 mg/dL; generally not > 12.7 to 12.9 mg/dL at peak within 3 to 5 days of life; usually resolves within 10 days; 50% full-term infants; higher incidence among preterm infants

       b. Breast-feeding hyperbilirubinemia

          (1) Breast feeding associated with prolonged physiologic hyperbilirubinemia in 30% breast-fed infants

          (2) True breast-milk hyperbilirubinemia

             (a) Begins by 4th day with peak bilirubin of 10 to 30 mg/dL by 10 to 15 days

        (b)   Incidence—1% to 2% breast-fed infants

   c.   Prolonged (non-physiologic) neonatal hyperbilirubinemia—associated with breast feeding, maternal diabetes, induced labor, prematurity, oriental ethnicity and male gender

   d.   Common in infancy

   e.   Less common in older children but associated with:

        (1)   Hemoglobinopathies

        (2)   Crigler-Najjar syndrome (type 1 glucuronyl transferase deficiency)—autosomal recessive disorder

        (3)   Gilbert syndrome—mild congenital defect in conjugation

2.   Conjugated (direct) types—caused by range of pathologic conditions (rare in newborns) including biliary obstruction, infection, drugs (aspirin, acetaminophen), and other metabolic disorders

   a.   Direct bilirubin > 1.5 to 2 mg/dL

   b.   Jaundice in first day of life

   c.   Total bilirubin > 12.9 mg/dL (full-term); > 15 mg/dL (preterm)

   d.   Persistence > 1 week (full-term); > 2 weeks (preterm)

   e.   More common in older children

- Signs and Symptoms: Yellow discoloration of skin, whites of eyes, gums and oral mucosa

- Differential Diagnosis

   1.   Transient neonatal hyperbilirubinemia

      a.   Physiologic

      b.   Breast-milk associated

      c.   Breast-milk jaundice

   2.   Infection

   3.   Hepatic disease

   4.   Intestinal obstruction

- Physical Findings

   1.   Clinical jaundice varies based on bilirubin level—5 mg/dL appears first on head, progresses down chest/abdomen as bilirubin increases; usually at least 15 mg/dL when noted on distal extremities

   2.   Hepatosplenomegaly

   3.   Edema

- Diagnostic Tests/Findings

1. Evaluate for pathologic causes for jaundice—sepsis, polycythemia
2. Coombs' test (DAT)
   a. Blood group incompatibilities—DAT usually positive
   b. Membrane disorders, red cell enzyme disorders, bacterial or viral sepsis, drug toxin—DAT usually negative
3. Bilirubin
   a. Indirect hyperbilirubinemia—unconjugated bilirubin increased
   b. Direct hyperbilirubinemia—conjugated bilirubin increased
4. Reticulocyte count—may be increased

- Management/Treatment: Based on etiology and age of child
   1. Indirect (unconjugated) hyperbilirubinemia
      a. Hydration and feeding
      b. Phototherapy
      c. Exchange transfusion
   2. Direct (conjugated) hyperbilirubinemia—treat underlying disease and/or refer as appropriate

Hemoglobinopathies

- Definition: Chronic hemolytic anemia resulting from production of abnormal hemoglobin due to inherited genetic mutation in globin genes
- Etiology/Incidence: Incidence associated with specific ethnic groups
   1. Beta (β) thalassemia
      a. β-chain synthesis decreased in β thalassemia intermedia; absent in β-thalassemia major (Cooley's anemia)
      b. Increased but ineffective erythropoiesis
      c. Shortened red cell life span
   2. Alpha (α) thalassemia
      a. α-chain production is impaired
      b. Increased but ineffective erythropoiesis
      c. Shortened red cell life span
   3. Hemoglobin C and E
      a. Amino acid substitution of lysine for glutamic acid
      b. Hemoglobin C—carrier state in 2% of African-Americans
      c. Hemoglobin E—prevalent in populations from Southeast Asia

4. Ethnic groups—individuals of African, Asian, and Mediterranean descent

- Signs and Symptoms

    1. β-thalassemia major and intermedia

        a. Pale skin or mucous membranes

        b. Weakness

        c. Facial deformities

    2. β-thalassemia minor (trait), α-thalassemia trait, Hemoglobin C, Hemoglobin E—usually asymptomatic

- Differential Diagnosis

    1. Iron deficiency anemia

    2. Lead poisoning

    3. Chronic infection

    4. Sideroblastic anemia

- Physical Findings

    1. β-thalassemia major and intermedia

        a. Splenomegaly, occasional hepatosplenomegaly (HSM)

        b. Jaundice, usually mild

        c. Abnormal facies secondary to extramedullary hematopoiesis— prominence of malar eminences, frontal bossing, depression of bridge of nose, exposure of upper incisors

        d. Growth retardation

    2. β-thalassemia minor, α-thalassemia trait, and hemoglobin C trait— physical examination normal

    3. Hemoglobin C and E—splenomegaly

- Diagnostic Tests/Findings

    1. β-thalassemia

        a. CBC with red cell indices

            (1) Hemoglobin—decreased

            (2) Hypochromia, microcytosis, low MCV, anisocytosis, target cells

            (3) Reticulocyte count—increased

        b. Hemoglobin electrophoresis

            (1) β^+ thalassemia

                (a) Hgb A—present

        (b) Hgb A_2—increased (usually > 3.6%, depending on laboratory)

        (c) Hgb F—normal or slightly increased

    (2) β^0 thalassemia

        (a) Hgb A—absent

        (b) Hgb A_2—increased (usually > 3.6%, depending on laboratory)

        (c) Hgb F—normal or slightly increased

2. β-thalassemia (minor or trait)—usually discovered on routine examination or in family investigation

    a. CBC with red cell indices

        (1) Hemoglobin—slightly decreased (9 to 11g/dL)

        (2) Hypochromic, microcytic cells, target cells, anisocytosis, basophilic stippling, low MCV, low MCH, normal RDW

    b. Hemoglobin electrophoresis

        (1) Hgb A_2—increased (usually > 3.6%, depending on laboratory)

        (2) Hgb F—may be mildly elevated

3. α-thalassemia trait

    a. CBC with red cell indices

        (1) Hemoglobin—may be slightly decreased

        (2) Microcytosis, hypochromia

    b. Hemoglobin electrophoresis—Hgb Barts on newborn screen; disappears by 1 to 3 months of age (2 gene deletion ~ 2%, 3 gene deletion ~ 2% to 6%)

4. Hemoglobin C and Hemoglobin E

    a. CBC with red cell indices

        (1) Hemoglobin—may be decreased

        (2) Hemoglobin C—target cells, spherocytes, increased reticulocytes

        (3) Hemoglobin E—target cells, microcytosis

    b. Hemoglobin electrophoresis

        (1) Hemoglobin C (Hgb C)—present

        (2) Hemoglobin E (Hgb E)—present

- Management/Treatment

1. β-thalassemia major

    a. Refer to hematologist

  b. Chronic transfusion protocol—to maintain hemoglobin, support growth, and prevent extramedullary hematopoiesis

  c. Chelation therapy (desferoxamine) after serum ferritin $\geq$ 2000 ng/mL—to remove excessive intracellular iron

  d. Splenectomy—may reduce transfusion requirements

    (1) Conjugate and polysaccharide pneumococcal vaccines as recommended by the American Academy of Pediatrics; should be given at least 2 weeks or longer prior to surgery, if possible, to increase the likelihood of eliciting a protective antibody response

    (2) Prophylactic penicillin 250 mg b.i.d. life long post-splenectomy

    (3) After splenectomy, increased risk for bacterial infections—for fever (> 101.5° F), immediate referral for blood cultures, empiric parenteral antibiotics active against encapsulated organisms

 2. β-thalassemia intermedia

  a. Observe hemoglobin

  b. Splenectomy may help

 3. β-thalassemia minor, α-thalassemia trait, hemoglobin C and E—no therapy

 4. Genetic counseling

Iron Deficiency Anemia

- Definition: A microcytic, hypochromic anemia caused by inadequate supply of iron
- Etiology/Incidence
  1. Causative factors
     a. Deficient dietary intake
     b. Increased demand—growth (low birth weight, prematurity, adolescence, pregnancy), cyanotic congenital heart disease
     c. Blood loss—GI tract is most common site
     d. Malabsorption—rare except for intestinal resection
  2. Incidence
     a. Most common nutritional deficiency in children
     b. Most common between 8 and 18 months of age and in adolescence
     c. Higher incidence in lower socioeconomic groups
- Signs and Symptoms: Vary with severity of anemia
  1. Mild anemia—usually asymptomatic

2. More severe anemia

   a. Fatigue

   b. Irritability

   c. Delayed motor development

   d. Eating nonnutrient substances such as ice, plaster, clay, paint, fabric (pica)

- Differential Diagnosis

  1. Hemoglobinopathy

  2. Lead poisoning

  3. Anemia of chronic disease or inflammation

- Physical Findings: Vary with severity of anemia

  1. Mild—normal physical examination

  2. More severe—pallor, tachycardia, systolic murmur, hepatomegaly, CHF

- Diagnostic Tests/Findings—see Table 1

- Management/Treatment

  1. Nutritional counseling—prevention

     a. Maintain breast feeding for 6 months if possible, supplemental iron drops or iron fortified cereal by 4 to 5 months of age

     b. Use iron fortified infant formula until 1 year of age

     c. Use iron fortified cereals from 6 to 12 months of age

     d. No cow's milk before 1 year of age, then limit to 18 to 24 oz/day

     e. Prescribe 2 to 3 mg/kg/day elemental iron in 1 to 2 doses/day for prophylaxis in low birth weight infants

  2. Oral iron medication

     a. Prescribe as elemental iron—3 to 6 mg/kg/day in 1 to 3 doses until hemoglobin normal, then 2 to 3 mg/kg/day for 4 months to replace iron stores

     b. See Table 1 regarding expected therapeutic response

     c. Failure to respond—consider the following reasons in this order

        (1) Failure or inconsistent administration of medication

        (2) Persistent or unrecognized blood loss

        (3) Incorrect diagnosis

        (4) Impaired GI absorption

  3. Parenteral iron-dextran—in cases of noncompliance, severe bowel disease, genuine intolerance, chronic hemorrhage, chronic diarrhea

Table 1

Diagnostic Tests for Iron Deficiency Anemia

Hemoglobin—< 3%tile for age[a]

Peripheral blood smear

- Hypochromic, microcytic red cells, confirmed by RBC indices MCV < 3%tile for age[a]

- Wide red cell distribution width (RDW) > 17

Serum ferritin—decreased

Serum iron and iron binding capacity

- Decreased serum iron

- Increased iron binding capacity (TIBC)

- Decreased iron saturation (16% or less)

Free erythrocyte protoporphyrin (FEP)—elevated

Therapeutic response to oral iron

- Reticulocyte with peak in 3 to 5 days after initiation of therapy

- Following peak reticulocytosis, hemoglobin level rises on average by 0.25 to 0.4 g/dL/day or hematocrit rises 1% per day

- Thereafter, hemoglobin rises more slowly—0.1 to 0.15 g/dL/day

[a] Refer to Dallman-Siimes algorithm (Figure 13-1, p. 286) *The Harriet Lane handbook* (16th ed.) by V. L. Gunn & C. Nechyba (Eds.), 2002, St. Louis: Mosby.
Note. From *Manual of pediatric hematology and oncology* (3rd ed., p. 43) by P. Lanzkowsky, 2000. Copyright 2000 by Academic Press. Adapted with permission.

4. Packed red cell transfusion—consider in debilitated children with infection, especially when signs of cardiac dysfunction are present and when the hemoglobin level is $\leq$ 4 g/dL

Sickle Cell Disease

- Definition: A group of hemoglobinopathies that include inheritance of two hemoglobins that sickle; these hemoglobins include Hgb S, C, O_{Arab}, D, G $_{Philadelphia}$, and α-chain mutant; transmitted as an autosomal recessive gene

- Etiology/Incidence

1. Hemoglobin S results from a single base pair substitution of valine for glutamic acid at the sixth position of the beta (β) globin gene; this results in red blood cells that become sickle shaped when deoxygenated; sickled shape of the RBCs leads to hemolysis and intermittent episodes of vascular occlusion that can cause tissue ischemia and acute and chronic organ dysfunction

2. Sickle cell disease occurs in individuals of African, Mediterranean, Indian, and Middle Eastern decent; incidence and clinical severity of sickle cell disease and trait in U.S. African-American population is listed in Table 2

Table 2

Differential Diagnosis and Incidence of Sickle Cell Disease and Sickle Cell Trait in U.S. African-Americans

Syndrome (Genotype)	Incidence	Clinical Severity	Hgb (g/dL)[a]	MCV (fl)[a]	Reticulocytes (%)[a]	Newborn Screening[b]	Electrophoresis (%)
Sickle cell anemia (SS)	1:400	Usually marked	6.5–9.5	> 80	5–20	FS	S 80–90 F 2–20 A_2 < 3.6
Sickle hemoglobin C (SC)	1:1000	Mild to moderate	9.5–13.5	75–95	5–10	FSC	S 45–55 C 45–55
Sickle beta plus (Sβ^+) thalassemia	1:4000	Mild to moderate	8.5–12.5	< 75	5–10	FSA or FS[c]	S 65–90 A 5–30 F 2–20 A_2 > 3.6
Sickle beta zero (Sβ^0) thalassemia	1:10,000	Marked to moderate	6.5–9.5	< 80	5–20	FS	S 80–92 F 2–10 A_2 > 3.6
Sickle cell trait (AS)	1:10	Asymptomatic	Normal	Normal	Normal	FAS	S 35–45% A 55–65%

[a] Hematologic values are approximate; results apply to older children
[b] Hemoglobins reported in order of quantity (e.g., FSA = F > S > A); F, fetal hemoglobin; S, sickle hemoglobin; C, hemoglobin C; A, hemoglobin A.
[c] Quantity of Hb A at birth; sometimes insufficient to quantitate
(AAP, 2002, NIH, 2002)

Table 3
Associated Problems of Sickle Cell Disease

Hemolysis

    Chronic anemia

    Jaundice

    Aplastic crisis[a]

    Cholelithiasis

    Delayed growth and sexual maturity

Vaso-occlusion

    Recurrent acute pain (e.g., dactylitis, musculoskeletal, abdominal)

    Functional asplenia (bacterial infections[a])

    Splenic sequestration[a]

    Acute chest syndrome[a]

    Stroke[a]

    Hyposthenuria and enuresis

    Papillary necrosis of kidneys

    Chronic nephropathy

    Priapism

    Avascular necrosis of humeral heads, femoral heads

    Proliferative retinopathy

    Leg ulcers

[a] Potential cause of mortality. (AAP, 2002, NIH, 2002)

- Signs and Symptoms: Vary with associated problems (see Table 3)
    1. Infection (peak incidence between 1 and 3 years of age)
        a. Fever
        b. Malaise
        c. Anorexia
        d. Poor feeding
    2. Acute painful events—"pain crisis", "vaso-occlusive crisis"
        a. Pain—most often in bones; but can occur in any part of body (chest, stomach, hands and/or feet, back, etc.); in children < 2 years of age usually in hands and/or feet (dactylitis)
        b. Swelling—sometimes seen at site of pain
        c. Low grade fever—sometimes occurs
    3. Splenic sequestration

a. Weakness

b. Irritability

c. Unusual sleepiness

d. Paleness

e. Large spleen

f. Fast heart rate

g. Pain in the left side of the abdomen—does not always occur

4. Aplastic crisis (is associated with parvovirus B19)

a. Pale

b. Malaise

c. Headache

d. Fever

e. Mild upper respiratory infection symptoms

- Differential Diagnosis

1. Infection

a. Septicemia

b. Meningitis

c. Pneumonia

d. Osteomyelitis

e. Viral illness

2. Acute painful events

a. Bone pain

(1) Bone infarct

(2) Osteomyelitis

(3) Rheumatoid arthritis

(4) Leukemia

b. Abdominal pain

(1) Cholelithiasis—right upper quadrant

(2) Splenic infarct—left upper quadrant

(3) Functional abdominal pain

(4) Gas pain

3. Splenic sequestration—chronic splenomegaly

4. Aplastic crisis—other viral illnesses

- Physical Findings: Sometimes but not always present

    1. Jaundice

    2. Cardiac murmur

    3. Splenomegaly

    4. Pallor

- Diagnostic Tests/Findings

    1. Prenatal diagnosis—can be done by analysis of DNA obtained through chorionic villus sampling (9 to 11 wks gestation) or amniocentesis (11 to 17 wks gestation)

    2. Usual diagnostic hemoglobin electrophoresis and hematologic results in infants and adults with sickle cell disease are presented in Table 2

    3. "Sickle prep" (metabisulfite solution)—should not be used as diagnostic test; does not distinguish among sickle cell anemia, other forms of sickle cell disease, and sickle cell trait or common interacting hemoglobinopathies such as Hgb C or thalassemia

    4. Splenic sequestration

        a. Hemoglobin—below baseline (steady state)

        b. Platelets—decreased

    5. Aplastic crisis

        a. Hemoglobin—below steady state

        b. Reticulocyte count— < 1.0%

- Management/Treatment

    1. Infection secondary to functional asplenia

        a. Prevention

            (1) Immunizations as recommended by American Academy of Pediatrics including conjugate pneumococcal and HIB vaccines

            (2) Polysaccharide pneumococcal vaccine—at 2 and 5 years of age

            (3) Prophylactic penicillin—in children with sickle cell anemia and sickle β^0 thalassemia; initiate before 3 months of age and continue until at least 5 years of age; oral penicillin VK 125 mg twice daily up to age 3 years, then 250 mg twice daily

            (4) Family education regarding increased risk of infection due to functional asplenia and need to seek medical attention promptly for evaluation of febrile illnesses

        b. Febrile illness (T $\geq$ 101.5° F) in children with sickle cell anemia, sickle β^0 thalassemia, sickle C disease (> 5 years of age or if spleen surgically removed)—

immediate referral for blood culture and empiric parenteral antibiotics active against encapsulated organisms such as *Streptococcus pneumoniae* and *Haemophilus influenzae*

2. Acute painful events

    a. Prevention—education regarding factors that may precipitate painful events, i.e., dehydration, hypoxia, fever, exposure to extreme temperatures; how to manage mild to moderate pain; and how to recognize signs of serious problems

    b. Home-based management

        (1) Oral intake of at least 150 cc/kg/day of fluids

        (2) For mild pain—acetaminophen or ibuprofen

        (3) For more severe pain—codeine should be alternated with NSAIDs

    c. Emergency department (ED) management—if home trial of oral opioids and NSAIDs fail, parenteral opioids (preferably morphine) may be used

    d. Inpatient management—if pain not reduced by ED management, hospitalization for hydration, parenteral opioids, and concomitant NSAID

    e. Nonpharmacologic measures such as heat, massage to area of pain, and distraction

3. Management of other problems associated with sickle cell disease— consultation with or referral to a pediatric hematologist

4. Frequent reinforcement of education regarding fever and pain management, spleen palpation

5. Anticipatory guidance regarding developmental issues such as toilet training, school attendance, delayed growth and development (SS and Sβ^0 thalassemia)

6. Genetic counseling

Lead Poisoning (Plumbism)

- Definition: A chronic disease particularly among young children due to the accumulation of toxic amounts of lead absorbed by the body; expert panel convened by Centers for Disease Control and Prevention (CDC) recommended a cut-off definition of lead poisoning as a whole blood lead level (BLL) $\geq$ 10 μg/dL

- Etiology/Incidence

1. Ingestion or inhalation of lead or lead compounds; transplacental transmission may also occur

2. Sources of lead exposure

    a. Lead-based paint in older homes built prior to 1978, especially housing built before 1950

  b. Lead contaminated soil and dust from automobile emissions (decreasing with use of lead-free gasoline)

  c. Lead contaminated drinking water (lead or lead-soldered pipes)

  d. Certain Mexican and Indian lead-containing folk remedies

 3. Highest prevalence among poor, inner-city children living in older, deteriorating housing

 4. Children between 1 and 3 years of age at greatest risk; 9 out of every 10 children with lead poisoning have history of pica

 5. Prevalence estimates have shown progressive declines in elevated blood lead levels (BLL); most recent data reports incidence of elevated BLL among U.S. children 1 to 5 years decreased from 88.2% (1976-1980) to 4.4% (1991-1994) (AAP, 1998)

 6. Lead toxicity may contribute to neurobehavioral, as well as cognitive, morbidities of childhood

- Signs and Symptoms: Vary with degree of exposure, usually none

 1. Mild acute lead poisoning—resembles gastroenteritis, e.g., anorexia, nausea, vomiting, constipation or diarrhea, and abdominal pain; other possible symptoms are sleep disturbances, metallic taste in mouth, limb pain, and headaches

 2. Severe lead poisoning—lethargy, difficulty walking, tingling

- Differential Diagnosis

 1. Iron deficiency anemia

 2. Alpha or beta thalassemia

- Physical Findings

 1. May see bluish discoloration of gingival border (Burtonian blue lines)

 2. Bradycardia

 3. Neuropathy

 4. Papilledema

 5. Ataxia

- Diagnostic Tests/Findings

 1. CDC revised guidelines (2002) no longer recommend universal screening

  a. Target screening based on well-child surveillance of risk

   (1) Living or regular contact with housing built before 1950 or built before 1978 and being renovated

   (2) Contact with children who have history of lead poisoning

  b. Universal screening for children living in high risk environments

   (1) Available data indicating areas with ≥ 27% of housing built before 1950

      (2)   Available data indicating areas with $\geq$ 12% of children between 1 and 2 years of age with elevated BLL (EBLL)

   c. American Academy of Pediatrics endorsed new CDC guidelines (AAP, 1998)

  2. Whole blood lead level test (BLL) by categories of risk

     a. Lead level < 10 μg/dL—not considered blood poisoning

     b. Lead level of 10 to 14 μg/dL—considered borderline (venipuncture confirmation within 3 mo)

     c. Lead level of 15 to 19 μg/dL (venipuncture confirmation within 3 mo)

     d. Lead level of 20 to 44 μg/dL (venipuncture confirmation within 1 wk to 1 mo)

     e. Lead level of 45 to 69 μg/dL (diagnostic venous blood testing within 24 to 48 hr)

     f. Lead level of > 70 μg/dL (medical emergency, retest immediately)

- Management/Treatment

  1. Follow-up BLL monitoring—frequency determined based on whether low or high risk and BLL obtained

     a. Lead level < 10 μg/dL—if high risk, retest in 6 mo; if low risk, no further testing needed

     b. Lead level of 10 to 14 μg/dL—at risk for lead poisoning; early follow-up within 3 mo, if follow-up level is 15 to 19 μg/dL or higher 3 mo apart, retest every 1 to 2 mo until results < 15 μg/dL for a least 6 mo, then every 6 to 9 mo

     c. Lead level of 15 to 19 μg/dL—at risk for lead poisoning; early follow-up within 2 mo, if follow-up level is > 15, retest every 1 to 2 mo until results < 15 μ/dL for at least 6 mo, then every 3 mo until child is 36 mo old; include educational and nutritional counseling

     d. Lead level of 20 to 44 μg/dL—early follow-up in 1 to 2 mo for BLLs 20 to 24 μg/dL, 2 wk to 1 mo for BLLs 25 to 44 μg/dL retest every 1 to 2 mo until results < 15 μg/dL for a least 6 mo, then every 3 mo until child is 36 mo old

     e. Lead level of 45 to 69 μg/dL—early follow-up as soon as possible retest every mo until results < 15 μg/dL for a least 6 mo, then every 3 mo until child is 36 mo old

     f. Lead level of > 70 μg/dL—early follow-up as soon as possible retest every mo until results <15 μg/dL for at least 6 mo, then every 3 mo until child is 36 mo old

  2. For blood lead level > 20 μg/dL, refer for further medical evaluation, interventions and follow-up

     a. Test for iron deficiency

    b. Environmental assessment and removal of known sources of lead in environment

    c. Medical evaluation for symptoms and possible pharmacologic management

        (1) Lead level of 20 to 44 μg/dL may require pharmacologic management

        (2) Lead level of > 45 μg/dL may require chelation therapy

  3. Primary prevention

    a. Outreach education regarding nutrition and avoidance of exposure

    b. Assessment of potential risk with specific environmental and health questions during routine well-child visits

Glucose-6-Phosphate Dehydrogenase (G-6-PD) deficiency

- Definition: X-linked autosomal recessive disorder in which activity of red cell enzyme G-6-PD is decreased or absent

- Etiology/Incidence

  1. Lack of G-6-PD decreases the ability to deal with oxidative stress and results in hemolysis; episodes of hemolysis may be induced by the following:

    a. Drugs such as aspirin, sulfonamides, antimalarials

    b. Fava beans, ingestion or exposure to pollen from the bean's flower (occurs in Mediterranean and Canton type deficiencies)

    c. Infection (in more susceptible individuals)

  2. Many genetic variants described with altered enzyme levels which determines the severity of disorder

    a. A Type—enzyme activity decreases with age of cell; hemolyzes only old RBC; occurs in 11% African-American males; 2% African-American females

    b. Mediterranean Type—associated with severe deficiency of enzyme

    c. Canton Type—severe disease in Asians

  3. Most common among individuals of African or Mediterranean descent

- Signs and Symptoms: Symptoms develop 24 to 48 hours after ingestion of substance having oxidant properties

  1. Weakness

  2. Pale appearance

  3. With severe cases

    a. Blood in the urine

    b. Yellow discoloration of skin, whites of eyes, and gums or inside of mouth

- Differential Diagnosis
    1. Other causes of hemolytic anemia
    2. Hemoglobinopathies
- Physical Findings
    1. Neonatal jaundice—usually associated with Mediterranean and Canton individuals
    2. Jaundice during episodes
- Diagnostic Tests/Findings
    1. G-6-PD fluorescence-based screen (may give false negative)
    2. Red blood cell indices during or just after hemolytic episode
        a. Heinz bodies present
        b. Fragmented cells and blister cells
    3. Reticulocytosis
    4. Hemoglobin—usually normal between episodes of hemolysis; may be decreased in Mediterranean or Canton
    5. Acute self-limiting hemolytic anemia with hemoglobinuria (Type A variant)
    6. Acute life-endangering hemolysis often leads to acute renal failure (all other variants)
- Management/Treatment
    1. Generally mild symptoms require minimal intervention
    2. Identification and avoidance of foods and drugs that cause hemolysis
    3. Transfusion for severe hemolysis
    4. Genetic counseling; routine screening not generally recommended

Bleeding Disorders

Hemophilia

- Definition: Bleeding disorder caused by congenital deficiency of either clotting factor VIII or IX
- Etiology/Incidence
    1. Hemophilia A (factor VIII deficiency, classical hemophilia)
        a. Third most common X-linked disorder, but 20% to 30% by spontaneous mutation
        b. Approximately 1:5000 male births
        c. 10% to 30% of patients develop antibodies against the functional activity of factor VIII

Table 4
Relationship of Factor Levels to Severity of Clinical Manifestations of Hemophilia A and B

Type	% Factor VIII/IX	Type of Hemorrhage
Severe	< 1	Spontaneous hemarthrosis and deep tissue hemorrhages
Moderate	1–5	Gross bleeding following moderate trauma; some hemarthrosis; rare spontaneous hemorrhage
Mild	6–49	Severe hemorrhage only following moderate to severe trauma or surgery

    d. Factor VIII deficiency is 4 times more common than factor IX deficiency

    2. Hemophilia B (factor IX deficiency, Christmas disease)—X-linked disorder, but 20% to 30% by spontaneous mutation

- Signs and Symptoms: Vary based on severity of factor deficiency

  1. Easy bruising at injection sites

  2. Prolonged bleeding following circumcision—not all severe hemophiliacs bleed post circumcision

  3. Excessive bruising after child begins walking

  4. Prolonged bleeding in any part of the body

  5. May have pain at the site of the bleed

- Differential Diagnosis

  1. Thrombocytopenia

  2. von Willebrand disease

  3. Vitamin K deficiency

  4. Disseminated intravascular coagulation (DIC)

  5. Child abuse

- Physical Findings: With acute bleeds, swelling, warmth and decreased range of motion may be present at the site

- Diagnostic Tests/Findings

  1. Prenatal diagnosis—can be done by fetal blood sampling (periumbilical blood sampling [PUBS]) (18 to 20 wks gestation) through fetoscopy or by analysis of DNA obtained through chorionic villus sampling (9 to 11 weeks gestation) or amniocentesis (11 to 17 wks gestation)

  2. Diagnostic test—direct assay of plasma factor activity level for hemophilia A and B—see Table 4

  3. Screening tests

     a. Activated partial thromboplastin time (APTT)—prolonged

b. Prothrombin time (PT)—normal

c. Bleeding time (not indicated)—normal

- Management/Treatment

    1. Collaborative interdisciplinary approach facilitated by regional hemophilia treatment center

    2. Factor replacement therapy

        a. Hemophilia A—factor VIII concentrate intravenously

        b. Hemophilia B—factor IX concentrate intravenously

        c. If development of inhibitor, consultation with hemophilia treatment center regarding factor replacement

    3. Prophylaxis

        a. Primary prophylaxis—regular infusions of factor VIII or IX given to prevent joint hemorrhage

        b. Secondary prophylaxis—started after a joint has developed a pattern or repeated bleeding; used to prevent further bleeding into the joint

    4. Desmopressin intranasally or intravenously—for mild factor VIII deficiency

    5. Antifibrinolytic therapy—for oral mucosal bleeds

    6. Physical therapy—for musculoskeletal bleeds

    7. Surgery—synovectomy, arthroscopic or with use of isotopes

    8. Anticipatory guidance regarding developmental issues such as discipline, child care, and schooling

    9. Genetic counseling

von Willebrand Disease (VWD)

- Definition: An inherited hemorrhagic disorder characterized by defective primary hemostasis and due to a quantitative or qualitative abnormality in von Willebrand factor (VWF)

- Etiology/Incidence:

    1. The most common congenital bleeding disorder

    2. Six variant types

        a. Type 1—previous Type I

        b. Type 2A—previous Type I B

        c. Type 2M—previous Type B

        d. Type 2B—previous Type II B

        e. Type 2N—previous Type Normandy

        f. Type 3—previous Type III

3. Affects at least 1% of the population

- Signs and Symptoms: Great variation in frequency, severity, and bleeding manifestations

  1. Nosebleeds

  2. Bleeding gums

  3. Heavy menstrual bleeding

  4. Prolonged oozing from cuts

  5. Increased bleeding after trauma or surgery

- Differential Diagnosis

  1. Thrombocytopenia

  2. Hemophilia

  3. Vitamin K deficiency

  4. Disseminated intravascular coagulation

- Physical Findings

  1. Easy bruising

  2. Multiple sites of bruising

  3. Oozing or bleeding at trauma or surgical site

- Diagnostic Tests/Findings

  1. Variation in findings by specific type of VWD as well as within same patient over time

  2. Bleeding time—usually prolonged

  3. von Willebrand factor—usually decreased or absent

  4. von Willebrand factor antigen—usually decreased or absent

  5. Blood group—VWF factor decreased in type O

- Management/Treatment

  1. Desmopressin acetate—used to treat bleeding complications or as preoperative preparation for Type 1; contraindicated in the treatment of Type 2 B

  2. Alternative treatment if desmopressin not indicated or effective—treatment with factor concentrates with intact von Willebrand factor should be considered

  3. Antifibrinolytic agents—particularly effective in areas where fibrinolysis appears to contribute to bleeding, i.e., in mucous membranes (nose, mouth, throat, and menorrhagia), trauma, and dental procedures and surgery

Idiopathic Thrombocytopenia (ITP)

- Definition: Immune-mediated disorder characterized by production of antiplatelet antibodies

1. Acute ITP—platelet count returns to normal (> 150,00/mm³) within 6 months

2. Chronic ITP—platelet count low beyond 6 months; approximately 10% of children with ITP

3. Recurrent or relapsing ITP—the platelet count decreases again after having returned to normal levels (rare)

- Etiology/Incidence

   1. Cause unknown, often appears to be related to sensitization by viral infection

   2. 4 to 5.3 cases/100,000 children

   3. Most prevalent during early to mid-childhood and in older adults, although it affects all ages

   4. Chronic ITP—more common in children > 7 years of age; more prevalent in females (3:1 ratio)

- Signs and Symptoms

   1. Bruising

   2. Nose bleeds

   3. Bleeding of gums and lips

   4. Except for bleeding, child appears well

- Differential Diagnosis

   1. Thrombocytopenia of other causes

      a. Bone marrow infiltration

      b. Septicemia

      c. Aplastic anemia

   2. Disseminated intravascular coagulation (DIC)

   3. Hemolytic uremic syndrome

   4. Acute leukemia

   5. In young child

      a. Congenital amegakaryocytic thrombocytopenia-absent radius syndrome

      b. Wiskott-Aldrich syndrome

   6. In older child, especially those with chronic symptoms

      a. Systemic lupus erythematosus

      b. HIV infection

      c. Lymphoma

- Physical Findings
  1. Petechiae, purpura, and ecchymosis
  2. Hemorrhages in mucous membranes
  3. Pallor usually not present (unless there has been significant bleeding)
- Diagnostic Tests/Findings
  1. CBC—generally the only required test
  2. Hemoglobin—normal or slightly reduced with prior bleeding; can drop with bruising only
  3. Platelet count
     a. $\leq$ 20,000/mm^3 (diagnostic for acute ITP); often $\leq$ 10,000/mm^3
     b. < 100,000/mm^3 for > 6 months (diagnostic for chronic ITP)
  4. WBC—normal; if active infection, may have increased neutrophils, lymphocytes, or atypical mononuclear cells
  5. Bleeding time test (unnecessary)—always abnormal if platelets < 50,000 mm^3
- Management/Treatment: Controversial
  1. Acute ITP
     a. Treatment usually not indicated if platelet count > 50,000/mm^3
     b. Treatment usually considered if platelet count < 20,000/mm^3, especially with extensive cutaneous (and especially mucosal) bleeding or if protective environment cannot be assured
     c. With severe nosebleeds (lasting longer than about 30 minutes), gastrointestinal, or intracranial bleeding require therapy.
     d. Pharmacologic management
        (1) Corticosteroids (prednisone 2 to 5 mg/kg/day orally for 1 to 3 weeks) may accelerate recovery in acute ITP but does not change outcome
        (2) Intravenous gamma globulin (IVGG)—regimens of 400, 800, 1000 mg/day for 2 or 5 days will increase platelet count in 2 to 3 days in most patients; total dose 2g/kg; lasts only 21 to 28 days; may require re-treatment
        (3) Methylprednisolone 30mg/kg/day for 3 days
        (4) Intravenous anti-D immunoglobulin (45 to 50 μg/kg)
  2. Chronic ITP
     a. Referral to a hematologist.
     b. Pharmacologic management—when thrombocytopenia worsens during viral illness or prior to elective surgery, prednisone or IVGG can be administered

c. Prolonged use of high dose steroids should be avoided

d. Splenectomy—treatment of choice when severe or symptomatic chronic ITP interferes significantly with child's lifestyle

   (1) Conjugate and polysaccharide pneumococcal vaccines as recommended by the American Academy of Pediatrics; should be given at least 2 weeks or longer prior to surgery, if possible, to increase the likelihood of eliciting a protective antibody response

   (2) Prophylactic penicillin 250 mg b.i.d. for at least 1 to 2 years postoperatively

   (3) After splenectomy, at increased risk for bacterial infections—for fever (T ≥ 101.5° F), immediate referral for blood culture and empiric parenteral antibiotics active against encapsulated organisms

3. Patient/family education

   a. Avoid all competitive contact sports that could result in head trauma

   b. Avoid aspirin and aspirin containing medications and ibuprofen

Cancers

Leukemias

- Definition: A malignant neoplasm of bone marrow characterized by proliferation of immature white cells

- Etiology/Incidence

  1. Etiology is usually unknown

  2. Accounts for 25% to 30% of all childhood cancers

  3. Acute leukemia constitutes 97% of all childhood leukemias and includes most common types:

     a. Acute lymphocytic leukemia (ALL)—75%; survival rate is 60% to 80%

     b. Acute myleloid leukemia (AML), also known as acute non-lymphocytic leukemia (ANLL)—20%; survival rate is 40% to 60%

  4. Chronic myelogenous leukemia (CML) constitutes 3% of childhood leukemia

  5. 1 per 25,000 of population up to 14 years of age

  6. Peak incidence between 2 and 5 years of age

- Signs and Symptoms

  1. Fatigue, headache

  2. Bruising

  3. Fever

    4. Nose bleeds

    5. Bone pain, limp

- Differential Diagnosis

    1. Chronic infections such as Epstein-Barr virus (EBV) or cytomegalovirus (CMV)

    2. ITP

    3. Transient erythroblastopenia of childhood

    4. Aplastic anemia

    5. Juvenile rheumatoid arthritis

- Physical Findings

    1. Pallor

    2. Purpura, ecchymosis

    3. Organomegaly, adenopathy

- Diagnostic Tests/Findings

    1. CBC—presence of blast cells on peripheral blood smear highly suggestive; needs confirmatory bone marrow examination

    2. Bone marrow aspiration/biopsy (required for diagnosis)—bone marrow replaced by > 30% blasts, usually 80% to 100%

- Management/Treatment

    1. Combination chemotherapy

    2. CNS prophylaxis

        a. Radiation therapy (for high risk patients)

        b. Combined intrathecal chemotherapy

    3. Patient/family education regarding side effects of therapy, anticipatory guidance on coping

    4. For relapse following chemotherapy—second course of chemotherapy may provide cure; for AML, bone marrow transplant is treatment of choice

    5. Long term follow-up for delayed effects of chemotherapy and/or radiation

Neuroblastoma

- Definition: Tumor mass along the neural pathway

- Etiology/Incidence

    1. Etiology—possible genetic factors; familial predisposition

    2. Most common malignancy in infancy, accounts for 7% of all childhood malignancies

    3. Metastases at onset in 70% to 75% of cases

4. 10 per 1 million live births annually

5. Survival rate for patients < 1 year of age, 82%; for 1 to 2 years of age, 32%; over 2 years, 10%

- Signs and Symptoms: Dependent on primary site, presence of metastases

    1. Listlessness

    2. Poor feeding

    3. Pale

    4. Weight loss

    5. Abdominal pain

    6. Weakness

    7. Irritability

- Differential Diagnosis

    1. Trauma

    2. Lymphadenopathy

    3. Leukemia

    4. Lymphoma

    5. Wilms tumor

- Physical Findings: Related to site of primary tumor

    1. Lymph node enlargement

    2. Hepatomegaly

    3. Abdominal or flank mass

    4. Periorbital ecchymoses (raccoon eyes)

    5. Scalp nodules

- Diagnostic Tests/Findings

    1. CT and/or MRI scan to determine site and location of any suspected masses

    2. Tissue biopsy to confirm diagnosis

    3. Bone marrow aspiration and biopsy to evaluate for infiltrating tumor

    4. Serum or urine catecholamine levels—increased

- Management/Treatment: Based on stage and site of tumor

    1. Treatment of emergent symptoms

    2. Surgery

        a. Staging excision of tumor

        b. Evaluation of treatment

3. Radiation therapy

4. Combination chemotherapy

5. Bone marrow transplant in some cases

6. Patient/family education regarding side effects of therapy

7. Anticipatory guidance on developmental issues such as sleep, toileting, discipline, and child care

8. Long term follow-up for delayed effects of chemotherapy and/or radiation

Retinoblastoma

- Definition: Congenital malignant intraocular tumor
- Etiology/Incidence
  1. Abnormal fetal neural crest cell maturation
     a. Hereditary—germinal mutation (40%); siblings and subsequent offspring at risk
     b. Acquired—somatic mutations
  2. Most common intraocular childhood tumor
     a. 1:10,000 live births
     b. Slightly higher incidence in males
     c. Accounts for 7% of all childhood cancers; 15% childhood cancer mortality
  3. Majority diagnosed before 5 years—$\frac{1}{3}$ are bilateral; usually diagnosed in first year
  4. Prognosis varies with age and tumor staging
     a. Overall survival rates > 90%
     b. Highest survival for children < 1 year and > 6 years
     c. High incidence of secondary malignancies may limit survival into third or fourth decade of life
- Signs and Symptoms
  1. Squinting
  2. Eyes turning inward or outward
  3. Painful red eye
- Differential Diagnosis
  1. Cataract
  2. Retinal detachment
  3. Persistent hyperplastic primary vitreous
  4. Coloboma

5. Retinopathy of prematurity

- Physical Findings
    1. Leukocoria—yellow-white pupillary reflex
    2. Strabismus
    3. Hyphema may be present
- Diagnostic Tests/Findings
    1. Fundoscopic examination under anesthesia or sedation—findings may include:
        a. Creamy-pink mass
        b. White avascular tumor mass
    2. CT of the orbits to evaluate extent of tumor and to determine optic nerve or bony structure involvement
    3. MRI to assess for optic nerve invasion
- Management/Treatment: Determined by stage and extent of disease
    1. Surgery
        a. Resection
        b. Enucleation
    2. Radiation therapy
    3. Chemotherapy—palliative
    4. Patient/family education regarding side effects of therapy
    5. Anticipatory guidance on developmental issues such as sleep, toileting, discipline, and child care
    6. Long term follow-up for recurrence or delayed effects of chemotherapy and/or radiation

Lymphomas

- Definition: Malignant disorders characterized by proliferation of cells usually restricted to lymphoid cells but may be found in bone marrow; includes Hodgkin's (HL) and non-Hodgkin's (NHL) lymphomas
- Etiology/Incidence
    1. Etiology unknown—possible etiologic factors
        a. Genetic predisposition
        b. Environmental exposures
        c. Epstein-Barr virus
        d. Immunologic disorders

2. Third most common childhood cancer—10%

    a. HL—1:100,000 children

        (1) Peak age—bimodal age incidence curve

            (a) 15 to 35 years

            (b) > 50 years

        (2) Survival—stages I to II, most are cured; stage III, 75% to 90%; stage IV, 60% to 80%

    b. NHL—15:100,000 children between 5 to 10 years

        (1) Peak age—5 to 15 years

        (2) Survival—stages I to II ~ 90%; stages III to IV ~ 70%

- Signs and Symptoms

  1. Hodgkin's

    a. Painless swelling of lymph nodes

    b. Fatigue

    c. Decreased appetite and weight loss

    d. Fever

    e. Night sweats

  2. Non-Hodgkin's

    a. Asymptomatic if not disseminated

    b. Difficulty swallowing or breathing

    c. Swelling in neck, face, upper extremities

    d. Abdominal pain

- Differential Diagnosis

  1. Other malignancy

  2. Lymphadenopathy associated with infection

- Physical Findings

  1. Hodgkin's

    a. Affected nodes—firm, non-tender, discrete; cervical and supraclavicular areas most common

    b. Splenomegaly

  2. Non-Hodgkin's

    a. Similar to Hodgkin's

    b. May vary depending on degree of involvement

- Diagnostic Tests/Findings
    1. Hodgkin's
        a. Chest radiograph—to explore possibility of mediastinal involvement and examine airway patency
        b. Biopsy—tumor giant cells (Reed-Sternberg cells)
        c. CBC with red cell indices
            (1) Hemoglobin—decreased
            (2) Normocytic and normochromic or microcytic and hypochromic
        d. Serum copper—increased
        e. Serum ferritin—increased
        f. Sedimentation rate (ESR)—increased
    2. Non-Hodgkin's—tissue diagnosis necessary before treatment is started, findings vary based on specific histiologic type
        a. Isolated peripheral nodes—excisional or fine-needle biopsy
        b. Mediastinal mass—thoracotomy or mediastinoscopy, parasternal fine-needle biopsy, or thoracentesis (if associated pleural effusion)
        c. Abdominal mass—open biopsy usually necessary
- Management/Treatment: Plan developed based on stage of involvement
    1. Multiagent chemotherapy
    2. Radiation
    3. Patient/family education regarding side effects of therapy
    4. Long term follow-up for delayed effects of chemotherapy and/or radiation

Wilms' tumor (Nephroblastoma)

- Definition: A primary malignant renal tumor
- Etiology/Incidence
    1. Etiology unknown; predisposing factors
        a. Genetic factors
            (1) Associated with aniridia, Beckwith-Wiedeman syndrome
            (2) Familial predisposition
        b. Environmental factors—chronic chemical exposure (hydrocarbons, lead)
    2. 6% of all cancer in children; 9:1 million Caucasian children/year
    3. Equal frequency in males and females
    4. 78% diagnosed between 1 and 5 years of age; peak incidence 3 to 4 years of age

   5.   Survival rate—70% to 90%

- Signs and Symptoms

   1.   May be asymptomatic

   2.   Abdominal mass—usually non-painful

   3.   Occasionally abdominal pain

   4.   Malaise, fever, loss of appetite

   5.   Vomiting

   6.   Blood in urine

- Differential Diagnosis

   1.   Hydronephrosis

   2.   Polycystic kidney disease

   3.   Neuroblastoma

   4.   Rhabdomyosarcoma

   5.   Lymphoma

- Physical Findings

   1.   Abdominal mass—usually asymptomatic

   2.   Hypertension

   3.   Associated congenital anomalies—aniridia, hemihypertrophy, genitourinary anomalies

- Diagnostic Tests/Findings

   1.   CBC and urine analysis for anemia, hematuria

   2.   CT of abdomen to evaluate:

      a.   Presence and function of opposite kidney

      b.   Evidence of bilateral involvement

      c.   Evidence of involvement of blood vessels of tumor

      d.   Lymph node involvement

      e.   Liver involvement

   3.   Abdominal ultrasound—may indicate that the tumor is intrarenal

   4.   Chest radiograph, CT of chest to evaluate for metastasis to lung

- Management/Treatment: Plan developed based on stage of involvement

   1.   Surgical excision

      a.   If unilateral—complete nephrectomy

      b.   If bilateral—nephrectomy of more involved site, excision biopsy/partial nephrec-tomy of smaller lesion in remaining kidney; or no surgery with radiation

2. Multiagent chemotherapy

3. Radiation therapy

4. Patient/family education regarding side effects of therapy

5. Long term follow-up for disease recurrence and delayed effects of chemotherapy and/or radiation

Osteosarcoma

- Definition: A solid tumor of the bone in which malignant spindle cell stroma produce osteiod; most common form of bone cancer in children

- Etiology/Incidence

  1. Etiology unknown

  2. Associated factors

     a. Genetic factors and family predisposition

        (1) Increased risk with hereditary retinoblastoma

        (2) Increased risk with chromosome 13 abnormalities

     b. Environmental factors—increased risk associated with previously irradiated bone

     c. Increased risk with taller children

  3. Incidence—7 teenagers per one million

     a. Peak incidence during adolescent growth spurt between 15 to 19 years of age

     b. Male incidence slightly higher than females

- Signs and Symptoms

  1. Local pain

  2. Local swelling

  3. Mass at end of long bone

  4. Decreased range of motion

- Differential Diagnosis

  1. Growing pains

  2. Trauma

  3. Osteomylelitis

  4. Tendonitis

  5. Septic arthritis

  6. Leukemia

- Physical Findings
    1. Pain over involved site
    2. Palpable mass
    3. Swelling
    4. Decreased range of motion of affected extremity
- Diagnostic Tests/Findings
    1. Radiograph of affected bone
    2. Computed tomography (CT) or magnetic resonance imaging (MRI) of affected bone
    3. Biopsy of area
- Management/Treatment
    1. Multiagent chemotherapy
    2. Surgery—amputation/limb sparing surgery
    3. Patient/family education regarding side effects of therapy, anticipatory guidance on coping
    4. Long term follow-up for delayed effects of chemotherapy

Immune deficiencies

Definition: A group of immune defects that can be classified according to
    1. Deficiency of immunoglobulin
    2. Deficiency of cell-mediated immunity
    3. Deficiency of both antibodies and cell-mediated immunity

Common Variable Immunodeficiency (CVID, "Acquired" Hypogammaglobulinemia)

- Definition: An immune disorder resulting from deficiency of all immunoglobulin (Igs)
- Etiology/Incidence: Genetic defect
- Signs and Symptoms (specific to manner of presentation): Recurrent or severe bacterial infections of respiratory tract (sinusitis, otitis, pneumonia) or skin (cellulitis, abscesses)
- Differential Diagnosis: Other immune deficiencies
- Physical Findings: Specific to manner of presentation
    1. Sinusitis—fever (T ≥ 101.5° F), periorbital edema, tenderness on percussion over sinuses
    2. Otitis—hyperemic, opaque, bulging tympanic membrane with poor mobility
    3. Pneumonia—retractions, flaring nares, diminished breath sounds, fine and crackling rales on affected side

4. Cellulitis or abscess—erythema, swelling, purulent drainage

- Diagnostic Tests/Findings: Serum immunoglobulin

1. IgG—decreased

2. IgA—decreased

3. IgM—decreased

- Management/Treatment: Intravenous immunoglobulin G (IgG) replacement (IVIG)

X-linked Agammaglobulinemia (Bruton's Tyrosine Kinase or BTK)

- Definition: Absent or inadequate gammaglobulins caused by B cell defect

- Etiology/Incidence

1. Inherited, X-linked disorder of B lymphocytes

2. Affected male infants usually asymptomatic for 3 to 6 months due to passive transmission of maternal antibodies then show frequent infections and failure-to-thrive

3. Incidence rates unknown

- Signs and Symptoms: (specific to manner of presentation)—recurrent or severe bacterial infections of the respiratory tract (sinusitis, otitis, pneumonia) or skin (cellulitis, abscesses)

- Differential Diagnosis: Other immune deficiencies

- Physical Findings: Specific to manner of presentation

1. Sinusitis—fever (T ≥ 101.5° F), periorbital edema, tenderness on percussion over sinuses

2. Otitis—hyperemic, opaque, bulging tympanic membrane with poor mobility

3. Pneumonia—retractions, flaring nares, diminished breath sounds, fine and crackling rales on affected side

4. Cellulitis or abscess—erythema, swelling, purulent drainage

- Diagnostic Tests/Findings

1. Serum immunoglobulins

   a. IgG—decreased

   b. IgA—decreased

   c. IgM—decreased

2. Blood T and B Lymphocytes—B cells decreased and T cells normal

- Management/Treatment

1. Intravenous immunoglobulin G (IgG) replacement (IVIG)

2. Prophylactic antibiotics

3. Antibiotic therapy for recurrent infections

Thymic Hypoplasia (DiGeorge Syndrome)

- Definition: A syndrome that includes T cell dysfunction secondary to hypoplasia of the thymus

- Etiology/Incidence

    1. Dysmorphogenesis occurs during embryogenosis resulting in hypoplasia of the thymus and parathyroid glands; may also have cardiac defects, abnormal facies, cleft palate, and hypocalcemia

    2. Occurs in males and females equally

    3. Presentation usually results from cardiac failure or, after 24 to 48 hours of age, from hypocalcemia

    4. Sometimes diagnosed during cardiac surgery when no thymus is found in mediastinum

    5. Increased susceptibility to viral, fungal, and bacterial infections

- Signs and Symptoms: Specific to manner of presentation

- Differential Diagnosis: Other immune deficiencies

- Physical Findings

    1. Characteristic features—hypertelorism; shortened lip frenulum; lowset, notched pinnae; and nasal cleft

    2. Other physical findings—specific to manner of presentation

- Diagnostic Tests/Findings:

    1. Routine chest radiograph may reveal absent thymus

    2. Blood T and B lymphocytes

        a. Lymphopenia

        b. Decreased T cells

        c. B cells normal

- Management/Treatment

    1. Prophylactic antibiotics

    2. Antibiotic therapy for recurrent infections

    3. Thymus transplant if donor available

    4. Bone marrow transplant

Wiskott-Aldrich Syndrome (WAS)

- Definition: X-linked disorder characterized by thrombocytopenia, eczema, and progressive deterioration of thymus-dependent cellular immunity
- Etiology/Incidence
    1. X-linked recessive inheritance; carrier detection is possible
    2. Specific defect unknown
    3. Incidence— ~ 4 per one million male births
- Signs and Symptoms
    1. Neonatal—bloody diarrhea, prolonged bleeding from circumcision
    2. Later—eczema and frequent infections
- Differential Diagnosis: Usually made during neonatal period due to thrombocytopenia
    1. Other causes of chronic diarrhea
    2. Other immune deficiencies
- Physical Findings: Specific to manner of presentation
- Diagnostic Tests/Findings
    1. Serum immunoglobulins
        a. IgG—normal
        b. IgA—increased
        c. IgM—decreased
    2. Blood T and B Lymphocytes
        a. B cells—normal
        b. T cells—decreased
    3. CBC—thrombocytopenia, small platelets
- Management/Treatment
    1. Platelet transfusions for bleeding
    2. IV Immunoglobulins
    3. Prophylactic antibiotics and antibiotic therapy for recurrent infections
    4. Splenectomy—may increase platelet count
        a. Conjugate and polysaccharide pneumococcal vaccines as recommended by the American Academy of Pediatrics; should be given at least 2 weeks or longer prior to surgery, if possible, to increase the likelihood of eliciting a protective antibody response

   b. Prophylactic penicillin 250 mg b.i.d. for at least 1 to 2 years post-splenectomy

   c. Increased risk for bacterial infections post-splenectomy—for fever (T ≥ 101.5° F) immediate referral for blood culture and empiric parenteral antibiotics against encapsulated organisms

5. Bone marrow transplant if HLA-matched donor is available

Questions
Select the best answer

1. Baseline management of all neonates with ABO incompatibility includes:

   a. Phototherapy
   b. Serial monitoring of bilirubin levels
   c. Exchange transfusion
   d. Simple transfusion

2. Which of the following is not associated with Rh incompatibility?

   a. Mother Rh negative, baby Rh positive
   b. Mother Rh positive, baby Rh negative
   c. More severe in subsequent sensitized pregnancies
   d. Hemolysis may occur up to 6 weeks or more

3. Clinical jaundice of the distal extremities would be noted at a bilirubin level of:

   a. < 5 mg/dL
   b. 5 mg/dL
   c. 10 mg/dL
   d. ≥ 15 mg/dL

4. β-chain synthesis is absent in:

   a. β-thalassemia minor
   b. β-thalassemia intermedia
   c. β-thalassemia major
   d. α-thalassemia trait

5. Which of the following are most often associated with Hemoglobin C

   a. Growth retardation
   b. Hepatosplenomegaly
   c. Usually asymptomatic
   d. Frontal bossing

6. Diagnostic findings consistent with β-thalassemia are:

   a. Hemoglobin—normal
   b. Reticulocytes—normal
   c. Hgb $A_2 < 3.6$
   d. Hypochromia, microcytosis

7. Asplenic children are at increased risk for which of the following?

   a. Bacterial infections
   b. Fungal infections

    c. Viral infections

    d. Parasites

8. Which of the following is not considered preventive management for iron deficiency anemia?

    a. Iron fortified cereal from 6 to 12 months of age

    b. Iron fortified formula until 6 months of age

    c. No cow's milk until 1 year of age

    d. If breast feeding, supplemental iron drops or iron fortified cereal by 4–5 months of age

9. The expected clinical severity of hemoglobin sickle C disease (Hgb SC) is:

    a. Asymptomatic

    b. Marked to moderate

    c. Mild to moderate

    d. Severe

10. The expected hemoglobin range for sickle cell anemia is:

    a. 6.5–9.5 g/dL

    b. 13.5–16.5 g/dL

    c. 8.5–12.5 g/dL

    d. 9.5–13.5 g/dL

11. Prophylactic penicillin should be initiated in children with sickle cell anemia by:

    a. 3 years of age

    b. 12 months of age

    c. 2–3 months of age

    d. 9 months of age

12. Hemolysis does not contribute to which of the problems associated with sickle cell disease?

    a. Chronic anemia

    b. Splenic sequestration

    c. Aplastic crisis

    d. Delayed growth

13. The following blood lead level is not considered lead poisoning:

    a. < 10 μg/dL

    b. 10–14 μg/dL

    c. ≥ 15 μg/dL

    d. > 25 μg/dL

14. Which of the following is not a precipitating factor for hemolysis in G-6-PD deficiency?

    a. Drugs

    b. Exposure to extreme temperatures

c. Ingestion of Fava beans

d. Infection

15. What percent of Factor VIII/IX is associated with severe hemophilia A and B?

    a. < 1

    b. 1–5

    c. 5–25

    d. 30–50

16. What type of hemorrhage would be expected with severe Factor VIII deficiency?

    a. Severe hemorrhage following moderate to severe trauma

    b. Gross bleeding following mild to moderate trauma

    c. Gynecologic hemorrhage

    d. Spontaneous hemarthrosis

17. Which of the following is the most common type of congenital bleeding disorder?

    a. Hemophilia A

    b. Hemophilia B

    c. von Willebrand Disease

    d. Idiopathic thrombocytopenia purpura

18. Which of the following medications should be avoided in a child with ITP?

    a. Decongestants

    b. Aspirin

    c. Acetaminophen

    d. Sulfa drugs

19. The following test is required to diagnose leukemia:

    a. CBC with differential

    b. Bone marrow aspiration/biopsy

    c. Chest radiograph

    d. Biopsy of an enlarged lymph node

20. Which of the following is not included as part of the initial therapy for ALL?

    a. Chemotherapy

    b. Radiation therapy

    c. Bone marrow transplant

    d. Intrathecal chemotherapy

21. Which malignancy is associated with genitourinary anomalies?

    a. Acute lymphocytic leukemia

    b. Chronic myleogenous leukemia

   c. Osteosarcoma
   d. Wilms' tumor

22. The peak incidence of Wilms' tumor is:

   a. 3–4 years of age
   b. 5–8 years of age
   c. 9–12 years of age
   d. 15–19 years of age

23. The peak incidence of osteosarcoma is:

   a. 4–7 years of age
   b. 8–11 years of age
   c. 12–14 years of age
   d. 15–19 years of age

24. The following type of infection is not associated with hypogammaglobulinemia:

   a. Sinusitis
   b. Pneumonia
   c. Urinary tract infection
   d. Cellulitis

25. The following diagnostic finding is consistent with X-linked agammaglobulinemia:

   a. IgG—normal
   b. B cells—decreased
   c. T cells—decreased
   d. IgA—normal

26. The following is not a characteristic feature of DiGeorge syndrome:

   a. Hypertelorism
   b. Cleft palate
   c. Cardiac defects
   d. Frontal bossing

27. The following diagnostic finding is consistent with Wiskott-Aldrich syndrome:

   a. IgG—normal
   b. IgA—decreased
   c. IgM—increased
   d. B cells—decreased

28. Management of a patient with a splenectomy does not include:

   a. Pneumococcal vaccines at least 2 weeks prior to surgery
   b. Prophylactic penicillin
   c. Blood culture and parenteral antibiotics for febrile illnesses
   d. Treating fever with antipyretics only and observing for resolution

Answers

1. b	11. c	20. c
2. b	12. b	21. d
3. d	13. a	22. a
4. c	14. b	23. d
5. c	15. a	24. c
6. d	16. d	25. b
7. a	17. c	26. d
8. b	18. b	27. a
9. c	19. b	28. d
10. a		

Bibliography

Abshire, T. C. (2001). Sense and sensibility: Approaching anemia in children. *Contemporary Pediatrics, 18(9)*, 104–113.

American Academy of Pediatrics (1994). Practice parameters: Management of hyperbilirubinemia in the healthy newborn. (Provisional Committee for Quality Improvement and Subcommittee on Hyperbilirubinemia). *Pediatrics, 94*, 558–565.

American Academy of Pediatrics (2002). Health supervision for children with sickle cell disease. *Pediatrics, 109*, 526-535.

Baggott, C. R., Kelly, K. P., Fochtman, D., & Foley, G. V. (Eds.). (2002). *Nursing care of the child and adolescents with cancer* (3rd ed). Philadelphia: W. B. Saunders Company.

Behrman, R. E., Kliegman, R. M., & Jensen, H. B. (Eds.), (2004). *Nelson textbook of pediatrics* (17th ed). Philadelphia: W.B. Saunders Company.

Buchanan, G. R. (2000). ITP: How much treatment is enough? *Contemporary Pediatrics, 17*, 112–121.

Centers for Disease Control and Prevention. (2002). *Managing elevated blood lead levels among young children: Recommendations from the Advisory Committee on Childhood Lead Poisoning Prevention.* Atlanta, GA: Author.

Christie, B. A. (Ed). (2002). *Nurses' guide to bleeding disorders.* New York: National Hemophilia Foundation.

Dunn, A. M., Burns, C., & Sattler, B. (2003). Environmental health in children. *Journal of Pediatric Health Care, 17*, 223–231.

Gunn, V. L., & Nechyba, C. (Eds.). (2002). *The Harriet Lane handbook* (16th ed.). St. Louis: Mosby.

Hay, W. W., Haywood, A. R., Levin, M. J., Sondheimer, J. M. (Eds.). (2002). *Current pediatric diagnosis & treatment* (16th ed.) Stamford, CT: McGraw-Hill/Appleton & Lange.

Hockenberry-Eaton, M. J. (Ed.). (1998). *Essentials of oncology nursing: A core curriculum.* Glenville, IL: Association of Pediatric Oncology Nurses.

Hoeklman, R. A., Adam, H. M., Nelson, N. M., Weitzman, M. L., & Wilson, M. H. (Eds.). (2001). *Primary pediatric care* (4th ed.). St. Louis: Mosby.

Jackson, P. L., & Vessey, J. A. (Eds.). (2000). *Primary care of the child with a chronic condition* (3rd ed.). St. Louis: Mosby.

Lane, P. A. (1996). Sickle cell disease. *Pediatric Clinics of North America, 43*, 639–664.

Lanzkowsky, P. (2000). *Manual of pediatric hematology and oncology* (3rd ed.). New York: Churchill Livingstone.

National Institutes of Health. (2002). *Management of sickle cell disease* (4th ed.) (NIH Publication No. 20-2117) Washington, DC: U.S. Government Printing Office.

Pickering, L. T. (Ed.) (2003). *Red Book: 2003 Report of the committee on infectious diseases in children* (26th ed.). Elk Grove Village, IL: American Academy of Pediatrics.

Werner, E. J. (1996). von Willebrand disease in children and adolescents. *Pediatric Clinics of North America, 43*, 683–707.

Yetman, R. J. (2003). Evaluation and management of childhood idopathic (immune) thrombocytopenia. *Journal of Pediatric Health Care, 17*, 261–263.

Endocrine Disorders

Jacalyn Peck Dougherty

Thyroid Disorders

Hypothyroidism

- Definition
    1. Congenital or acquired metabolic disorder resulting in absent or insufficient production of thyroxin by thyroid gland
    2. May be familial or sporadic; possibly associated with enlargement (goiter) of thyroid gland (Foley, 2001)
    3. Depending on cause, may progress as permanent or transient disorder (Foley, 2001)
    4. Congenital vs. acquired
        a. Congenital—may affect fetus as early as 1st trimester; in children with mild hypothyroidism missed by newborn (NB) screening, symptoms may present in later infancy or childhood
        b. Juvenile-acquired—may have onset within 1st year of life but usually onset occurs in childhood or adolescence
    5. Primary vs. secondary
        a. Primary—disease or disorder of thyroid gland (thyroid gland failure)
        b. Secondary—disease or disorder of hypothalamus or pituitary gland compromises thyroid gland function
- Etiology/Incidence
    1. Congenital hypothyroidism
        a. Absence (athyreosis), underdevelopment (dysgenesis) or ectopic gland most common
        b. Inherent dysfunction in transport or assimilation of iodine or in synthesis or metabolism of thyroid hormone (e.g., thyroid enzyme defects, familial dyshormonogenesis)
        c. Maternal disease adversely affecting fetal thyroid development and function (prenatal exposure to iodine-containing or goitrogenic drugs and agents, e.g., thiouracil, methimazole, iodines; maternal exposure to radioactive iodine; placental crossing of maternal antibodies to fetal thyroid gland)
        d. Iodine deficiency causing endemic goiter and cretinism
        e. Hypothalamic or pituitary disorder (e.g., pituitary agenesis, anencepahly)
        f. Affects 1 infant in every 4000 live births (Foley, 2001; Weinzimer, Lee, & Moshang, 1997)
        g. Higher incidence in Hispanic and Native-American infants (AAP, 1993)
        h. Higher incidence in areas with endemic iodine deficiency
    2. Juvenile-acquired hypothyroidism (Foley, 2001; Rogers, 1994)

a. Chronic lymphocytic thyroiditis (Hashimoto's, autoimmune) most common cause beyond perinatal period

b. Late manifestation of congenital absence, underdevelopment (dysgenesis), or atrophy of thyroid gland

c. Late manifestation of congenital defects in synthesizing or metabolizing thyroid hormone

d. Ablation of thyroid through medical procedures (e.g., surgery, irradiation, radioactive iodine)

e. Exposure to iodine-containing drugs and agents; drug-induced (e.g., antithyroid drugs, excessive iodide, lithium, cobalt); exposure to naturally occurring goitrogens in foods, water pollutants

f. Disease of hypothalamus or pituitary (e.g., pituitary tumors, trauma), rare; child will show other signs of hypothalamic or pituitary disease

g. Endemic goiter from nutritional iodide deficiency—most common thyroid disease worldwide

- Signs and Symptoms

1. Affects multiple systems; many nonspecific, insidious signs and symptoms; severity depends on age of onset and degree of thyroid deficiency; symptoms vary for infants vs. children

2. May be familial history of thyroid and pituitary diseases; may have maternal prenatal history of thyroid disease or ingestion of antithyroid medications or foods

3. May be associated with other autoimmune disease or syndromes (e.g., Down, Turner's)

4. Neonates/infants

   a. Infants may have no obvious symptoms during first month of life

   b. History of lethargy, poor feeding, prolonged elevated bilirubin (>10 mg/dL > 3 days of age)

   c. May be post-mature; increased birth weight (> 4000 g)

5. Older infants, children, adolescents

   a. History of poor growth, intolerance to cold, poor appetite, constipation

   b. Mental and physical sluggishness, developmental delay

- Differential Diagnosis

1. Differentiate primary hypothyroidism due to intrinsic thyroid gland defects from secondary thyroid deficiency caused by pituitary or hypothalamic disorders

2. Congenital thyroxine-binding globulin (TBG) deficiency or "euthyroid sick syndrome" seen in small or sick newborns or in children with acute or chronic severe illnesses, surgery, trauma, or malnutrition

- Physical Findings

  1. Affects multiple systems; severity of findings depends on age of onset and degree of thyroid deficiency

  2. Neonates/infants

     a. Prolonged jaundice; poor feeding

     b. Growth deceleration

     c. Hypothermia, skin mottling

     d. Large fontanels, especially posterior; wide sutures; hirsute forehead; coarse facial features; dull expression; facial edema; nasal discharge; macroglossia

     e. Normal, slightly enlarged or goitrous thyroid gland; if thyroid ectopic, may see mass at base of tongue or in midline of neck

     f. Hoarse cry

     g. Axillary, prominent supraclavicular fat pads

     h. Respiratory distress in term infant

     i. Bradycardia (< 100 beats/min.)

     j. Distended or protuberant abdomen, umbilical hernia, constipation

     k. Lumbar lordosis, hypotonia

  3. Infants, children, and adolescents

     a. Increased weight for height, myxedema with hypothyroidism of long duration

     b. Linear growth retardation or growth deceleration; delayed bone maturation, dentition, tooth eruption

     c. Developmental delay; poor motor coordination, dull appearance

     d. Delayed puberty, occasionally precocious puberty or pseudoprecocity; menstrual disorders

     e. Skin cool, pale, gray, mottled, thickened, increased pigmentation, carotenemia

     f. Hair dry, brittle; lateral thinning of eyebrows

     g. Possible enlarged thyroid gland (goiter); may feel cobblestone-like

     h. Galactorrhea, constipation

     i. Myopathy, muscular hypertrophy, poor muscle tone; prolonged relaxation phase of deep tendon reflexes (DTR)

     j. Delayed bone age

     k. If advanced hypothyroidism and myxedema, may be "chubby" and have periorbital edema

- Diagnostic Tests/Findings

    1. Newborn screening for congenital hypothyroidism is routine in all 50 states

        a. Abnormal newborn screen—repeat thyroid screen for confirmatory diagnosis with thyroid stimulating hormone (TSH) and thyroxine (T_4)

        b. Elevated serum TSH and low T_4 diagnostic of transient or permanent primary hypothyroidism

        c. Positive TSH receptor-blocking antibodies (TRBAb)—diagnostic for transient congenital hypothyroidism

        d. Additional thyroid function tests—serum thyroxine-binding globulin (TBG); tri-iodothyronine resin uptake (T_3RU) (Weinzimer, Lee & Moshang, 1997)

    2. Acquired hypothyroidism secondary to pituitary or hypothalamic disorders (Foley, 2001; Weinzimer, Lee & Moshang, 1997)

        a. Low free (unbound) thyroxine (free T_4), usually normal TSH; and low thyroxine-binding globulin (TBG)

        b. Abnormal pituitary function tests

    3. Euthyroid sick syndrome (non-thyroidal illness syndrome) secondary to coexisting acute or chronic illness—low T_4 level with normal TBG; low T_3; normal TSH; free T_4 and reverse T_3 levels high normal or elevated

    4. Autoimmune (Hashimoto's) thyroiditis (with goiter present)—normal T_4 and TSH; elevated serum thyroid peroxidase or thyroglobulin antibody titers

    5. Repeat thyroid function tests if clinical suspicion of hypothyroidism, history of thyroid disease in pregnancy; positive history of thyroid dyshormonogenesis (AAP, 1993)

    6. May have abnormal thyroid scan, ultrasound, imaging, or bone age results

- Management/Treatment

    1. Physician consultation or referral to pediatric endocrinologist for suspected or confirmed hypothyroidism

    2. For congenital hypothyroidism, rapid and adequate thyroid hormone replacement critical to avoid irreparable neurologic impairment and mental retardation; treat within first month of life for best prognosis for optimal intellectual development

    3. Drug of choice daily oral levothyroxine (L-thyroxine); after treatment initiated for hypothyroidism in infancy, monitor T_4 and TSH levels monthly during first year of life, every other month during second year, quarterly during third year, and biannually thereafter (Rogers, 1994); monitor additionally as needed whenever dose adjusted

    4. Recommended dosages of levothyroxine (T_4) vary by age; dosage/kg/day decreases over time with age

5. In older children and adolescents, increase thyroid dose gradually to full replacement dose to avoid undesirable side effects and clinical symptoms of thyrotoxicosis (e.g., headaches, abrupt personality changes)

6. Once older children and adolescents in euthyroid state, monitor adequacy of levothyroxine therapy with regular, periodic T_4 and TSH levels

7. Give levothyroxine an hour before meals to prevent reduced absorption, especially for infants; iron may interfere with absorption

8. Educate parents and child about disease, treatment regimen, and routine monitoring; with thyroid replacement, child will be livelier, less docile, may lose water weight, hair of normal texture will replace dry hair, may have transient stomach or head aches (Weinzimer, Lee, & Moshang, 1997)

9. Genetic counseling may be indicated if familial etiology

10. Trial off of medication may be indicated at age 3, if possibility child had transient congenital hypothyroidism

Hyperthyroidism

- Definition: Excessive production and secretion of thyroid hormone (TH) by thyroid gland (thyrotoxicosis) resulting in increased basal metabolism, goiter, autonomic nervous system disorders, and problems with creatinine metabolism

- Etiology/Incidence

  1. Caused by excess production of thyroid hormone (e.g., Graves' or autoimmune hyperthyroidism, pituitary tumor) or excess release of thyroid hormone (e.g., subacute thyroiditis, Hashimoto's toxic thyroiditis, iodine-induced hyperthyroidism) (Rogers, 1994)

  2. Most common cause is autoimmune response (Graves')—body produces thyroid stimulating immunoglobulins (TSI) which stimulate TSH receptors in thyroid gland, causing overproduction of TH and thyroid hypertrophy; has genetic predisposition

  3. If mother is thyrotoxic prenatally or has history of Graves', infants may have transient congenital hyperthyroidism (neonatal Graves') since thyroid-stimulating immunoglobulins (TSI) cross placenta to fetus; rare

  4. Graves more common in girls than boys (5 or 6:8) (Gotlin & Chase, 1997; Jospe, 2001), highest incidence between 12 and 14 years; rare before 10 years

- Signs and Symptoms

  1. May have family history of thyroid disorder (e.g., Graves') or maternal history of antithyroid drug ingestion for treatment of Graves' during pregnancy

  2. Neonates/infants (Rogers, 1994; Jospe, 2001; Van Vliet, 2003)

     a. In neonate, signs and symptoms usually present shortly after birth or may present days or weeks later; not common, but can have severe consequences if untreated; diagnosis rarely made in newborn period

    b. Prematurity, low birth weight, poor weight gain, weight loss

    c. Restlessness, irritability

    d. Fever, flushing

3. Child/adolescent

    a. Weight loss, although increased appetite; may have accelerated growth and advanced bone age with long-term illness

    b. Nervousness; irritability; decreased attention span; behavior problems; decline in school performance; emotional lability; restlessness; fatigue; weakness; heat intolerance; increased perspiration

    c. Sleeplessness or sleep restlessness, insomnia, nightmares

    d. Visual disturbances, e.g., increased lacrimation, diplopia, photophobia, blurring

    e. Palpitations

    f. Frequent urination and loose stooling, may have enuresis

    g. Amenorrhea

- Differential Diagnosis

  1. Neonates—systemic illness, sepsis, and narcotic withdrawal

  2. Children and adolescents

         a. Nodular thyroid disease

         b. Thyroid cancer

         c. Euthyroid goiter

         d. Chronic disease, e.g., pituitary disease, severe anemia, leukemia

         e. Thyroiditis

         f. Accidental or deliberate excessive thyroid hormone or iodine ingestion

         g. Chorea

         h. Psychiatric illness, e.g., anxiety disorder, anorexia

- Physical Findings

  1. Neonates and infants

         a. May be small for gestational age

         b. Lid retraction, proptosis, periorbital edema

         c. Face may be flushed

         d. Enlarged thyroid (goiter)

         e. Tachycardia without underlying heart disease

         f. Increased gastrointestinal motility

g. Severely affected neonates may have jaundice, microcephaly, frontal bossing, craniosynostosis, ophthalmopathy, exophthalmia, thrombocytopenia, cardiac problems, hepatosplenomegaly, other signs of severe illness (Zimmerman & Gan-Gaisano, 1990; Jospe, 2001)

2. Children and adolescents (Jospe, 2001)

a. Warm, moist, smooth, diaphoretic skin; face may be flushed

b. Eye findings, e.g., proptosis, exophthalmos, upper lid lag with downward gaze, lid retraction, stare appearance, periorbital and conjunctival edema

c. Variable-size enlarged, tender or nontender, spongy or firm thyroid with palpable border; may have thyroid bruit or thrill

d. Tachycardia, systolic hypertension, increased pulse pressure

e. Proximal muscle weakness, diminished fine motor control, tremor, short DTR relaxation phase

f. Advanced skeletal maturation radiographically

- Diagnostic Tests/Findings

1. If signs or symptoms of thyrotoxicosis or enlarged thyroid, do confirmatory laboratory thyroid function tests

2. Thyroiditis indicated by elevated T_4, free T_4, T_3 resin uptake (T_3RU) and low serum cholesterol

3. Circulating thyroid simulator immunoglobulin (TSI) and other thyroid antibody tests including thyrotropin receptor antibody (TRAb) titers may be positive

4. May have moderate leukopenia, hyperglycemia, and glycosuria (Gotlin & Chase, 1997)

5. Graves' Disease—elevated T_4 and low TSH; advanced bone age

6. Radioactive iodine uptake scan shows increased uptake if excess TH production; if increased release of TH only, will have decreased radioactive iodine uptake

7. High plasma T_4 does not necessarily indicate hyperthyroidism as there is a physiological transient peak of plasma T_4 on day two of life, diagnosis of true hyperthyroidism requires low or undetectable TSH with high T_4 and/or T_3 (Van Vliet, 2003, p. 354)

- Management/Treatment

1. Physician consultation or referral to pediatric endocrinologist for suspected or confirmed hyperthyroidism

2. Treatment dictated by identified etiology for hyperthyroidism and degree of thyrotoxicity

3. Prompt diagnosis and treatment especially important in neonates as condition may be life-threatening

4. Treatment goal is prompt return to euthyroidism with use of:

    a. Antithyroid drugs to inhibit thyroxine (T_4) synthesis and conversion of T_3 to T_4, e.g., propylthiouracil, methimazole

    b. Antithyroid drugs or radioiodine treatment of thyroid gland (ablative therapy)

    c. Beta-adrenergic receptor blockers to control nervousness and cardiovascular symptoms, e.g., propranolol, atenolol

    d. Thyroid surgery no longer considered primary form of treatment except in pregnancy under certain circumstances (Kappy, Steelman, Travers & Zeitler, 2003; Jospe, 2001)

5. Restricted physical activity if hyperthyroidism severe or in preparation for surgery

6. Educate parent and child about disease, duration of treatment, side effects of medications or complications if surgery required, adherence to treatment regimen, and, if Graves' disease, need for lifelong monitoring; advise of complications, e.g., thyrotoxicosis

7. Genetic counseling may be indicated if familial etiology

Thyroiditis

- Definition: Inflammation of thyroid gland caused by autoimmune response to the thyroid gland (chronic lymphocytic thyroiditis, [Hashimoto's]); infectious agents (acute suppurative and subacute nonsuppurative); or from exposure to radiation or trauma; occasionally idiopathic

- Etiology/Incidence (Kappy, Steelman, Travers & Zeitler, 2003)

    1. Acute suppurative thyroiditis with bacterial etiology—e.g., group A streptocci, pneumococci, *S. aureas,* and anaerobes; rare

    2. Subacute nonsuppurative thyroiditis caused by viruses—e.g., mumps, influenza, echovirus, coxsackie, Epstein-Barr, adenovirus; rare in U.S.

    3. Chronic lymphocytic thyroiditis (chronic autoimmune or Hashimoto thyroiditis)—non-infectious autoimmune inflammatory disease of thyroid most common cause of goiter and hypothyroidism in childhood; highest incidence in children 8 to 15 years; more common in females than males (4:1); increasing incidence may be associated with rising incidence of Type 1 diabetes (Kappy, Steelman, Travers & Zeitler, 2003; Dallas & Foley, 2003)

- Signs and Symptoms

    1. With infectious thyroiditis, may have recent history of or concurrent upper respiratory illness

    2. With chronic autoimmune thyroiditis, may have family history of autoimmune thyroid disease

    3. Onset in acute thyroiditis rapid; insidious onset in subacute and chronic lymphocytic thyroiditis

4. Fever, malaise; may feel quite ill with acute suppurative or subacute thyroiditis, particularly with former

5. With acute and subacute thyroiditis, pain and tenderness of thyroid with radiation to other areas of neck, ear, chest; with acute suppurative thyroiditis, severe pain with neck extension; no tenderness with chronic lymphocytic thyroiditis

6. Complaints of unilateral or bilateral swelling of the thyroid, complaints of fullness in anterior neck; sensation of tracheal compression

7. May have sore throat, hoarseness, dysphagia

8. May have nervousness, irritability, other symptoms of mild hyperthyroidism

- Differential Diagnosis

   1. Infectious toxic thyroiditis must be distinguished from chronic lymphocytic autoimmune thyroiditis; simple goiters due to inborn errors of T_4 synthesis; and chronic autoimmune thyroiditis (Hashimoto's) associated with adolescence in girls; and thyroglossal duct abscesses (Kappy, Steelman, Travers & Zeitler, 2003)

   2. Goiters induced by drugs—(e.g., from iodine, lithium, para-amino salicylic acid, thionamides, white turnip plants); by transplacental exposure to TH by breast feeding of newborns when mothers on antithyroid therapy (Weinzimer, Lee & Moshang, 1997)

   3. Cancerous or cystic thyroid nodules

- Physical Findings

   1. Findings variable depending on etiology—i.e., infectious vs. autoimmune

   2. May be toxic-appearing if infectious etiology but not necessarily thyrotoxic

   3. In infectious thyroiditis—thyroid gland unilaterally or bilaterally enlarged, tender, firm

   4. In chronic lymphocytic thyroiditis, usually symmetric, nontender, firm, freely moveable, diffusely enlarged "pebbly" goiter

- Diagnostic Tests/Findings (Kappy, Steelman, Travers & Zeitler, 2003)

   1. Laboratory findings variable depending on etiology

   2. In acute suppurative thyroiditis—usually no consistently associated endocrine disturbances; moderate to marked shift to left in differential; elevated sedimentation rate

   3. Subacute nonsuppurative thyroiditis—radioiodine uptake usually reduced; serum TH levels normal or elevated

   4. In chronic lymphocytic thyroiditis—usually normal T_4, free T_4, T_3 RU, but may be elevated or depressed; thyroid autoantibodies usually present, abnormal thyroid scan, surgical or needle biopsy diagnostic but rarely indicated

- Management/Treatment
    1. Physician consultation or referral to pediatric endocrinologist for suspected or confirmed thyroiditis
    2. Specific antibiotic therapy required for acute suppurative thyroiditis and may be needed for subacute nonsuppurative thyroiditis since latter is difficult to distinguish from former; acetylsalicylic acid or other anti-inflammatory drugs
    3. Treatment for automimmune chronic lymphocytic thyroiditis controversial; levothyroxine may be used to decrease goiter but efficacy in preventing progression of hypothyroidism in long term not supported (Kappy, Steelman, Travers & Zeitler, 2003)
    4. Adolescents with autoimmune chronic lymphocytic thyroiditis need lifelong monitoring since development of hypothyroidism is possible, subacute thyroiditis self-limiting
    5. Genetic counseling may be indicated for familial etiology

Pituitary Disorders

Diabetes Insipidus (DI)

- Definition: Excretion of large amounts of dilute urine due to insufficient function of antidiuretic hormone (ADH, arginine vaspopressin, disorder in ADH receptors in kidney, primary renal disease, or, rarely in children, to primary polydipsia; compromised ability to concentrate urine)
- Etiology/Incidence
    1. Central (hypothalamic, neurogenic, vasopressin-sensitive) DI caused by hypofunction of hypothalamus/posterior pituitary or increased vasopressin metabolism resulting in ADH deficiency (Muglia & Majzoub, 2002)
        a. Genetic—familial autosomal dominant trait, rare
        b. Congenital—e.g., anatomic defects in brain
        c. Acquired secondary to accidental or surgical trauma, infection, cerebral anoxia, neoplasm, or infectious disease; trauma following removal of hypothalamic area tumors major cause
        d. Secondary to autoimmune or infiltrative disease, e.g., histiocytosis, lymphocytic hypophysitis
        e. Idiopathic
        f. Other—brain death, increased vasopressin metabolism, drugs, e.g., ethanol
    2. Nephrogenic (vasporessin-resistant) DI caused by reduced renal responsiveness to ADH (not CNS mediated)
        a. Familial—X-linked inherited disorder of ADH receptor sites in kidney in

males primarily; females rarely affected, less common etiology but more severe

b. Acquired

(1) Renal failure, e.g., obstructive uropathy, polycystic kidney disease

(2) Electrolyte disorders (hypercalcemia, hypokalemia)

(3) Nephrotoxic drugs, e.g., lithium, demeclocycline, amphotericin, methicillin, rifampin

(4) Other illness, e.g., sickle cell

- Signs and Symptoms

1. Symptoms vary depending on etiology, age, anterior pituitary function, preservation of normal thirst, diet (Bode, Crawford & Danon, 1996)

2. Central (neurogenic) DI

a. May have family history of congenital ADH deficiency

b. Generally rapid onset; disease may be masked as failure-to-thrive

c. History of poor weight gain, deficient growth if long duration

d. Unexplained fever, irritability

e. Intense thirst, polydipsia, desire for cold drinks, preference for cold water; irritable when fluid withheld; unable to sleep through night without water intake

f. Vomiting, constipation; unexplained fever in infants

g. Tendency to avoid diets high in protein and salt

h. Polyuria, nocturia, enuresis in previously toilet-trained child; clear urine; unable to concentrate urine after fluid restriction

i. May have symptoms of intracranial tumor (headaches, strabismus, double vision vomiting, precocious puberty)

j. May follow intracranial surgical procedures or trauma; CNS disease; rarely idiopathic (Goepp & Ackerman, 2001)

3. Nephrogenic DI (Muglia & Majzoub, 2002; Majzoub & Muglia, 2003)

a. Genetic or acquired causes—may have family history of congenital nephrogenic DI or maternal history of polyhydramnios; infants may do well on breast feeding until weaning, infection, or introduction of solids, then may fail to thrive; often present with fever, vomiting, dehydration

b. Female carriers of trait have varying severity of disease

c. Poor weight gain, deficient growth if long duration; may be malnourished

d. Increased thirst, polydipsia, history of large water intake, poor food intake because of preference for water over milk or solids

e. Dehydration, absence of tears, perspiration; if dehydration severe, may have seizures

f. Irritability; may have poor attention span, poor school performance

g. Vomiting; polyuria, nocturia

- Differential Diagnosis

1. Distinguish DI caused by suppression of vasopressin secretion (congenital vs. acquired central DI) from DI caused by reduced renal responsiveness to arginine vasopressin (congenital vs. acquired nephrogenic DI)

2. Psychogenic polydipsia (compulsive water drinking) and other causes of polyuria (e.g., drug-induced polydipsia [e.g., thioridazine, tricyclics]; hypokalemia; hypercalcemia [including hypervitaminosis D]; primary and secondary renal disease; diabetes mellitus)

- Physical Findings

1. Central (neurogenic) DI (Kappy, Steelman, Travers & Zeitler, 2003)

a. Variable levels of dehydration; if disease unrecognized, infants may have high fever, vomiting, seizures, circulatory collapse

b. Poor weight gain, deficient growth if long duration; may be malnourished

c. Irritability; may have poor attention span

d. May have symptoms of brain tumor (e.g., strabismus, nystagmus)

2. Nephrogenic DI

a. Variable levels of dehydration; dry skin, no tears, no perspiration; if severe, infants may have high fever, convulsions, circulatory collapse

b. Failure to thrive, malnourished; if long duration, may have growth retardation, delayed sexual maturation, CNS damage

c. Fever, irritability

d. Large or distended bladder except immediately after voiding; nonobstructive hydonephrosis, hydroureter

- Diagnostic Tests/Findings (Kappy, Steelman, Travers & Zeitler, 2003, p. 944; Majzoub & Muglia, 2003)

1. History of pathological polydipsia and polyuria (> 2 L/m^2/day)

2. Urine specific gravity (< 1.010; osmolality < 300 mOsm/kg)

3. Inability to concentrate urine after fluid restriction

4. Hyperosmolality of plasma

5. Hypernatremia (> 160 mEq/L) (Bode, Crawford, & Danon, 1996)

6. Positive water deprivation test—to establish diagnosis of DI and differentiate central vs. nephrogenic DI

    a. Serum osmolality > 300 mOsm/kg, and urine osmolality < 300 mOsm/kg diagnostic of DI (Majzoub & Muglia, 2003)

    b. ADH administration (vasporessin) differentiates central vs. nephrogenic DI

       (1) Central DI—decreased urine volume and increased urine osmolality

       (2) Nephrogenic DI—no further changes in urine volume or osmolality

7. With MRI, absence or diminished "bright spot" in posterior pituitary; diminished blood flow to posterior pituitary (Majzoub & Muglia, 2003)

8. Low serum ADH concentration in central DI; high serum ADH level in nephrogenic DI

- Management/Treatment

1. Immediate physician consultation or referral to pediatric endocrinologist for suspected or confirmed DI

2. Careful adequate rehydration to avoid seizures, intellectual impairment due to CNS damage from hypernatremia and dehydration, particularly in infants who may not be able to make known their need for water or to obtain water necessary to quench thirst (Majzoub & Muglia, 2003); early recognition and management needed to avoid sequelae of stunted growth and cognitive impairment

3. Treat treatable underlying causes of nephrogenic DI, e.g., hypokalemia, drug-induced, obstructive uropathy

4. Treatment of choice for diabetes insipidus—intranasal desmopression acetate (DDAVP); infants sometimes given extra free water rather than DDAVP for normal hydration (Kappy, Steelman, Travers & Zeitler, 2003); with nephrogenic DI, may need diuretics, e.g., thiazides, prostaglandin synthesis inhibitors, e.g., indomethacin

5. Breast feeding preferable; adequate calories for growth; with nephrogenic DI, water allowed as demanded, sodium intake restricted (Lum, 2003); teach regarding avoidance of severe dehydration

6. Genetic counseling may be indicated for familial etiology

7. Treat other identified causes, e.g., germinomas, histiocytosis, craniopharyngiomas (Kappy, Steelman, Travers & Zeitler, 2003)

Growth disturbances

Short stature

- Definition

1. Variation from average pattern of growth (Gotlin & Chase, 1997); associated with normal variants of growth and pathologic conditions

2. Growth adequacy determined by consideration of both growth rate and absolute height; severe form of short stature defined as height > 3 standard deviations below the mean

3. Revised CDC growth chart should be used to evaluate growth of children (www.cdc.gov/growthcharts) (Lifshitz & Boteco, 2003)

- Etiology/Incidence

    1. Multiple etiologies—genetic, constitutional, physiologic, environmental, psychosocial

        a. Normal growth variations (most common)

            (1) Familial or genetic normal variant of average growth pattern which is familial, racial, or genetic; child "constitutionally small" and remains small as adult

            (2) Constitutional delay of growth with delayed growth pattern resulting in delayed physical maturity but normal final adult height

        b. Pathologic causes of short stature (Kappy, Steelman, Travers & Zeitler, 2003)

            (1) Nutritional—hypocaloric, gastrointestinal disorders

            (2) Endocrine—growth hormone (GH) deficiency; occurs in 1:4000 children

                (a) Hereditary—rare gene deletion

                (b) Idiopathic—about 66% cases caused by suspected deficiency or impairment in hypothalamic secretion of human growth hormone-releasing (hGH) hormone

                (c) Acquired—secondary to pituitary/hypothalamic disease, CNS infection, trauma, intracranial tumors

            (3) Other endocrine disturbances—hypothyroidism, hypopititarism, excess cortisol, precocious puberty

            (4) Chromosomal defects (Turner's, Down syndrome)

            (5) Intrauterine growth retardation (IUGR)—sporadic or associated with syndromes, e.g., De Lange syndrome, Russell-Silver syndrome; infections; placental abnormalities, maternal abnormalities, e.g., drug use, malnutrition

            (6) Bone development disorders—achondroplasia, skeletal disorders

            (7) Metabolic—storage diseases, inborn errors of metabolism

            (8) Systemic and chronic diseases and congenital defects— e.g., liver, hematologic, respiratory, cardiovascular, renal, CNS disease or tumors

            (9) Associated with chronic systemic diseases, birth defects, mental retardation, cancers

            (10) Psychosocial factors, e.g., deprivation dwarfism

            (11) Chronic drug intake, e.g., glucocorticoids

- Signs and Symptoms

    1. Normal growth variations

    a. Familial short stature—usually small at birth (≤ 3%) but consistent with family pattern

    b. Constitutional growth delay—usually normal size at birth with declining height and weight to < 5% between 1 and 3 years of age; delayed pubesence; family history of similar growth pattern in parents or other family members

2. Pathologic growth variations

    a. History of poor nutritional intake, malabsorption syndromes

    b. Symptoms of GH deficiency—failure to grow, headaches, delayed dental development, visual field defects, polyuria, polydipsia, delayed sexual maturation, CNS abnormalities, history of trauma, infection, radiation to CNS

    c. Signs and symptoms of other endocrine disorders—fever, lethargy, irritability, developmental delay, dull appearance, FTT, increased weight for height, polyuria, polydipsia, constipation, delayed sexual maturation, CNS symptoms, CNS surgery

    d. Intrauterine growth retardation (IUGR) and low birth weight (LBW); normal BW or normal growth pattern with subsequent onset of decelerated or delayed growth; history of premature aging

    e. Symptoms of other systemic or chronic illness—FTT, congenital defects including intrinsic diseases of bone

    f. Dysmorphism at birth, chromosomal abnormalities, syndromes, congenital skeletal defects or anomalies, e.g., abnormal upper to lower body ratio; abnormal or disproportionate features

    g. Signs and symptoms of neglect, emotional maltreatment; abnormalities in psychosocial development; parents may be overwhelmed or disorganized and not intentionally neglectful or abusive

    h. Chronic drug intake, e.g., glucocorticoids, high doses of estrogens, androgens

- Differential Diagnosis: Distinguish normal variants of familial short stature and constitutional growth delay from pathologic causes

- Physical Findings

1. Familial or constitutional short stature—height, weight, occipital-frontal circumference (OFC) growth curve patterns generally consistent, symmetric

    a. Familial—growth chart showing BW ≤ 3% but consistent with family pattern; follows growth curve; normal physical examination; radiographic bone age consistent with chronological age

    b. Constitutional delay—growth chart showing normal size at birth with declining height and weight throughout 1 to 3 years to < 5%; normal physical examination; bone maturation 2 to 3 years behind chronological age

2. Pathologic short stature

    a. GH deficiency—BW may be normal, birth length 50% that of normal child;

height and weight growth deficits; infantile fat distribution; youthful facial features; midfacial hypoplasia; visual field defects; small hands and feet; newborn may have microphallus (stretched penile length of < 2.5 cm vs. normal mean length of 4 cm [Styne, 1996]); may have CNS findings

  b. Primordial short stature

    (1) IUGR—BW and birth length below normal for gestational age, OFC normal or < 3rd percentile; subsequent growth parallel to or < 3rd percentile

    (2) Primordial dwarfism with premature aging—child appears older than age

    (3) Short stature with and without dysmorphism—height, weight < 3rd percentile, may have normal physical examination other than small size or may have various abnormal physical findings, e.g., microcephaly

  c. Short stature associated with chromosomal abnormalities—may have dysmorphism or stigmata of specific congenital or familial disorders, e.g., Turner's syndrome (webbed neck, small jaw, prominent ears, epicanthal folds, low posterior hairline, broad chest, cardiac defects) or Down syndrome

  d. Short stature associated with bone or cartilage development disorders, e.g., skeletal dysplasia, short extremities with normal size head and trunk, frontal bossing, abnormal upper to lower body ratios, abnormal or disproportionate features, rickets, leg bowing

  e. Short stature associated with symptoms of endogenous cortisol excess, e.g., Cushing's disease with moon facies, hirsutism, "buffalo hump," striae, hypertension, fatigue, voice deepening, obesity, amenorrhea

  f. Chronic drug intake, e.g., glucocorticoid excess with hypertension, plethora, moon facies, purple striae, interscapular fat pad, truncal obesity, muscle wasting

  g. Abnormalities in psychosocial development; neglectful parents

- Diagnostic Tests/Findings (Weinzimer, Lee, & Moshang, 1997; Kappy, Steelman, Travers & Zeitler, 2003, p. 943)

  1. Abnormalities in previous sequential, consistent recordings of height, weight, and OFC plotted on age-standardized growth charts

  2. In familial short stature and constitutional delay, height may be < 3rd percentile but growth rate normal; careful family history of familial growth patterns may elucidate familial vs. constitutional delay as etiology of short stature

  3. In growth failure, slower than normal growth rate results in flattened growth curve or decrease in growth parameter percentiles

  4. May have abnormal complete and segmental growth measurements and upper to lower body ratio measurements

5. Laboratory tests to confirm diagnosis based on clinical findings and to rule out systemic disease or hormonal deficiency; findings depend on etiology

   a. Abnormal CBC—chronic anemia, infection, leukemia

   b. Elevated sedimentation rate—collagen-vascular disease, cancer, chronic infection

   c. Abnormal biochemical profiles—adrenal insufficiency, renal disease

   d. Abnormal stool examination—inflammatory bowel disease, severe parasitism

   e. Abnormal thyroid function studies—hypothyroidism

   f. Low serum human growth hormone (hGH), insulin growth factor (IGF-1), IGF-binding protein—growth hormone deficiency (GHD) (Kappy, Steelman, Travers & Zeitler, 2003)

   g. Abnormal urinalysis—renal disease

6. Delayed maturity on radiographic bone age indicates constitutional delay (generally 2 to 3 years behind chronological age), GH deficiency, hypothyroidism, severe systemic illness; normal bone age found in familial short stature

7. Nutritional evaluation may show inadequate calories

8. Abnormal home/social evaluation may suggest psychosocial etiology

9. Abnormalities on skull radiograph, CT, MRI of cranium if intracranial lesion

10. Karyotype analysis in short girls with pubertal delay may indicate Turner syndrome

- Management/Treatment

  1. Physician consultation or referral to appropriate pediatric specialists for children with other than familial or constitutional growth delay

  2. If familial or constitutional growth delay, only periodic monitoring of growth pattern needed; reassurance

  3. If marked psychosocial problems arise in boys because of pubertal delay, short-term testosterone may initiate sexual development (Weinzimer, Lee, & Moshang, 1997)

  5. Optimize treatment for other endocrine or systemic or chronic illnesses to minimize compromised growth; adequate calories for growth

  6. GH may be indicated for children with known GH deficiency (controversial)

Excessive growth

- Definition: Variation from average pattern of growth in linear height with height > 2 SD above the mean; excess height for age

- Etiology/Incidence (Frasier, 1996, 2003; Gotlin & Chase, 1997)

  1. Normal variation in growth—constitutional tall structure (familial, genetic) most common, familial tendency to mature early

  2. Pathologic variations in growth

a.   Endocrine disorders

   (1)   Infant of diabetic mother (IDM)

   (2)   GH excess—usually due to pituitary adenoma

   (3)   Precocious puberty—androgen or estrogen excess prior to puberty from CNS disorder, adrenal or gonadal disorder, e.g., excess of androgens, estrogens, or both, or idiopathic cause leads to accelerated linear growth, early bone and sexual maturation, and adult short stature; more common in females than males; males have more pathologic etiologies, e.g., CNS disease, females have more idiopathic precocious puberty

b.   Genetic causes

   (1)   Marfan syndrome—autosomal dominant, connective tissue disorder

   (2)   Chromosomal abnormalities (e.g., Klinefelter syndrome in males with $\geq$ 2 X chromosomes with usual normal adult stature), XYY, XXYY

c.   Other

   (1)   Idiopathic or exogenous obesity—early puberty with accelerated growth; usually adult height not beyond expected genetic potential

   (2)   Homocystinuria—inherited inborn error of metabolism

   (3)   Cerebral gigantism (Sotos syndrome)—possible hypothalamic dysfunction; adult stature normal to excessive

   (4)   Beckwith-Weidemann syndrome

- Signs and Symptoms

   1.   Concern about tall stature or excessive growth primarily with adolescent girls/parents

   2.   Symptoms accompanying tall stature variable depending on underlying etiology

   3.   Familial or constitutional tall stature—length normal at birth, tall stature evident by 3 to 4 years; growth rate slows after 4 or 5 years with curve then parallel to normal curve (Frasier, 1996)

   4.   IDM—history of maternal diabetes, large for gestational age (LGA)

   5.   Beckwith-Wiedemann—LGA, rapid growth in childhood; concern about height; symptoms of hypoglycemia

   6.   GH excess—symptoms vary depending on age when excess GH secretion occurs; concern about height, other symptoms of GH excess (e.g., headache, excessive perspiration, visual impairment, coarsening of facial features, enlargement of nose, ears, jaw, increases in hand and feet, galactorrhea, menstrual irregularity, polyuria, polydipsia, joint pain)

   7.   Precocious puberty—concern about height, increase in growth rate, and early development of pubic hair common presenting signs

a.   True precocity of familial or idiopathic origin—causes early secondary sex characteristics with testicular enlargement and spermatogenesis in boys, menarche and mature ova in girls

b.   Incomplete or pseudoprecocity—adrenal or gonadal tumor or dysfunction causes early secondary sex characteristics but no testicular enlargement, no ovulation

c.   CNS disorders/tumors—more common in males, may have seizures

8.   Marfan's—concern about height, vision problems

9.   Klinefelter's syndrome—concern about height, school and behavior problems, lowered verbal IQ, vision problems, delayed adolescent development, testes before puberty normal or small

10.   Obesity—normal height, weight at birth

11.   Homocystinuria—concern about height, mental retardation, vision problems, CNS symptoms, back pain

12.   Cerebral gigantism (Sotos)—concern about height; normal height at birth, rapid growth first year of life (> 97% height at 1 year) to 3 to 4 years, feeding problems, developmental delay

- Differential Diagnosis: Normal variants of constitutional tall structure need to be distinguished from pathologic causes; distinguish pseudoprecocity from true sexual precocity; cause of testicular enlargement may be testicular tumor; ovarian tumor may cause early menarche

- Physical Findings

1.   Constitutional tall stature—variant of normal; 2 to 4 SD above average height for age; normal body proportions; normal physical examination and appropriate pubertal development and timing (Frasier, 2003)

2.   Endocrine disorders

a.   IDM—LGA at birth; > 90% for height and weight

b.   GH excess—tall; soft tissue growth; prominent mandible; supraorbital ridge; large nose; space between teeth; hypertension; heart failure; large hands and feet, thickened bones, overgrowth of joints of extremities; visceral enlargement; osteoporosis, kyphosis, may have signs of CNS symptoms

c.   Precocious puberty—tall stature; in males, secondary sexual development before age 9 years (Styne, 2003); in females, breast development before 8.0 years, sexual pubic hair before 9.0 years or menses before 9.5 years (Rosenfield, 2002)

3.   Genetic disorders

a.   Marfan's—tall stature, dolicocephaly, abnormal body proportions, thin extremities, increased arm and leg length, lowered upper/lower segment ratio, increased arm span, arachnodactyly, myopia and other visual abnormalities, external ear abnormalities, pectus excavatum, heart murmur, scoliosis or kyphosis, laxity and hyperextension of joints, hypotonicity

    b. Klinefelter syndrome—tall stature, underweight for height and age, mental retardation, long legs, low upper/lower body segment ratio, gynecomastia, normal penile size and pubic hair but small, firm testes with decreased sensitivity to pressure, cryptorchidism, hypospadias

4. Other causes of tall stature

    a. Obesity—accelerated height and weight, generally normal examination otherwise

    b. Homocystinuria—tall stature, myopia and other ocular problems, CNS symptoms, possible convulsions, mental retardation, osteoporosis, vertebral collapse

    c. Cerebral gigantism (Sotos syndrome)—large BW and height, dysmorphic features, abnormal body proportions with increased arm span, mental retardation, macrocephaly, dolichocephaly, prominent forehead, hypertelorism with other ocular abnormalities, high arched palate, pointed chin, CNS findings, poor motor coordination

    d. Beckwith-Weidemann syndrome—large BW and height, oomphalocele, umbilical hernia, accelerated growth in childhood, macroglossia, high arched palate, mid-face hypoplasia, hemihypertrophy

- Diagnostic Tests/Findings

1. Previous sequential, consistent recordings of height, weight, and OFC plotted on age-standardized growth charts show height > 2 SD above mean for age

2. Careful family history of tall growth patterns may elucidate familial etiology of tall stature; growth rate normal, growth curve parallels normal curve in familial tall stature

3. Laboratory tests to confirm diagnosis based on clinical findings and to rule out endocrine disease (Weinzimer, Lee & Moshang, 1997)

    a. GH excess—low ACTH, FSH, LH; high or normal GH; abnormal GTT

    b. Cerebral giantism—normal GH secretion

    c. Klinefelter—high pituitary gonadotropin, LH, FSH; azoospermia

    d. True precocious puberty—elevated basal LH, FSH concentrations; pubertal LH response to GnRH

    e. Beckwith-Weidemann—low blood glucose (hyperinsulinemia)

4. Radiographic bone age not advanced in constitutional tall stature; advanced in cerebral gigantism, obesity, precocious puberty

5. Abnormal echocardiogram with Marfan's; may have abdominal mass on ultrasound with precocious puberty

6. Abnormalities on skull radiograph, CT, or MRI of cranium with intracranial lesion

   7.   Karyotype analysis may indicate chromosomal abnormalities, syndromes

- Management/Treatment

   1.   Physician consultation or referral to appropriate pediatric specialists for children with other than constitutional tall stature

   2.   Pharmacologic management controversial; if marked concern about calculated predicted adult height, endocrinologist may accelerate epiphyseal closure with gonadal steroids; if precocious puberty, may slow growth with GnRH agonist

   3.   Homocystinuria—restrict dietary methionine, supplement dietary cystine

   4.   GH excess from CNS tumor or adrenal or gonadal tumor—surgery as indicated

   5.   Management of endocrine disease associated with tall stature

   6.   Beckwith-Wiedemann—treat excess insulin production

Adrenal Gland Disorders

Adrenocortical Insufficiency

- Definition: Inadequate production and secretion of adrenal hormones caused by failure of adrenals to secrete glucocorticoids, mineralocorticoids, and adrenal androgen (primary adrenal insufficiency, Addison's) or deficient secretion of ACTH from pituitary (secondary adrenal insufficiency)

- Etiology/Incidence

   1.   Primary adrenal insufficiency

      a.   Congenital adrenal hyperplasia (CAH)—hereditary

      b.   Chronic adrenal insufficiency (hypoadrenocorticism, Addison's disease) with destruction of adrenals from infection or hereditary autoimmune disease or adrenal calcification

      c.   Congenital absence or underdevelopment of adrenals; newborn adrenal hemorrhage (with complicated or traumatic delivery)

      d.   Malignancy (adrenal tumor)

   2.   Secondary adrenal insufficiency

      a.   Hypopituitarism—deficient secretion of ≥ 1 pituitary hormones due to congenital brain malformations, head trauma, histiocytosis, infection, tumors, radiation

      b.   Cessation of glucocorticoid therapy after prolonged large-dose administration of glucocorticoids (e.g., asthma, nephrosis, leukemia)

      c.   Other—post-surgical, infants of steroid-treated mothers, respiratory distress syndrome, anencephaly, pituitary defects

- Signs and Symptoms

   1.   Acute adrenal insufficiency (Adrenal crisis)

    a. Known or unknown diagnosis of Addison's—crisis may be first presentation of illness

    b. Recent or concurrent infection or febrile illness; surgery; exposure to excessive heat in susceptible individuals

    c. History of abrupt withdrawal of large-dose steroid therapy

    d. Weight loss, fever, fatigue, nausea, vomiting, diarrhea, dehydration, abdominal pain, anorexia, salt craving despite anorexia, symptomatic hypoglycemia, muscle weakness

  2. Chronic adrenal insufficiency—poor weight gain, weight loss, fatigue, weakness, lethargy, exercise intolerance, headache, anorexia, nausea, vomiting which may be forceful or projectile, diarrhea, dehydration, salt craving, increased pigmentation, hypotension

- Differential Diagnosis

  1. Differentiate acute adrenal insufficiency from severe acute infections, diabetic coma, CNS disturbances, acute poisoning; in newborn, distinguish from respiratory distress, intracranial hemorrhage, sepsis (Kappy, Steelman, Travers & Zeitler, 2003, p. 968)

  2. Differentiate chronic adrenal insufficiency from anorexia nervosa, muscular disorders (e.g., myasthenia gravis), nephritis, chronic infection (e.g., TB); consider chronic form of disease if patient has recurrent spontaneous hypoglycemia

- Physical Findings

  1. Acute adrenal insufficiency (adrenal crisis)—moribund, fever followed by hypothermia, cachexia, acutely dehydrated, vomiting, hypotension, confusion, coma, weakness, abdominal pain, nausea; increased skin pigmentation

  2. Chronic adrenal insufficiency (Addison's)—lethargy, dehydration, poor weight gain, weight loss, vomiting, hypotension, small heart size on radiograph, bronze skin pigmentation, especially of areola, mucous membranes, hand creases, axilla and groin, extensor surfaces of joints, and surgical scars

- Diagnostic Tests/Findings (Kappy, Steelman, Travers & Zeitler, 2003)

  1. Laboratory studies—decreased serum sodium and bicarbonate, $PaCO_2$, blood pH, and blood volume; hyperkalemia, and increased BUN; urinary sodium and sodium to potassium ratio elevated relative to degree of hyponatremia; eosinophilia; moderate neutropenia

  2. Confirmatory tests to assess functional capacity of adrenal cortex

    a. Lack of response in plasma cortisol and aldosterone to ACTH stimulation testing

    b. Increased baseline serum ACTH in primary adrenal failure

    c. Decreased urinary free cortisol and 17-hydroxycorticosteroid excretion

    d. Metyrapone test (in hospital)—non-elevation of morning 11-deoxycortisol level after midnight dose of metyrapone

    e. Corticotropin-releasing-hormone (CRH) test abnormal

- Management/Treatment

1. Immediate treatment of life-threatening acute adrenal crisis

2. Referral to endocrinologist for suspected or confirmed adrenal insufficiency

3. Pharmacologic—after initial stabilization, chronic corticosteroid replacement with glucocorticoids (e.g., hydrocortisone), mineralocorticoid, (e.g., fluorocortisone) and/or sodium chloride (table salt); increased dosages may be needed during severe illness, trauma, stress, or surgery

4. Monitor for steroid excess, particularly for decreasing height and weight; monitor for insufficient glucocorticoid treatment (headache, weight loss, nausea, hypotension); monitor blood glucose, ACTH, sodium and potassium

5. Avoid abrupt withdrawal of corticosteroids to avoid adrenal crisis

6. Education regarding risk of acute episodes; Medic Alert tag; consider emergency hydrocortisone injection kit for use in accident or severe stress (New, del Balzo, Crawford & Speiser, 1990)

Adrenocortical Hyperfunction

- Definition: Excessive production and secretion by the adrenal gland of cortisol, adrenocortical androgens, estrogen, and/or aldosterone

- Etiology/Incidence (Migeon & Lanes, 2003)

1. Hypercortisolism (Cushing's)—excess cortisol (ACTH) secretion by adrenals

    a. Adrenal tumors (Cushing syndrome)—relatively rare but occurs in all ages

    b. Pituitary adenomas (Cushing disease)

    c. Chronic exposure to glucocorticoids to treat inflammation and for immunosuppression (iatrogenic hypercortisolism)

    d. Ectopic ACTH-secreting tumors—nonpituitary tumors stimulate the adrenal cortex, causing excess ACTH secretion, rare; usually seen in children < 12 years

2. Adrenogenital syndrome—virilizing adrenal tumor causes elevated adrenal androgen secretion

3. Feminizing adrenal tumors—causes elevated adrenal estrogen secretion

4. Hyperaldosteronism

    a. Secondary—physiologic attempts to maintain homeostatis with serum electrolytes and fluid volume due to renal compromise or physiologic response to severe illness

    b. Primary—due to adrenal tumor or hyperplasia

- Signs and Symptoms

    1. Ubiquitous effects of adrenal hormones lead to multiple and varied signs and symptoms

    2. Hypercortisolism (Cushing's)—slowed growth and development, obesity, emotional lability (depression and euphoria), delayed pubertal onset, easy bruising, increased appetite, back pain

    3. Adrenogenital syndrome—increase in linear growth rate and muscle development, acne, premature pubarche, development of secondary sex characteristics in boys, enlarged and erectile clitoris in females, menstrual irregularities in older girls

    4. Feminizing adrenal tumors—rapidly increasing height, development of secondary sex characteristics in girls with possible breakthrough vaginal bleeding; gynecomastia in males

    5. Hyperaldosteronism—in infants, FTT, vomiting, weakness; may have history of recent diarrhea, increased sweating, heat exposure; history of renal or liver disease (e.g., cirrhosis, nephritis, renal ischemia); in primary hyperaldosteronism, muscle weakness, unusual periodic paralysis; paresthesias, tetany; polyuria; polydipsia

- Differential Diagnosis

    1. Hypercortisolism should be distinguished from exogenous obesity; virilizing adrenal tumors from virilizing gonadal tumors; and feminizing adrenal tumors from premature thelarche and idiopathic sexual precocity

    2. Hyperaldosteronism due to physiologic response to maintain homeostasis in severe illness vs. pathology (e.g., renal disease, adrenal tumor) should be determined

- Physical Findings

    1. Ubiquitous effects of adrenal hormones lead to multiple and varied clinical findings

    2. Hyperadrenocorticism—poor growth rate may precede obesity or other symptoms; relatively short stature; obesity; purple striae; truncal obesity; "buffalo type" adiposity of face, neck, and trunk; fat pad in interscapular area; plethoric or "moon" facies; delayed onset of secondary sex characteristics; muscle weakness; may have virilism; may have hemihypertrophy; delayed skeletal maturation; osteoporosis, especially of spine

    3. Adrenogenital syndrome—increase in linear growth rate; hirsutism; acne; deepening voice; increased muscle mass; masculinization of prepubertal children (boys with pubic, axillary, and sometimes facial hair with adult-size penis, frequent erections, pre-pubertal or slightly enlarged testes) (girls with pubic and axillary hair with enlarged and erectile clitoris); advanced bone age

    4. Feminizing adrenal tumor—increase in linear growth rate; gynecomastia in males; prepubertal testes, pubic hair; breast development in females, may have pubic hair; advanced bone age

5. Primary hyperaldosteronism—in infants, FTT; weakness; dehydration; tetany; hypertensive or normotensive; nocturnal enuresis; muscle weakness, unusual periodic paralysis

- Diagnostic Tests/Findings (Migeon & Lanes, 2003; Kappy, Steelman, Travers & Zeitler, 2003)

   1. Various confirmatory tests are used to determine specific etiology of adrenal hyperfunction

   2. Plasma cortisol concentrations elevated; may be loss of normal diurnal variation in cortisol secretion

   3. Low serum chloride and potassium levels; may have elevated sodium, pH, CO_2

   4. Serum ACTH slightly elevated with adrenal hyperplasia (Cushing disease), decreased with adrenal tumor, and very elevated with ACTH-producing pituitary or ectopic (extra-pituitary) tumors

   5. Low eosinophil counts; leukocyte count with polymorphonuclear leukocytosis with lymphopenia, possibly elevated RBC

   6. Elevated urinary free cortisol and urinary 17-hydroxycorticosteroid excretion; abnormal urinary 17-ketosteroid excretion; may have glycosuria

   7. Abnormal patterns of dexamethasone suppression and abnormal CRH stimulation tests

   8. Adrenogenital syndrome—androgen secretion not suppressed by dexamethasone administration; advanced bone age

   9. Feminizing adrenal tumor—elevated adrenal steroids in urine; elevated urinary and plasma estrogen levels; advanced bone age

   10. Hyperaldosteronism—hypokalemia, high aldosterone; may have low or elevated plasma renin level; may have increased chloride, potassium, and prostaglandin excretion in urine

   11. CT and MRI to assess for adrenal tumors; pituitary imaging to assess for pituitary tumor

- Management/Treatment

   1. Referral to pediatric endocrinologist for management of suspected or confirmed adrenocortical hyperfunction

   2. Surgery indicated for adrenal tumors, pituitary adenomas, ectopic ACTH-producing tumors

   3. ACTH pre- and postoperatively to stimulate nontumerous contralateral adrenal cortex

   4. Discontinuance of excessive glucocorticoid therapy if adrenocorticol hyperfunction

Miscellaneous

Hypoglycemia

- Definition: Symptoms provoked by abnormally low blood glucose levels occurring when child with diabetes receives excessive insulin, fails to eat, or exercises too strenuously; in children without diabetes, blood glucose level must be < 40 mg/dL and < 30 mg/dL in newborns (Gotlin & Chase, 1997)

- Etiology/Incidence

    1. Transient neonatal hypoglycemia

        a. SGA infants with decreased production of blood sugar due to physiologic immaturity or inadequate glycogen stores

        b. LGA infants of diabetic mothers (IDM) with hyperplasia of beta cells of pancreas due to chronic intrauterine exposure to elevated maternal blood sugar

        c. Increased glucose use from physiologic stressors secondary to asphyxia, anoxia, respiratory illness, heart disease, infection, cold injury, or starvation

    2. Hypoglycemia of childhood

        a. Hyperinsulinism—caused by abnormalities of beta cells (e.g., adenoma, islet cell hyperplasia); most common cause of persistent, recurrent hypoglycemia in first year; peak onset in first year and after age 3 years

        b. Functional fasting hypoglycemia ("ketotic hypoglycemia")— occurs between 1 and 5 years of age; peaks at 2 years; more common in SGA infants, males, and children with BW < 2500 g; associated with fasting in past 24 hours; episodes may occur periodically and with less frequency; rare after 5 years (Orlowski, 2001)

        c. Associated with CNS disorders

        d. Metabolic disorders and endocrine insufficiency, e.g., deficiency; galactosemia, hypopituitarism, congenital hypothyroidism, adrenal insufficiency; usually apparent in first 2 years of life

        e. Severe malnutrition states, e.g., chronic diarrhea, liver disease

        f. Other—drug ingestion, drug toxicity (alcohol, aspirin, oral hypoglycemic agents); associated with accidental ingestion or deliberate administration

- Signs and Symptoms

    1. Neonatal hypoglycemia—findings variable depending on degree of hypoglycemia; irritable, jittery, refusal to feed; tend to be small or large for gestational age

    2. Childhood hypoglycemia

        a. Findings variable depending on degree and etiology of hypoglycemia; may have mood changes, nervousness, weakness, hunger, epigastric pain, vomiting

        b. May have history of diabetes with recent history of excessive insulin, failure to eat, strenuous exercise; complaints of hunger; intentional or accidental ingestion of oral hypoglycemic agents, alcohol, salicylate

    c. May have known personal or familial history of inherited metabolic disorder or inherited hormonal deficiency; may have symptoms of metabolic disorder or hormonal deficiency

    d. Functional fasting ("ketotic hypoglycemia")—history of vomiting, anorexia, failure to eat previous 24 hours, often have URI; may have early morning seizures

- Differential Diagnosis: Distinguish among various possible etiologies of hypoglycemia (e.g., functional ketotic vs. inherited metabolic and endocrine disease) because of underlying implications for management

- Physical Findings

    1. Neonatal hypoglycemia—variable findings

        a. Cachexic or macrosomic infant

        b. Irritability, lethargy, weak cry

        c. Hypothermia, cyanosis, diaphoresis; pallor

        d. Uncoordinated eye movements, eye-rolling

        e. Apnea, irregular breathing, tachycardia

        f. Twitching, jitteriness, convulsions, semiconsciousness or coma

    2. Childhood hypoglycemia

        a. Signs as above

        b. May have diminished growth, difficulty talking, signs of other systemic illness, abdominal or pelvic masses, unsteady gait, concurrent illness

- Diagnostic Tests/Findings

    1. Transient neonatal hypoglycemia—routine Dextrostix on all newborns after birth; if high risk for hypoglycemia, e.g., SGA, IDM, Dextrostix frequently; if Dextrostix ≤ 45 mg/dL, do immediate quantitative blood glucose; hypoglycemic if:

        a. Whole blood glucose level < 35 mg/dL in first 24 hours or < 40 mg/dL thereafter *or*

        b. Plasma glucose level < 40 mg/dL in first 24 hours or < 45 mg/dL thereafter (Gilmore & Marks, 2001)

    2. Low blood glucose levels during hypoglycemic episode; consistent and repeated levels below 40 mg/dL with associated signs and symptoms need further confirmatory tests (Gotlin & Chase, 1997, p. 758)

    3. In hyperinsulinemia, serum insulin levels may be inappropriately elevated when compared with glucose level obtained at same time (Gotlin & Chase, 1997, p. 758)

- Management/Treatment
    1. Consultation with or referral to physician or endocrinologist for delineation of etiology and management
    2. Treat hypoglycemic episodes promptly and adequately to prevent CNS injury; especially important for younger children
    3. Hypoglycemic reactions in children with diabetes—see diabetes mellitus in this chapter
    4. Surgery for pancreatic adenoma, partial pancreatomy if insulin secretion suppression unsuccessful
    5. Children with functional (fasting, ketotic) hypoglycemia—treat with liberal carbohydrate diet with bedtime snacks, moderate restriction on ketogenic foods; avoid prolonged fasting, especially if child ill; parents may need to check urinary ketones

Hyperglycemia

- Definition: Common hereditary metabolic and endocrine disorder characterized by insulin deficiency resulting in abnormal metabolism of carbohydrate, protein, and fat (type 1, formerly termed insulin dependent diabetes mellitus [IDDM]) or may have specific carbohydrate intolerance causing insulin resistance at tissue level (type 2 diabetes, formerly termed Non-insulin Dependent Diabetes Mellitus [NIDDM])

- Etiology/Incidence: Hyperglycemia results from mechanisms that cause failure of pancreatic beta-cell function or other processes not directly involving beta cells; frequency of diabetes mellitus (DM) is rising, increases with age, average age of onset decreasing
    1. Type 1—destruction of beta islet cells of pancreas; uncommon in infancy and toddlerhood, increases until adolescence, then drops sharply; peaks occur between 5 and 7 years and at time of puberty; boys and girls equally affected; more frequently diagnosed in winter, especially with adolescents; environmental factors may increase or decrease expression of diabetes in susceptible individuals; multifactorial, associated with genetic predisposition and environmental factors including viruses (e.g., mumps, coxsackie, congenital rubella), environmental toxins, nutrition, and physical and emotional stress (Escobar, Becker & Drash, 2003; Rosenblum & Silverstein, 2003; Sperling, 2002)
        a. Type 1A—immune-mediated (previously termed juvenile diabetes or insulin-dependent diabetes); most common type of diabetes in those < 40 years
        b. Non-type 1—non-immune-mediated insulin-deficient diabetes; frequently found in overweight teens and in black and Hispanic children who develop diabetes
    2. Type 2—non-insulin-dependent, non-immune mediated; associated with being overweight; not being prone to ketosis and insensitivity to insulin (Chase & Eisenbarth, 2003); insulin resistance associated with childhood obesity, onset most often > 10

years of age; more likely in children and adolescents of predominantly Native American, Hispanic, African American origins; rapidly increasing form of diabetes; includes Maturity-Onset Diabetes of Youth (MODY) characterized by slow onset; treatment with diet and exercise and oral hypoglycemics after initial treatment with insulin (Chase & Eisenbarth, 2003; Stoffers, 2000), less severe symptoms, and autosomal dominant inheritance pattern (Chase & Eisenbarth, 2003; Stoffers, 2000)

3. Other—associated with administration of high doses of steroids (e.g., in renal disease, rheumatoid arthritis, asthma, leukemia) or anti-leukemia drugs; excessive endogenous cortisol production; CNS tumors, pheochromocytoma; cystic fibrosis

- Signs and Symptoms
    1. May present with very mild symptoms or in diabetic ketoacidosis
    2. Symptoms of type 1 diabetes mellitus
        a. Polyuria, polydipsia, polyphagia (primary complaints)
        b. Weight loss or failure to gain weight; variable decrease in linear growth
        c. Behavioral changes, headache, emotional lability, fatigue, recent "flu-like" illness
        d. Abdominal pain, nausea, vomiting, constipation, nocturia, enuresis
        e. History of recent illness, stress, missed insulin if known diabetic
    3. Symptoms of type 2 diabetes mellitus
        a. Many of the above symptoms but generally less severe than in type 1 diabetes mellitus
        b. Mild to moderate polyuria and polydipsia
        c. Weight loss
        d. History of high caloric intake and sedentary lifestyle
        e. Positive family history of type 2 diabetes mellitus
- Differential Diagnosis
    1. Diabetes insipidus
    2. Non-diabetes causes of polyuria, e.g., psychogenic polydipsia, CNS injury, tumors
    3. Other causes of fatigue, weight loss, behavioral change, e.g., Hashimoto's hypothyroidism, systemic illness
- Physical Findings
    1. Type 1 diabetes mellitus
        a. Dehydration, irritability
        b. Weight loss
        c. Visual disturbances

d. Fatigue, muscular weakness, declining physical performance

e. Long-term complications—joint contractures, diabetic retinopathy, compromised renal function

2. Type 1 diabetes with diabetic ketoacidosis

a. Marked dehydration, irritability, lethargy, drowsiness, stupor, coma

b. Tachycardia, cardiac arrhythmias, Kussmaul breathing (long, deep, labored breathing)

c. Dry mucous membranes, cherry-red lips, hypotension, rapid and thready pulse, hyperventilation, low temperature, "fruity" acetone breath

d. Vomiting, abdominal spasm, tenderness

3. Type 2 maturity onset diabetes of youth (MODY)

a. Marked obesity

b. Acanthosis nigracans

c. Vaginal candidiasis in females

- Diagnostic Tests/Findings

1. Glycosuria; urinary ketones

2. Elevated blood glucose—random blood glucose level > 300 mg/dL or fasting blood glucose levels > 200 mg/dL sufficient to make diagnosis of type 1 diabetes (Chase & Eisenbarth, 2003, p. 979)

3. Elevated plasma glucose—repeated findings of fasting plasma glucose level > 126 mg/dL or plasma glucose level > 200 mg/dL when taken either randomly (with symptoms of diabetes) or two hours after oral glucose load (Chase & Eisenbarth, 2003)

4. Elevated glycosylated hemoglobin (HbA_{1c})

5. In mild diabetic ketoacidosis (DKA) venous blood pH 7.2 to 7.3; moderate DKA venous blood pH 7.10 to 7.19; severe DKA venous blood pH < 7.10 (Chase & Eisenbarth, 2003)

6. Possible positive antibody tests—HLA, islet cell; insulin autoantibody (Gotlin & Chase, 1997); in type 2 diabetes, negative islet cell antibodies

- Management/Treatment

1. Immediate hospitalization if severe diabetic ketoacidosis

2. Consultation with physician or referral to pediatric endocrinology team for diagnostic evaluation, initial care and management and/or for confirmation/management of associated diseases, e.g., hypothyroidism; referral as needed for treatment by ophthalmologist and for emotional/behavioral disorders

3. After initial stabilization, for children with type 2 diabetes, slow gradual weight loss, exercise regimen, education stressing lifestyle changes to achieve weight loss,

oral hypoglycemic agents following insulin if insulin initially needed to stabilize blood glucose levels

4. After initial stabilization, children with type 1 diabetes generally treated with combination of short- and long-acting-insulin; types, onset, peak action, and duration of insulin varies (see Table 1)

5. Critical goal of treatment to maintain blood glucose levels at near normal to prevent acute complications (e.g., hypoglycemia and ketoacidosis), intermediate complications (e.g., lipoatrophy and lipohypertrophy, limited joint mobility, growth failure, pubertal delay), and chronic complications (e.g., retinopathy, nephropathy, and neuropathy) (Rosenbloom & Silverstein, 2003)

6. Educate child and parents regarding disease; self-monitoring of blood glucose 4 times daily; insulin types, timing, dosages, adjustments, optimal nutrition; need for consistency in meal and snack time and in moderate, regular exercise; need for increased insulin during illness or stress; prompt treatment of infection; signs and symptoms of hypoglycemia and ketoacidosis; urine testing; complications of poor blood glucose management; availability of glucose and glucagon for acute hypoglycemic episodes (0.3 mg for children < 10 years, 0.5 mg sc or IM for older children) (Gotlin & Chase, 1997)

7. Encourage parents to obtain user-friendly resources for helping them to better understand the disease and its management (e.g., *Understanding diabetes* (10th ed.) by H. P. Chase (2002) in English and Spanish and coloring books about diabetes available from The Guild of the Children's Diabetes Foundation (1 (800) 695-2873)

Table 1

Bioavailability characteristics of the insulins

	Human Insulin Type	Onset	Peak Action	Duration
Short-acting	Regular Actrapid,® Velosulin®	30 – 45 min	2 – 4 hr	5 – 7 hr
	Semilente, Semitard®	30 – 60 min	4 – 6 hr	6 – 8 hr
Intermediate-acting	Lente, Lentard,® Monotard®	2 – 4 hr	8 – 10 hr	15 – 18 hr
	NPH, Insulatard,® Protaphane®	2 – 4 h	8 – 10 hr	12 – 14 hr
Long-acting	Ultralente, Ultratard®	4 – 5 hr	8 – 14 hr	15 – 18 hr

From "Endocrine and metabolic disorders" by R. W. Gotlin and H. P. Chase (p. 749). In *Handbook of Pediatrics* (18th ed.) by G. B. Merenstein, D. W. Kaplan, & A. A. Rosenberg (Eds.), 1997, Stamford, CT: Appleton & Lange. Copyright by The McGraw-Hill Companies. Reprinted with permission.

8. Supportive care of patient and family through stages of grieving following diagnosis; emphasize normalcy, view of child as "child with diabetes" vs. "diabetic child"

9. Recognize phases of diabetes—development of clinical symptomatology; clinical remission or "honeymoon" period of variable duration due to improved beta cell function after initial therapy started; relapse with progressive increase in insulin requirement

10. Ideal fasting blood glucose level (when without food for 2+ hours) varies with age of child (Chase & Eisenbarth, 2003)

    a. $\leq$ 4 years, 80 to 200 mg/dL

    b. 5 to 11 years, 70 to 180 mg/dL

    c. $\geq$ 12 years, 70 to 150 mg/dL

11. Treatment of insulin reactions (Chase, 2002, p. 38)

    a. Mild reaction (hunger at unusual time, shakiness or irritability)—do blood sugar test if possible; if blood sugar < 60 mg/dL, give a glass of milk, small glass of juice, or 4 oz. sugared soda; wait 10 minutes for sugar to absorb, then give solid food (crackers, sandwich, fresh fruit, etc.); if blood sugar > 60 mg/dL, give just solid food

    b. Moderate reaction (very confused, very pale, very shaky)—give Insta-Glucose, Reactose™, Monojel™, or any source of simple sugar, like sugared soda or juice; do blood sugar test as soon as possible, repeat blood test after 10 minutes to make sure blood sugar is > 60 mg/dL; if blood sugar is not > 60 mg/dL, repeat initial treatment and wait another 10 minutes; once blood sugar is > 60 mg/dL, give solid food

    c. Severe reaction (loss of consciousness, seizure, convulsion)—give glucagon and do blood sugar level as soon as possible; if person does not improve after 10-20 minutes, may need to call 911 or get extra help; a second dose of glucagon can also be given

12. Glycosylated hemoglobin (HbA_{1c}) blood test every 3 months to assess overall blood sugar levels and to help in ascertaining compliance with treatment regimen; gives reliable measurement of long-term glycemic control during preceding 3 months; normal HbA_{1c} values vary by laboratory but are usually < 6.2%; desired levels for children vary by age; children $\geq$ 12 years should be < 7.8%, children 5 to 11 years should be < 8.5%, and children < 5 years should be between 7.5% and 9% (Gotlin & Chase, 1997, p. 750; Chase & Eisenbarth, 2003, p. 982); higher levels are allowed in younger children to reduce risk of effects of hypoglycemia on developing brains

13. Sexually-active adolescents need instruction regarding pregnancy prevention; oral contraceptives are acceptable if blood pressure is normal

14. Explore with parents additional topics such as use of insulin pumps (Chase, 2003) and insulin pens (Fleming, 2000), obtaining medical alert bracelets, communication

with extended family and school personnel about child's illness, and the research directed at diabetes prevention research (e.g., The Diabetes Prevention Trial: Type 1, 1 (800) 425-8361)

Disorders of Pubertal Development

- Definition: Abnormal development or delay in initiation of secondary sexual characteristics

- Etiology/Incidence: Abnormalities in pubertal development associated with CNS or gonadal disorder or dysfunction; includes temporary and permanent delays of pubertal onset or true (complete) or pseudoprecocious (incomplete) puberty

    1. Intersex—ambiguous genitalia or inappropriate for gonadal sex due to endocrinopathy

    2. Precocious pubertal development—in males, secondary sexual characteristics before 9 years (Kappy, Steelman, Travers & Zeitler, 2003); in females, onset of breast development before 8 years, sexual pubic hair before 9.0 years or menses before the age of 9.5 years (Rosenfield, 2002); however, breast and pubic hair development in females may occur normally for a small percentage of younger girls

        a. True (complete) precocious puberty is mediated by pituitary gonadotropin secretion involving all secondary sex characteristics

        b. Pseudoprecocious (incomplete) puberty involves one type of secondary sexual characteristic (e.g., premature thelarche [breast development] or pubarche [pubic hair development]; mediated by excessive estrogen/androgen stimulation for age from ovaries/testes, adrenal cortex, or exogenous sources

    3. Hypogonadism—causes lack of secondary sexual characteristics (sexual infantilism)

        a. In boys, lack of secondary sexual characteristics after 17 years suggests abnormal testicular maturation; may be due to testicular failure or dysfunction (primary failure due to anorchia, castration, Klinefelter's, mumps, radiation, trauma, tumor, endocrinopathies, etc.) or to pituitary/hypothalamic dysfunction (panhypopituitarism, empty sella syndrome, gonadotropin deficiency, LH, FSH deficiencies, endocrinopathies, etc.)

        b. In girls, may have lack of onset of secondary sex characteristics and amenorrhea due to primary ovarian failure (due to gonadal dysgenesis, enzyme defects, infection, surgery, radiation, chemotherapy, etc.) or to secondary ovarian failure (hypothalamic disorder or dysfunction, CNS irradiation, eating disorders, excessive exercise, chronic illness, etc.)

- Signs and Symptoms

    1. If intersex, history of confusion of sex assignment at birth

    2. May have normal growth and development through childhood; at puberty, may have abnormal sexual development; females may have virilization, primary amenorrhea; males may have incomplete virilization

3. May have history of underlying disease, dysfunction, or systemic illness causing delay in or premature pubertal onset; history of exposure to radiation, drugs, etc.

4. May have history of early development of one or all secondary sex characteristics, tall stature, symptoms of endocrine disease (e.g., hypothyroidism, congenital adrenal hyperplasia), intracranial disease (e.g., visual disturbances), abdominal disease (e.g., adrenal or gonadal tumor) or dysfunction (see growth disturbances this chapter)

5. May have delayed development of secondary sex characteristics and symptoms of metabolic or endocrine disturbances (e.g., constipation); intracranial disease (e.g., failure to grow, seizures); syndrome stigmata (e.g., developmental delays); abdominal disease (abdominal enlargement) or dysfunction (see growth disturbances and adrenal gland disorders this chapter)

- Differential Diagnosis

    1. Ambiguous genitalia or suspected intersex—distinguish true hermaphroditism (both ovarian and testicular tissue present), female pseudohermaphroditism (female genotype, only ovaries), and male pseudohermaphroditism (genotype male, only testes)

    2. Structural abnormalities of genital tract and associated intracranial, endocrine, abdominal, or pelvic disease (Rosenfield, 2002)

    3. Precocious puberty—distinguish between true (complete) precocious puberty mediated by pituitary gonadotropin secretion involving all secondary sex characteristics vs. pseudoprecocious (incomplete) puberty involving one type of secondary sexual characteristics

    4. Premature sexual development—distinguish normal variants of premature thelarche (isolated premature breast development) and pubarche (early pubic hair development) in girls from pathologic causes; distinguish normal variants of premature adrenarche in boys (adrenal maturation with pubic hair and body odor) from pathologic causes

- Physical Findings

    1. May have normal or abnormal physical examination depending on underlying etiology of pubertal disorder (e.g., normal examination in constitutional delay, findings of chronic or systemic illness or midfacial defects in pathologic pubertal delay, tall stature in Klinefelter's, etc.)

    2. May have normal or abnormal genitalia depending on underlying etiology of pubertal disorder and timing (e.g., genitalia may be ambiguous in congenital adrenal hyperplasia; may have cryptorchidism in sexual infantilism or in pituitary insufficiency; may have abdominal mass or testicular mass in gonadal tumor; may have microphallus in human GH deficiency, may have small testes in testicular failure, may have abnormal pelvic examination, etc.)

    3. With precocious puberty, may have tall stature, premature secondary sex characteristics

4. With contrasexual pubertal development may have gynecomastia in males due to hypogonadism from Klinefelter's; excessive virilization of prepubertal girls with pubic hair, oily skin, acne, clitoromegaly, hirsutism

5. With delayed pubertal development for age (constitutional delay of puberty), may have normal examination except for delayed growth and development (short stature but low normal growth rate) during childhood; delayed bone age; relatively short legs for height or greater upper/lower body ratio; descended normal testes that are prepubertal in size, consistency (Lee, 2003)

6. With delayed or interrupted pubertal development may have findings consistent with endocrine disorder (e.g., anisomia, the lack of ability to smell, and micropenis in gonadotropin abnormalities; hirsutism and dry hair and skin in hypothyroidism, etc.)

- Diagnostic Tests/Findings

  1. Tanner staging of breast, genitals, pubic hair development

  2. Laboratory findings variable depending on etiology of pubertal disorder; tests may include plasma or serum LH, FSH; GH, electrolytes, thyroid tests; blood and urinary pH, urine specific gravity, sedimentation rates, BUN, creatinine, etc.

  3. Tests of hormonal function as needed (e.g., GnRH to differentiate hypogonadotropic hypogonadism and constitutionally delayed puberty)

  4. CT, MRI, or ultrasound as needed to rule in or rule out central CNS, adrenal, renal, gonadal, or thyroid disease; bone age

  5. Other laboratory tests as needed—karyotype if ambiguous genitalia or Klinefelter's suspected

- Management/Treatment

  1. Physician consultation or referral to pediatric endocrinologist for suspected pathologic cause of pubertal delay or abnormal development

  2. Treatment dictated by identified etiology for pathologic cause of pubertal delay or abnormality in pubertal development (e.g., hormonal therapy may be immediate, as with congenital adrenal hyperplasia, or at puberty with testosterone for testicular failure)

  3. Management of underlying endocrine disorders and diseases and systemic illness (e.g., hypothyroidism, poorly controlled diabetes, anorexia, inflammatory bowel disease, etc.)

Gynecomastia

- Definition: Visible or palpable glandular enlargement of the male breast occurring commonly in healthy adolescent males (pubertal gynecomastia); occasionally indicative of underlying disease (pathologic gynecomastia); seen frequently in newborns (neonatal gynecomastia)

- Etiology/Incidence

  1. Neonatal gynecomastia—due to cross-placental transfer of maternal hormones; usually resolves by 2 to 3 weeks

  2. Pubertal gynecomastia—influence of too little androgen and/or too much estrogen on mammary tissue; transient, may occur in 40% to 66% of normal boys during puberty (Lee, 2003; Styne, 2002); onset between 10 and 12 years, peak occurrence 13 and 14 years, usually resolves by 16 to 17 years of age (Braunstein, 1996)

  3. Pathologic gynecomastia—secondary to drug side effects (e.g., cimetadine, digitalis, phenothiazine, treatment with hCG, testosterone, or estrogen), underlying disease or syndromes (e.g., Klinefelter's), injury to the nervous system, chest wall or testes; or, may be idiopathic

- Signs and Symptoms—breast development in other than pubertal females

- Differential Diagnosis:

  1. Transient pubertal gynecomastia from obesity (lipomastia) and pathologic causes—tumor (lipoma, neurofibroma, cancer)

  2. Breast infection

  3. Fat necrosis due to injury

  4. Drugs (estrogens, anabolic steroids, marijuana)

  5. Klinefelter's, gonadal dysfunction

- Physical Findings

  1. Neonatal—usually bilateral, often asymmetric breast tissue enlargement; resolves within 1 to 2 weeks

  2. Pubertal (physiologic) gynecomastia—breast tissue enlargement glandular, movable, disk-shaped, below areola, non-adherent to skin or underlying tissue; typically breasts unequal in size and < 3 cm in diameter; breasts may be tender, nipples irritated due to rubbing on clothing; if tissue ≥ 4 to 5 cm/diameter and breasts dome-shaped, macrogynecomastia present; Tanner stages II to IV pubertal development with testes ≥ 3 cm length (Mahoney, 1990)

  3. Pathologic gynecomastia—malnourishment, lymphadenopathy, delayed sexual maturity with undermasculinization, signs of chronic disease (e.g., goiter, liver or renal disease, endocrinopathies, cancer, colitis, CF, AIDS); breast tissue ≥ 3 cm/diameter, asymmetric, hard, fixed, indurated, not directly beneath areola; may have absent, underdeveloped or asymmetric testes

- Diagnostic Tests/Findings

  1. Endocrinology studies as indicated

  2. Imaging techniques as appropriate—ultrasonography of testes to identify impalpable testicular tumor; CT, MRI of abdomen to identify adrenal tumors

  3. Karyotyping if Klinefelter's suspected

- Management/Treatment

    1. Neonatal—parent education and reassurance about etiology, transience, and normalcy of condition

    2. Pubertal (physiologic) gynecomastia < 4 cm—explanation, reassurance, and observation; regression usually spontaneous, within a few months, rarely beyond 2 years

    3. Physiologic macrogynecomastia (≥ 4 cm mass)—medical or surgical treatment usually required as regression rare, especially if gynecomastia present for > 4 years; pharmacologic therapy (e.g., tamoxifen, danazol, testosterone) sometimes used

    4. Gynecomastia usually very upsetting to adolescent but often not discussed because of embarrassment; reassure about transience and spontaneous regression

Menstrual Disorders: Amenorrhea

- Definition

    1. Primary amenorrhea—failure of onset of menarche in females who are 16 years and have normal pubertal growth and development; 14 years with absence of normal pubertal growth and development; or in girls who have not begun menstruation 2 years after completed sexual maturation (Polaneczky & Slap, 1992)

    2. Secondary amenorrhea—absence of menstruation for > 3 cycles or at least 6 months after menstruation established (Polaneczky & Slap, 1992)

- Etiology/Incidence

    1. Primary amenorrhea

        a. Constitutional/familial (common)

        b. Obstructions of menstrual flow (e.g., fusion or stenosis of labia, imperforate hymen)

        c. Estrogen deficiency

            (1) Primary ovarian insufficiency—organic or functional ovarian failure (e.g., anatomic anomalies, pelvic irradiation, enzyme defects, autoimmune disease, infection)

            (2) Secondary ovarian insufficiency—organic or functional ovarian failure from hypothalamic/pituitary disorders (e.g., decreased gonadotropin secretion, effects of chronic diseases such as DM, CF, anorexia; excessive exercise; endocrine disease)

        d. Androgen excess (e.g., polycystic ovaries, adrenal androgen excess [Cushing's])

        e. Ovarian tumors

    2. Secondary amenorrhea; many causes same as primary amenorrhea

        a. Pregnancy (most common)

   b. Hypothalamic, pituitary, and adrenal disorders or tumors; chromosomal abnormalities (e.g., Turner's); endocrinopathies; chronic illness, especially those causing severe weight loss or malnutrition; conditions affecting gonadal function

   c. Pharmacologic agents (discontinuance of birth control pills, use of tranquilizers)

   d. Significant emotional stress or strenuous exercise programs, especially with runners, ballet dancers, and gymnasts; major weight loss

   e. Uterine dysfunction after abortion, infection, C-section

   f. Hysterectomy

- Signs and Symptoms

   1. Primary amenorrhea—no history of menses in adolescence; may have symptoms of marked psychosocial stress, adrenal dysfunction or gonadal disease, pituitary or hypothalamic disease, chronic illness including eating disorders, chromosomal abnormalities, pregnancy; may have cyclic abdominal pain without menstruation in pseudoamenorrhea

   2. Secondary amenorrhea—sudden or gradual cessation of menses; symptoms vary depending on underlying etiology; may exercise excessively. See primary amenorrhea in this chapter

- Differential Diagnosis

   1. Determine if underlying etiology due to chronic illness, CNS disease, endocrinopathy

   2. Distinguish primary amenorrhea due to constitutional or familial etiology from pregnancy

   3. Distinguish secondary amenorrhea due to pregnancy, underlying disease or disorder

   4. Determine amenorrhea vs. ''pseudoamenorrhea'' (menstruation occurs but obstruction prevents release of menstrual blood)

- Physical Findings

   1. May have normal physical examination or signs of chronic, systemic illness or syndromes (e.g., underweight, CNS tumor or dysfunction, endocrinopathies, autoimmune disease, anorexia, malnourishment, unusually tall or short stature); may show signs of pregnancy

   2. May have lack of development of secondary characteristics or normal sexual development

   3. Pelvic examination may show pregnancy, reproductive system abnormalities (e.g., cervical atresia, imperforate hymen)

- Diagnostic Tests/Findings

   1. Pregnancy test

2. Careful family history to rule out constitutional/familial delay, then consultation with physician and/or referral to specialists as needed

- Management/Treatment

1. Constitutional/familial primary amenorrhea—education, reassurance, monitoring

2. Amenorrhea associated with other etiologies requires further evaluation, physician consultation or referral to appropriate specialist (e.g., reproductive endocrinologist, surgeon, pediatric neurologist, obstetrician, psychologist)

3. Treatment directed at management or correction of underlying cause of abnormal menstrual processes (e.g., surgery if imperforate hymen, adrenal tumors)

4. Sensitivity to significant concern of delayed development by child and family very important

5. Parent and child education regarding amenorrhea and adherence to any treatment regimen

6. Genetic counseling may be indicated if genetic etiology

Questions
Select the best answer

1. Secondary hypothyroidism results from:

   a. Excess release of thyroid hormone beyond the newborn period
   b. Intrauterine exposure to thyrotoxic drugs
   c. Disease or disorder of the thyroid gland itself
   d. Disease or disorder of the hypothalamus or pituitary gland compromising thyroid function

2. Congenital hypothyroidism has a higher incidence in which of the following populations?

   a. African-Americans
   b. Hispanic and Native-Americans
   c. Asian-Americans
   d. Euro-Americans

3. Which of the following is not a sign or symptom of congenital hypothyroidism?

   a. Hoarse cry
   b. Frequent stooling
   c. Coarse features
   d. Lethargy

4. The most common cause of hyperthyroidism in children and adolescents is:

   a. Graves' (autoimmune) disease
   b. Thyroid cancer
   c. Thyroid nodules
   d. Pituitary tumor

5. Which of the following is not found in an adolescent with untreated Graves' disease?

   a. Behavioral problems
   b. Sleep disturbances
   c. Tendency to gain weight easily
   d. Tachycardia

6. In which one of the following children would you most suspect hyperthyroidism?

   a. A 16-year-old male who complains about restlessness
   b. A 14-year-old adolescent female who is heat intolerant and has amenorrhea
   c. A male pre-teen with behavior problems
   d. A six-year-old female who complains of tiredness

7. The most common thyroiditis is:

   a. Subacute thyroiditis caused by a viral infection of the gland
   b. Acute suppurative thyroiditis caused by bacterial infection

   c. Caused by exposure to radiation or trauma

   d. Hashimoto's or chronic autoimmune thyroiditis

8. Nephrogenic, or vasopressin-resistant, diabetes insipidus:

   a. Is caused by anatomic defects in the brain causing hypofunction of the pituitary or hypothalamus

   b. Results from damage to the hypothalamus or pituitary from surgical trauma or infection

   c. Is caused by reduced renal responsiveness to antidiuretic hormone (ADH)

   d. Has oliguria as a primary presenting symptom

9. An infant with polydipsia, polyuria, irritability, and failure to thrive, should be evaluated for:

   a. Diabetes insipidus

   b. Homocystinuria

   c. Growth hormone deficiency

   d. Hyperglycemia

10. Which one of the following is not characteristic of constitutional growth delay?

   a. There is generally no history of a similar growth pattern in other family members

   b. The child usually remains constitutionally small as an adult

   c. Final adult stature tends to be normal

   d. Weight and height at birth are generally in the lower percentiles

11. A newborn or infant with birth length < 50% and microphallus should be suspected of having:

   a. Growth hormone deficiency

   b. Congenital hypothyroidism

   c. Primordial short stature

   d. Down syndrome

12. An adolescent male who fails to develop secondary sex characteristics at puberty and who has small, underdeveloped testes should be suspected of having:

   a. Adrenal hyperplasia

   b. Klinefelter's syndrome

   c. Marfan's syndrome

   d. Cerebral gigantism (Sotos syndrome)

13. Individuals with chronic adrenal insufficiency often have:

   a. Frequent otitis media

   b. High energy levels

   c. Love for physical activity

   d. A craving for salt

14. In the newborn period, infants of diabetic mothers (IDMs) are particularly at risk for:

    a. Small size for gestational age
    b. Intrauterine growth retardation (IUGR)
    c. Disorders in bone development
    d. Hypoglycemia

15. Which statement is true about true (complete) precocity or incomplete (pseudoprecocity)?

    a. True precocity occurs because of hormonal stimulation from the pituitary or hypothalamus causing gonadal maturation and fertility
    b. Pseudoprecocity does not involve development of any secondary sex characteristics
    c. Incomplete precocity is caused by adrenal or gonadal tumor or dysfunction and results in increased linear growth but no development of secondary sex characteristics
    d. Incomplete or pseudoprecocity leads to testicular enlargement and ovulation

16. An adolescent who has tall stature, increased arm span, arachnodactyly, laxity of joints, pectus excavatum, and an abnormal echocardiogram would be suspected of having:

    a. Turner's
    b. Beckwith-Wiedemann syndrome
    c. Marfan's
    d. Klinefelter's syndrome

17. Which one of the following is not found in children with growth hormone excess?

    a. Tall stature
    b. Prominent mandible and supraorbital ridge
    c. High or normal plasma growth hormone
    d. Short stature

18. A pathognomonic skin finding in children with chronic adrenal insufficiency (Addison's) is:

    a. Purple striae
    b. Increased pigmentation in the axilla, groin, areola, hand creases and in surgical scars
    c. Dry, thickened skin
    d. Increased perspiration

19. Which of the following findings is not characteristic of children and infants with hyperadrenocorticism?

    a. Advanced skeletal maturation
    b. "Moon" facies
    c. Delayed onset of secondary sex characteristics
    d. "Buffalo type" adiposity of face, neck, and trunk

20. Transient neonatal hypoglycemia is:

    a. Most common in AGA infants
    b. Low in premature SGA infants

    c. Most common in LGA infants

    d. Least common in LGA infants

21. Regular insulin:

    a. Has a quicker onset of effect and longer duration than NPH

    b. Has a slower onset of effect and shorter duration than NPH

    c. Has a quicker onset of effect and shorter duration than NPH

    d. Has the longest duration of the insulins available

22. The preferred name now for insulin-dependent diabetes mellitus (IDDM) is:

    a. Maturity-onset diabetes

    b. Type 1 diabetes

    c. Type 2 diabetes

    d. Insulin resistance syndrome

23. Blood glucose levels of children 5 to 11 years with diabetes should be maintained between:

    a. 70 to 180 mg/dL

    b. 100 to 200 mg/dL

    c. 60 to 80 mg/dL

    d. Slightly over 200 mg/dL

24. Blood glucose levels of younger children with diabetes are maintained at slightly higher levels than blood glucose levels of older children because:

    a. Children have a greater need for available glucose in the blood system

    b. Younger children tend to be more active

    c. Younger children become more irritable than do older children

    d. Lowering the risk of hypoglycemia in younger children is particularly important in order to avoid the potential for hypoglycemia with consequent neurological system damage

25. Glucagon should be used to treat:

    a. Children with mild hypoglycemia

    b. Children with moderate hypoglycemia

    c. Children with severe hyperglycemia

    d. Children with severe hypoglycemia

26. Which finding is not a sign or symptom of diabetes onset in children?

    a. Alopecia

    b. Glycosuria

    c. Polydipsia

    d. Polyuria

27. Abdominal pain and vomiting are particularly critical to monitor in children with diabetes because these findings may represent the onset of:

    a. Ketoacidosis
    b. Gastrointestinal infection
    c. Hyperglycemia
    d. Autoimmune response to the pancreas

28. Which of the following statements is not true about type 1 diabetes?

    a. The "honeymoon" period post-diagnosis is of variable duration
    b. Diabetes is a relatively common disease in childhood
    c. Children with type 1 diabetes can switch to oral insulin agents once they reach adulthood
    d. Three factors influence a child's potential to develop diabetes—genetic predisposition, autoimmune response, and exposure to viral or chemical agents

29. Precocious pubertal development is defined as the development of secondary sexual characteristics in boys before age ___ years and menses in girls before the age of ___ years.

    a. 10 years; 10 years
    b. 6 years; 8 years
    c. 9 years; 9.5 years
    d. 6 years; 9 years

30. In boys, lack of secondary sexual characteristics after 17 years suggests:

    a. Castration
    b. Abnormal testicular function
    c. True hermaphroditism
    d. Pituitary adenoma

31. The peak incidence for adolescent gynecomastia occurs at age:

    a. 10 years
    b. 13-14 years
    c. 16 years
    d. 18 years

32. The most common cause of primary amenorrhea is:

    a. Obstructions of menstrual flow
    b. Primary ovarian insufficiency
    c. Secondary ovarian insufficiency
    d. Constitutional or familial

Answer key:

1. d	12. b	22. b
2. b	13. d	23. a
3. b	14. d	24. d
4. a	15. a	25. d
5. c	16. c	26. a
6. b	17. d	27. a
7. d	18. b	28. c
8. c	19. a	29. c
9. a	20. c	30. b
10. c	21. c	31. b
11. a		32. d

Bibliography

American Academy of Pediatrics (1993). Newborn screening for congenital hypothyroidism: Recommended guidelines. *Pediatrics*, 91(6), 1203-1209.

Becker, D. J. (2003). Complications of insulin-dependent diabetes mellitus in childhood and adolescence. In F. Lifshitz (Ed.), *Pediatric endocrinology* (4th ed., pp. 669-682). NY: Marcel Dekker, Inc.

Bode, H. H., Crawford, J. D., & Danon, M. (1996). Disorders of antidiuretic hormone homeostasis: Diabetes insipidus and SIADH. In F. Lifshitz (Ed.), *Pediatric endocrinology* (3rd ed., pp. 731-751). NY: Marcel Dekker, Inc.

Braunstein, G. D. (1996). Pubertal gynecomastia. In F. Lifshitz (Ed.), *Pediatric endocrinology* (3rd ed., pp. 197-205). NY: Marcel Dekker, Inc.

Chase, H. P. (2002). *Understanding diabetes* (10th ed.). Denver, CO: Barbara Davis Center for Childhood Diabetes.

Chase, H. P., & Eisenbarth, G. S. (2003). Diabetes mellitus. In W. W. Hay, Jr., A. R. Hayward, M. J. Levin, & J. M. Sondheimer (Eds.), *Current pediatric diagnosis and treatment* (16th ed., pp. 978-985). NY: Lange Medical Books/McGraw-Hill.

Dallas, J. S., & Foley, T. P., Jr. (2003) Thyromegaly. In F. Lifshitz (Ed.), *Pediatric endocrinology* (4th ed., pp. 393-406). NY: Marcel Dekker, Inc.

Drash, A. L. (1996). Management of the child with diabetes mellitus. In F. Lifshitz (Ed.), *Pediatric endocrinology* (3rd ed., pp. 617-629). NY: Marcel Dekker, Inc.

Escobar, O., Becker, D., & Drash, D. L. (2003). Management of the child with diabetes mellitus. In F. Lifshitz (Ed.), *Pediatric endocrinology* (4th ed., pp. 653-668). NY: Marcel Dekker, Inc.

Fisher, D. A. (2002). Disorders of the thyroid in childhood and adolescence. In M. A. Sperling, *Pediatric endocrinology* (2nd. ed., pp 187-210). Philadelphia: W.B. Saunders.

Fleming, E. R. (2000). Mightier than the syringe. *American Journal of Nursing*, 100(11), 44-48.

Foley, T. P., Jr. (2001). Hypothyroidism. In R. L. Hoekelman, H. M. Adam, N. M. Nelson, M. L. Weitzman, & M. H. Wilson (Eds.). *Primary pediatric care* (4th ed., pp. 1561-1565). St. Louis: Mosby.

Frasier, S. D. (1996). Tall stature and excessive growth syndromes. In F. Lifshitz (Ed.), *Pediatric endocrinology* (3rd ed., pp. 163-174). NY: Marcel Dekker, Inc.

Frasier, S. D. (2003). Tall stature and excessive growth syndromes. In F. Lifshitz (Ed.), *Pediatric endocrinology* (4th ed., pp. 133-146). NY: Marcel Dekker, Inc.

Gilmore, M. M., & Marks, K. H. (2001). Critical neonatal illnesses. In R. L. Hoekelman, H. M. Adam, N. M. Nelson, M. L. Weitzman, & M. H. Wilson (Eds.), *Primary pediatric care* (4th ed., pp. 600-610). St. Louis: Mosby.

Gotlin, R. W., & Chase, P. (1997). Endocrine and metabolic disorders. In G. B. Merenstein, D. W. Kaplan, & A. A. Rosenberg (Eds.), *Handbook of pediatrics* (18th ed., pp. 708-762). Stamford, CT: Appleton & Lange.

Jospe, N. (2001). Hyperthyroidism. In R. L. Hoekelman, H.M. Adam, N. M. Nelson, M. L.

Weitzman, & M. H. Wilson (Eds.), *Primary pediatric care* (4th ed., pp. 1554-1557). St. Louis: Mosby.

Kappy, M. S., Steelman, J. W., Travers, S. H., & Zeitler, P. S. (2003). Endocrine Disorders. In W. W. Hay, Jr., A. R. Hayward, M. J. Levin , & J. M. Sondheimer (Eds.), *Current pediatric diagnosis and treatment* (16th ed., pp. 937-977). NY: Lange Medical/McGraw-Hill.

Lee, P. A. (2003). Puberty and its disorders. In F. Lifshitz (Ed.), *Pediatric endocrinology* (4th ed., pp. 211-238). NY: Marcel Dekker, Inc.

Lifshitz, F., & Botero, D. (2003). Worrisome growth. In F. Lifshitz (Ed.), *Pediatric endocrinology* (4th ed., pp. 1-46). NY: Marcel Dekker, Inc.

Lum, G. (2003). Kidney & urinary tract. In W. W. Hay, Jr., A. R. Hayward, M. J. Levin, & J. M. Sondheimer (Eds.), *Current pediatric diagnosis and treatment* (16th ed., pp. 693-716). NY: Lange Medical Books/McGraw-Hill.

Mahoney, C. P. (1990). Adolescent gynecomastia - Differential diagnosis and management. *Pediatric Clinics of North America*, 37(6), 1389-1404.

Majzoub, J. A,. & Muglia, L. J. (2003). Disorders of water homeostasis. In F. Lifshitz (Ed.), *Pediatric endocrinology* (4th ed., pp. 755-785). NY: Marcel Dekker, Inc.

Migeon, C. J., & Lanes, R. L. (2003). Adrenal cortex: Hypo- and hyperfunction. In F. Lifshitz (Ed.), *Pediatric endocrinology* (4th ed., pp. 147-173). NY: Marcel Dekker, Inc.

Muglia, L. J., & Majzoub, J. A. (2002). Disorders of the posterior pituitary. In M. A. Sperling, *Pediatric endocrinology* (2nd ed., pp. 289-322). Philadelphia: W.B. Saunders.

New, M. I., del Brazo, P., Crawford, C., & Speiser, P. (1990). The adrenal cortex. In S. A. Kaplan (Ed.), *Clinical pediatric endocrinology* (pp. 181-234). Philadelphia: W. B. Saunders Company.

Orlowski, C. C. (2001). Hypoglycemia. In R. L. Hoekelman, H. M. Adam, N. M. Nelson, M. L. Weitzman, & M. H. Wilson (Eds.), *Primary pediatric care* (4th ed., pp. 1985-1991). St. Louis, MO: Mosby.

Polzaneczky, M. W., & Slap, G. G. (1992). Menstrual disorders in the adolescent: Amenorrhea. *Pediatrics in Review*, 13(2), 43-48.

Rogers, D. G. (1994). Thyroid disease in children. *American Family Physician*, 50(2), 344-350.

Rosenbloom, A. L., & Silverstein, J. H. (2003). Diabetes mellitus in the child and adolescent. In F. Lifshitz (Ed.), *Pediatric endocrinology* (4th ed., pp. 611-651). NY: Marcel Dekker, Inc.

Rosenfeld, R. G., & Cohen, P. (2002). Disorders of growth hormone/Insulin-like growth factor secretion and action. In M. A. Sperling (Ed.), *Pediatric endocrinology* (2nd ed., pp. 211-288). Philadelphia: W.B. Saunders.

Rosenfield, R. L. (2003). Puberty in the female and its disorders. In M. A. Sperling (Ed.), *Pediatric endocrinology* (2nd, pp. 455-518). Philadelphia: Saunders.

Sperling, M. A. (2002). Diabetes mellitus. In M. A. Sperling (Ed.), *Pediatric endocrinology* (2nd ed., pp. 323-366). Philadelphia: Saunders.

Stoffers, D. A. (2000). Maturity-onset diabetes of the young (MODY): The past, present, and future. *Growth Genetics and Hormones*, 16(3), 37-41.

Styne, D. M. (2002). The testes: Disorders of sexual differentiation and puberty. In M. A. Sperling (Ed.), *Pediatric endocrinology* (2nd, pp. 565-628). Philadelphia: Saunders.

Van Vliet, G. (2003). Thyroid disorders in infancy. In F. Lifshitz (Ed.), *Pediatric endocrinology* (4th ed., pp. 347-358). NY: Marcel Dekker, Inc.

Weinzimer, S. A., Lee, M. M., & Moshang, T., Jr. (1997). In M. W. Schwartz, T. A. Curry, A. J. Sargent, N. J. Blum, & J. A. Fein (Eds.), *Pediatric primary care: A problem-oriented approach* (3rd ed., pp. 529-541). St. Louis: Mosby.

Zimmerman, D., & Gan-Gaisano, M. (1992). Hyperthyroidism in children and adolescents. *Pediatric Clinics of North America*, 37(6), 1273-1288.

Multisystem and Genetic Disorders

Alison W. Schultz
Virginia Richardson

Introduction

All disorders addressed in this chapter occur relatively rarely, but for the involved child, family, and caregivers, each presents life-long challenges in health care, adaptation, and coping. In general, when one of these disorders is suspected or diagnosed, the PNP should refer the child and family to the most appropriate specialty center for consultation and collaborative management. Knowledge about each condition and its management is rapidly expanding, and personnel at such centers are most current in this essential practice foundation.

The Pediatric Nurse Practitioner (PNP), however, remains responsible for assisting the child and family with all primary care issues, some of which will be disorder specific. The PNP also is a central contact for the child and family for issues of care coordination and community-based interventions, advocacy, assistance with stress management and promotion of positive adaptation and coping. PNPs working with children who have any of these disorders must become familiar with the issues commonly confronting such children and their families, legislation protecting the rights of individuals who have chronic illness or disability, and support organizations and agencies that can be helpful to caregivers and families. Among the most helpful are the 65 University Affiliated Programs (UAPs) for Developmental Disabilities in the United States and territories, and the Federal, State and local divisions of the Maternal Child Health Bureau (MCHB). Information about UAPs can be obtained by calling the American Association of UAPs at 301-588-8252. Information about MCHB programs is usually available in your local telephone book, or can be obtained by calling 301-443-2350. Also, many support organizations and other information about these disorders can be found on the Internet, using the disorder's name as the key word. The Alliance of Genetic Support Groups, (800) 336-4363 and http://www.geneticalliance.org is a comprehensive resource for conditions with genetic basis.

Where possible, information about disorder specific support organizations is included in the management sections of this chapter. *Exceptional Parent* magazine, 1170 Commonwealth Avenue, Boston MA 02134-4645, (617) 730-5800 www.exceptionalparent.com provides a wealth of information for parents of children who have various special health care needs. The March of Dimes Birth Defects Foundation, 1275 Mamaroneck Avenue, White Plains NY 10605, (888) 663-4637 www.marchofdimes.com provides information about congenital diseases and disorders, and the National Information Center for Children and Youth with Disabilities (NICHCY), PO Box 1492, Washington DC 20013 www.nichcy.org provides information on all disabling conditions.

Congenital Diseases

Acquired Immune Deficiency Syndrome (AIDS)

- Definition: Advanced stage of illness in individuals infected with the Human Immunodeficiency Virus (HIV); CDC case definition of HIV classifies children according to presence or absence of clinical signs and symptoms and according to status of immune function and clinical findings. Refer to most current edition of the *AAP Red Book* for details.

- Etiology/Incidence

  1. In children, primarily (90%) maternal to infant perinatal HIV transmission; breast feeding is primary postnatal vertical maternal to infant transmission route

  2. National infant cord blood seroprevalence of HIV 0.17%; rates vary widely, up to 8%; most seroprevalence is maternal antibody; 13% to 40% of perinatally exposed infants acquire disease if mother is untreated during pregnancy and with no chemoprophylaxis during labor or for the newborn

- Signs and Symptoms: Median onset for infants with perinatal infection is 12 to 18 months; HIV, however, can be latent for years

  1. Prematurity

  2. Low birth weight

  3. Recurrent serious bacterial or viral infections—especially oral thrush

  4. Failure to thrive

  5. Recurrent fevers

  6. Chronic diarrhea

  7. Diminished activity

  8. Developmental delays

- Differential Diagnosis

  1. Infectious disease or other associated conditions without underlying HIV

  2. Other immune deficiencies of infancy

- Physical Findings

  1. Falling ratio of head circumference to height and weight, due to encephalopathic direct effect on brain growth

  2. Lymphadenopathy—≥ 0.5 cm at more than 2 sites; bilateral at one site

  3. Hepatosplenomegaly

  4. Parotitis, nephropathy, CNS disease

- Diagnostic Tests/Findings

  1. Detection of HIV—DNA from anticoagulated whole blood or by Polymerase Chain Reaction (PCR) from peripheral blood mononuclear cells

2. For adolescents ≥ age 13, documentation of HIV infection with one or more of 26 clinical conditions such as multiple or recurrent serious bacterial infections (AAP, 2000, p. 327)

3. Cases of HIV meeting AIDS criteria are reportable

- Management/Treatment

    1. Risk reduction through prevention of maternal infection, assuring clean blood and tissue supplies, prevention of STD and needle sharing

    2. Reduction of risk of perinatal HIV—through treatment of pregnant mother and perinatal chemoprophylaxis of mother and infant

    3. Monitoring of CD4$^+$ lymphocyte count and percentage, CBC, differential, platelet count

    4. Antiretroviral therapy in consultation with HIV management specialists

    5. Treatment of infections and other associated conditions

    6. Early intervention for developmental delay

    7. Maximum supportive care for child and family

    8. *CDC National Prevention Information Network*
       P.O. Box 6003
       Rockville MD 20849-6003
       (800) 458-5231
       http://www.cdcnpin.org

Chlamydia (Refer to Gu/Gyn chapter)

- Definition: A group of intracellular parasites with three known species, *C. trachomatis, C. psittaci* and *C. pneumoniae*

- Etiology/Incidence

    1. 40% to 70% of infants born to women infected with chlamydia will develop infection at one or more sites

    2. Transmission occurs from cervical maternal infection to infant during vaginal delivery

    3. Prevalence among sexually active women about 5%; among adolescents may be as high as 20%

    4. *Chlamydia trachomatis*—most prevalent sexually transmitted disease in the U.S.

- Signs and Symptoms: *Chlamydia trachomatis* in the neonate

    1. Neonatal conjunctivitis—mild to severe

        a. 5 days to several weeks after delivery, usually vaginal

        b. Conjunctival injection

        c. Mucoid eye discharge, ocular edema

2. Neonatal pneumonia

   a. 2 to 19 weeks of age

   b. Persistent "staccato" cough with congestion

- Differential Diagnosis

   1. Nonchlamydia conjunctivitis

      a. Chemical reaction to silver nitrate

      b. Infections due to gonorrhoeae, *Staphylococcus aureus, Haemophilus influenzae,* streptococcus, herpes simplex, enteric bacteria

   2. Bronchitis/Pneumonia—respiratory syncytial virus, other viral, bacterial causes

- Physical Findings

   1. Neonatal conjunctivitis

      a. Injected conjunctiva with exudate within first weeks of life

      b. Pseudomembrane

      c. Friable conjunctiva

   2. Neonatal pneumonia

      a. Afebrile

      b. Tachypnea

      c. Rales, but rarely wheezes

- Diagnostic Tests/Findings

   1. Chest radiograph shows hyperinflation, no consolidation, bilateral diffuse infiltrates

   2. Peripheral eosinophilia (> 300 cells/mL)

   3. Elevated serum immunoglobulins

   4. Isolation of organism by tissue culture; culture must contain epithelial cells

      a. In addition to eye and respiratory tract, *Chlamydia trachomatis* may be found in rectal, vaginal and nasopharyngeal secretions of infants born to infected mothers; infants often not symptomatic, but may shed organism for up to three years

      b. Frequently isolated from vagina, and sometimes from rectum of children who have been sexually abused; sometimes difficult to know whether infection related to child abuse or congenital transmission

- Management/Treatment: Infants, oral erythromycin suspension, 50 mg/kg/ day for 10 to 14 days, repeated once if needed; approximately 20% of infants need second course of treatment

Gonococcal Infection (Refer to Gu/Gyn chapter)

- Definition: Infections caused by acquisition of *Neisseria gonorrhoeae*
- Etiology/Incidence: Maternal transmission to neonate from contact with vaginal secretions during birth
- Signs and Symptoms
    1. Ophthalmia; injected, swollen conjunctiva with exudate
    2. Fever, irritability, rapid respiration, rapid heart rate
    3. Purulent exudate or secretions from any orifice
- Differential Diagnosis
    1. Conjunctivitis
        a. Chemical reaction to silver nitrate
        b. Infections due to chlamydia, *Staphylococcus aureus, Haemophilus influenzae,* streptococcus, herpes simplex, or enteric bacteria
    2. Bronchitis/pneumonia—respiratory syncytial virus (RSV), other viral, bacterial causes
    3. Skin, oropharyngeal, arthritic, vaginal, urethral, rectal, systemic infection
    4. Other causative organisms
    5. Allergy
- Physical Findings
    1. Gonococcal ophthalmia neonatorum—conjunctivitis, appearing 2 to 5 days after birth, occasionally up to 25 days
        a. Thin, clear discharge from eye that becomes thick, mucoid, sometimes bloody
        b. Edema of lids, conjunctiva
        c. Untreated, may progress to edema and ulceration of cornea, globe perforation and blindness, and/or may become systemic infection
    2. Other—scalp abscesses (neonate); purulent vaginal, urethral, or rectal secretions; exudative pharyngitis or tonsillitis; cough; rales; fever; rash; multiple joint swelling
- Diagnostic Tests/Findings:
    1. Initial evaluation—microscopic identification of gram-negative intracellular diplococci in smears of exudate
    2. Culture in approved laboratory against strict CDC standards
- Management/Treatment: **Follow current CDC guidelines**
    1. Ophthalmia neonatorum prophylaxis—silver nitrate 1% aqueous; erythromycin ophthalmic ointment 0.5%; tetracycline ophthalmic ointment (1%)
    2. Hospitalize infected neonates

3. Ceftriaxone IM or IV is drug of choice for gonococcal infections in children; dose varies by age of child and site of infection; ceftriaxone given as prophylaxis to asymptomatic infants of mothers with untreated gonococcal infections

Congenital Syphilis (Refer to Gu/Gyn chapter)

- Definition: Systemic infection of transplacental or perinatal acquisition resulting in a non-random association of clinical findings

- Etiology/Incidence
    1. *Treponema pallidum*—mother with history of syphilis whose treatment is not documented as complete with full follow-up
    2. Incidence rising, especially among children of women of lower socioeconomic status; often coexistent with HIV

- Signs and Symptoms
    1. 60% of infants with congenital infection have no symptoms in the first week of life, but will develop symptoms if not immediately treated; initial presentation up to 2 years of age
    2. Low birth weight/prematurity
    3. Bone pain or tenderness; decreased movement
    4. Rhinitis, coryza
    5. Syphilitic rash (maculopapular, bullous, followed by desquamation)

- Differential Diagnosis
    1. Any of the ''TORCH'' congenital conditions
    2. Rash stage—pityriasis rosea, scabies, tinea

- Physical Findings
    1. May be asymptomatic at birth
    2. Hepatomegaly
    3. Splenomegaly
    4. Lymphadenopathy

- Diagnostic Tests/Findings
    1. Direct visualization of spirochete by dark field microscopy; direct fluorescent antibody test for *Treponema pallidum*
    2. Nontreponomel tests—Venereal Disease Research Laboratory microscopic slide test (VDRL); Rapid plasma reagin (RPR)
    3. Treponemal tests—fluorescent treponemal antibody absorbed; microhemagglutination assay for antibody to *Treponema pallidum*
    4. Elevated LFT; positive VDRL in CSF

5. Anemia, thrombocytopenia

6. Radiographic changes (''moth eaten'' metaphysis)

- Management/Treatment

    1. Prevention of sexually transmitted diseases; treat all infected individuals, especially sexually active women and partners

    2. Screen serum of all mothers before infant is discharged; treat all neonates ≤ 4 weeks of age of seropositive mothers, who meet criteria, with aqueous penicillin G 100,000 to 150,000 U/kg/day IV for 10 to 14 days (AAP, 2000, p. 555)

    3. Older infants and children—aqueous penicillin G 200,000 to 300,000 U/kg/day IV for 10 days

    4. Follow-up to determine appropriately falling titers

Herpes (Refer to Gu/Gyn chapter)

- Definition: Group of infectious diseases caused by the Herpes simplex virus (HSV) Type I or II

- Etiology/Incidence

    1. Infection through direct contact of virus with host mucous membrane or abraded skin

    2. Neonatal incidence—1:3000 to 1:20,000 live births

- Signs and Symptoms

    1. Neonatal skin-eye-mouth (SEM) disease

        a. Usually presents in first two weeks of life

        b. Blisters, most often on presenting part, frequently at site of abraded skin

    2. Neonatal CNS disease

        a. Ill infant in second to third week of life

        b. Seizures

        c. Apneic episodes

    3. Neonatal disseminated disease

        a. Acutely ill infant during first week of life

        b. Seizures, lethargy, appears ill

        c. Unresponsive to antibiotic therapy

- Differential Diagnosis: ''TORCH'' diseases—toxoplasmosis, other agents (HIV, *listeria,* syphilis, gonococcus, group B streptococcus, varicella-zoster, malaria), rubella, cytomegalovirus inclusion disease, herpes simplex

- Physical Findings

    1. Neonatal skin-eye-mouth (SEM) disease

        a. Vesicles with erythematous base, clear or cloudy fluid, sometimes appearing pustular, limited to skin, eyes and mouth

        b. Transient fever, malaise (low acuity)

    2. Neonatal CNS disease

        a. Herpetic skin lesions in 60% of cases

        b. Cranial nerve abnormalities

        c. Bradycardia

    3. Neonatal disseminated disease

        a. Seizures, lethargy, often on first day of life

        b. Fever, tachypnea, labored breathing with onset of HSV pneumonitis

        c. Clinical signs of hepatitis—hepatomegaly

- Diagnostic Tests/Findings

    1. Virus isolation from skin, mucous membranes, urine, blood, stool or CSF

    2. Detection of fluorescent antibodies (especially when skin lesions are active)

    3. Polymerase chain reaction (PCR)—helpful in CNS infection

    4. Serology rarely useful in acute HSV infection

    5. Increased CSF protein and pleocytosis

    6. Pulmonary radiograph reveals bilateral, patchy infiltrates from 3 to 10 days of neonatal disseminated disease

    7. Abnormal liver function test results

- Management/Treatment:

    1. Parenteral acyclovir treatment of choice for neonatal HSV infection

    2. Infants with ocular involvement add topical ophthalmic drug treatment.

    3. Refer to APA, 2003, p. 347

Cytomegalic Inclusion Disease (CMV)

- Definition: Congenital infectious disease caused by prenatal infection with cytomegalovirus, a member of herpes virus family

- Etiology/Incidence

    1. During maternal infection with CMV, virus crosses placenta and spreads via fetal blood stream, mainly affecting CNS, liver and eyes

    2. Most common intrauterine infection, affecting 1% of newborns; approximately 10%

are symptomatic; about half present with classic cytomegalic inclusion disease; remainder can shed virus for months, but may never show sequelae

- Signs and Symptoms
  1. Early global developmental delay
  2. Mental retardation
  3. Growth retardation

- Differential Diagnosis
  1. Congenital toxoplasmosis
  2. Rubella
  3. Herpes

- Physical Findings: Classic congenital CMV manifestations are: (Stamos & Rowley, 1994)
  1. Small for gestational age (SGA)
  2. Petechiae, purpura, thrombcytopenia
  3. Hepatosplenomegaly
  4. Jaundice
  5. Microcephaly
  6. Chorioretinitis
  7. Intracranial calcification
  8. Hearing impairment
  9. Intrauterine growth retardation

- Diagnostic Tests/Findings: Isolation of CMV from infant urine, pharynx or peripheral blood leukocytes within first three weeks of life

- Management/Treatment
  1. Primary prevention in women of child-bearing age and younger, since both initial infection and reactivation during pregnancy can cause fetal infection
  2. Congenitally affected infants—refer to developmental disabilities center for interdisciplinary management of complex disabilities
  3. Asymptomatic infants with congenital CMV
     a. Refer to audiology for periodic sensorineural hearing evaluation
     b. Screen frequently for growth retardation and emerging developmental delays
     c. Refer to ophthalmology—emerging chorioretinitis
     d. Refer to dentistry—defective tooth enamel
     e. Monitor for hepatosplenomegaly

4. Neonatal acquisition—often presents as afebrile pneumonia after 8 week incubation period; test suspect infants

5. Seek specialist consultation regarding use of anti-viral drugs; use is not routinely recommended at this time

Congenital Rubella Syndrome (CRS) (Refer to Infectious Disease chapter)

*   Definition: Non-random association of congenital abnormalities associated with maternal infection with rubella virus during first 16 weeks of fetal gestation

*   Etiology/Incidence

    1. Maternal to fetal transmission of rubella virus

    2. 1:10,000 births in areas where vaccination rates are high; higher in areas of low vaccination; serologic surveys reveal 10% of young adults are susceptible

*   Signs and Symptoms

    1. Intrauterine growth retardation

    2. Developmental delays/mental retardation

    3. Deafness

    4. Blindness

    5. Failure to thrive, related to heart defects

*   Differential Diagnosis

    1. Congenital CMV

    2. Syphilis

    3. Toxoplasmosis

*   Physical Findings

    1. Congenital heart defects

    2. Cataracts, retinopathy, glaucoma

    3. Petechial or purpuric rash

    4. Sensorineural defects

    5. Microphthalmia

*   Diagnostic Tests/Findings

    1. Viral culture of nasopharyngeal secretions; laboratory must be notified of suspected rubella

    2. Serology

*   Management/Treatment

    1. Isolate infants with CRS from pregnant/potentially pregnant women for one full year

2. Two-thirds of infants with CRS show no symptoms at birth; if maternal infection known or suspected, obtain cultures to determine if infant is shedding virus

3. Early intervention for developmental stimulation

4. Refer to cardiology, ophthalmology, audiology for evaluation

5. Psychosocial support to child and family

6. Ensure appropriate school placement and supports

7. Rubella is a reportable disease

Hepatitis B (Refer to Gastrointestinal Disorders chapter)

- Definition: Incurable infectious disease affecting the liver resulting in chronic carrier state; can cause serious complications such as hepatocellular carcinoma or chronic liver disease; complications fatal for 4000 to 5000 people annually in U.S.

- Etiology/Incidence

    1. Person to person transmission of hepatitis B virus via close personal contact, saliva and other secretions, blood and blood products through wound exudates or sexual contact with infected individuals; perinatal vertical transmission from infected/carrier mother to infant

    2. 22,000 carrier mothers deliver annually; 70% to 90% of newborns infected, 80% if mother had clinical hepatitis during third trimester; chronic carrier state ensues for up to 90%; approximately 25% die of chronic liver disease as adults

- Signs and Symptoms

    1. Long incubation period—40 to 160 days; average is 90 days

    2. Skin rash

    3. Arthralgia

    4. Moderate fever, nausea, vomiting in some cases

    5. Loss of appetite

- Differential Diagnosis

    1. Hepatitis A, Hepatitis C, Hepatitis D, Hepatitis E

    2. Cystic fibrosis, Wilson disease, metabolic liver disease

    3. Infectious causes such as CMV, toxoplasmosis, echovirus, Epstein Barr virus

- Physical Findings

    1. Neonatal infection usually results in "healthy" chronic carrier state

    2. Later, progression to liver disease with:

        a. Liver enlargement, tenderness

        b. Jaundice

    c. Arthralgia or arthritis

    d. Rash or urticaria

- Diagnostic Tests/Findings

  1. Presence of surface antigen HBsAg, HBeAg antigen, or antibodies to either of these or HBcAg (core antigen)

  2. Aminotransferase elevation—peaks at about one month

  3. Bilirubin elevation

  4. Elevated WBC; elevated serum alpha-fetoprotein concentration

- Management/Treatment

  1. No specific therapy for HBV infection yet available

  2. Perinatal exposure—HBIG 0.5 mL + vaccination in first 12 hours of life

  3. Prevention—universal child HBV immunization, with adolescent "catch up"

  4. Supportive care during acute phase

  5. Monitor for hepatic failure (rare), hospitalize if occurs, restrict protein intake

Toxoplasmosis

- Definition: Communicable parasitic infection

- Etiology/Incidence

  1. Placenta to fetus transmission of *Toxoplasma gondii* in mother with primary infection during pregnancy

  2. 1:1000 to 1:10,000 live births; about 40% of infants of mothers with primary infection will become infected

- Signs and Symptoms

  1. Severe

    a. Immediate—microcephaly, seizures, jaundice, fever

    b. Later—developmental delays, cerebral palsy, visual problems, hearing impairment/deafness

  2. Subclinical (later signs)

    a. Visual impairment

    b. Hearing impairment

    c. Poor coordination

    d. Developmental delays

- Differential Diagnosis

  1. Cytomegalovirus

    2. Syphilis

    3. Rubella

    4. Hemolytic disease of the newborn

- Physical Findings

    1. Severe

        a. Retinal lesions on fundoscopic examination

        b. Splenomegaly, hepatomegaly

        c. Lymphadenopathy

        d. Jaundice

        e. Thrombocytopenia

        f. Growth failure

    2. Subclinical (later signs)—retinal lesions on fundoscopic examination

- Diagnostic Tests/Findings

    1. Pre-natal—fetal blood or tissue analysis; ultrasonography for bilateral, symmetrical ventriculomegaly

    2. Polymerase chain reaction assay (PCR)—detection of genomic material

    3. Visual detection of tachyzoites in newborn CSF, ventricular fluid, blood, bone marrow, brain or placental tissue, or detection 1 to 6 weeks after mouse innoculation

    4. Detection of antitoxoplasma IgM in umbilical cord or newborn serum

    5. Persistent high IgG titers

    6. Ventricular dilitation

    7. Cerebrospinal fluid abnormalities

    8. Intracerebral calcifications

- Management/Treatment

    1. Congenital—one year treatment with pyrimethamine with sulfadiazine and folinic acid supplement; corticosteroids for acute inflammation

    2. Spiramycin for primary infection during pregnancy if no evidence of fetal infection; pyrimethamine and sulfonamide after fetal infection has occurred

    3. Offer consideration of selective termination of pregnancy if evidence of severe effects on fetus early in pregnancy

Fetal Alcohol Syndrome (FAS)

- Definition: Non-random grouping of congenital anomalies in persons whose mothers ingested alcohol during pregnancy

- Etiology/Incidence

1. Dose related (*dose necessary to cause FAS unknown*) teratogenic effect of maternal prenatal alcohol ingestion; alcohol and its metabolite acetaldehyde cross placenta and are believed to:

   a. Decrease protein syntheses

   b. Impair cellular growth and migration

   c. Decrease production of neurotransmitters

   d. Inhibit nerve myelination

2. Differential effects according to trimester

   a. First trimester—physical defects and mental retardation

   b. Second trimester—growth retardation and mental retardation

   c. Third trimester—mental retardation without physical defects or growth retardation

3. Most common cause of mental retardation in U.S.

4. Incidence of FAS 2:1000; incidence of fetal alcohol effects (FAE) at least 2 to 3 times higher

- Signs and Symptoms

  1. Alcoholic mother

  2. Infant alcohol withdrawal symptoms (irritability, hyperactivity, jitteriness) and alcohol odor to amniotic fluid if alcohol abuse during last days of pregnancy

  3. Term birth, but small for gestational age

  4. Slow growth

  5. Mental retardation

- Differential Diagnosis: Other congenital disorders causing atypical appearance and mental retardation (e.g., Down syndrome, Fragile X syndrome)

- Physical Findings

  1. Small head circumference

  2. Widely spaced eyes with narrow lids and epicanthal folds

  3. Short, upturned, or beak like nose with broad nasal bridge

  4. Thin upper lip-vermilion border

  5. Absent or flattened philtrum

  6. Micrognathia

  7. Dental malocclusion

  8. Congenital heart defects

  9. Hip subluxation or dislocation

10. Seizure disorder

11. Attention deficit disorder

12. Ophthalmologic disorders—myopia/strabismus

13. Hearing impairment

14. Below average height and weight for age

15. Cleft palate

- Diagnostic Tests/Findings

    1. IQ usually in 60 to 80 range, stable throughout life

    2. History of maternal alcohol abuse during pregnancy

- Management/Treatment

    1. No known treatment to reverse primary defects

    2. Promote stable, supportive home environment

    3. Ensure appropriate education with necessary support services

    4. Identify and treat associated health conditions (e.g., seizures, congenital heart defects, vision problems)

    5. Prophylactic antibiotics for subacute bacterial endocarditis (SBE), if cardiac effects present

    6. National Organization on Fetal Alcohol Syndrome
       216 G Street N.E.
       Washington, DC 20002
       (800) 666-6327

Genetic Syndromes

Trisomy 18 (Edwards' Syndrome)

- Definition: Autosomal chromosomal disorder with karyotype 47 XY or XX + 18, trisomy of chromosome 18; associated with severe mental retardation and other congenital defects; 5% to 10% survive beyond first year of life

- Etiology/Incidence

    1. Nondisjunction during meiotic division resulting in trisomy of chromosome #18

    2. Second most common autosomal chromosome disorder

    3. 1:3500 to 8000 live births; 3:1 female predominance

    4. 90% die by 1 year

- Signs and Symptoms

    1. Small for gestational age

2. Severe global developmental delays

3. Feeding problems/growth failure

- Differential Diagnosis: Trisomy 13; other rare chromosomal aberrations

- Physical Findings

  1. Apnea

  2. Microcephaly

  3. Low set ears

  4. Heart murmur

  5. Clenched hands with over-riding fingers and crossed thumb

  6. Severe failure to thrive (FTT)

- Diagnostic Tests/Findings

  1. Karyotype

     a. Fluorescent in-situ hybridization (FISH) analysis

     b. Results usually available within 48 hours

  2. Echocardiogram to detect congenital cardiac defects

  3. Chorionic villi sampling or amniocentesis with subsequent pregnancies

- Management/Treatment

  1. Genetic counseling

  2. Psychosocial support to parents and family

  3. Refer to cardiology

  4. Support nutritional needs; may require gastric feedings

  5. Prophylactic antibiotics to prevent subacute bacterial endocarditis (SBE), if cardiac effects present

  6. Enroll in early intervention program for habilitative therapies

  7. Assist family with management of special needs child—may require in-home nursing

  8. Support Organization for Trisomy 18, 13, and Related Disorders (SOFT),
     2982 S. Union Street
     Rochester, NY 14624
     (800) 716-SOFT (7638)

Down Syndrome (DS) (Trisomy 21)

- Definition: A recognizable grouping of congenital physical malformations, coupled with mental retardation and karyotype 47 XY or XX + 21; also known as Trisomy 21

- Etiology/Incidence
  1. Presence of critical lower region of a third #21 chromosome, usually contributed due to nondisjunction in maternal zygote formation
  2. 1:700 births
  3. Affects males and females equally
  4. Increased risk with advanced maternal age, though most infants with DS are born to younger mothers due to higher birth rates among younger women
- Signs and Symptoms
  1. Mental retardation, mild to severe
  2. Typical phenotypic signs at birth
     a. Flattened, hypoplastic mid-face
     b. Small mouth with high, narrow palate
     c. Tongue large for mouth
     d. Small ears
     e. Inner epicanthal folds
     f. Upward slanting palpebral fissures
     g. Hypotonia
     h. Sometimes brachydactyly, single transverse palmar crease
     i. Flattened occiput
     j. History of seizures—up to 13%
- Differential Diagnosis: Other genetic or chromosomal syndromes
- Physical Findings
  1. Phenotype as above
  2. Signs of congenital heart disease—50%, e.g., murmur, abnormal heart rate, rapid respiratory rate, labored respirations, cyanosis
  3. Signs of hypothyroidism and other endocrine problems—15%
  4. Signs of esophageal or duodenal atresia—12%
  5. Ligamentous laxity—100%
  6. Vision or hearing impairments—up to 90%
  7. Obesity—50% by early childhood
- Diagnostic Tests/Findings
  1. Pre or postnatal chromosome analysis reveals 47 XY or XX + 21 karyotype
  2. CBC with differential to identify those with leukemia; 10 to 15 fold increased risk

3. Radiographic finding of atlantoaxial instability—10%

- Management/Treatment

    1. Primary prevention via education re: risk factors; secondary prevention via prenatal diagnosis

    2. Early intervention by PT, OT, speech therapists

    3. Genetic counseling for parents and older siblings

    4. Periodic full history and physical with sensory and developmental evaluations

    5. Nutritional support

    6. Prophylactic antibiotics to prevent SBE, if cardiac effects

    7. Prompt consultation and referral for specialist treatment of associated conditions

    8. Association for Children with Down Syndrome
       2616 Martin Avenue
       Bellmore, NY 11710

       National Down Syndrome Congress
       7000 Peachtree-Dunwood Road N.E.
       Lake Ridge 400 Office Park Bldg 5
       Suite 100
       Atlanta, GA 30328
       (800) 232-NDSC

       National Down Syndrome Society
       666 Broadway, Suite 800
       New York, NY 10012
       (800) 221-4602
       http://www.ndss.org

Fragile X Syndrome

- Definition: Nonrandom association of clinical signs and symptoms including recognizable phenotype of subtle physical abnormalities, mental retardation of varying degrees, behavioral abnormalities, and karyotype showing fragile site on X chromosome

- Etiology/Incidence

    1. Genetic anomaly, labeled FMR1, on X chromosome at Xq27.3, the same position as the fragile site

    2. Atypical X-linked recessive inheritance pattern

    3. Affected individuals—1:1000 males; 1:2000 to 1:2500 females

    4. Carrier females—1:700

    5. Approximately 20% of males asymptomatic, but can transmit gene resulting in symptomatic offspring

6. Most common inherited cause of mental retardation (MR); second most common genetic cause of MR

- Signs and Symptoms

    1. Developmental delay

    2. Hyperactivity

    3. Speech delay; perseverative speech; echolalia

    4. Poor gross motor coordination

    5. Stereotypies, e.g., talking to self, spinning, hand flapping

    6. Gaze aversion

    7. History of seizures—17% to 50%

- Differential Diagnosis

    1. Autism, Asperger syndrome, or pervasive developmental disorder

    2. Mental retardation with nonspecific etiology

    3. Klinefelter syndrome, Sotos syndrome

    4. Attention deficit hyperactivity disorder

- Physical Findings

    1. Macrocephaly

    2. Prominent forehead with long thin face and prominent jaw, especially in adolescence

    3. Macro-orchidism in adolescent males; may be seen as early as age 5

    4. Protuberant, large ears, long or wide

    5. Soft, smooth skin

    6. Heart murmur or apical midsystolic click

    7. Serous otitis media

    8. Strabismus—40%

    9. Joint laxity (especially fingers), hip subluxation, occasionally club foot

- Diagnostic Tests/Findings

    1. DNA analysis from whole blood in approved laboratory to confirm diagnosis

    2. Prenatal testing from chorionic villus or amniocentesis sample

- Management/Treatment

    1. Psychosocial support to parents, child and family

2. Genetic counseling—no spontaneous mutations have been found for Fragile X syndrome; all family members should undergo genetic testing to identify transmitting males, carrier females, and affected individuals

3. Regular well-child examination with attention to:

   a. Cardiac auscultation—if click or murmur heard, obtain echocardiogram, consider referral to cardiologist for possible mitral valve prolapse

   b. Otoscopic evaluation—serous otitis media

   c. Ophthalmologic evaluation—strabismus (40%), myopia

   d. Developmental evaluation—mild to severe delays, (usually moderate)

   e. Anticipatory guidance

4. Enroll in early intervention as soon as delays are recognized; speech/language therapy and sensory/motor integration therapy thought to be most helpful

5. Ensure appropriate educational placement with necessary supports

6. Prophylactic antibiotics with dental care and all surgeries for SBE, mitral valve prolapse

7. National Fragile X Foundation
   P.O. Box 190488
   San Francisco, CA 94119
   (800) 688-8765
   http://www.nfxf.org

Turner's Syndrome (XO Karyotype)

- Definition: Chromosomal anomaly resulting in 45,XO (female) karyotype, with predictable associated signs and symptoms

- Etiology/Incidence

   1. Nondisjunction during meiotic division, usually maternal; more than half have a mosaic chromosomal complement (45,XO/46/XX)

   2. 1:1500 to 1:2500 live births; most common sex-chromosome anomaly affecting females; many affected embryos do not survive to term

- Signs and Symptoms

   1. Short stature with "square" appearance

   2. Low hairline

   3. Chronic ear infections

   4. Learning disabilities

   5. Lack of development of secondary sexual characteristics

- Differential Diagnosis

   1. Congenital lymphedema without Turner's karyotype

2. Coarctation of aorta without Turner's karyotype

- Physical Findings
    1. Neonatal—lymphedema, webbed neck, low hairline, swelling of hands and feet
    2. Widely spaced, often inverted nipples with "shield" shaped chest
    3. Heart murmur
    4. Ear deformities
    5. Strabismus, amblyopia, ptosis
    6. Scoliosis (10%)
    7. Nail dysplasia
    8. Defective dentition
    9. High blood pressure

- Diagnostic Tests/Findings
    1. Cytogenetic testing for Karyotype 45 XO
    2. Cardiac ultrasonography or MRI for:
        a. Coarctation of aorta (20%)
        b. Bicuspid aortic valve (50%)
    3. Renal ultrasound to detect renal anomalies
    4. Thyroid function tests to detect low T_4, high TSH indicating hypothyroidism
    5. Abdominal and pelvic ultrasound to detect gonadal dysgenesis
    6. Plasma gonadotropin studies to detect low levels of normal female hormones

- Management/Treatment
    1. Refer to endocrinology
        a. Growth hormone therapy beginning when growth falls below 5th percentile on normal female child growth chart
        b. Hormone (estrogen) replacement therapy beginning about 14 years of age
        c. Monitor for hypothyroidism
    2. Genetic counseling
    3. Psychosocial support
    4. Assistance in school for learning disabilities
    5. Referral to cardiology for cardiac anomaly diagnosis and treatment
    6. Prophylactic antibiotics for SBE if cardiac effects present
    7. Referral to ENT, orthopedics, urology, ophthalmology, pediatric dentist as needed

8. Turner's Syndrome Society of the U.S.
   14450 T. C. Jester
   Suite 260
   Houston, TX 77014
   (800) 365-9944

Klinefelter Syndrome (XXY Karyotype)

- Definition: Nonrandom association of physical characteristics and learning and behavioral disorders seen in males with the 47,XXY karyotype

- Etiology/Incidence
  1. Maternal meiotic nondisjunction resulting in contribution of two X chromosomes to maternal zygote (ova); when ova is fertilized by sperm containing one Y chromosome, resulting embryo has Klinefelter karyotype
  2. 1:1000 live births
  3. Most common cause of hypogonadism and infertility in men

- Signs and Symptoms
  1. Tall male, especially at adolescence and beyond
  2. Slow, incomplete pubertal development
  3. Behavioral and psychiatric disorders (shy, immature, anxious, aggressive, antisocial)
  4. Thin child
  5. Language impairment

- Differential Diagnosis
  1. Marfan syndrome
  2. Sotos syndrome
  3. Trisomy 8p

- Physical Findings
  1. Tall for age, with disproportionate lower limb length
  2. Gynecomastia
  3. Small, firm testes
  4. Cryptorchidism
  5. Small phallus
  6. Hypospadias

- Diagnostic Tests/Findings
  1. Chromosome analysis yields 47, XXY karyotype
  2. High FSH, LH and low testosterone levels

- Management/Treatment

    1. Early intervention for learning disorders

    2. Counseling/therapy for behavioral disorders

    3. Psychosocial support for family

    4. Genetic counseling

    5. Refer to endocrinology for consideration of testosterone therapy at age 11 or 12

    6. Screen for breast cancer (4%)

    7. Reduction mammoplasty for severe gynecomastia

    8. American Association for Kleinfelter Syndrome
        Information and Support
        2945 W. Farwell Ave.
        Chicago, IL 60645-2925
        (888) 466-5747

Tay-Sachs Disease

- Definition: Inborn error of metabolism resulting in neurologic degenerative disease and death, usually by 3 years of age

- Etiology/Incidence

    1. Autosomal recessive single gene disorder; deficiency of hexosaminidase A (hex A) which is necessary for breakdown of ganglioside G_{m2}; as glycoside accumulates in neurons, axons degenerate and demyelination occurs

    2. 3:10,000 live births; mainly in Ashkenazic Jewish population; gene carrier frequency in U.S. 1:27 among Jews and 1:380 among non-Jews

- Signs and Symptoms

    1. Normal development until age 3 to 6 months, then progressive deterioration

    2. Listlessness

    3. Muscle weakness

    4. Slow neurological development, loss of developmental milestones

    5. Feeding problems

    6. Frequent upper respiratory infections

    7. Apathy, irritability

    8. Seizures

    9. Deafness/blindness

- Differential Diagnosis

    1. Other inborn errors of metabolism

2. Leukodystrophies

3. Muscular dystrophy

- Physical Findings

  1. Hypotonia, followed by spasticity and paralysis

  2. "Cherry red" spot on retina

  3. Translucent skin, delicate pink coloring

  4. Abnormal increase in head size due to cerebral gliosis

  5. Dysphagia

  6. Decerebrate posturing

  7. Eventual vegetative state

- Diagnostic Tests/Findings: Serum enzymatic assay yields deficiency of hexosaminidase A

- Management/Treatment

  1. Genetic counseling

  2. Primary prevention via carrier screening

  3. Secondary prevention via prenatal diagnosis and elective termination of pregnancy

  4. No known treatment for underlying metabolic deficiency

  5. Supportive/comfort care for child; assist to obtain home nursing services as disease progresses and care burden increases

  6. Psychosocial support for parents and family

  7. The National Tay-Sachs and Allied Diseases Association
     2001 Beacon Street, #204
     Brookline, MA 02146
     (617) 277-4463

Marfan Syndrome

- Definition: Inherited disorder of connective tissue; affects the skeletal, cardiovascular and ocular systems

- Etiology/Incidence

  1. Autosomal dominant inheritance of defective fibrillin gene (FBN1 mapped to chromosome 15 [15q21.1]); 15% sporadic mutation

  2. Incidence is 1:20,000

- Signs and Symptoms

  1. Skeletal—tall stature; long, thin extremities, long fingers, narrow facies

2. Rapid heart rate, chest pain; palpitations or syncope suggestive of mitral valve prolapse

3. Vision impairment

4. Normal intelligence with learning disorders, attention deficit hyperactivity disorder (40%)

- Differential Diagnosis

    1. Beals syndrome (congenital contractural arachnodactyly)

    2. Homocystinuria

- Physical Findings

    1. Skeletal

        a. Loose joints

        b. Scoliosis (60%)

        c. Pectus excavatum or carinatum

        d. Narrow palate

        e. Dolichomorphism—elongation of tubular bones, as evidenced by increased upper limb span, low upper to lower segment ratio, hand length exceeding 11% of height, foot length exceeding 15% of height

    2. Murmur indicative of mitral valve prolapse

    3. Ocular—upwardly dislocated lens, retinal detachment

    4. Myopia

- Diagnostic Tests/Findings

    1. Diagnosis based on clinical manifestations; must document involvement of at least one of the three systems—cardiovascular, ocular, skeletal

    2. Positive family history plus one or more systems (as above) conclusive

    3. Cardiac evaluation (chest radiograph, electrocardiogram, echocardiogram)—mitral valve prolapse common; signs of dilatation of aortic root or dissecting aortic aneurysm

    4. Ocular evaluation—slit-lamp examination

    5. Skeletal evaluation—scoliosis screening; trunk/extremities ratio

- Management/Treatment

    1. Refer to cardiology for periodic echocardiogram to detect dissecting aortic aneurysm, mitral valve prolapse in severe cases, surgical graft repair of the ascending aorta and aortic valve has been successful

    2. Propanolol to reduce effect of ventricular ejection on ascending aorta

3. Refer to ophthalmology for treatment of myopia, lens subluxation, cataracts, glaucoma, retinal detachment

4. Refer to endocrinology for hormonal treatment to curtail height, valuable psychological effect; prevention of scoliosis and kyphosis; prevention of secondary problems of feet

5. Psychosocial support for patient and family

6. Genetic counseling

7. Ensure mainstream or inclusive school placement with any necessary supports, with attention to physical activity limitations if cardiovascular involvement

8. National Marfan Foundation (NMF)
   382 Main Street
   Port Washington, NY 11050
   (800) 862-7326
   http://www.marfan.org

Hurler Syndrome (MPS IH)

- Definition: Inborn mucopolysaccharidosis metabolic disorder in which dermatan and heparan sulfate accumulate and are excreted in urine; typically, death occurs by 10 years of age

- Etiology/Incidence

    1. Deficiency of enzyme α-L-iduronidase; autosomal recessive inheritance

    2. 1:100,000 incidence

- Signs and Symptoms

    1. Coarse facial features with enlarged tongue, full lips, flat nasal bridge; mild at birth, progressing with growth

    2. Developmental peak at age 2, followed by deterioration

    3. Recurrent upper respiratory tract infections

    4. Recurrent inguinal hernia

    5. Vision and hearing impairments

    6. Joint limitations and contractures

    7. Short stature

- Differential Diagnosis: Other progressive neuropathies and inborn errors of metabolism, particularly other mucopolysaccharidoses and thyroid deficiency

- Physical Findings

    1. Skeletal abnormalities, including spinal anomalies/gibbus formation

    2. Macrocephaly, scaphocephaly

    3. Hepatosplenomegaly

4. Clouded corneas

5. Inguinal/umbilical hernia

6. Valvular heart disease; coronary artery disease

- Diagnostic Tests/Findings

    1. Prenatal diagnosis with amniocentesis or chorionic villus sampling and enzyme analysis

    2. Postnatal via serum and urine enzyme analysis

- Management/Treatment

    1. Genetic counseling

    2. Psychosocial support

    3. Anticipatory guidance

    4. Early intervention; appropriate school placement with supports as needed

    5. Bone marrow transplantation in selected cases, especially after early diagnosis and with human leukocyte antigen (HLA) matched sibling donor

    6. Refer to audiology and opthalmology for evaluation and treatment, as indicated

    7. To date, enzyme replacement therapy not effective

    8. National MPS Society, Inc.
       102 Aspen Drive
       Downingtown, PA 19335
       (601) 942-0100

Prader-Willi Syndrome

- Definition: Congenital disorder characterized by voracious, uncontrollable appetite and obesity

- Etiology/Incidence

    1. Usually sporadic mutation; when detectable (about 50%) mutation at same location of chromosome 15 as the mutation for Angelman syndrome, although conditions are very dissimilar due to phenomenon of genetic imprinting

    2. 1:10,000 to 1:15,000 incidence

- Signs and Symptoms

    1. Voracious appetite during childhood and beyond, resulting in severe obesity

    2. Mental retardation

    3. Behavior problems

    4. Hypontonia, poor suck and feeding problems in infancy; resolution with time

- Differential Diagnosis: Other neurological and musculoskeletal disorders with early hypotonia (including cerebral palsy) and developmental delay

- Physical Findings
    1. Obesity
    2. Small hands and feet
    3. Small genitalia
    4. Cryptorchidism
    5. Short stature
    6. Scoliosis
- Diagnostic Tests/Findings
    1. In 50% of cases, chromosome analysis detects aberration of chromosome 15 section 15q11 to 15q13
    2. Remainder of cases are diagnosed by clinical signs and symptoms
    3. Growth Hormone deficiency frequent, but not universal
- Management/Treatment
    1. Behavioral therapy for control of eating and other problem behaviors
    2. Genetic counseling
    3. Early intervention and appropriate school placement with supports
    4. Psychosocial support for child and family
    5. Refer to endocrinology for evaluation and management of Growth Hormone deficiency
    6. Prader Willi Syndrome Association
       5700 Midnight Pass Road
       Sarasota, FL 34242
       (800) 926-4797
       http://www.pwsausa.org

Multisystem Disorders

Cerebral Palsy (CP)

- Definition
    1. Disorders of motion and posture related to static injury to the developing brain
    2. Types
        a. Spastic (diplegia, tetraplegia, hemiplegia) **most frequent**
        b. Dyskinetic
        c. Ataxic
        d. Mixed

- Etiology/Incidence
  1. CNS insult may be congenital, hypoxic, traumatic or ischemic; may occur prenatally, perinatally, postnatally
  2. Birth asphyxia associated with only 3% to 13% of cases
  3. High association with prematurity and very low birth weight
  4. Apgar score of 3 or less at 20 minutes associated with 250 times increased risk
  5. Tetraplegia associated with serious intrauterine infections, fetal encephalopathies and perinatal hypoxia
  6. Prevalence 2.7:1000 at school entry; most common pediatric physical disability
  7. Hereditary spastic type CP—rare
- Signs and Symptoms
  1. Movement or posture abnormality that evolves with growth, but is not itself progressive
  2. Delays in reaching developmental milestones, especially motor
  3. Infancy
     a. Abnormal or retained primitive reflexes
     b. Poor muscle tone in first few weeks
     c. Some irritability, lethargy
     d. Weak suck, difficulty swallowing
     e. Oral hypersensitivity
     f. Fisted hands, even at rest
  4. Later infancy/toddler
     a. Scissoring
     b. Toe to toe gait if ambulatory
     c. "W" sitting
     d. "Bottom scoot" in place of crawl
     e. Resistance to spoon feeding/table foods
     f. Tonic bite, tongue thrust
     g. Early hand preference
  5. Vision impairment (50%)
  6. Hearing impairment (10%)
  7. Seizures (35% to 50%)
  8. Mental retardation (50% to 75%); more common with greater physical disability

- Differential Diagnosis
    1. Neurodegenerative disorders such as Duchenne muscular dystrophy
    2. Inborn errors of metabolism
    3. Spinal cord tumor/syrinx
    4. Brain tumor
    5. Hydrocephalus
    6. Subdural hematoma
    7. Dystonias
- Physical Findings
    1. Abnormal muscle tone (hypo or hypertonia)
    2. Infancy—retained primitive reflexes
    3. Hyperactive tendon and heightened stretch reflexes; positive Babinski
    4. Restricted joint range of motion
    5. Hip click or clunk on Barlow maneuver or Ortolani test
    6. Movement related muscle spasms
    7. "Clasp-knife" limb muscle stretch response
    8. Low weight for height
    9. Neuromuscular scoliosis
- Diagnostic Tests/Findings
    1. Developmental evaluation—delays in gross motor, fine motor, speech, according to type of CP and presence of mental retardation
    2. Brain MRI—periventricular leukomalacia
- Management/Treatment
    1. Coordinate interdisciplinary management to promote optimum health and function
    2. Enroll in early intervention services
    3. Identify and treat associated conditions (e.g., seizures, visual impairment, hearing impairment, gastroesophageal reflux)
    4. Prevent secondary conditions (e.g., failure to thrive, skin breakdown, dental caries)
    5. Functional therapies to build on strengths and promote compensation for physical impairments
    6. Parent/family support for positive coping and stress relief
    7. Spasticity relief

      a. Enteral medication—lioresal, diazepam, dantrium sodium, tizanidine hydrochloride

      b. Botulinum toxin IM to major affected muscles, or nerve block injections

      c. Intrathecal lioresal

      d. Selective dorsal root rhizotomy

8. Nutritional support

9. Ensure appropriate education with supportive services and therapies

10. United Cerebral Palsy Association, Inc.
    1660 L Street, N.W.
    Suite 700
    Washington, DC 20036-5602
    (800) USA-5UCP
    (800) 872-5827

Spina Bifida

- Definition: Congenital multisystem defect resulting from failure of neural tube closure during early embryonic development; one of several "neural tube defects"

- Etiology/Incidence

    1. Multifactorial inheritance pattern; environmental contribution not well understood, although addition of folic acid to dietary intake reduces occurrence probability by one-half

    2. Spina bifida occulta—incidence up to 10% of population

    3. Myelomeningocele—1:1000; decreasing, probably due to folic acid supplementation and prenatal diagnosis with selective termination, (not proven)

- Signs and Symptoms

    1. Urinary "dribbling", unable to achieve urinary continence

    2. Frequent urinary tract infections

    3. Chronic constipation, difficulty with bowel continence

    4. Motor developmental delays, especially lower extremity related gross motor delays

    5. Intelligence in normal range, but with learning disorders, often with attention deficit hyperactivity disorder (AD/HD)

- Differential Diagnosis: Syndromes of which spina bifida is associated, e.g., Meckel-Gruber syndrome

- Physical Findings

    1. Spina bifida occulta—usually benign; may have sacral dimple, hairy patch at base of spine, uneven gluteal folds

2. Arnold-Chiari Type II CNS malformation (nearly 100%)—associated with progressive hydrocephalus, difficulty swallowing, hypoventilation, apnea

3. Meningocele or Myelomeningocele—signs at birth include lesion at some point along thoraco-lumbar-sacral spine, often with a cyst-like structure protruding; neural elements may be apparently absent or may be easily visualized within the sac

4. Widely spaced cranial sutures, bulging fontanel, macrocephaly (with hydrocephalus)

5. Lack of typical lower extremity function, sometimes with orthopedic deformity (club foot, dislocated or subluxed hip, tibial torsion)

6. Abnormal deep tendon reflexes in lower extremities

7. Abnormal neonatal reflexes in lower extremities

8. Decreased or absent anal wink

9. Atrophied lower extremity/hip muscles

10. Scoliosis, kyphosis

11. Obesity in older children and adolescents (> 50%)

12. Neurogenic bowel and bladder

13. Latex sensitivity (> 40%)

- Diagnostic Tests/Findings

   1. Prenatal diagnosis possible by maternal serum screening for elevated alpha-fetoprotein, followed by ultrasound diagnostics for spinal anomaly and head "lemon sign"

   2. Postnatal diagnosis made on clinical basis

   3. Hydrocephalus after birth, increasing head circumference out of proportion to other growth parameters

- Management/Treatment

   1. Infants diagnosed prenatally should be referred to tertiary center with appropriate supports for birth (possible planned C-section) and immediate neonatal intensive care

   2. Refer to multidisciplinary treatment center for specialty management—assistance from orthopedist, urologist, neurosurgeon, developmental pediatrician, orthotist, physical and occupational therapists, nutritionist, advanced practice nurse and social worker

   3. Enroll infant in early intervention program as soon as medically stable

   4. Monitor for urinary tract infections; expect less common organisms

   5. Monitor for shunt malfunction if presence of shunted hydrocephalus; baseline head CT scan; follow-up if increased intracranial pressure suspected; refer to neurosurgeon for evaluation of suspected shunt malfunction or tethered card

   6. Monitor for development of orthopedic problems, especially scoliosis and unilateral hip subluxation or dislocation; baseline and follow-up radiographic studies

7. Monitor for skin breakdown

8. Nutritional and behavioral intervention to prevent obesity

9. Test for latex sensitivity (skin or RAST); latex precautions

10. Anticipatory guidance for development, safety

11. Psychosocial support to family and child

12. Assistance finding least restrictive school placement and other community supports—restrict from heavy contact sports only; otherwise full inclusion should be encouraged

13. Genetic counseling

14. All women of child-bearing age should consume 0.4 mg folic acid daily to help prevent neural tube defects; women at high risk should consult obstetrician for higher dose, 4.0 mg/day recommended

15. Spina Bifida Association of America (SBAA)
    4590 MacArthur Blvd., Suite 250
    Washington, DC 20007-4226
    (202) 944-3283
    (800) 621-3141

Toxic Shock Syndrome (TSS)

- Definition: Acute, life-threatening, multisystem infectious disorder leading to shock and multiple organ failure; CDC case definition (Sagraves, 1995)

- Etiology/Incidence:

  1. *Staphylococcus aureus; Streptococcus pyogenes* (Group A streptococci); association with staph or strep infections and use of tampons during menstruation

  2. 0.5:100,000 with wide geographic variations

- Signs and Symptoms:

  1. Headache

  2. Sore throat

  3. Abdominal cramps

  4. Vomiting

  5. Watery, non-bloody diarrhea

  6. Muscle tenderness, weakness

  7. Confusion, disorientation

  8. Generalized erythroderma

- Differential Diagnosis:

  1. Stevens-Johnson syndrome

   2. Kawasaki disease

   3. Scarlet fever

   4. Measles

   5. Leptospirosis

   6. Rocky mountain spotted fever

   7. Septic shock

   8. Systemic lupus erythrematosus

- Physical Findings

   1. Inflamed mucous membranes

   2. Erythroderma or scarlitinaform rash

   3. Edematous hands and feet

   4. Hyperemic conjunctiva, non-purulent drainage

   5. CDC diagnostic criteria for *S. aureus* TSS include:

      a. Fever at least 38.9° C (102° F)

      b. Hypotension

      c. Rash

      d. Desquamation of rash

      e. Involvement of at least three major organ systems

- Diagnostic Tests/Findings:

   1. Culture *S. aureus* from nasopharynx, vagina, or wound; or isolation of Group A streptococci

   2. Other findings include:

      a. Leukocytosis

      b. Anemia, thrombocytopenia

      c. Abnormal renal, liver, metabolic and musculoskeletal findings as condition progresses to affect many organ systems

      d. Negative blood, CSF cultures

- Management/Treatment

   1. Hospitalization

   2. Maximum supportive care

   3. Aggressive treatment of hypotension and fluid and electrolyte imbalances

   4. Remove infected foreign bodies (tampons); drain, irrigate infected wounds

5. IV antibiotics at maximum dose for age/weight for *S. aureus* or *S. pyrogenes* as appropriate

6. Surgical consult for necrotizing fasciitis

7. Intravenous immune globulin (IVIG) for nonresponding illness

Sudden Infant Death Syndrome (SIDS)

- Definition—''The sudden death of an infant under 1 year of age that remains unexplained after a thorough case investigation, including performance of a complete autopsy, examination of the death scene, and review of the clinical history'' (Brooks, 1997, p. 1622)

- Etiology/Incidence

  1. Unknown cause

  2. 1.1:1000 live births, twofold greater incidence in African-American infants; somewhat higher in Native-Americans; lower in Asians

  3. Peak incidence 2 to 4 months; uncommon before 2 weeks and after 6 months

- Signs and Symptoms: Infant unexpectedly found lifeless after a period of sleep

- Differential Diagnosis

  1. Meningitis

  2. Intracranial hemorrhage

  3. Myocarditis

  4. Accidental trauma

  5. Child abuse

- Physical Findings

  1. Full cardiorespiratory arrest

  2. Unresponsive to resuscitation

- Diagnostic Tests/Findings: Diagnosis of exclusion, with autopsy and investigation failure to find adequate cause of death

- Management/Treatment

  1. Risk reduction

     a. Promote excellent prenatal care

     b. Supine or side sleeping position for normal healthy infants

     c. Avoid maternal and passive smoking

     d. Separate sleeping place for infants

     e. Avoid soft bedding

     f. Maintain comfortable room temperature

g. Avoid heavy blankets, over bundling

h. Apnea monitoring for high risk infants

    (1) Premature with persistent apnea

    (2) Infant born after two previous siblings with SIDS

    (3) Post-apparent life threatening event (ALTE) requiring stimulation

    (4) Infants with central hypoventilation syndrome

2. After infant's death

a. Maximum support to family, others

b. Provide factual information

c. Assist with necessary tasks

d. Assist nursing mother with abrupt cessation of breast feeding

3. National SIDS Resource Center
2070 Chain Bridge Road
Suite 450
Vienna, VA 22182
(703) 821-8955
http://www.circsol.com/SIDS/

Reye's Syndrome

- Definition: Acute, noninflammatory hepatic encephalopathy, which often follows a viral infection

- Etiology/Incidence

    1. Unknown; association with viral infection (especially varicella and influenza) and aspirin use, but not universal

    2. Decreased occurrence with increased education regarding danger in use of aspirin with viral illness

- Signs and Symptoms

    1. Sudden development of protracted vomiting, delirium, stupor, inappropriate behavior 5 to 7 days after onset of viral infection; often after signs of recovery

    2. Progressive neurological deficit, leading to coma

    3. Headache

    4. Confusion

    5. Lethargy

- Differential Diagnosis

    1. Inborn errors of metabolism

    2. Infections of the CNS

3. CNS effects of poisoning, especially with aspirin, acetaminophen, valproic acid, antiemetics

- Physical Findings

    1. Hepatomegaly without jaundice

    2. Papilledema

- Diagnostic Tests/Findings

    1. Fatty infiltration in liver, CNS tissues, heart, pancreas, kidneys

    2. Elevation of liver enzymes

    3. Low serum glucose

    4. Elevated ammonia

- Management/Treatment

    1. Usual cause of death is cerebral edema and herniation

    2. Hospitalization for maximum supportive therapy to decrease cerebral edema, maintain serum glucose, correct electrolyte imbalances, and correct significant coagulopathy

    3. National Reye's Syndrome Foundation, Inc.
       P.O. Box 829
       Bryan, OH 43506-0829
       (800) 233-7393

Questions
Select the best answer

1. Which of the following is not among the physical signs of Fragile X syndrome in adolescent males?

   a. Protruding ears
   b. Macro-orchidism
   c. Hypertonia
   d. Prominent jaw

2. Which of the following physical stigmata are common in newborns with Down syndrome?

   a. Microcephaly, large ears and mouth, flattened philtrum
   b. Hypotonia, large appearing tongue and small mouth, upward slant to eyes
   c. Fair mottled skin, large hands and feet, broad stocky neck
   d. Funnel or pigeon-breasted chest, brushfield spots, extra digits

3. A two month-old-infant, who had a small sacral myelomeningocele repaired shortly after birth, is brought in by her mother for her well-child check. Her head circumference, which had been along the 75th percentile, was measured and plotted to be at the 97th percentile today. Your most appropriate *first* action would be to:

   a. Order a head CT scan
   b. Refer Kathleen to neurosurgery for placement of VP shunt to manage hydrocephalus
   c. Discount that measurement as a "fluke" and recheck it at the next well-child visit
   d. Recheck and replot the child's head circumference yourself at this visit

4. The diagnosis of Down syndrome in the newborn nursery:

   a. Can be made on the basis of clinical findings, making other studies unnecessary
   b. Indicates concern for associated Wilm's tumor
   c. Indicates need for confirmatory chromosomal studies
   d. Always means the child will have a heart defect

5. The parents of a child who recently died of Edwards' Syndrome (Trisomy 18) ask about their chances of having another child with Edwards' syndrome. Your best response is:

   a. They should not worry, since Edwards' syndrome is so rare
   b. They have a 1 in 4 chance, since this condition has an autosomal recessive inheritance pattern
   c. They should seek genetic counseling for the best answer to this question
   d. They should not have more children

6. Your 20-month-old-patient has a confirmed diagnosis of Hurler's syndrome, and is being seen for an upper respiratory illness. Anticipatory guidance should include:

   a. Recurrent upper respiratory infections are common in children who have Hurler's syndrome
   b. Development will progress well until at least age 6, and then deteriorate

    c. Genetic counseling is not advisable, since the chances of these parents having another child with Hurler's are extremely small

    d. Vision and hearing evaluation is unnecessary

7. Young infants with cerebral palsy often show:

    a. Voracious appetite and weight gain

    b. Increased muscle tone in the first weeks of life

    c. Hypotonia in the first weeks of life

    d. Unusually severe reactions to their first immunizations

8. A child born at 28 weeks gestation now has mild spastic diplegia. The child is under the care of a pediatric orthopedist, but does not attend an early intervention program, nor a referral center for the care of children with cerebral palsy. Which evaluations are especially needed before entering a mainstreamed preschool?

    a. The Stanford Binet IQ Test

    b. Vision and speech

    c. CBC with differential

    d. Chromosome studies

9. Children with Marfan syndrome:

    a. Rarely have ophthalmologic problems

    b. Should be evaluated for scoliosis throughout childhood and adolescence

    c. Should not be mainstreamed due to fragile medical status

    d. Usually are retarded

10. Which of the following is a *conclusive indicator* for the use of an infant apnea monitor?

    a. Symptomatic premature infants

    b. Infants of opiate or cocaine abusing mothers

    c. A child who has had one sibling die of SIDS

    d. A child who required no stimulation to recover from an apnea episode

11. Which of these factors is not closely associated with SIDS?

    a. Infants between 12 to 14 months of age

    b. Infants who sleep prone

    c. Infants of mothers who smoke

    d. Infants who are over bundled

12. Congenital HIV infection:

    a. Is diagnosed through finding maternal antibodies in infant serum

    b. Does not respond to antiretroviral therapy

    c. May be latent for years before clinical signs develop

    d. Does not include lymphadenopathy as a physical finding

13. Usual features of Fetal Alcohol Syndrome do not include:

    a. Widely spaced eyes with narrow lids
    b. Strabismus
    c. Taller and heavier than other children, beginning at about age 4
    d. Broad nasal bridge

14. It is known that Fetal Alcohol Syndrome (FAS) is caused by maternal alcohol ingestion during pregnancy. Which of the following statements is true?

    a. There is no concern for FAS in infants of mothers who report having only one or two drinks during their first trimester
    b. FAS is dose dependent. Therefore, if a woman drinks only once a day during her pregnancy, she should not be worried
    c. Heavy maternal drinking during the third trimester places the baby at greatest risk for the most abnormalities
    d. The "dose" of alcohol that causes FAS is not known

15. HIV infection can be diagnosed by:

    a. Antigen antibody detection
    b. Detection of HIV DNA from whole blood or by PCR of DNA from peripheral blood mononuclear cells
    c. Diagnosis of one or more conditions in the CDC AIDS definition
    d. Diagnosis of AIDS in the mother

16. Which of the following infant diseases is not associated with exposure in the first trimester of pregnancy?

    a. Cytomegalic inclusion disease (CMV)
    b. Chlamydia conjunctivitis
    c. Toxoplasmosis
    d. Rubella

17. Hepatitis B is a serious chronic disease which:

    a. Is curable with acyclovir therapy
    b. Is transmitted only by blood and blood products
    c. Results in recognizable disease in the first six weeks of life
    d. Can be prevented in perinatally exposed infants by giving HBIG and hepatitis immunization

18. Which of the following facts does not apply to Turner's syndrome?

    a. Their child will be a daughter, but will not develop secondary sexual characteristics without medical intervention
    b. Their child will be mentally retarded
    c. With appropriate growth hormone treatment by an endocrinologist, their daughter will show improved growth approximating more typical stature
    d. Their daughter has a relatively high chance of having a congenital heart defect

19. Joshua is the infant son of Mr. and Mrs. Abrahamson, who are of Askenazic Jewish descent. At his 9 month well-child check, his parents express concerns because he has stopped rolling over, seems listless, and is becoming quite irritable. Within your work-up to rule out Tay-Sachs disease, which of the following would not indicate probable Tay-Sachs?

    a. Hypotonia
    b. Retinal detachment
    c. "Cherry red" spot on retina
    d. Transluscent appearance and delicate pink coloring to skin

20. Prader-Willi Syndrome is a congenital genetic disorder characterized by:

    a. Failure to thrive
    b. 100% detection rate with chromosome analysis for a 15q deletion
    c. Emergence of spasticity during toddler years
    d. Voracious appetite and development of obesity

21. Stephanie, age 16, is brought to your office having suddenly become acutely ill with headache, sore throat, abdominal cramps, vomiting, watery, non-bloody diarrhea, and confusion. Her skin is clear. She is menstruating. Which of the following would immediately be a high priority in your differential diagnosis?

    a. Rotavirus
    b. Irritable bowel syndrome
    c. Toxic shock syndrome
    d. Marfan syndrome

22. Reye's syndrome is an acute illness that mainly affects the:

    a. Renal system
    b. Musculoskeletal system
    c. Liver and CNS
    d. Gastrointestinal system

23. Individuals who have spina bifida are at high risk for allergy to:

    a. Eggs
    b. Pollens
    c. Latex
    d. Dust mite feces

24. Gonococcal infections in children are best treated with:

    a. Penicillin
    b. Doxycycline
    c. Quinolones
    d. Ceftriaxone

25. Which of the following does not apply to neonatal disseminated herpes disease?

    a. Hyperactive newborn with apparent spasticity
    b. Clinical picture consistent with sepsis
    c. Infant acutely ill during the first week of life
    d. Unresponsive to antibiotic therapy

Answers

1. c	10. a	18. b
2. b	11. a	19. b
3. d	12. c	20. d
4. c	13. c	21. c
5. c	14. d	22. c
6. a	15. b	23. c
7. c	16. b	24. d
8. b	17. d	25. a
9. b		

Bibliography

American Academy of Cerebral Palsy & Developmental Medicine. (2002). *Developmental medicine and child neurology.* 91, 2-51.

American Academy of Pediatrics. (2003). In L. K. Pickering (Ed.). *Red Book 2003: Report of the committee on infectious diseases (26th ed).* Elk Grove Village, IL: Author.

American Academy of Pediatrics committee on pediatrics AIDS. (1999). *Pediatric human immunodeficiency virus (HIV) infection—a compendium of AAP guidelines on pediatric HIV infection.* Elk Grove Village, IL: Author

American Academy of Pediatrics committee on substance abuse and committee on children with disabilities. (2000). Fetal alcohol syndrome and alcohol related neurodevelopmental disorders. *Pediatrics, 106*(2), 358–61.

American Academy of Pediatrics task force on infant sleep position and sudden infant death syndrome. (2000). *Pediatrics, 105*(3), 650–6.

Glasgow, J., & Middleton, B. (2001). Reye syndrome—insights on causation and prognosis. *Archives of Diseases in children,* 85(5), 351-353.

Hoekelman, R. A., Adam, H. M., Nelson, N. M., Weitzman, M. L., & Wilson, M. H. (Eds.). (2001). *Primary pediatric care* (4th ed.). St. Louis: Mosby Year Book.

Jorde, L. (2003). *Medical genetics* (3rd ed.). St. Louis: Mosby.

Advanced Practice, Role Development, Current Trends and Health Policy

Leanne C. Busby
Mary A. Baroni

Introduction

Advanced practice registered nurses (APRN) must remain informed regarding role development, current issues and trends related to their practice as well as changes in health care policy, as each has an impact on the evolving practice environment. Although current information is presented, the reader is encouraged to contact local and State regulatory bodies for variations in practice requirements.

Advanced Practice Nursing

- Definition of Advanced Practice Registered Nursing (APRN)
  1. National Council of State Boards of Nursing (NCSBN)—"practice... based on knowledge and skills acquired in basic nursing education; licensure as a registered nurse; graduation from or completion of a graduate level APRN program accredited by a national accrediting body and current certification by a national certifying body in the appropriate APRN specialty. Practice as an advanced practice registered nurse means an expanded scope of nursing, with or without compensation or personal profit, and includes but is not limited to:
     a. Assessing clients, synthesizing and analyzing data, and understanding and applying nursing principles at an advanced level.
     b. Analyzing multiple sources of data, identifying alternative possibilities as to the nature of a health care problem and selecting appropriate treatment.
     c. Making independent decisions in solving complex client care problems.
     d. Developing a plan that establishes diagnoses, sets goals to meet identified health care needs, and prescribes a regimen of health care.
     e. Performing acts of diagnosing, prescribing, administering and dispensing therapeutic measures, including legend drugs and controlled substances, within the advanced practice registered nurse's focus os practice.
     f. Managing clients' physical and psychosocial health-illness status.
     g. Providing for the maintenance of safe and effective nursing care rendered directly or indirectly.
     h. Promoting a safe and therapeutic environment.
     i. Providing expert guidance and teaching.
     j. Participating in client and health systems management.
     k. Advocating for clients, and communities by attaining and maintaining what is in the best interest of the client or group.
     l. Evaluating responses to interventions, the effectiveness of the plan of care and the health regimen.
     m. Communicating and working effectively with clients, families and other members of the health care team.

    n. Utilizing research skills and acquiring and applying critical new knowledge and technologies to practice domain.

    o. Teaching the theory and practice of advanced practice nursing.'' (NCSBN, 2003, p. 3-4).

2. ''Advanced practice registered nurse (APRN) should be used as an umbrella term to include nurse anesthetists, nurse midwives, nurse practitioners and clinical nurse specialists to designate appropriately credentialed nurses who assume primary responsibility for the direct care of clients'' (NCSBN, 2002).

3. ''The term advanced nursing practice shoul be used to describe advanced clinical practice...there are certainly other types of specialized roles in the profession, notably educators, administrators, and researchers and these roles are vital to the profession's continued development...Some of these nurses possess advanced practice knowledge and skills as well. However, if they do not have a patient-family focused clinical practoce, they are not considered APNs by this definition.'' (Hamrick, Spross & Hanson, 2000).

4. American Nurses Association (ANA)—''registered nurse who has met advanced educational and clinical practice requirements beyond the 2 to 4 years of basic nursing education required of all RNs.'' (ANA, 2003, p. 1).

5. National Association of Pediatric Nurse Practitioners, (formerly known as the National Association of Pediatric Nurse Associates and Practitioners) (NAPNAP)—a PNP is an advanced practice registered nurse who provides patient care to children and young adults. To function in this role, the PNP must have completed a formal educational program specializing in pediatric health care and have met the State Board of Registered Nursing regulations that govern their practice (2003)

    a. 1992 Position statement on entry into practice endorsed the master's level for PNP preparation

    b. Curricular content includes growth and development, pathophysiology, physical, developmental, family and cultural assessments, laboratory skills, and the diagnosis and management of common childhood illnesses and behavioral problems

Role Development

- First NP program established in 1964 prepared pediatric nurse practitioners (PNP) through collaborative efforts of Loretta C. Ford, EdD, RN and Henry K. Silver, MD at the University of Colorado

    1. PNP role development provided a model for other emerging nurse practitioner (NP) specialties

    2. Original support of PNP role as ''physician extender'' to improve access concerns due to shortage of primary care providers

    3. Most early PNP education occurred within certificate and/or continuing education

programs; e.g., Colorado program included 4 months didactic study followed by 18 months clinical practicum training

4. Early research focused on quality of care, cost-effectiveness, productivity, clinical decision-making skills and role satisfaction of the PNP

5. National Association of Pediatric Nurse Practitioners (NAPNAP) organized in 1973 to establish PNP practice guidelines

6. Early resistance to NP role as too much of a "medical model" from mainstream graduate nursing education, that focused on "nursing model" of Clinical Nurse Specialist (CNS) role development

7. During 1980 to 1989 more physicians resulted in less need for nurse practitioner (NP)

8. During 1990 to 1998 increased emphasis on primary care resulted in decreased need for specialty care; NP seen as viable, cost effective member of healthcare delivery team

- Majority of NP programs currently at the Master's degree level within mainstream nursing education

  1. By 1989, 85% federally funded NP programs were graduate level

  2. Distinction between NP and CNS roles in practice have blurred

  3. Blended NP/CNS programs focusing on Advanced Practice Nursing (APN) are emerging within graduate nursing education

  4. Advantages/disadvantages of blended NP/CNS role remains controversial

  5. Most current programs require 2 years of full-time or 3 to 4 years of part-time graduate study

- Curriculum Guidelines and Content.

  1. Association of Faculties of Pediatric Nurse Practitioner and Associate Programs (AFPNP/AP)—first published terminal competencies (1981) later updated in 1996

  2. National Association of Nurse Practitioner Faculties (NONPF)—published curriculum guidelines and standards for NP education (1990) later updated in 1995

  3. Core graduate nursing content includes: Nursing theory and research, organizational/leadership theory, ethical/legal issues, multicultural care, economics, community based care, managed care, and health care delivery systems

  4. Advanced practice core content includes: Advanced health assessment, pharmacology, physiology, advanced pathophysiology or other related sciences depending on the APRN specialty; clinical decision making process, advanced nursing interventions/therapeutics, health promotion/disease prevention, community based practice, role differentiation, and interpersonal and family theory

  5. APRN specialty content includes information that is unique to type of APRN role, information that is unique to health care needs of respective specialty population, information that supports standards and competencies established by professional spe-

cialty organizations, clinical decision making applied to specialty practice, and faculty supervised clinical practice experience (NONPF, 1997)

- Conceptual Models For Advanced Practice Nursing
    1. Benner's model of expert practice (1985)
    2. Calkin's model of advanced nursing practice (1984)
    3. Shuler's model of NP practice (1993; 1998)
        a. Holistic patient needs
        b. NP/Patient interaction
        c. Self-care
        d. Health prevention
        e. Health promotion
        f. Wellness

Advanced Practice Trends and Issues

- Components of Advanced Practice Registered Nursing Role
    1. Coordinator of care
    2. Patient advocate
    3. Accountable for patient outcomes and cost effectiveness
    4. Direct care giver
    5. Educator
    6. Administrator
    7. Researcher
    8. Consultant
    9. Case manager
    10. Change agent
- Standards and Scope of Practice
    1. Standards of practice
        a. Described by ANA (1998) as authoritative statements by which to measure quality of practice, service or education
        b. Establishes minimum levels of acceptable performance
        c. Provides consumer with means to measure quality of care received (Hawkins & Thibodeau, 2002)
        d. Both generic and specific specialty standards exist

  e. Specialty groups have also developed standards, including: National Association of Pediatric Nurse Practitioners (NAPNAP), Association for Women's Health, Obstetric, and Neonatal Nurses (AWHONN)—formerly NAACOG

  f. PNP relevant standards of practice

   (1) American Nurses Association (ANA) Maternal-Child Health (MCH) Standards—first published in 1983

   (2) NAPNAP Standards—first published in 1987

   (3) AWHONN Standards

  g. Can be used to provide legal expectations of practice but were not designed to define standards of practice for clinical or legal purposes

2. Scope of practice

  a. Based on what is legally allowable in each State under its Nurse Practice Act

  b. Provides guidelines vs. specific mandates for nursing practice

  c. Is not mandated

  d. Varies widely from State to State (Hawkins & Tibodeau, 2002) and over time

  e. Often based on legal requirements within State and national standards

  f. NAPNAP first published Scope of Practice for PNPs in 1983 with updated statements published in 1990 and 2000

  g. Fluid and evolving (Hamric, Spross & Hanson (2000)

3. Nurse practice acts

  a. Authorizes Boards of Nursing in each State to establish statutory authority for licensure of registered nurse (RN)

  b. Authority includes use of title, authorization for scope of practice, and disciplinary grounds (Bosna, 1997)

  c. Evolves from statutory law which, after interpretation, becomes regulatory language

  d. NCSBN website—(http://www.nesbn.org) has full text state practice acts for 31 states

4. Clinical practice guidelines or protocols

  a. Definition: "Systematically developed statements to assist practitioner and patient about appropriate care for specific clinical outcomes" (IOM, 1990)

  b. Need/requirements for guidelines/protocol development

   (1) Standards for PNP practice include the collaborative development of appropriate pediatric protocols (NAPNAP, 1987)

   (2) Variable requirements depending on individual State nurse practice act and standards of practice

      (3) Protocol requirements may be met with recognized reference books and published clinical guidelines

  c. Examples of pediatric related practice guidelines for preventive care

      (1) Bright futures (MCHB)

      (2) Guidelines for Adolescent Preventive Services (AMA)

      (3) Guide to Clinical Preventive Services

  d. Examples of pediatric related practice guidelines for illness management

      (1) Asthma (NIH, AAP)

      (2) Hearing Screening (NIH, AAP)

      (3) HIV—Agency for Healthcare Research and Quality (AHRQ), formerly Agency for Health Care Policy and Research (AHCPR)

      (4) Otitis media with effusion (AHRQ)

      (5) Pain (AHRQ)

      (6) Sickle Cell disease (AHRQ)

- Regulation Of Advanced Nursing Practice

  1. Credentialing—regulatory mechanism(s) to insure accountability for competent practice

    a. Mandates accountability/responsibility for competent practice

    b. Validation of required education, licensure, and certification

    c. Necessary to assure public of safe health-care provided by qualified individuals

    d. Necessary to assure compliance with federal and State laws related to nursing practice

    e. Acknowledges APRN advanced scope of practice

    f. Should provide appropriate avenues for public or individual practice complaints

    g. Allows profession to be accountable to public and its members by enforcing professional standards for practice (Hickey, Ouimette, & Venegoni, 2000)

    h. Tension between certification bodies, State Boards of Nursing, and nursing education accrediting organizations regarding role and responsibility for credentialing intensified in the 1990s with the proliferation of NP programs

    i. National task force on quality nurse practitioner education convened in 1995 with broad-based representation

      (1) National Organization of Nurse Practitioner Faculties (NONPF)

(2)   American Academy of Nurse Practitioners (AANP)

(3)   American Association of Colleges of Nursing (AACN)

(4)   American Nurses Credentialing Center (ANCC)

(5)   National Association of Neonatal Nurses (NANN)

(6)   The National Association of Nurse Practitioners in Women's Health (NPWH) (formerly the National Association of Nurse Practitioners in Reproductive Health)

(7)   National Association of Pediatric Nurse Practitioners (NAPNAP)

(8)   National Certification Board for Pediatric Nurse Practitioners and Nurses (NCBPNPN)—Pediatric Nursing Certification Board (PNCB) as of 2003

(9)   National Certification Corporation (NCC)

(10) National League for Nursing (NLN)

(11) National League for Nursing Accrediting Commission (NLNAC)

j. Nurse practitioner credentialing remains within the domain of nongovernmental professional agencies with oversight of accreditation standards by the Nationsl Commission for Certifying Agencies (NCCA) http://www.noca.org/ncca/ncca.htm

k. NP credentialing currently available through NCCA recognized certifying agencies:

(1)   Pediatric Nursing Certification Board (PNCB)—formerly NCBPNPN
800 South Frederick Avenue, Suite 104
Gaithersburg, MD 20877-4250
(301-330-2921) (1-888-641-2767)

(a)   PNP

(b)   Pediatric acute care NP—in developmental stages

(2)   American Nurses Credentialing Center (ANCC)
600 Maryland Avenue, SW Suite 100 West,
Washington DC 20024-2572
(1-800-284-2378)

(a)   Adult Nurse Practitioners

(b)   Family Nurse Practitioners

(c)   Several types of other nurse practitioner specialties

(3)   American Academy of Nurse Practitioners (AANP)
Certification Administration
P.O. Box 12926
Austin, TX 78711
(512-442-4262)

      (a) Family Nurse Practitioners

      (b) Adult Nurse Practitioners

2. Certification

   a. Definition—process by which nongovernmental agency or association confirms that an individual licensed professional has met certain predetermined standards as specified by that profession for specialty practice

   b. Purpose—to assure the public that an individual has mastered a body of knowledge and acquired skills in a particular specialty

   c. May be required for State licensure and reimbursement

   d. Required for APRN practice in some states (Hickey, Ouimette, & Venegoni, 2000)

3. Prescriptive authority

   a. Some level of prescriptive authority for NP and Certified Nurse-Midwives (CNM) since mid-1970s

   b. As of 1998, all states have approved and/or implemented some degree of prescriptive authority; Illinois legislation passed with statutory authority pending

   c. Required pharmacology education within graduate program and continuing education to maintain authority—specific requirements vary by State

   d. Scope of prescriptive authority varies by State; full scope includes ability to obtain federal DEA registration number

4. Multi-state Nurse Licensure Compact

   a. Since 1998, 17 states have passed legislation to recognize nursing RN licensure among participating states.

   b. In 2000, Wisconsin became the first state to include advanced practice nurses within legislation on multi-state compacts

   c. NCSBN and NP stakeholders developed a position paper in 2000 to guide multistate recognition of APRN licenses/authority to practice

   d. http://www.ncsbn.org/regulation/nlc_licensure_aprn.asp

5. Clinical privileges

   a. Possibility of hospital staff membership opened to nonphysician providers by Joint Commission on Accreditation of Health Care Organizations (JCAHO) in 1983

   b. Current issue for APRN practice

- Practice Issues

   1. Collaborative practice

    a. Definition: ANA's *Nursing: A Social Policy Statement* (2003) describes collaboration as "true partnership" in which all players have and value power, recognize and accept separate and combined areas of responsibility and activity, and share common goals

    b. Purpose—to enhance quality of care and improve patient outcomes through ongoing continuity and coordination of care (Hickey, Ouimette, & Venegoni, 2000)

    c. Interdisciplinary teams—examples of collaborative practice

2. Case management

    a. Definition—"A collaborative process which assesses, plans, implements, coordinates, monitors, and evaluates options and services to meet an individual's health needs through communication and available resources to promote quality cost-effective outcomes." (Case Management Society of America, 1994)

    b. Purpose—to mobilize, monitor and control resources that patient uses over course of an illness while maintaining a balance between quality and cost (Hickey, Ouimette, & Venegoni, 2000)

    c. Components of role

        (1) Planning care for cost effectiveness and optimal outcomes

        (2) Procuring and coordinating care

        (3) Monitoring and evaluating outcomes

        (4) Performing physical assessments

        (5) Selecting laboratory and other tests

        (6) Prescribing medications (Hawkins & Thibodeau, 1999; Synder, 1999)

        (7) Requires that provider have strong communication skills and clinical expertise

        (8) Provides care along continuum, decreases fragmentation of services, enhances patient and family quality of life, and contains costs

    d. Key features associated with case management models:

        (1) Standardized appropriate use of resources aimed at identified outcomes within appropriate time frames

        (2) Promotes collaborative practice among disciplines

        (3) Promotes coordinated continuity of care over course of illness

        (4) Promotes job satisfaction for providers

        (5) Promotes patient and provider satisfaction with care delivery while minimizing cost to institution (Hickey, Ouimette, Venegoni, 2000)

    e. Populations appropriate for case management

        (1) Those for whom course of treatment is costly and unpredictable

    (2) Those who experience frequent or chronic readmissions to hospital

    (3) Those involved with multiple providers or multiple disciplines (Hickey, Ouimette, & Venegoni, 2000)

3. Quality improvement (QI)

    a. Definition—Organized creation of beneficial change...the attainment of unprecedented levels of performance (Juran, 1999)

    b. Alternative terms—Total Quality Management (TQM); Continuous Quality Improvement (CQI); differs from Quality Assurance (QA) in being continuous rather than episodic process

    c. Systematic, organized structures, processes, and expected outcomes focus on defining excellence and assuring accountability for quality of care

    d. Provides framework for ongoing evaluation of practice through identification of norms, criteria, and standards that measure program effectiveness and minimize liablity

    e. QI mechanisms and strategies

        (1) Peer review

            (a) Recognize and reward nursing practice

            (b) Leads to higher standards practice

            (c) Discourages practice beyond scope of legal authority

            (d) Improves quality of care (Cherry & Jacob, 2002)

            (e) Provides for accountability and responsibility

        (2) Other methods of evaluation

            (a) Audit—retrospective measurement of quality

            (b) Interviews and questionnaires

            (c) Patient satisfaction surveys or interviews

4. Risk management

    a. Systems and activities designed to recognize and intervene to decrease risk of injury to patients and subsequent claims against healthcare providers; based on assumption that many injuries to patients are preventable

    b. Evaluates sources of legal liability in practice such as:

        (1) Patients

        (2) Procedures

        (3) Quality of record keeping

    c. Areas of liability risk

        (1) Practitioner-client relationship

       (2)   Communication and informed consent

       (3)   Clinical expertise

       (4)   Self-evaluation by professionals of need to stay current

       (5)   Documentation

       (6)   Consultation and referral

       (7)   Policies, procedures, and protocols

       (8)   Supervision of others

   d.   Includes educational activities that decrease risk in identified areas

5. Malpractice

   a.   Professional misconduct, unreasonable lack of skill; infidelity in professional or fiduciary duties; illegal, immoral conduct resulting in patient harm

   b.   Alleged professional failure to render services with degree of care, diligence and precaution that another member of same profession in similar circumstances would render to prevent patient injury

   c.   Malpractice insurance

       (1)   Does not protect APRN from charges of practicing medicine without a license if APRN is practicing outside legal scope of practice for that State

       (2)   National Practitioner Data Bank collects information on adverse actions against health care practitioners, including nurses

       (3)   Types of coverage

           (a)   Occurrence coverage—covers malpractice event which occurred during policy period, regardless of date of discovery or when claim filed

           (b)   Claims made coverage—covers only claims filed during policy coverage period, regardless of when event occurred; optional tail coverage contract extends the coverage of a claims made policy into the future to cover all claims filed after the basic claims made coverage period

6. Negligence—failure of individual to do what a reasonable person would do that results in injury to another

7. Reimbursement

Whether working independently, sharing a joint practice with a physician, or practicing within a hospital, or managed care system, APRNs must be reimbursed appropriately. Standards that determine private pay insurance mechanisms are often modeled after federal policies such as Medicaid and Medicare. However, even when the federal government establishes mandates that encourage direct payment of nonphysi-

cian healthcare providers, barriers to reimbursement are often encountered in State level rules and regulations
(Hamric, 2000)

a. Medicaid

    (1) Authorized in 1965 as Title XIX of Social Security Act

    (2) Federal/State matching program with federal oversight

    (3) Financed through federal and State taxes, with between 50% and 83% of total Medicaid costs covered by federal government

    (4) Does not cover all people below federal poverty level, but State Medicaid programs are required by federal government to cover certain categories such as:

        (a) Recipients of Aid to Families with Dependent Children (AFDC)—States set own eligibility requirements for AFDC

        (b) People over 65, blind, or totally disabled who are eligible for cash assistance under federal Supplemental Security Income (SSI) program

        (c) Pregnant women (for pregnancy-related services only) and children under six with family incomes up to 133% of federal poverty level

        (d) Children born after September 1983 in families whose income is at or below federal poverty level

    (5) States can choose to cover "medically needy"

    (6) Coverage required for certain services

        (a) Hospital and physician services

        (b) Laboratory and radiographic services

        (c) Nursing home and home health care services

        (d) Prenatal and preventive services

        (e) Medically necessary transportation

    (7) States can add services to list and can place certain limitations on federally mandated services

    (8) Although Medicaid recipients cannot be billed for services, States can impose nominal copayments or deductibles for certain services (Bodenheimer, 2002)

b. Medicare

    (1) Federally mandated program established in 1965, provides health insurance for aged and disabled individuals

(2) Eligibility covers hospital service, physician services, and other medical services

(3) Income level does not impact eligibility

(4) Medicare Part A

    (a) Those 65 years of age and older who are eligible for Social Security are automatically enrolled, whether or not they are retired—persons are eligible for Social Security when they (or their spouses) have paid into Social Security system through employment for 40 quarters or more

    (b) Those who have paid into system for less than 40 quarters can enroll in Medicare Part A by paying monthly premium

    (c) Those who are under age 65 and are totally and permanently disabled may enroll in Medicare Part A after receiving Social Security disability benefits for 24 months

    (d) Those with chronic renal disease requiring dialysis or transplant may also be eligible for Part A without a two year waiting period

    (e) Services covered include some hospitalization costs; some skilled nursing facility costs, although custodial care is not covered; home health care—100% for skilled care; 80% of approved amount for medical equipment; and hospice care—100% for most services

    (f) Payment for hospitalization is based on projected costs of caring for patient with given problem—each Medicare patient admitted to a hospital is classified according to a diagnosis-related group (DRG); the hospital is then paid a predetermined amount for each patient admitted with the given DRG, if hospital costs are above payment rate, the hospital must absorb loss; if costs are below payment rate, hospital allowed to keep a percentage of excess

    (g) APRN not paid directly for services delivered in a hospital

(5) Medicare Part B—Supplementary Medical Insurance (SMI)

    (a) Monthly premium is charged

    (b) Some-low income people are eligible to have monthly premium paid by Medicaid

    (c) Financed by general federal revenues and by Part B monthly premiums

    (d) Covers all medically necessary services—80% of an approved amount after annual deductible; includes physician services, physical, occupational, and speech therapy; medical equipment and diagnostic tests, and some preventative care such as Pap tests, mammograms, hepatitis B, pneumococcal and influenza vaccines can be included in medical expenses

c. APRN—Medicaid/Medicare coverage

    (1) Omnibus Budget Reconciliation Act (OBRA) 1989—mandated Medicaid reimbursement for certified pediatric and family nurse practitioners began July 1, 1990; providers required to practice within the scope of State law and do not have to be under supervision or associated with a physician or other provider

        (a) Level of payment determined by States—reimbursement rates range from 70% to 100% of fee-for-service physician Medicaid rate (Pearson, 2003)

        (b) Pediatric and family nurse practitioners may bill Medicaid directly after attaining provider number from State Medicaid agency

        (c) States can elect to pass laws allowing them to extend Medicaid payment to other types of NP not identified in federal statutes

    (2) Legislation (1997) has expanded direct Medicare reimbursement for APRN in all geographic locations

        (a) APRN reimbursement at 85% of physician fee schedule when billing independently using APRN billing number; direct physician supervision not required

        (b) When APRN is employed by physician, the physician practice may receive 100% of customary physician charge, according to "Incident to" rules (Buppert, 1998)

        (c) APRN must be RN currently licensed to practice in the State in which services are rendered; must meet requirements for NP practice in State in which services are rendered; must be currently certified as a primary care NP; must have successfully completed a formal advanced practice educational program of at least one academic year that includes at least four months of classroom instruction and awards a degree, diploma, or certificate OR, have successfully completed a formal advanced practice educational program and have been performing in that expanded role for at least 12 months during the 18-month period immediately preceding February 8, 1978, the effective date for the provision of services of NP as reflected in the conditions for certification for rural health clinics

        (d) NP covered services are limited to services an NP is legally authorized to perform under the State law in which the NP practices and must meet training, educational and experience requirements prescribed by the Secretary of Health and Human Services

(3) NP services covered under Part B if service would be considered physician's services if furnished by MD or Doctor of Osteopathy (DO); if NP is legally authorized to perform services in the state in which they are performed; if services are performed in collaboration with MD/DO (collaboration specified as a process whereby NP works with physician to deliver health care within scope of NP expertise with medical direction and appropriate supervision as provided for in jointly developed guidelines or other mechanisms defined by federal regulations and law of the state in which services are performed); and services are otherwise precluded from coverage because of one of the statutory exclusions

(4) "Incident to" refers to services provided as an integral, yet incidental, part of the physician's personal, professional services in the course of diagnosis or treatment of injury or illness—these services must occur under direct personal supervision of a physician, and the APRN must be an employee of the physician group; services must occur during the course of treatment where the physician performs an initial service and subsequent services in a manner that reflects the physician's active participation and management of the course of treatment—direct personal supervision does not mean that the physician must be in the same room as the APRN, however, the physician must be present in the office suite and available for assistance and direction while the APRN provides patient care (Buppert, 1998)

(5) When APRN performs "incident to" service in physician's office, billing must be submitted to Medicare by employing physician, under the physician's name, provider number and CPT code—payment is made at full physician rate and is paid to physician or physician practice

(6) When APRN provides service in skilled nursing facility, or nursing facility located in urban area as defined by law, Medicare payment can be obtained—medicare reimbursement is also available for APRN services in skilled nursing facilities (SNF) in nonrural areas on a reasonable charge basis; this amount may not exceed physician fee schedule amount for service and payment is made to the APRN's employer

(7) Centers for Medicare and Medicaid Services (CMS)

    (a) Formerly Health Care Financing & Administration (HCFA)

    (b) Oversight of several federal programs including Medicare, Medicaid, State children's health insurance program (SCHIP), HIPPA and CLIA

    (c) Website: http://cms.hhs.gov

d. Other third party payors

(1) Private insurer reimbursement is contract specific per State insurance commission

(2) Civilian Health and Medical Program of the United States (CHAMPUS)

(a) Federal health plan for military personnel, including surviving dependents, families, and retirees

(b) APRN reimbursement for services

(3) Federal Employees Health Benefit Program (FEHBP)

(a) One of largest employer sponsored group health insurance programs

(b) APRN recognized as designated health care provider

e. Methods of payment for advanced practice nurses

(1) Fee-for-service model

(a) Unit of payment by visit or procedure

(b) Can occur with utilization review in which case payor has right to authorize or deny payment of expensive medical interventions such as hospital admission, extra hospital days, and surgery

(2) Episodic model

(a) One sum is paid for all services delivered during a given illness

(b) DRG fee payment

(3) Capitation model, PPO, and HMO are covered in section on Managed Care in this chapter

- Professional Organizations

1. Purpose and benefits

a. Establish practice standards

b. Collective voice to promote nursing and quality of care

c. Monitor and influence policy and legislative initiatives

d. Position papers on practice issues

e. Disseminate information

2. Examples

a. American Nurses Association (ANA)

b. National Association of Pediatric Nurse Practitioners (NAPNAP)

c. National Conference of Gerontological Nurse Practitioners

d. National Organization of Nurse Practitioner Faculties (NONPF)

e. American Academy of Nurse Practitioners (AANP)

f. American College of Nurse Practitioners (ACNP)

g. Nurse Practitioner Associates for Continuing Education (NPACE)

h. National Association of School Nurses

    i.   Association for Women's Health, Obstetrics, and Neonatal Nurses (AWHONN)

    j.   The National Association of Nurse Practitioners in Women's Health (NPWH) (formerly the National Association of Nurse Practitioners in Reproductive Health [NANPRH])

- Research in Advanced Practice: "Practice-based research is essential to the development of advanced practice nursing for the future." (NONPF, 1995, p. 84)

    1.   Major trend is outcome studies

    2.   Sources of federal funding

        a.   Agency for Healthcare Research and Quality (AHRQ)

            (1)   Formerly the Agency for Health Care Policy and Research (AHCPR)

            (2)   *http://www.ahcpr.gov/*

        b.   National Institutes of Health (NIH)

            (1)   Includes the National Institute for Nursing Research (NINR)

            (2)   *http://www.nih.gov/*

        c.   Maternal and Child Health Bureau (MCHB)

            (1)   Functions within Health Resources and Services Administration (HRSA)

            (2)   *http://www.mchb.hrsa.gov/*

    3.   Sources of research findings

        a.   Conferences

        b.   Scholarly publications

        c.   Distribution of summaries of research studies (Hawkins & Thibodeau, 1996)

    4.   Use of research in practice setting

        a.   Develop research-based clinical pathways

        b.   Track clinical outcomes and variances

        c.   Demonstrate quality and cost effectiveness of care

        d.   Give structure to demonstration projects

        e.   Persuade lawmakers of NP value and contributions in today's health care system

        f.   Improve quality and patient outcomes

    5.   Benefit of research for patients

        a.   Provides thorough understanding of patient situation

        b.   Provides more accurate assessment of situations

        c.   Increases effectiveness of interventions

    d. Increases provider sensitivity to patient situations

    e. Assists providers to more accurately determine need for and effectiveness of interventions (Hickey, Ouimette, & Venegoni, 2000)

6. Barriers to research utilization

    a. Time and cost of conducting research studies

    b. Resistance to change in work setting

    c. Lack of rewards for using research findings

    d. Lack of understanding or uncertainty regarding research outcomes (Hickey, Ouimette, & Venegoni, 2000)

7. Strategies to overcome barriers to research utilization

    a. Creation of organizational culture that values and uses research

    b. Creation of environment where questions are encouraged, critical thinking is appreciated, and nursing care is evaluated

    c. Support for research through time allocation and financial commitment (Hickey, Ouimette & Venegoni, 2000)

Health Policy

- Policy Influences

    1. Healthy People 2000

        a. Published in 1990 by U.S. Department of Health and Human Services; mid-course review of progress published in 1995; subsequent review of progress published in December 1999

        b. Purpose—committed nation to obtain three broad goals

           (1) Increase span of healthy life for all Americans

           (2) Reduce health disparities among Americans

           (3) Achieve access to preventive services for all Americans (DHHS, 1990)

        c. Contained 300 specific objectives based on 22 priority areas leading to socially and economically productive lives

        d. Objectives focused on equal access, acceptability, availability, continuity, cost and quality of care

        e. Objectives organized within broad categories of health promotion, health protection, and preventive services

        f. Identified priority of systematic collection, analysis, interpretation, dissemination, and use of data to understand national health status and plan effective prevention programs

        g. Individuals, communities and organizations were responsible for determining how they would achieve the goals by the year 2000 (Hickey, Ouimette & Venegoni, 1996)

h. Progress (1998–1999) towards meeting Healthy People 2000 goals

    (1) Fifteen percent of objectives met in areas of nutrition, maternal and child health, heart disease and mental health

        (a) There were 17 maternal\infant health objectives; progress made on 8 of the 17 including

            (i) Perinatal/infant mortality—although U.S. ranks 25th among industrialized countries for infant mortality

            (ii) Screening for fetal abnormalities and genetic disorders

        (b) No progress on four or movement away on five of the target goals for problems including fetal alcohol syndrome and low birth weight

    (2) Forty-four percent of objectives, including those related to childhood immunizations, breast feeding, regular dental visits, mammography screening and consumption of fruits and vegetables per day are proceeding on track (DHHS, 1999)

2. Healthy People 2010

    a. Released in 2000 by U.S. Department of Health and Human Services

    b. Builds on initiatives set in Healthy People 2000

    c. Purpose—designed to achieve two broad-based goals

        (1) Increase quality and years of healthy life

        (2) Eliminate health disparities

    d. Contains 467 objectives with twenty-eight focus areas

    e. Objectives focus on partnering for health improvements; eliminating health disparities; increasing quality and years of healthy living; and harnessing technology for health

    f. Objectives categorized into the following focus areas

        (1) Physical activity and fitness

        (2) Nutrition

        (3) Tobacco use

        (4) Educational\community-based programs

        (5) Environmental health

        (6) Food Safety

        (7) Injury\violence prevention

        (8) Occupational safety and health

    (9)   Oral health

   (10)   Access to quality health services

   (11)   Family planning

   (12)   Maternal, infant and child health—fetal, infant, child and adolescent deaths; maternal deaths and illnesses; prenatal care; obstetrical care; risk factors; developmental disabilities and neural tube defects; prenatal substance exposure; breastfeeding, newborn screening and service systems for children with special health care needs

   (13)   Medical products safety

   (14)   Public health infrastructures

   (15)   Health communication

   (16)   Prevention and health promotion

   (17)   Disability and secondary conditions

   (18)   Heart disease and stroke

   (19)   Kidney disease

   (20)   Mental health and mental disorders

   (21)   Respiratory diseases

   (22)   Sexually transmitted diseases

   (23)   Substance abuse

g. Ten ''leading health indicators'' (LHI)—physical activity; overweight and obesity; tobacco use; substance abuse; responsible sexual behavior; mental health; injury and violence; environmental quality; immunizations; access to health care

h. Written for States and communities to tailor health objectives to their specific needs (DHHS, 1999)

    (http://www.healthypeople.gov)

3. Prevention guidelines

   a. ''Put Prevention Into Practice''—campaign established by U.S. Public Health Service to enhance delivery of preventive care in primary care practice

   b. *Clinicians Handbook of Preventive Services: Put Prevention Into Practice,* (1998)—provides practical and comprehensive reference on preventive services to primary care providers including:

    (1)   Health screening schedules for early disease detection and immunization

    (2)   Disease prophylaxis issues

    (3)   Risk factor counselling techniques

(4) Educational resources on preventive care (Hickey, Ouimette & Venegoni, 2000)

http://www.ahcpr.gov/clinic/ppiphand.htm

c. *Guide to Clinical Preventive Services* (U.S. Preventive Services Task Force, 1996) presents national clinical preventive services guidelines for practice and educational settings

(1) Age and gender specific

(2) Suggests targeted examinations, immunizations and health counseling that should be part of periodic health visits

4. Nursing's Agenda for Health Care Reform (ANA, 1991)

a. Supports creation of a health care system that assures access, quality, and services at affordable costs

b. Supports ongoing primary care

c. Calls for basic core of essential health services to be available to all, and for restructured health care system focusing on consumers and their health and health care delivery in familiar, convenient sites

d. Proposes shift from focus on illness and cure to orientation on wellness and caring

e. Supports provisions for long-term care and insurance reforms to assure improved access to coverage

f. Calls for establishment of public/private sector review of resource allocations, cost reduction plans, and fair and consistent reimbursement for all providers

• Utilization of Health Policy

1. Shifting trend toward primary care and early preventive measures; supports need for APRN

2. Four major factors influencing health care delivery services

a. Payors—individual health care consumers, businesses that pay for health insurance for employees, and government through public programs and entitlement programs such as Medicare and Medicaid

b. Insurers—take money from payors, assume risks, and pay providers

c. Providers—includes hospitals, physicians, nurses, APRN, physician assistants, pharmacies, home health agencies, and long term care facilities

d. Suppliers—pharmaceutical and medical supply industries

3. Legislative strategies and political involvement

a. Professional organizations monitor policy issues and keep membership informed—e.g., NAPNAP legislative newsletter

b. Local networks of APRN develop practice guidelines and advocate for policies to enhance practice

- Types of Health Care Delivery Systems

1. Primary health care

   a. Definition: "Primary care is the provision of integrated, accessible health care services by clinicians who are accountable for addressing a large majority of personal health care needs, developing a sustained partnership with patients, and practicing in the context of family and community (Institute of Medicine, Committee on Future of Primary Care, 1994)"

   b. Activities and/or functions define boundaries of primary care, such as curing or alleviating common illnesses and disabilities

   c. Entry point to a system that includes access to secondary and tertiary care

   d. Attributes include care that is accessible, comprehensive, coordinated, continuous, and accountable

   e. Strategy for organizing health care system as a whole; gives priority and allocates resources to community-based rather than hospital-based care

   f. Categories of primary care providers (PCP) and nature of care

      (1) Medical specialties—family medicine, general internal medicine, general pediatrics, obstetrics and gynecology as specified in the Clinton administration's Health Security Act

      (2) Other experts have included NP and physician assistants (PA) as primary care providers (PCP)

   g. Many definitions stress self-responsibility for health (Hickey, Ouimette, & Venegoni, 2000)

2. Managed care

   a. Definition: "An integrated network that combines financing and delivery of health care services to covered individuals." (Mahn & Spross, 1996, pg. 446)

      (1) Network connects consumers, sponsors, providers, and third party payors

      (2) Initial managed care organization was Kaiser Health Plan (California) established in 1930s (Bodenheimer, 2002)

   b. Objectives

      (1) Manage use and price of health care delivery system

      (2) Control type, level and frequency of treatment

      (3) Restrict level of reimbursement for services

   c. Type of health insurance plan designed to control costs while assuring quality care

   d. Obligation to manage is shared among providers, consumers and payers

      (1) Providers no longer dictate price of care delivery; must assume more financial risk for population assigned to them for care

      (2) Consumers have fewer choices of coverage, providers and greater financial responsibility

      (3) Payors manage health care dollars through benefit design, selective contracting, and shifting financial risk to providers (Hickey, Ouimette, & Venegoni, 2000)

   e. Types of managed care plans

      (1) Health Maintenance Organizations (HMO)

         (a) Most common type

         (b) By 1994, enrollment at 52 million (20.3% of population)

         (c) Offer pre-established benefit package—including preventive, inpatient and outpatient care

         (d) HMO contracts with providers to provide care to enrollees

         (e) Providers at financial risk resulting in incentive to provide high quality, cost effective care

         (f) Enrollees select a primary care provider (PCP) who manages total care by authorizing specialty visits, hospitalization, and other services

         (g) PCP may be MD, APRN or PA providers; serving as "gatekeepers"

      (2) Preferred Provider Organizations (PPO)

         (a) Compromised managed care option that is alternative between indemnity and HMO insurance

         (b) Uses financial incentives to influence consumer and provider behaviors

         (c) Refers to variety of arrangements between insurers, providers, and third-party payers rather than standard plan

         (d) Often owned by large insurance companies such as Prudential, Travelers and Aetna

         (e) Available primarily to employed commercial population

      (3) Point of Service Plans (POS)

         (a) Consumers decide whether to use a provider network, or seek care outside the network

        (b)   If variation of HMO plan, PCP coordinates care for enrollees; if variation of PPO plan, enrollees may choose lower cost options outside of provider network

        (c)   Most rapidly growing type of managed care

    (4) Integrated delivery systems

        (a)   Vertical integration of services across levels of care into seamless system with improved access for enrollees

        (b)   Capitated payment—financial risk shifts from payor to provider; unit of value is cost per member per month (PMPM); providers receive age and sex adjusted budget to cover services to maintain wellness of specific target population

        (c)   Emphasis on provision of appropriate but not unlimited care with financial benefit of keeping population healthy through systematic preventive services

f.   Reimbursement under managed care

    (1) Providers accept financial risk for care provided to specific population of enrollees

    (2) Capitated payment

        (a)   Provider receives payment in advance

        (b)   Payment level reflects expected utilization by enrolled population for which provider is responsible

    (3) Provider must control volume and cost

    (4) Efficiency usually rewarded through bonus payments for operating within budget and meeting goals for quality and efficiency

g.   Monitoring, evaluation and accreditation in managed care

    (1) Health plan employer data and information set (HEDIS)—provides quality measures and compares with benchmark standards and goals

    (2) National committee for quality assurance (NCQA)

        (a)   Major accreditation body for managed care organizations

        (b)   Standards in six critical areas are evaluated—quality management, utilization management, credentialing, preventive health services, medical records, members rights/responsibilities

    (3) NCQA reported reviews of 30% of the 554 HMOs in the U.S. as of 1995; 31% received full accreditation; 56% received one year or provisional accreditation; 12% were denied accreditation (Mischler & Quinn, 1995)

h.   Challenges and opportunities of managed care for APRN

    (1) Need for balance between quality of care and costs inherent in diagnosis/management per client visit

        (a) Educational programs must incorporate managed care content into curriculum

        (b) APRN must combine strong clinical and financial skills to determine cost of providing care to target population

        (c) Success in managed care environment requires systems-thinking skill to complement primary care skills; blended NP/CNS models may provide this necessary linkage with added focus on case management, utilitization/resource management, quality improvement, and client education/advocacy within systems of care

    (2) APRN strategies for success within evolving managed care environment

        (a) Determine strategies to increase efficiency without sacrificing quality of client-provider interactions; e.g., group well-child visits

        (b) Lobby for APN inclusion on provider panels

        (c) Maintain partnerships with APRN educational programs for collaborative study and documentation of APRN effectiveness

- Health Insurance Portability and Accountability Act of 1996 (HIPPA)

  1. Health Insurance Reform—addresses preexisting conditions and provides portability of health insurance when an employee changes or loses their job

  2. Administrative simplification

    a. Electronic transactions and code set standards

    b. Unique identifiers

    c. Privacy

    d. Security

  3. Centers for Medicare & Medicaid Services (CMS) responsible for oversight and compliace with administrative simplification mandates except for Privacy provisions which is iverseen by the Office of Civil Rights (OCR)

  4. Target dates for implementation and compliance with Administrative Simplification

    a. Electronic transactions & code set standards—October 2003

    b. Unique identifiers—July 2004

    c. Privacy—April 2003

    d. Security—April 2005

    e. Small health plans have an additional year for full compliance for unique identifiers, privacy, and security provisions

5. "Covered entities"
   a. Health plans
   b. Health care clearinghouses
   c. Health care providers who conduct any electronic transitions of health related information

6. Website information
   a. CMS website www.cms.hhs.gov/hipaa/hipaa2
   b. OCR website www.hhs.gov/ocr/hipaa

Questions
Select the best answer

1. If the two broad-based goals of Healthy People 2010 are met, the nation will:

   a. Increase quality of healthy, years of healthy life span and eliminate health disparities
   b. Increase healthy life span, increase access and improve economics related to health for all Americans
   c. Increase healthy life span, reduce health disparities, and improve economics related to the health of all Americans
   d. Reduce health disparities, increase access to health care services and make life more socially acceptable for all Americans

2. Which of the following objectives from Healthy People 2000 has not made progress towards achieving its targeted goal?

   a. Low birth weight
   b. Infant mortality
   c. Fetal mortality
   d. Screening for genetic disorders

3. Preventive health guidelines include references to:

   a. Immunizations, health screening, disease prophylaxis, education and infection control
   b. Immunizations, counseling, health screening, disease prophylaxis and education
   c. Health screening, disease prophylaxis, counseling and CPR
   d. Health screening, disease prophylaxis, education, immunizations and CPR

4. Nursing's Agenda for Health Care Reform:

   a. Is supportive of equal access, cost effective, high quality care
   b. Is a mandate to all nurses in the U.S.
   c. Is a summary of nursing research related to health care reform
   d. Is a report of the status of nursing in the 1990s

5. The nurse practitioner role was initially established to:

   a. Improve access to care and partially solve physician shortage
   b. Reduce the nursing shortage and improve access to care
   c. Improve working conditions of nurses while improving access to care
   d. Improve nursing's image through expansion of the role

6. Early nursing research focused on:

   a. The response of policy makers to the nursing shortage
   b. The effectiveness of the NP as a primary care giver
   c. An effort to demonstate quality and cost effectiveness of NP
   d. The role of the NP as a physician extender

7. Which of the following is not a major factor influencing health care delivery services?

    a. Provider
    b. Payors
    c. Insurers
    d. Agencies

8. All definitions of primary health care include:

    a. The concept of universal access and accountability
    b. The concept of universal access and AIDS prevention
    c. The concept of universal access and a focus on self-responsibility for health
    d. The concept of universal access and a focus on reimbursement for services rendered

9. Standards of practice are:

    a. Authoritative statements used to measure quality
    b. Used to measure outcome but are not authoritative
    c. Designed for legal purposes
    d. Not designed for legal purposes and cannot be used to measure quality

10. Quality improvement activities include:

    a. Patient satisfaction surveys only
    b. Peer review, patient satisfaction surveys, chart audits
    c. Defining four practice domains
    d. Systems to decrease risk of injury to patients

11. Most risk management programs are based on the assumption that:

    a. Many injuries to patients are preventable
    b. Most legal liability is a result of poor documentation
    c. Most injuries to patients are not preventable
    d. Malpractice insurance is generally unnecessary

12. If an APRN practices beyond his/her scope:

    a. Malpractice insurance will protect him/her from a charge of practicing medicine without a license
    b. Malpractice insurance will not protect him/her from a charge of practicing medicine without a license
    c. He or she is legally accountable to the certifying body
    d. The collaborating physician is legally accountable to the certifying body

13. Standards of practice may be used to:

    a. Establish minimal levels of performance
    b. Establish reimbursement schemes for APRN
    c. Mandate nursing practice across the nation
    d. Mandate nursing practice in certain States

14. Scope of practice:

    a. Is identical across the States
    b. Is determined by the federal government
    c. Is mandated by the federal government
    d. Varies from State to State

15. Medicaid provides health insurance coverage to:

    a. Certain categories of people whose personal income falls below the federal poverty level
    b. Anyone whose personal income falls below the federal poverty level
    c. Newborns, pregnant women and those over 65 whose personal income falls below the federal poverty level
    d. Those who are elderly

16. Medicaid reimbursement is available to an APRN:

    a. Practicing in federally designated areas
    b. At a rate that is between 70% and 100% of the physician rate
    c. Only if the APRN is in collaborative practice with a physician
    d. Practicing in nursing homes only

17. Medicare reimbursement for services:

    a. Is not dependent on the patient's income level
    b. Depends on the patient's income level
    c. Is not available to APRN under any circumstances
    d. Is only available to APRN who is in collaborative practice with a physician

18. Medicare Part A covers:

    a. Hospital, skilled nursing facility, and hospice care
    b. All medically necessary services
    c. Skilled nursing facility care only
    d. Hospice care only

19. Medicare Part B covers:

    a. All medically necessary services
    b. Inpatient hospital care
    c. Outpatient physician services only
    d. Skilled nursing facility and hospice care

20. To receive Medicare reimbursement, APRN must:

    a. Be nationally certified and maintain prescriptive privileges
    b. Maintain a current license in the State in which they are practicing
    c. Practice in a designated medically underserved area
    d. Practice with a physician

21. The term "incident to" refers to:

    a. The occasions when an APRN practices independently but occasionally consults with a physician
    b. The notion that the physician must be present in the office suite and immediately available to provide assistance in order for the APRN to bill for services rendered
    c. The notion that a physician must examine the patient along with the APRN if Medicare is to be billed for services rendered
    d. Medicaid only and is not pertinent to Medicare billing

22. "Incident to" billing is specific to:

    a. Medicare
    b. Medicaid
    c. Medicare and Medicaid
    d. Private insurance companies

23. The Civilian Health and Medical Program of the United States (CHAMPUS):

    a. Is a federal health plan which covers health care for military personnel and their families and recognizes APRN as reimbursable provider
    b. Is a federal health plan which covers health care for military personnel and recognizes APRN as reimbursable provider
    c. Is a federal health plan which covers health care for military personnel and their families but does not recognize APRN as reimbursable provider
    d. Only covers hospital expenses of military personnel and their families

24. The knowledge base of the APRN is based on:

    a. Medical content
    b. Theoretical content only
    c. Scientific content and theory
    d. Theory and research

25. The role of the APRN has traditionally focused on:

    a. The delivery of primary health care to all people
    b. The delivery of acute health care to all people
    c. Chronic care
    d. The medical model

26. The nurse practitioner role began:

    a. With the establishment of a pediatric nurse practitioner program in an effort to expand the role of the registered nurse in order to meet the needs of the children of the nation
    b. As a result of the new entitlement programs, Medicare and Medicaid
    c. When it was evident that the medical schools across the U.S. could not prepare enough family practitioners to meet the nation's need
    d. As an experimental program at Duke University Medical Center

27. Legal authority for APRN practice is granted by:

    a. Federal law
    b. Regulations from the Department of Health and Human Services
    c. State law and regulations
    d. The Board of Medicine in most States

28. Direct reimbursement to APRN has resulted in:

    a. Increased access to cost-effective, quality primary care
    b. Increased malpractice claims against APRN
    c. Decreased consumer choice of health care providers
    d. Proliferation of APRN in independent practice

29. Malpractice insurance:

    a. Protects an APRN from charges of practicing medicine without a license when they are practicing outside the legal scope of practice
    b. Does not protect an APRN from charges of practicing medicine without a license when they are practicing outside the legal scope of practice
    c. Does not pay for legal defense if the APRN is practicing beyond the legal scope of practice
    d. Is important, but should not be purchased if the facility in which the APRN is employed carries good coverage

30. Collaborative practice:

    a. Limits autonomy and not reasonable in current managed care environment
    b. Will enhance quality of care and improve patient outcomes
    c. Will limit consumer choice of providers
    d. Excludes the concept of interdisciplinary teams

31. Case management:

    a. Balances quality and cost of patient care
    b. Has not been found to be cost effective
    c. Decreases the autonomy of the APRN
    d. Is rarely used today

32. The major trend in health policy research today is:

    a. Outcome studies
    b. Primary care studies
    c. Studies that compare practice strategies of MD and NP
    d. Studies that compare patient satisfaction with care delivered by MD versus NP

33. Current prescriptive authority for APRN:

    a. Varies among the States
    b. Is fairly consistent among the States

    c. Provides DEA numbers for APRN

    d. Allows APRN to move freely from State to State

34. Managed care is a term that describes:

    a. An established system of health care delivery that is mandated by the federal government

    b. A network of providers who contract to provide services for a specific group of enrollees

    c. A system that does not recognize APRN as a primary provider

    d. A network of hospitals and nursing homes that provide care to chronically ill people

35. Certification is:

    a. A procedure through which the government appraises and grants certification to the APRN

    b. Granted by the individual States

    c. Governed by each State's Board of Nursing

    d. A process in which a non-governmental agency or group verifies that an APRN has met certain predetermined standards for specialty practice

36. Licensure:

    a. Is a federal process that is used to standardize health care facilities

    b. Is granted by a State government agency and grants permission to engage in the practice of a given profession

    c. Cannot be used to prohibit anyone from practicing a given profession

    d. Is a federal process that is used to standardize educational programs

37. Reimbursement under managed care:

    a. Requires that the provider accept the financial risk for the care provided to a specific population of enrolled patients

    b. Requires that the managed care organization accept the financial risk for the care provided to a specific population of enrolled patients

    c. Does not reward efficient care delivery

    d. Is not available to APRN

38. An integrated delivery system:

    a. Is one that delivers high quality care but is often not cost effective

    b. Delivers a vertical integration of services with capitated payment

    c. Does not include rationing of resources

    d. Does not include a capitated payment scheme

Answers

1. a	14. d	27. c
2. a	15. a	28. a
3. b	16. b	29. b
4. a	17. a	30. b
5. a	18. a	31. a
6. c	19. a	32. a
7. d	20. b	33. a
8. a	21. b	34. b
9. a	22. a	35. d
10. b	23. a	36. b
11. a	24. c	37. a
12. b	25. a	38. b
13. a	26. a	

Bibliography

American Association of Colleges of Nursing. (1996). *The essentials of master's education for advanced practice nursing.* Washington DC: AACN

American Nureses Association. (2003). *Nursing's social policy statement* (2nd ed.(. Washington, DC: American Nurses Publishing

American Nurses Association. (1991). Nursing's agenda for healthcare reform. Washington, DC: American Nurses Publishing

Association of Faculties of Pediatric Nurse Practitioner and Associate Programs. (1996). Philosophy, conceptual model, terminal competencies for the education of pediatric nurse practitioners. Cherry Hill, NJ: NAPNAP.

Bodenheimer, T. S. (2002). *Understanding health policy: A clinical approach. (3rd. ed.).* NY: McGraw-Hill.

Bosna, J. (1997). Using nurse practitioner certification for state nursing regulation: An update. *The Nurse Practitioner: The American Journal of Primary Health Care, 22*(6), 213–216.

Buppert, C. (1998). Reimbursement for nurse practitioner services. *The Nurse Practitioner: The American Journal of Primary Health Care, 23*(1), 67–81.

Cady, A. F. (2003). *The advanced practice nurse's legal handbook. Philadelphia: Lippincott Williams & Wilkins.*

Case Management Society of America. (2002). *CMSA's standards of practice for case management revised 2002.* Little Rock, AR: Case Management Society of America.

Cherry, B., & Jacob, S. R. (2002). *Contemporary nursing: Issues, trends and management* (2nd ed.). St. Louis: Mosby.

Hamric, A. B., Spross, J. A., & Hanson, C. M. (2000). *Advanced practice nursing: An integrative approach* (2nd ed.). Philadelphia: W. B. Saunders.

Hardy Havens, D. M., Ronan, J. P., & Hannan, C. (1996). Maintaining the nurse practitioner identity in a world of managed care. *Journal of Pediatric Health Care, 10,* 86–88.

Hawkins, J. W., & Thibodeau, J. A. (2002). *The advanced practice nurse: Current issues* (5th ed.). NY: Tiresias Press.

Hickey, J. V., Ouimette, R. M., & Venegoni, S. L. (2000). *Advanced practice nursing: Changing roles and clinical applications* (2nd ed.). Philadelphia: J. B. Lippincott, Williams & Wilkins.

IOM. (1990). *Clinical practice guidelines: Directions for a new program.* Washington, DC: National Academy Press.

Juran, M. (1999). *Juran's quality handbook* (5th ed.). New York: McGraw Hill.

Mezey, M. D., & McGivern, D. O. (1998). *Nurses, nurse practitioners: Evolution to advanced practice* (3rd ed.). Philadelphia: W. B. Saunders.

Mischler, N., & Quinn, N. (1995). Research report: National committee for quality assurance (NCQA) accreditation. Milliman & Robertson.

NAPNAP. (1987). *Standards of practice for PNP/As. Cherry Hill, NJ: Author.*

NAPNAP. (1989). Risk management for pediatric nurse practitioners. Cherry Hill, NJ: Author.

NAPNAP. (2000). *Scope of practice.* Cherry Hill, NJ: Author.

National Council of State Boards of Nursing. (2002). *Regulation of advanced practice nursing: 2002 National Council of State Boards of Nursing Position Paper: Retrieved 1/04 from http:// www.ncsbn.org*

National Organization of Nurse Practitioner Faculties Curriculum Guidelines Task Force. (1995). *Advanced nursing practice: Curriculum guidelines and program standards for nurse practitioner education.* Washington, DC: NONPF

National Organization of Nurse Practitioner Faculties. (1997). *Criteria for evaluation of nurse practitioner programs: A report of the national task force on quality nurse practitioner education.* Washington, DC.

Pearson, L. (2003). Fifteenth annual legislative update: How each state stands on legislative issues affecting advanced nursing practice. *Nurse Practitioner: The American Journal of Primary Care, 28*(1), 35-58.

Shuler, P. A., & Davis, J. E. (1993). The Shuler nurse practitioner model: A theoretical framework for nurse practitioner clinicians, educators, and researchers, Part I. *Journal of the American Academy of Nurse Practitioners, 5*(1), 11–18.

Shuler, P. A., & Davis, J. E. (1993) . The Shuler nurse practitioner model: Clinical application, Part 2. *Journal of the American Academy of Nurse Practitioners, 5*(2), 73–88.

Shuler, P. A., & Huebscher, R. (1998). Clarifying nurse practitioner's unique contributions: Application of the Shuler nurse practitioner practice model. *Journal of the American Academy of Nurse Practitioners, 10*(11), 491–499.

Snyder, M., & Mirr, M. P. (1999). *Advanced practice nursing: A guide to professional development* (2nd ed.). NY: Springer Publishing.

U.S. Department of Health and Human Services. (1990). *Healthy people 2000: National health promotion and disease prevention objectives* (DHHS Publication No. PHS 91-50213). Washington, DC: Agency for Health Care Policy and Research.

U.S. Department of Health and Human Services. (1998). *Clinicians handbook of preventative services: Put prevention into practice* (2nd ed.). Washington, DC: U.S. Government Printing Office.

U.S. Department of Health and Human Services. (1999). *Healthy people 2000 program review 1998–1999.* Washington, DC: U.S. Government Printing Office.

U.S. Department of Health and Human Services. (1999). *Healthy people 2010 fact sheet: Healthy people in healthy communities.* Washington, DC: U.S. Government Printing Office.

U.S. Department of Health and Human Services (2000). *Healthy people 2010* (2nd. ed.). Washington, DC: U. S. government printing office.

Index

001B/3/P